# Rate – Interval Conversion Table

| Rate (BPM) | Cycle length (ms) | Rate (BPM) | Cycle length (ms) |
|---|---|---|---|
| 20 | 3000 | 215 | 279 |
| 25 | 2400 | 220 | 273 |
| 30 | 2000 | 225 | 267 |
| 35 | 1714 | 230 | 261 |
| 40 | 1500 | 235 | 255 |
| 45 | 1333 | 240 | 250 |
| 50 | 1200 | 245 | 245 |
| 55 | 1091 | 250 | 240 |
| 60 | 1000 | 255 | 235 |
| 65 | 923 | 260 | 231 |
| 70 | 857 | 265 | 226 |
| 75 | 800 | 270 | 222 |
| 80 | 750 | 275 | 218 |
| 85 | 706 | 280 | 214 |
| 90 | 667 | 285 | 211 |
| 95 | 632 | 290 | 207 |
| 100 | 600 | 295 | 203 |
| 105 | 571 | 300 | 200 |
| 110 | 545 | 305 | 197 |
| 115 | 522 | 310 | 194 |
| 120 | 500 | 315 | 190 |
| 125 | 480 | 320 | 188 |
| 130 | 462 | 325 | 185 |
| 135 | 444 | 330 | 182 |
| 140 | 429 | 335 | 179 |
| 145 | 414 | 340 | 176 |
| 150 | 400 | 345 | 174 |
| 155 | 387 | 350 | 171 |
| 160 | 375 | 355 | 169 |
| 165 | 364 | 360 | 167 |
| 170 | 353 | 365 | 164 |
| 175 | 343 | 370 | 162 |
| 180 | 333 | 375 | 160 |
| 185 | 324 | 380 | 158 |
| 190 | 316 | 385 | 156 |
| 195 | 308 | 390 | 154 |
| 200 | 300 | 395 | 152 |
| 205 | 293 | 400 | 150 |
| 210 | 286 | | |

$$\text{Rate (BPM or min}^{-1}) = \frac{60{,}000}{\text{Cycle length (ms)}}$$

$$\text{Cycle length (ms)} = \frac{60{,}000}{\text{Rate (BPM or min}^{-1})}$$

W. Fischer · Ph. Ritter, Cardiac Pacing in Clinical Practice

Springer-Verlag Berlin Heidelberg GmbH

W. Fischer · Ph. Ritter

# Cardiac Pacing in Clinical Practice

With a Foreword by D. Hayes

With 324 Figures in 547 Parts, 8 Tables, and Glossary

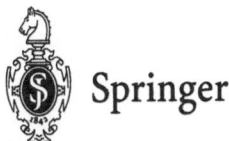

Springer

Dr. med. Wilhelm Fischer
Innere Abteilung, Krankenhaus Peißenberg
Hauptstraße 55–57, D-82380 Peißenberg

Dr. med. Philippe Ritter
Dept. de Stimulation Cardiaque d'Électrophysiologie
Centre Chirurgical Val d'Or, F-92210 Saint Cloud

Translator: Rodolphe Ruffy

Translation of the Second German Edition 1997, and of the French Edition 1997
W. Fischer, Ph. Ritter: Praxis der Herzschrittmacher-Therapie
2. Auflage 1997, ISBN 3-540-60264-X
Ph. Ritter, W. Fischer: Pratique de la stimulation cardiaque, Edition 1997
ISBN 978-3-642-63741-4


Library of Congress Cataloging-in-Publication Data
Fischer, Wilhelm. 1949– [Praxis der Herzschrittmachertherapie. English] Cardiac pacing
in clinical practice / W. Fischer, Ph. Ritter ; with a foreword by David Hayes ; [translator,
Rodolphe Ruffy]. – – 1st ed. p. cm.
"Translation of the second German edition 1997" – T. p. verso
Includes bibliographical references and index.
ISBN 978-3-642-63741-4     ISBN 978-3-642-58810-5 (eBook)
DOI 10.1007/978-3-642-58810-5
1. Cardiac pacing. I. Ritter, Ph., 1949– . II. Title. [DNLM: 1. Pacemaker, Artificial. 2. Car-
diac Pacing, Artificial. WG 26 F529p 1998a]
RC684.P3F5513   1998
617.4  120645--dcZT
DNLM/DLC for Library of Congress   98-12136 CiP

© Springer-Verlag Berlin Heidelberg 1998
Originally published by Springer-Verlag Berlin Heidelberg New York in 1998

The use of general descriptive names, registered names, trademarks, etc. in this publication
does not imply, even in the absence of a specific statement, that such names are exempt
from the relevant protective laws and regulations and therefore free for general use.

Product liability: The publisher cannot assume any legal responsibility for given data,
especially as far as directions for the use and the handling of chemicals and technical
devices are concerned. This information can be obtained from the instructions on safe
laboratory practice and from the manufacturers of chemical and laboratory equipment.

Cover Design: F. Steinen-Broo, eSTUDIO CALAMAR, E-17494 Pau
Typesetting: FotoSatz Pfeifer GmbH, D-82166 Gräfelfing

SPIN: 10769266     22/3111 – 5 4 3 2 1 – Printed on acid-free paper

*Dedicated to our families*

# Foreword

Pacemaker technology has evolved rapidly over the nearly 40 year history of the device. On several occasions over the past decade, I have heard individuals involved in some aspect of cardiac pacing, state that pacemaker technology had reached the end of it's developmental stage and no further improvements should be anticipated. Conversely, I've also heard many far-sighted individuals discuss potential pacemaker features and applications that seemed far-fetched. The latter group have been vindicated as pacemaker technology continues to advance. In such a dynamic field, it is crucial that state-of-the-art information exists and that it is provided in an understandable format.

In the course of our medical library acquisitions, many of us have purchased a medical textbook based upon the title that promises „state-of-the-art" information, only to be disappointed when the text fails to adequately deliver the expected information. Anyone who reads „Cardiac Pacing in Clinical Practice", whether cover-to-cover or used as a reference for management of clinical pacing problems, will find that the text fulfills all expectations. Drs. Ritter and Fischer have provided a comprehensive, understandable, state-of-the-art guide to clinical management of the pacemaker patient that can be appreciated by both physician and allied professional.

Preparation of such a comprehensive text by only two authors is an arduous task. However, the benefits of limited authorship is evident as one reads this book. There is a consistent style throughout in both text and graphics. This avoids redundancy and facilitates comprehension. In addition, the consistent writing style allows the authors to build on complexity from the beginning to end of each chapter. For example, the description of pacemaker system implantation encompasses the most basic portions, such as attaching the lead to the pulse generator, as well as less commonly encountered aspects such as pacemaker implantation in the cardiac transplant patient.

The extensive clinical experience of the authors is clearly evident. Every chapter is complete and up-to-date, from the description of the newer combipolar pacing configuration to new indications for pacing, and the extensive glossary and index makes it easy to seek answers to specific clinical questions. Readers who are involved in the day-to-day care of the pacemaker patient will find several chapters particularly helpful. The extensive discussion of pacing modes and their application allows a logical approach to individualizing pacemaker prescriptions. An exhaustive guide to patient follow-up and programming is provided. Thorough knowledge and understanding of this text should allow providers to avoid complications in their practice. However, in the event that a patient with a complication is referred for treatment, practical management guidelines for everything from hematoma formation to Accufix™ lead management is included.

It is highly likely that this text will prove to be an enduring source of information in the field of cardiac pacing, providing an inclusive guide with an international perspective. Those of us dedicated to providing expert care in the arena of cardiac pacing, are hopeful that many countries will eventually develop and apply standards of care for the paced patient. Ritter and Fischer provide a work that could serve as a basis for such standards.

*David L. Hayes, MD*

# Acknowledgements

This book is the result of an intensive collaboration between scientists, engineers, and physicians from separate institutions, cities, countries, and continents.

Ms. Monika Schrimpf of Springer-Verlag deserves a great deal of credit for her assistance and organization and Ms. Ursula Appl, Dipl.-Ing., for the excellent and expert translation she provided the authors with.

Furthermore, we gratefully acknowledge the invaluable assistance of Prof. Werner Irnich; both his counsel and his review of the whole book with regard to its physics and correct use of terminology are much appreciated.

We owe many thanks to Ulf H. Knabe, MD, for his helpful input and proofreading of the sections on surgery and to Martin R. Locher for his valuable editorial contributions to the German edition during its extensive revision.

Thanks are also due to Kaoru Kunisada, MD, Japan, for his fine cooperative efforts.

Special thanks also go to Bernard Dodinot, MD, Editor in Chief of *Stimucoeur Stimulography*, for giving us permission to reproduce a great number of the figures included in this book; to Rodolfo Ruffy, MD, Cardioscript International, for the very professional translation of this book from the German and French, and for his corrections and advice; to David Hayes, MD, for kindly writing the foreword; and to Jacques Mugica, MD, and Prof. Claude Daubert, MD, for their great help in making this work possible.

*Philippe Ritter*                                                 *Wilhelm Fischer*
St. Cloud                                                           Peissenberg

# Contents

## 9  Pulse Generator and/or Lead Replacement

# Abbreviations[1]

| | | | |
|---|---|---|---|
| A | A wave (in atrial electrogram); activation of the atrium | ERT | Elective replacement time |
| AC | Alternating current | ES | Extrasystole |
| Ah | Ampere-hour | H | Signal of His bundle (His electrogram) |
| AH | Interval between the atrial electrogram (A wave) and activation of the His bundle (His electrogram) | HOCM | Hypertrophic obstructive cardiomyopathy |
| AICD | Automatic implantable cardioverter/defibrillator | HV | Interval between the His bundle (His electrogram) and the ventricular electrogram |
| AMC | Automatic mode conversion | Hz | Hertz |
| AV | Atrioventricular | IC | Integrated circuit |
| AVD | AV delay; AV interval | ICD | Implantable cardioverter/defibrillator |
| BBB | Bundle branch block | ICHD | Intersociety Commission for Heart Disease Resources |
| BOL | Begin of life | | |
| BOS | Begin of service | IEC | International Electricotechnical Commission |
| BPEG | British pacing and electrophysiology group | INR | International normalized ratio |
| BPM | Beats per minute | IPG | Implantable pulse generator |
| BTS | Bradycardia-tachycardia syndrome | IS-1 | International standard no. 1 |
| CPU | Central processing unit | ISO | International Standards Organization |
| CPX | Cardiopulmonary stress testing | I.U. | International unit |
| CSM | Carotid sinus massage | i.v. | Intravenous |
| CSNRT | Corrected sinus node recovery time | $k\Omega$ | Kiloohm |
| CVTL | Conditional ventricular tracking limit | kV | Kilovolt |
| CWS | Chest wall stimulation | LAH | Left anterior hemiblock |
| DAB | Diagonal atrial bipolar | LBBB | Left bundle-branch block |
| DC | Direct current | LPH | Left posterior hemiblock |
| ECG | Electrocardiogram | mA | Milliampere |
| ELT | Endless loop tachycardia | $min^{-1}$ | Per minute: unit for rate |
| EMI | Electromagnetic interference | ms | Millisecond |
| EOL | End of life | MRI | Nuclear magnetic resonance imager |
| EOS | End of service | MSNRT | Maximal sinus node recovery time |
| EP | Evoked potential | MSR | Maximal sensor rate |
| ER | Evoked response | MSRI | Minimal sensor rate interval (according to MSR) |
| ERI | Elective replacement indicator | mT | Millitesla |

1 For abbreviations of the International Pacemaker Code, see foldout table at back of book. ECG uses the signals P–U in accordance with Einthoven; these abbreviations are not listed here. The symbols A, P, V, R are used in the terminology of cardiac pacing to distinguish the following: *A* atrial stimulus; *P* atrial spontaneous event; *V* ventricular stimulus; *R* ventricular spontaneous event

| | | | |
|---|---|---|---|
| mV | Millivolt | PVC | Premature ventricular contraction |
| MV | Minute ventilation | RAM | Random access memory |
| μA | Microampere | RBBB | Right bundle-branch block |
| μJ | Microjoule | ROM | Read only memory |
| μT | Microtesla | RRT | Recommended replacement time |
| NASPE | North American Society of Pacing and Electrophysiology | SACT | Sinoatrial conduction time |
| | | SNRT | Sinus node recovery time |
| NBG code | NASPE/BPEG generic pacemaker code | SR | Sinus rhythm |
| | | SSS | Sick sinus syndrome |
| $O_2$ | Oxygen | SVT | Supraventricular tachycardia |
| Ω | Ohm | TARP | Total atrial refractory period |
| PAC | Premature atrial contraction | UR | Upper rate |
| PMT | Pacemaker mediated tachycardia | URI | Upper rate interval |
| PPM | Pulses per minute | V | Volt |
| PSA | Pacer system analyzer | VA | Ventriculo-atrial |
| PTT | Partial thromboplastin time | VES | Ventricular extrasystole |
| PVARP | Postventricular atrial refractory period | VS-1 | Voluntary standard No. 1 |
| PVB | Premature ventricular beat | WPW syndrome | Wolff-Parkinson-White syndrome |

# Introduction

## A Short History of Cardiac Pacing

The history of pacemaker technology is characterized by a large number of data and facts whose selection must always be fragmentary, particularly in a brief outline. The selection here is restricted to the essentials.

427 – 347 B.C. *Plato:* Mentions the electric effect of the torpedo fish
1747 *Squires:* Cardiac resuscitation by electric stimuli
1761 *Morgagni:* Circulation-induced syncope
1800 *Bichat:* Electric stimulation of the heart in decapitated persons (Fig. 1)
1827 *Adams* and
1846 *Stokes:* Syndrome of bradycardia and syncope

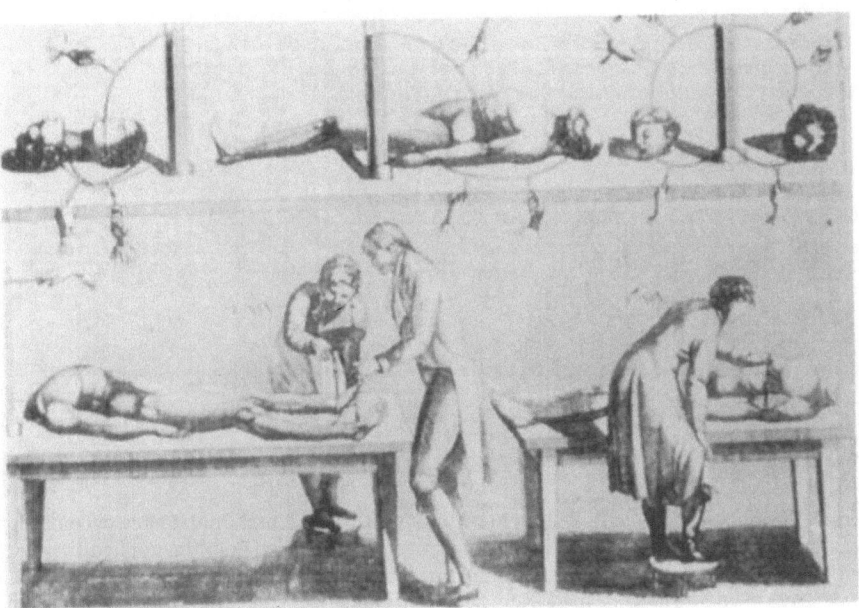

**Fig. 1.** In 1800 Bichat published his research work on the electrostimulation of the heart in decapitated persons. The French revolution had provided an abundant number of test objects (Medtronic document)

| 1882 | *Von Ziemssen:* Stimulation of the heart from outside upon partial resection of the chest wall |
| 1932 | *Hyman's* apparatus („artificial pacemaker" extracorporeal) |
| 1952 | *Zoll:* External electric stimulation of the heart by means of plate electrodes |
| 1956 | First extracorporeal pacemaker for long-term use |
| 1958 | *Furman* and *Robinson:* Transvenous access, aggregate still extracorporeal |
| 1958 | *Elmquist* and *Senning:* First implantable pacemaker with externally chargeable accumulator, pacemaker asynchronous (fixed-rate) (Fig. 2) |
| 1960 | *Chardack* and *Greatbatch:* Pacemaker with zinc-mercury batteries (two-year life) |
| 1962 | *Furman:* First implantation of an endocavitary pacemaker system |

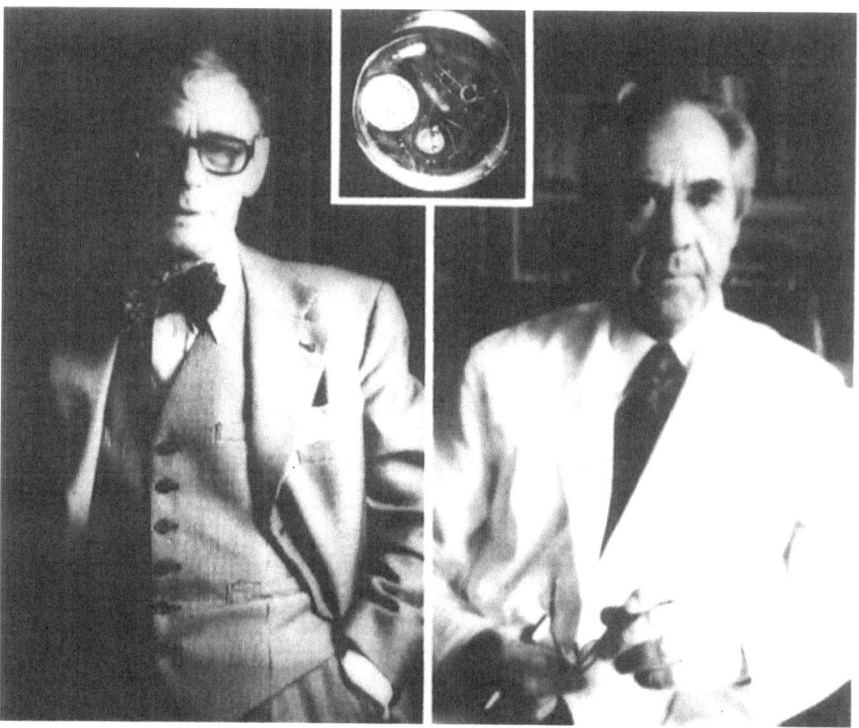

**Fig. 2.** Elmquist (*on the left*), Senning (*on the right*) and the first implantable pacemaker. 1958 was a historic date for cardiac pacing since Elmquist and Senning applied the first implantable pacemaker with an accumulator rechargeable from the outside. This pacemaker was asynchronous or fixed-rate, i.e. the stimulus was constantly released at a given rate without consideration of the cardiogenic action. The service life of these first pacemaker aggregates was between 15 and 20 min. It is a curiosity of medical history that Elmquist and Senning did not believe in the long-term success of this method at the time (document, Siemens Pacesetter)

| 1962 | *Nathan* and *Center:* First atrially synchronous pacemaker (VAT) with one electrode |
|------|------|
| 1963 | First programmable pacemaker |
| 1963 | *Lagergren:* Combination of transvenous access and subcutaneous battery-operated pacemaker |
| 1964 | *Castellanos, Sykosch:* First demand pacemaker in VVI mode |
| 1967 | *Laurens:* Nuclear-powered pacemaker |
| 1969 | *Berkovits:* AV-sequential pacing, first bifocal pacemaker (here DVI mode) |
| 1972 | Pacemaker operated by a lithium battery (Medico): SAFT battery LT 355 |
| 1972 | *Lowdry:* Encapsulation of pacemakers in titanium (Telectronics) |
| 1973 | *Parsonnet:* Introduction of porous electrodes |
| 1973 | *Meibom:* Introduction of the Vario function |
| 1974 | *Camilli:* Description of a pacemaker, rate modulated by the variations of blood pH |

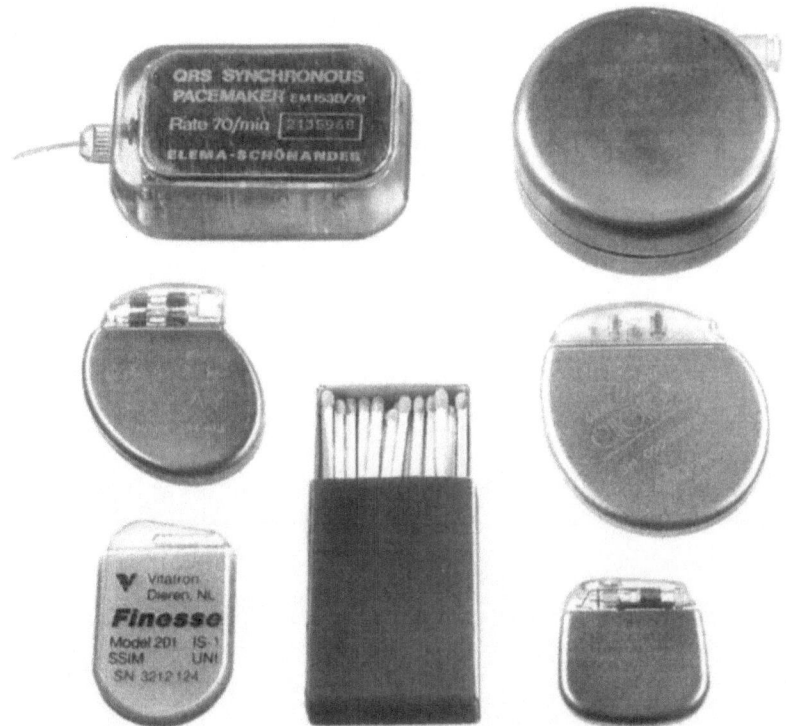

**Fig. 3.** Size changes of the implantable pacemaker over the course of time: two historic pacemakers (*upper row*), modern dual chamber pacemakers (*middle row*), and „Mini" single chamber pacemakers (*lower row*); matchbox provided for size comparison

| 1975 | *Irnich:* Proposal of DDD (universal) concept |
|------|------|
| 1977 | *Funke:* Introduction and first implantation of DDD pacemaker |
| 1978 | *Lemon:* Introduction of anchor leads |
| 1978 | *Mugica:* Proposal of a diagnostic pacemaker |
| 1979 | *Richter:* Introduction of carbon electrodes by Siemens |
| 1979 | Appearance of the first pacemaker, rate modulated by walking (RS4 CPI) |
| 1980 | Introduction of vitreous carbon (Ela) and pyrolytic (Sorin) electrodes |
| 1980 | *Mirowski:* automatic implantable cardioverter/ defibrillator (AICD) |
| 1980 | *Ripart* and *Jacobson:* Introduction of the software pacemaker concept |
| 1980 | *Antonioli:* Introduction of a new VAT single lead concept |
| 1982 | *Rederie:* Tests with merely diagnostic systems |
| 1983 | *Stokes:* Introduction of steroid electrodes |

The technical development is currently exponential. It depends today on the microprocessors which offer important memories permitting the automation of complex functions and the conservation of characteristic information. In the same way the energy consumption of circuits is in constant reduction.

Leads also show a great evolution due to a better knowledge of materials, the introduction of steroids on the tip of the lead, and their reduction of size. These elements contribute to the reduction of the energy consumption during pacing. Therefore it is possible to reduce the size of pacemakers (Fig. 3), a factor that we don't consider anymore as determinant in the selection of the model to implant.

# CHAPTER 1

# Brief Review of the Anatomy, Electrophysiology and Pathophysiology of the Cardiac Conduction System

## 1.1
## Anatomy and Electrophysiology

The formation and propagation of the electrical signal which signals the contraction of the heart muscle, stems from the activity of nodal tissue, made of distinct myocardial cells, organized within specialized anatomical structures (Figs. 1.1, 1.2).

## The Sinoatrial Node

In normal circumstances, the sinoatrial node is in charge of formation of the cardiac electrical impulse. It is located at the margin of the right atrium, near the superior vena cava, perfused by the sinoatrial artery which originates from the right coronary system in 70% of cases, and from the left in 30%. The collection of sinus nodal cells depolarizes regularly and triggers the propaga-

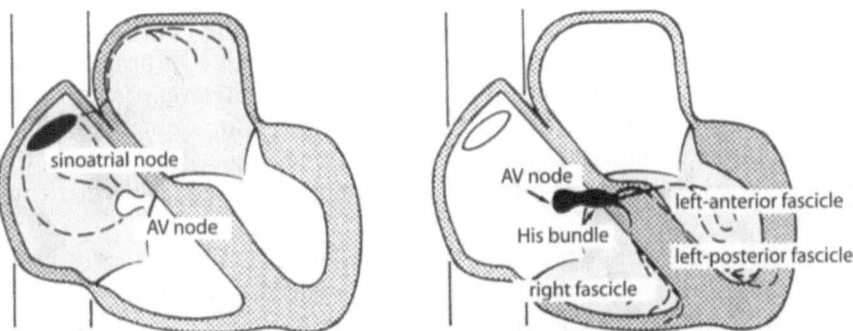

**Fig. 1.1.** The sinus node is located in the upper portion of the right atrium, between superior vena cava and the right atrial appendage. Three preferential „pathways" course from the sinus node to the atrioventricular node, and a fourth is headed toward the left atrium

**Fig. 1.2.** Past the bundle of His, the conduction system divides into right and left bundle branches. While the right bundle branch is quite distinct, the left bundle branch gives rise to two (anterior and posterior) hemibranches. This main bundle branch system is continued by the Purkinje network

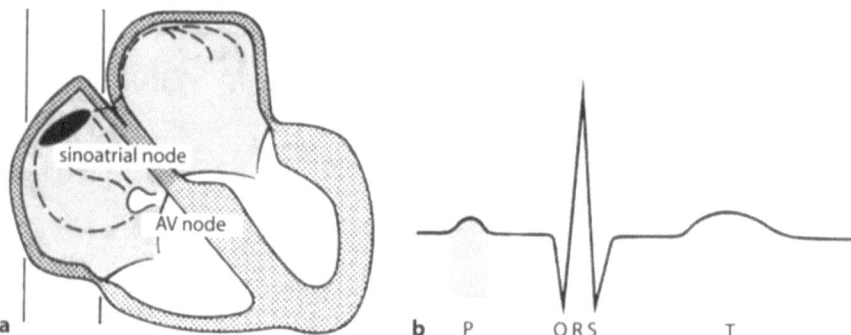

**Fig. 1.3.** The P wave of the surface electrocardiogram corresponds to the depolarization of the atrial myocardium

tion of the electrical impulse by contiguity to the remainder of the atrial myocardium. Conduction velocity is slow, on the order of 0.01–0.05 m/s. The sinoatrial node is the highest nodal automatic focus, and its activity is modulated by a sympathetic (accelerator) and parasympathetic (moderator) neural network.

The depolarization wavefront originating from the sinoatrial node spreads over three preferential pathways within the right atrium, and towards the roof of the left atrium by way of the Bachman bundle, to activate simultaneously both atria. The P wave of the surface electrocardiogram corresponds to depolarization of both atria (Fig. 1.3).

## The Atrioventricular Node

The activation front reaches the atrioventricular node, the only electrically conductive pathway between atria and ventricles. Its conductive properties are decremental, which means that all stimuli reaching the atrioventricular node, as during an atrial tachyarrhythmia (atrial fibrillation for example), will not be transmitted to the ventricles. In absence of pathologic atrial rhythm, the role of the atrioventricular node is to synchronize atrial and ventricular contractions.

The atrioventricular node is located near the tricuspid valve, on the right side of the interatrial septum. Its blood supply is provided by the atrioventricular nodal artery which originates from the right coronary system in 90% of cases, and from the left in 10%. It is also modulated by the sympathetic nervous system (which facilitates atrioventricular conduction) and parasympathetic system (which slows atrioventricular conduction).

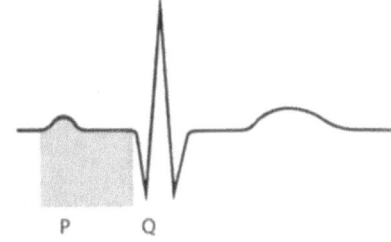

**Fig. 1.4.** The PR interval begins with the onset of the P wave and ends with the onset of the QRS

## The His Bundle

The His bundle originates from the atrioventricular node. Conduction velocity within this bundle is high (between 1 and 2 m/s), such that the signal to contract reaches the ventricular myocardial cells very rapidly. The His bundle bifurcates into two branches: the right bundle branch consisting of a single fascicle down to the Purkinje fibers, and the left bundle branch, which spreads in a tape-like fashion over the left surface of the interventricular septum, and which has been, from an electrophysiologic standpoint, subdivided into anterior and posterior hemibranches.

The electrical activity of the atrioventricular node and of the His bundle is not visible on the surface electrocardiogram and is a component of the PR interval (Fig. 1.4).

## The Purkinje Network

The right and left bundle branches are continued by the Purkinje fibers network which spreads widely over the ventricular endocardial surface and transmits the command of activation directly to the myocardial cells. This phase is expressed on the surface electrocardiogram as the QRS complex (Fig. 1.5).

Depolarization is followed by a phase of repolarization, of which only the ventricular part is visible, as the T wave, on the electrocardiogram.

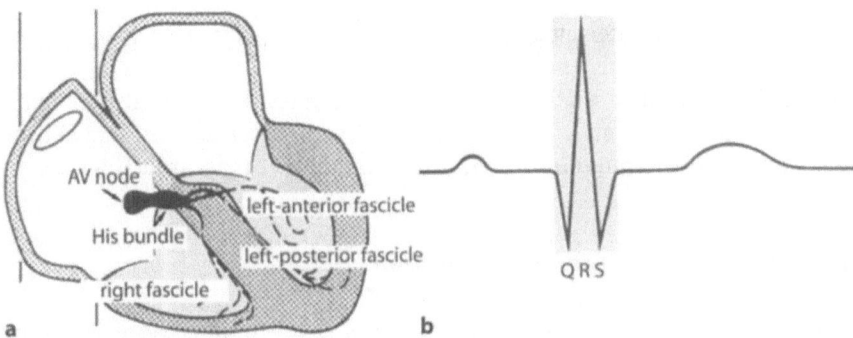

**Fig. 1.5.** Ventricular depolarization corresponds to the QRS complex on the surface electrocardiogram

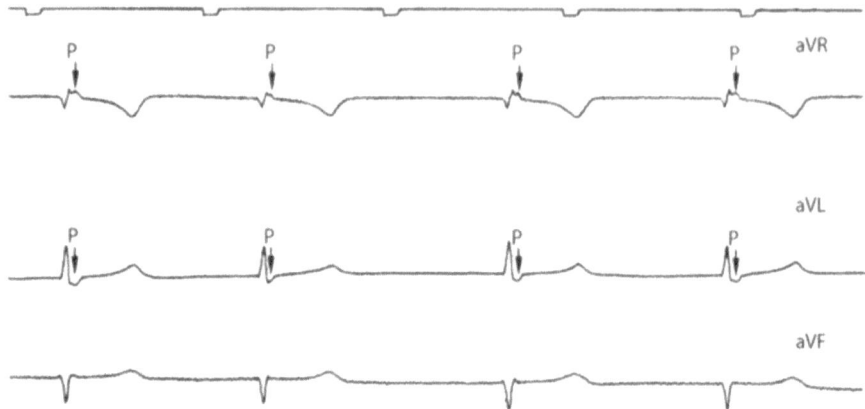

**Fig. 1.6.** In absence of sinus node activity (the dominant automatic focus), a secondary focus takes charge of the rhythm at the level of the atrioventricular node. The rate is slow and the QRS complex is followed by retrograde atrial conduction. The P wave appears behind the QRS and its polarity is reversed (positive in aVR and negative in aVL). *Arrows,* P

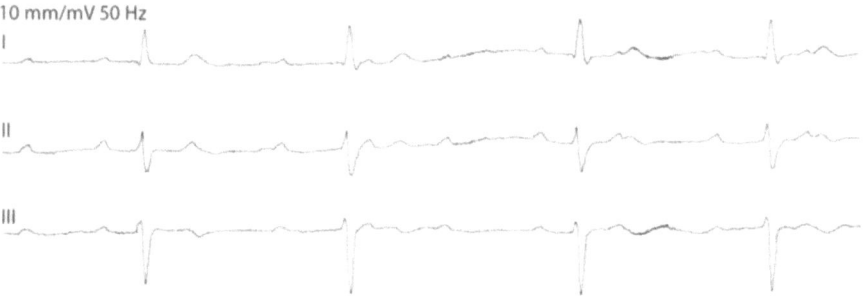

**Fig. 1.7.** Tracing showing third degree atrioventricular block. The ventricular rate is in the neighborhood of 35 BPM

## Automatic Foci

In case of failure of the sinoatrial node, the dominant automatic focus, secondary (the atrioventricular node) or tertiary (the His-Purkinje system) foci take control of the cardiac rhythm at slower escape rates: 40–60 beats per minute (BPM) for the atrioventricular node, and 20–40 BPM for the Purkinje network. Such substitute rhythms often cause symptoms due to bradycardia (Figs. 1.6, 1.7).

## Anterograde and Retrograde Conduction

Normal conduction, from atria to ventricles, is called anterograde. However, conduction may take place in the opposite direction, from a premature ventricular complex for example; it is then called retrograde. The presence of anterograde atrioventricular conduction block does not necessarily mean absence of retrograde conduction. This bi-directional conduction may be the source of rhythm disturbances and of a certain number of complications in cardiac pacing (see p. 89–91, 95–104, 359–561).

## Refractory Periods of the Heart

Myocardial depolarization is accompanied by a refractory period, which has been subdivided in an absolute and a relative refractory period. The duration of this refractory period varies depending on the type cardiac tissue being considered and on particular circumstances (Fig. 1.8).

### The Absolute Refractory Period

During the absolute refractory period, an electrical stimulus evokes no response. Thus, a ventricular pacemaker spike remains ineffective during the refractory phase of the ventricle. Consequently, on the surface electrocardiogram, a ventricular pacing spike falling during the refractory period does not modify the spontaneous ventricular activity. In addition, an arrhythmia cannot be triggered (Fig. 1.9).

### The Relative Refractory Period

The relative refractory period immediately follows the absolute refractory period. The myocardium is excitable, but only with a stimulation strength higher than the minimal strength for depolarization needed when the stimulus is delivered outside of the refractory periods. In healthy myocardium a stimulus 12 to 25 times stronger is needed to trigger a depolarization during this interval. This period, situated just before the peak of the T wave of the surface electrocardiogram, is often called the vulnerable period since an ectopic stimulus, from a pacemaker for example, may trigger a ventricular tachyarrhythmia if delivered during it (Fig. 1.10). A spontaneous, very premature extrasystole (R on T) may have the same effect.

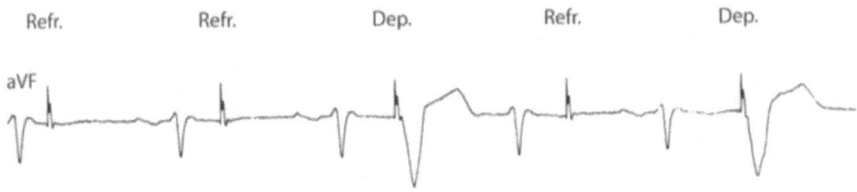

**Fig. 1.8.** A stimulus (V00 mode, asynchronous, fixed rate) delivered during the refractory period of the ventricular myocardium causes no depolarization (*Refr.*). In contrast, a stimulus falling just after the end of the absolute refractory period (of a spontaneous depolarization) is effective (*Dep.*)

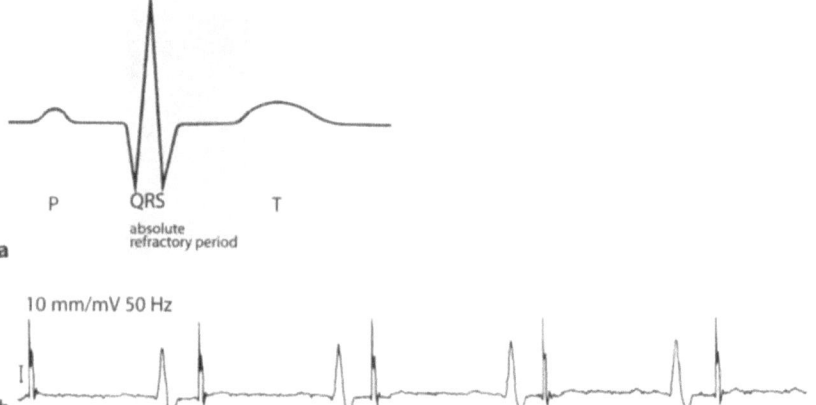

**Fig. 1.9. a** On the surface electrocardiogram, the absolute refractory period corresponds to the interval between the onset of the QRS complex and the early part of the T wave. Its duration depends on the heart rate and other individuals factors
**b** An electrical stimulus delivered during this period causes no ventricular depolarization

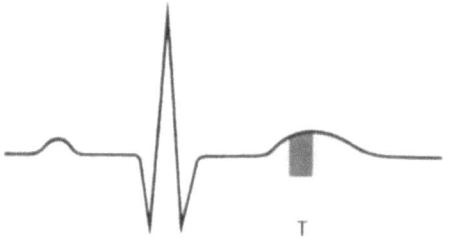

**Fig. 1.10.** The vulnerable period corresponds roughly to the T wave of the surface electrocardiogram, particularly the 30 ms preceding the peak of the T wave

### Refractory Periods in Various Cardiac Tissues

The refractory periods of atria, atrioventricular node, and ventricles have different durations. In abnormal myocardium, the risk of serious rhythm disturbances is considerably greater than when the heart is healthy. The dispersion of refractory periods is of great importance, at times associated with isolated areas of conduction block, abnormalities all susceptible to cause local reentry, the trigger of severe tachyarrhythmias. The risk is particularly high in ischemic myocardium, as well as during drug intoxication or electrolyte disturbances since the threshold for the development of life-threatening arrhythmias from a conventional pacing stimulus is much lower.

> In cardiac pacing, the term „refractory period" defines a time interval during which the pacemaker cannot sense an event within the cardiac chamber being considered; it has therefore an entirely different meaning than the natural refractory period of the heart.

## 1.2
## The Main Depolarization and Conduction Disorders

### Sinus Node Disease (the Sick Sinus Syndrome)

Sinus node dysfunction occurring within the node itself or at the interface between the node and the atrial myocardium is manifest either as sinus bradycardia, or as sinoatrial block of variable degree (Fig. 1.11) culminating as sinus arrest with escape rhythm from a subsidiary, slower automatic focus (in this case usually from the atrioventricular node), or as chronotropic incompetence.

### Chronotropic Incompetence

The recognition of chronotropic incompetence is based on one or several of the following findings (Fig. 1.12a):

- Absolute chronotropic incompetence: no increase in sinus rate with effort.
- Relative chronotropic incompetence: abnormal slow resting heart rate and/or delayed acceleration of heart rate during effort and/or inadequate maximal exercise heart rate and/or excessively rapid fall in heart rate following exercise.

The diagnosis of chronotropic incompetence may be difficult since its physiologic consequences may, in any given case, be quite variable.

### Atrial Tachyarrhythmias

These episodes of bradycardia may be complicated by bouts of tachycardia, resulting in a bradycardia – tachycardia syndrome, in which marked bradycardia alternates with periods of rapid rhythms, usually due to atrial fibrillation or flutter (Fig. 1.12b). Moreover, prolonged episodes of atrial bigeminy are often observed in these patients.

The diagnostic hinges on surface electrocardiographic recordings, particularly Holter (24 h ambulatory) recordings. Should this information remain inconclusive, intracardiac recordings, along with provocative maneuvers may be needed.

### Electrophysiological Testing

This requires a multi-channel amplifier and recorder, as well as a programmable external stimulator. The method involves the placement of bipolar or multipolar pacing and recording endocardial electrode catheters in the high right atrium,

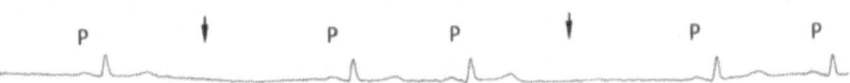

**Fig. 1.11.** A P wave is intermittently missing (*arrow*). This phenomenon is described as sino-atrial dysfunction or sinoatrial block

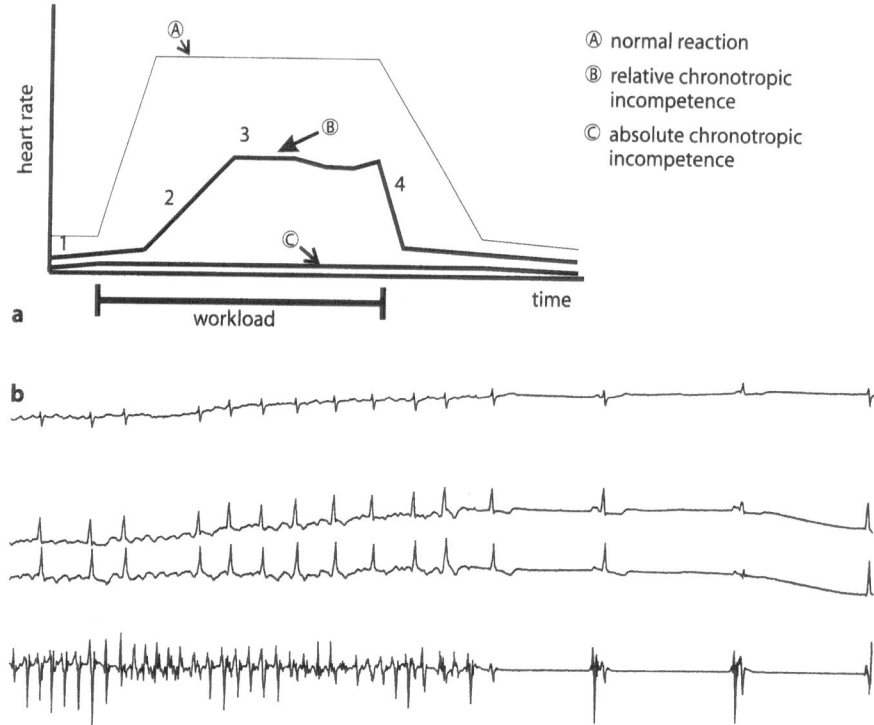

**Fig. 1.12. a** Different profiles of chronotropic incompetence: Absolute chronotropic incompetence: no increase in sinus rate with effort; Relative chronotropic incompetence: abnormal slow resting heart rate (*1*) and/or delayed acceleration of heart rate during effort (*2*) and/or inadequate maximal exercise heart rate (*3*) and/or excessively rapid fall in heart rate following exercise (*4*)
**b** Bradycardia-tachycardia syndrome. Upon cessation of atrial fibrillation, sinus rhythm is slow and a junctional escape rhythm emerges. The intracardiac atrial recording (*bottom tracing*) shows variability of the endocavitary signal during fibrillation

His bundle region, ventricular apex and coronary sinus, depending on the type of electrophysiologic study to be performed.

Several variables may be studied in the case of sinus node disease, including sinoatrial conduction, sinus node recovery time, findings pointing to an arrhythmogenic substrate and the inducibility of atrial arrhythmias.

*Sino atrial conduction time* is rarely measurable directly as the time interval between the onset of sinus node electrogram and the onset of the P wave on the surface electrocardiogram. Instead, either the Narula method (eight atrial events paced at a rate 10% faster than the spontaneous sinus rate and measurement of the subsequent sinus return cycle), or the Strauss method (delivery of a progressively earlier atrial extrastimulus after eight sinus beats and measurement of the subsequent sinus return cycle) can be applied toward this measurement. The difference between the sinus return cycle and the baseline sinus cycle corresponds to the sum of the retrograde (atriosinus) conduction time (entry of the stimulus into the node from the site of stimulation) and the anterograde (sinoatrial) conduction time (exit of the sinus impulse to the depolarization signal recorded at that same site).

The sinoatrial conduction time is, thus, the measured value of the return sinus cycle divided by 2, the upper limit of which should not exceed 175 ms.

*The sinus node recovery time*, more often used and more sensitive, is analyzed by the method of Mandel which measures the sinus return cycle following one minute of high right atrial stimulation at several decremental cycle lengths, beginning at 10 BPM above the baseline sinus cycle up to 200 BPM. The delay in sinus node recovery is corrected as a function of the baseline sinus cycle, and should not exceed 550 ms or 150% of the baseline cycle (Fig. 1.13). It is important to verify that the return cycle is indeed of sinus origin, and that so-called secondary pauses do not occur following a few sinus cycles of normal duration. These tests may be refined by blockade of the autonomic nervous system, allowing to distinguish between an extrinsic and an intrinsic origin of the observed abnormalities.

*The study of sinoatrial conduction and of sinus node function* is completed by looking for the presence of findings in favor of atrial vulnerability. The study of the atrial arrhythmogenic substrate includes measurements, at various paced cycle lengths, of the atrial refractory period and the recognition of its failure to adapt to changes in drive cycle length, the measurement of intra- and interatrial conduction in search of abnormally long time intervals, and an examination of native and evoked endocavitary electrograms in search of signal fragmentation.

*Testing the inducibility of arrhythmias* is done by way of provocative maneuvers consisting of introducing one, two, or three atrial extrastimuli during paced rhythm to attempt triggering atrial fibrillation or tachycardia, paying attention to whether or not it remains sustained.

These various tests may also be rendered more sensitive by the administration of certain drugs.

Ultimately, excluding the typical case of prolonged sinus pauses, an indication for pacing will often rely on the association of symptoms with several abnormalities of sinus node function. A finding of atrial vulnerability guides the choice of pacemaker to be implanted.

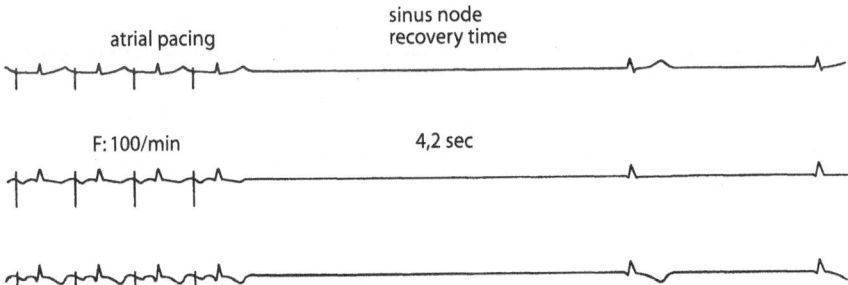

**Fig. 1.13.** Example of sinus node recovery time greater than 4200 ms. The spontaneous sinus rate before pacing was 60 BPM, i.e. an interval of 1000 ms. The corrected sinus node recovery time is, thus, markedly pathologic, measuring 4200 – 1000 = 3200 ms (actually it is even longer, because there are no spontaneous P waves visible)

## Atrioventricular and Intraventricular Conduction Disorders

### Atrioventricular Block (AVB)

This conduction disorder may occur at the level of the atrioventricular node, of the His bundle, or of the bundle branches, and presents in various degrees (Figs. 1.14, 1.15). *First degree atrioventricular block* is characterized by a lengthening of the PR interval on the electrocardiogram.

*Second degree AVB* presents in two varieties:

• In type I, also called Wenckebach phenomenon or Mobitz I, the PR interval progressively lengthens until a P wave is no longer followed by a QRS complex. Then the period resumes. This anomaly, commonly observed in young, healthy individuals, particularly during sleep, is often benign.

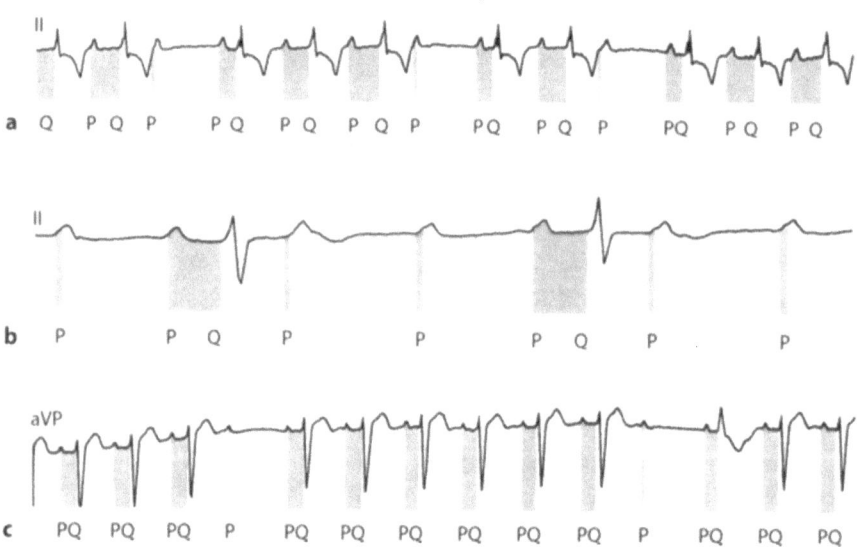

**Fig. 1.14. a** Mobitz I (Wenckebach periodicity) second degree atrioventricular block with typical gradual prolongation of the PR interval from one cycle to the next, until block of atrioventricular conduction
**b** Mobitz II second degree atrioventricular block. The PR interval is prolonged (280 ms), and only one out of three P waves is conducted (3 : 1 block)
**c** Mobitz II second degree atrioventricular block (all PR intervals are equal until block of the P wave occurs)

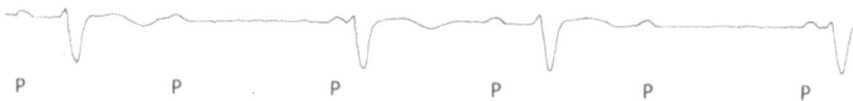

**Fig. 1.15.** „High degree" atrioventricular block. The third QRS is probably associated with the preceding P wave. The other P waves and QRS complexes are dissociated

- In type II, also called Mobitz II, a P wave is blocked without preceding lengthening of the PR interval (Fig. 1.14c). Several consecutive P waves may be blocked with a 3 : 1, 4 : 1, or higher degree of atrioventricular dissociation; the block is then called „high degree".

In *third degree AVB (complete AVB)*, conduction between atria and ventricles is completely interrupted. The ventricular rate is slow, driven by an automatic focus situated in the distal portion of the conduction system (His-Purkinje tissue), with dissociation of the more rapid atrial activity.

The type of block identified electrocardiographically does not invariably identify correctly the level of the conduction disorder, although the Wenckebach phenomenon generally occurs in the atrioventricular node and Mobitz II in the more distal conduction system. In presence of a narrow QRS complex, the block is most likely at the atrioventricular nodal level or, rarely, in the His bundle. In high degree AVB with a wide QRS complex and a slow ventricular rate, the level of block is a priori subhisian.

To pinpoint the level of block, one may proceed with the direct recording of atrial, His bundle and ventricular electrograms by placing a multipolar electrode catheter in the region of the His bundle. A *suprahisian* conduction disorder is defined as a prolongation of the interval between the atrial electrogram (A wave) and activation of the His bundle (His electrogram) or, in the worst case, conduction block between A and H, while the relationship between His and ventricular electrograms remains normal (HV interval no longer than 55 ms) (Fig. 1.16). An *intrahisian* conduction disorder is characterized by a prolongation or a splitting of the His bundle electrogram, with presence of an interval $H_1$-$H_2$, while A-$H_1$ and $H_2$-V remain normal. Finally, an *infrahisian* conduction abnormality causes a prolongation of the H-V interval, or a conduction block between H and V (Fig. 1.17).

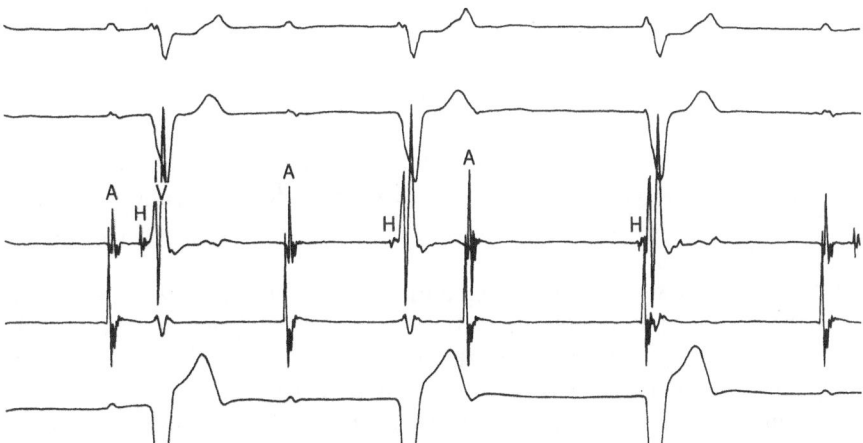

**Fig. 1.16.** Recording of complete atrioventricular block with atrioventricular dissociation. The *third trace* is from the His bundle region, and the *fourth trace* from the high right atrium. The block is suprahisian: there is block of conduction between the atrial electrogram (*A*) and activation of the His bundle (*H*). Recording speed 100 mm/s

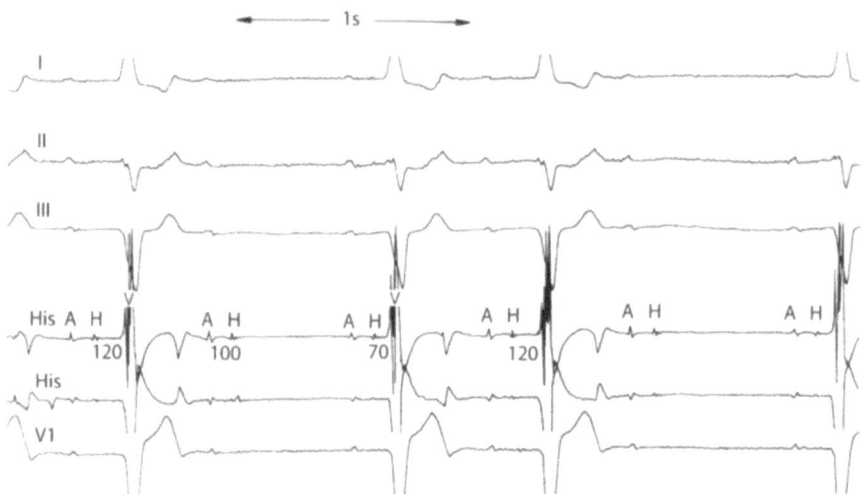

**Fig. 1.17.** Mobitz I second degree atrioventricular block with Wenckebach periodicity. The site of block is infrahisian with progressive lengthening of the HV interval until complete block (*fourth and fifth traces* are from the His bundle region). Though Mobitz I block most commonly occurs in the atrioventricular node, this example clearly shows an exception to the rule

The identification of the *Wenckebach point* (development of suprahisian conduction block during incremental atrial pacing) is important since it helps choosing the mode of pacing by providing further information with regard to the quality of anterograde atrioventricular nodal conduction. These tests may be rendered more sensitive by the administration of various drugs.

### Bundle Branch Blocks

From an electrophysiologic standpoint, three distinct divisions of the His bundle have been described that preserve conduction between atria and ventricles: the right bundle branch, the left anterior fascicle, and the left posterior fascicle, the last two being the constituents of the left bundle branch system. Consequently, a fascicular block may consist of block of the right bundle branch, of the left anterior fascicle (left anterior hemiblock), or of the left posterior fascicle (left posterior hemiblock) (Fig. 1.18).

*Bifascicular block* may consist of left bundle branch block, or of left anterior or posterior fascicular block in association with complete right bundle branch block. *Trifascicular block* involves all three fascicles (Fig. 1.19), and will appear as complete AVB if block is complete over all three fascicles.

Certain electrocardiographic findings allow the anticipation of a later evolution towards high degree AVB (Fig. 1.20). These include alternating bundle branch block (complete right bundle branch block alternating with complete left bundle branch in absence of extrasystoles), first degree AVB in presence of right bundle branch block and left posterior fascicular block, and first degree AVB in

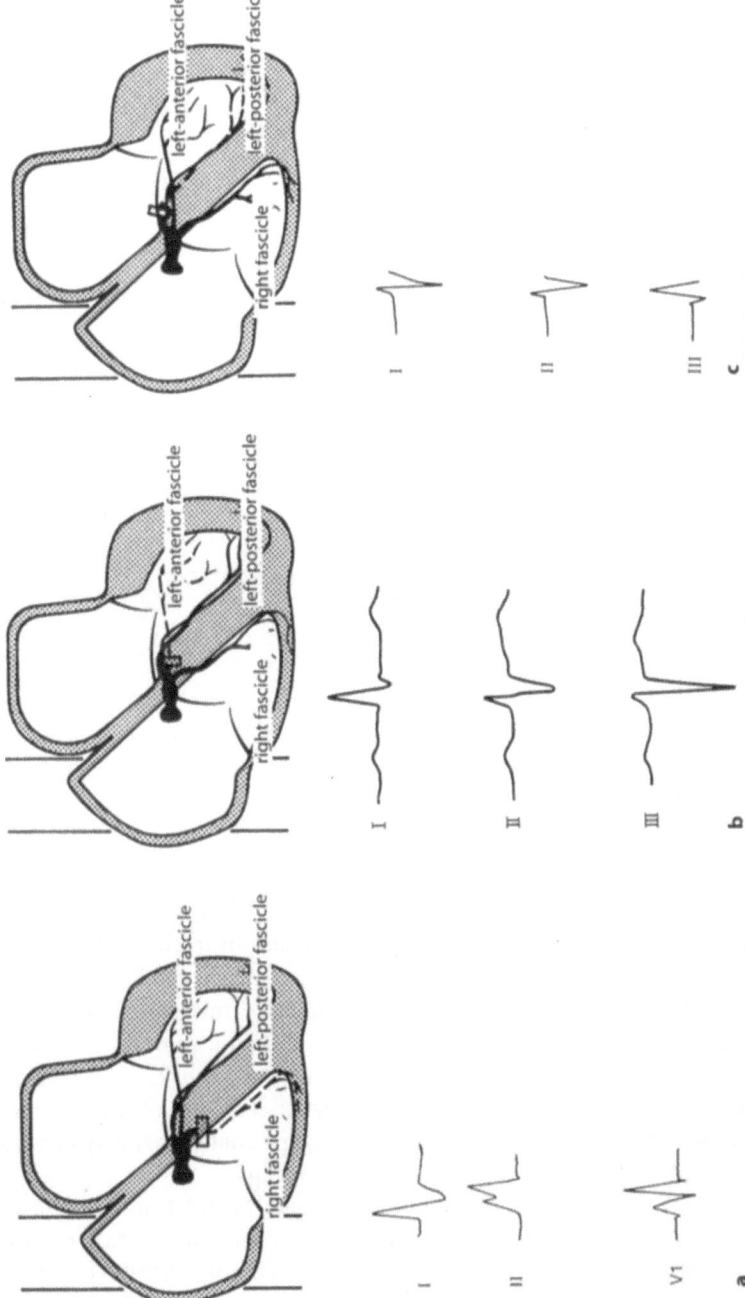

**Fig. 1.18. a** Complete right bundle branch block. **b** Left anterior fascicular block with axis deviation of the QRS beyond $-30°$ **c** Left posterior fascicular block with axis deviation of the QRS beyond $+120°$

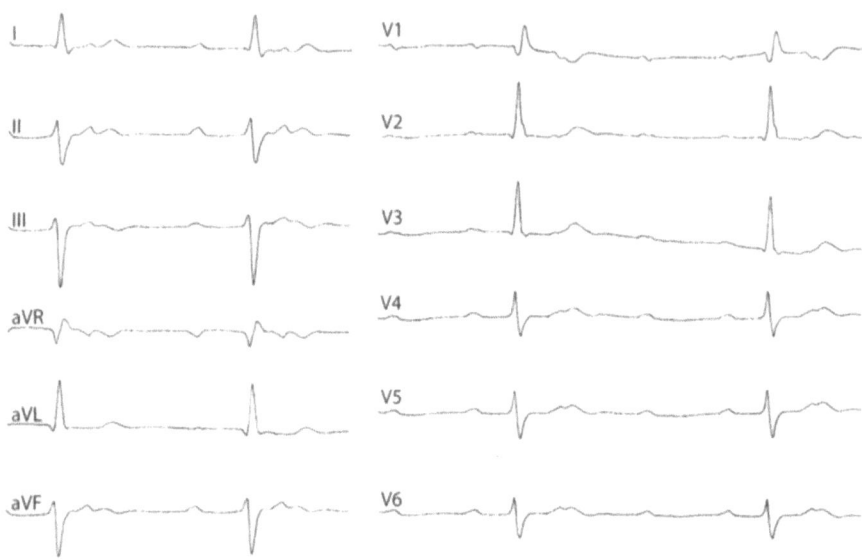

**Fig. 1.19.** Electrocardiographic findings in trifascicular block (right bundle branch block, left anterior fascicular block and prolonged PR interval, *left panel*) complicated by periods of „high degree" atrioventricular block (3 : 1, *right panel*)

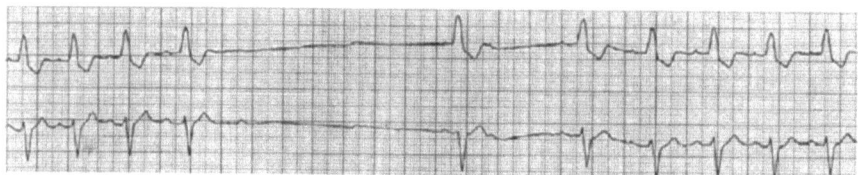

**Fig. 1.20.** Paroxysmal third degree atrioventricular block during vaso-vagal reaction in the background of first degree atrioventricular block and left bundle branch block

presence of left bundle branch block. First degree AVB with left anterior fascicular block, right bundle branch block and left posterior fascicular block, isolated left bundle branch block, and isolated left posterior fascicular block are intermediate predictors. In presence of such abnormalities, intracardiac recordings as described earlier may be performed, depending on the clinical presentation, to assess more precisely the risk of complete conduction block. In such cases, certain maneuvers (rapid atrial stimulation, abrupt cessation of rapid ventricular pacing, carotid sinus massage, and pharmacologic challenges) may increase the sensitivity obtained from simple baseline recordings.

In contrast, right bundle branch block coupled with left anterior fascicular block, isolated right bundle branch block, isolated left anterior fascicular block, and first degree AVB in presence of a narrow QRS complex, are not considered to be predictors of risk in absence of telltale symptoms.

# CHAPTER 2

# General Technical Concepts

The myocardial cellular membrane may be viewed as an electrical capacitor. When an electrical stimulus is applied to it, an action potential is triggered. Given a sufficient current strength, above the depolarization threshold, activation will propagate by contiguity to the entire myocardium and provide the signal for myocardial contraction. Thus, cardiac stimulation requires the formation of a localized and transient electrical field to depolarize a few cells in the vicinity of the electrode. This role is assumed by the pacing system which consists of a battery, interfaced with an electronic circuitry which delivers electrical current to the myocardium via a lead whose extremity includes an electrode in contact with endocardium or epicardium.

The pacemaker (pulse generator) delivers the stimulus necessary to activate the myocardium and senses the heart's intrinsic activity. The electronic circuits modulate the pacemaker's behavior according to the programs loaded in its memory and to the heart's spontaneous electrical activity. The electronics and power supply are contained in a can consisting of titanium alloy or of stainless steel.

The lead usually contains a multifilar bi-directional conductor (from pacemaker to heart and vice-versa) insulated in silicone or polyurethane, a connector interfacing with the pulse generator, and one or more electrode(s) in contact with the cardiac tissue. Through the lead, the pacemaker can stimulate the heart as well as sense its spontaneous activity.

## 2.1
## How to Stimulate the Heart

Myocardial cells are normally polarized at rest, with a transmembrane potential which depends on the activity of membrane ionic pumps allowing the maintenance of differences in transmembrane concentrations of these ions. Consequently, there are more sodium ions outside than inside the cells; conversely, there are more potassium ions inside than outside. The resulting resting potential difference is approximately 90 mV, and this value remains stable throughout the resting period in the working myocardial tissue. Upon cellular stimulation, whatever the nature of the stimulus and if the resting potential is brought to the depolarization threshold, a sudden reversal of the potential occurs as a result of

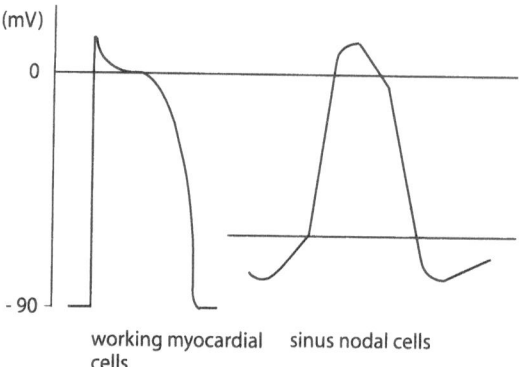

(mV)

0

- 90

working myocardial    sinus nodal cells
cells

**Fig. 2.1.** The action potential of working myocardial cells and that of nodal tissue have different characteristics. The former maintain a stable diastolic potential and can only be depolarized by an external stimulus, whatever its kind (electrical, chemical or mechanical), while nodal cells reach the depolarization threshold automatically in enddiastole

a sudden ion flux, with massive entry of sodium into the cell, and entry of calcium ions followed by exit of potassium ions. In the case of nodal cells, capable of generating the electrical impulse governing the signal of myocardial contraction, the transmembrane potential is not stable as a result of the progressive passage of ions across the membrane during diastole, causing the voltage across the membrane to drift until it reaches the threshold of depolarization (Fig. 2.1).

In the context of permanent pacing, the site of stimulation is the negative electrode, that is in contact with the myocardium. The positive pole is either the proximal pole of a bipolar electrode or, in the case of unipolar stimulation (for unipolar versus bipolar stimulation, see p. 48 – 52) the pacemaker can itself. Since the negative electrode is located in the extracellular space, the pacing stimulus can only modify the transmembrane potential by modifying the ionic behavior within that space, probably causing a sizable movement of sodium ion towards the electrode and a decrease in transmembrane potential in its vicinity. As soon as the depolarization threshold has been reached, an action potential is triggered in the cells neighboring the electrode, with subsequent propagation by contiguity.

## Basic Principles of Electricity

The units of the various parameters to be discussed are those commonly used in the field of cardiac pacing. The pacing stimulus is defined by its strength (amplitude of stimulation) and duration (width). The voltage thus generated by the pacemaker induces an electrical current towards the heart. The energy, expressed in microjoules (mJ), delivered by each stimulus is defined by the following formulas:

Energy delivered by each stimulus (in µJ) = voltage (V) × current (I) × stimulus duration (t) = $V^2$ stimulus duration (t) / resistance (R).

**Fig. 2.2.** Energy is the product of power multiplied by duration. Power is the product of voltage multiplied by delivered current: Energy = VIT (energy in joules, V in volts, I in amperes, T in seconds). In cardiac pacing this formula can be used to calculate the energy necessary to cause depolarization. This relationship may also be expressed by way of Ohm's law: V = RI, or I = V/R; hence energy = (V²T/R), where V is the stimulus amplitude, T its duration and R the tissue resistance. From this formula, one may deduce the energy consumed by the pacemaker which varies with the square of V and is directly proportional to T

**Energy** = work performed

$$E = V \cdot I \cdot T$$

From Ohm's law $V = R \cdot I$ one derives:

$$E = \frac{V^2 \cdot T}{R}$$

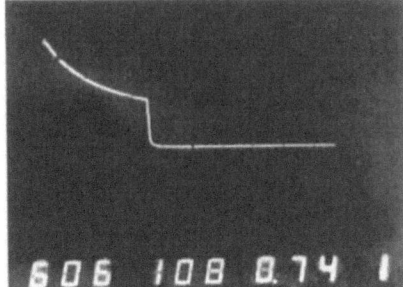

**Fig. 2.3.** Example of photoanalysis of stimulus spike. There is a time dependent drop in voltage. *Numbers* at the bottom of the illustration indicate from left to right: the pacing interval, the voltage (in mV) on the ECG lead recorded, the pulse duration (in ms), and the ECG lead recorded

Hence, delivered energy varies proportionally to the voltage squared, and proportionally to the duration of the stimulus (Fig. 2.2).

Voltage drops over time because of the phenomenon of polarization of the electrode (see Appendix), a phenomenon which has important practical consequences (Fig. 2.3). More details regarding basic principles of cardiac stimulation can be found in the Appendix (pp. 388–392).

## Pacing Threshold

The pacing threshold (or threshold of stimulation) is defined as the weakest electrical stimulus capable of triggering a cardiac depolarization in diastole, when delivered past the end of all natural refractory periods (Fig. 2.4). It can be expressed variably in current, charge, energy and voltage. It is classically expressed in current (mA), which remains independent of the resistance at the electrode-tissue interface. Likewise, charge (in mC) is a good way of expressing threshold since its unit (current time) is the same as that used to determine the charge of the pacemaker battery (ampere hour). Voltage is a less satisfactory way of expressing threshold since it decreases over time during delivery of the stimulus because of the phenomenon of polarization. However, for convenience, threshold is usually expressed in V since pacemakers currently available deliver pulses with constant voltages. The same applies to energy (in mJ) since it is a function of voltage (current voltage time).

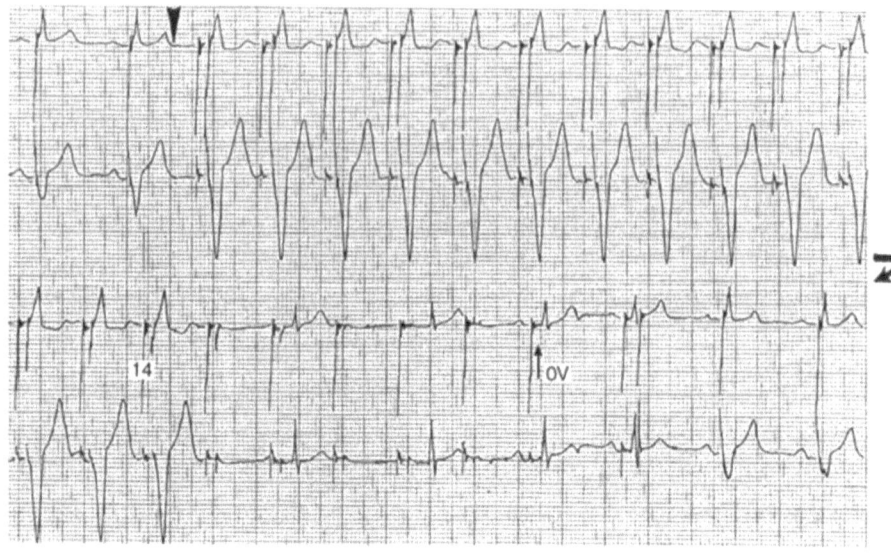

**Fig. 2.4.** Measurement of pacing threshold is performed by gradually decreasing the voltage delivered until capture failure. The ventricular pulse amplitude of this dual-chamber pacemaker is decreased with each cycle by 0.25 V from 4.75 V by an automatic function instructed by the programmer. The 14th, but not the 15th pulse captures the ventricle. The threshold is therefore at 1.5 V

These various values vary with pulse duration according to different mathematical relations. The most classical curve is that of Lapicque, or voltage – duration, also known as chronaxie – rheobase which describes the relation between threshold voltage and stimulus duration (Figs. 2.5, 2.6.). The curve is not linear. The threshold pulse amplitude increases significantly with a decrease in pulse duration. All points defined by their pulse duration and voltage situated above the curve are associated with myocardial depolarization, as opposed to all points below the curve. The rheobase is the least voltage needed to depolarize the heart at an infinite pulse duration. The chronaxie is the shortest pulse duration required to depolarize the heart at a voltage twice the rheobase.

The energy consumed at the pacing threshold is the least for a pulse duration measured at chronaxie (Fig. 2.7). Chronaxie and rheobase determine the quality of the electrical characteristics of a pacing electrode. The pacing threshold value is usually lower by 0.1 to 0.2 V when it is determined by a decremental (from higher to lower pulse strength) than by an incremental method. This is known as the Wedensky phenomenon.

In clinical practice, the determination of the pacing threshold is critical, since the programming of the pacing parameters (pulse duration and amplitude) determines the safety margin of pacing as well as the energetic efficiency of the system. It is generally recommended to set this safety margin at 100% with respect to the pacing threshold.

**Fig. 2.5.** The pacing threshold corresponds to the minimal voltage which results in depolarization. This curve defines the pacing threshold at various pulse durations. Beyond 1 ms, threshold is stable. In contrast, at pulse durations shorter than 0.25 ms, threshold increases significantly. Programmed values of pulse strength and duration programmed above the curve (beyond the pacing threshold) cause myocardial depolarization. Conversely, pulse strengths programmed in the area under the curve will be ineffective

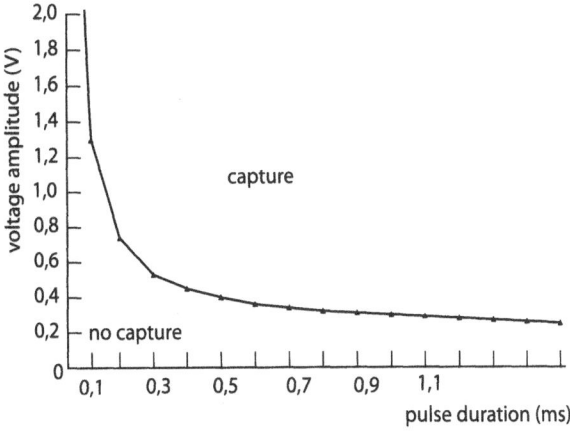

**Fig. 2.6.** Two particular measurements can be made from the pacing threshold curve: the rheobase is defined as the voltage resulting in myocardial depolarization at an infinite pulse duration (in this case 0.2 V). The chronaxie is measured from the rheobase. It represents the pulse duration at threshold at a voltage twice the rheobase (in this case 0.5 ms)

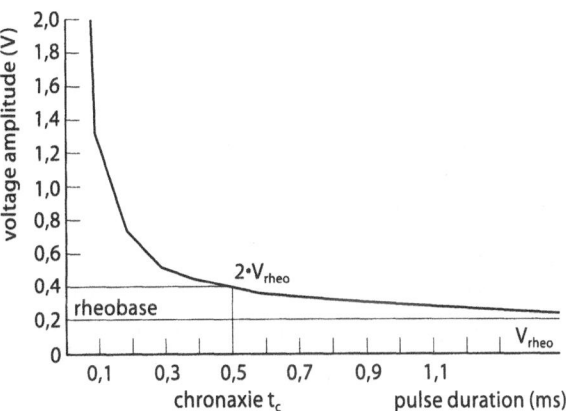

However, it may be difficult to determine accurately this safety margin because circadian physiologic variations in the threshold charge may reach 50%, occasionally more in some individuals, as a result of changing conditions such as sleep, physical activity, meals, fever, etc. Therefore, it is advised to program the charge at twice threshold to obtain a safety margin of 100%. This margin may need to be even greater in the post implantation period because of the rise in threshold caused by an early inflammatory reaction (Fig. 2.8.).

In the chronic phase, after the threshold has stabilized (at least 3–6 months after implantation of the electrode), programming aims at guaranteeing effective pacing while minimizing energy consumption to optimize the battery's life expectancy. The best compromise is to set the pulse duration near chronaxie, a zone where variations in energy, charge, voltage and current are relatively small, and to double the threshold voltage measured at that pulse duration. One must remember that the 100% safety margin has to be verified from a measure of the charge, and that, at constant pulse duration, a doubling of the voltage will guar-

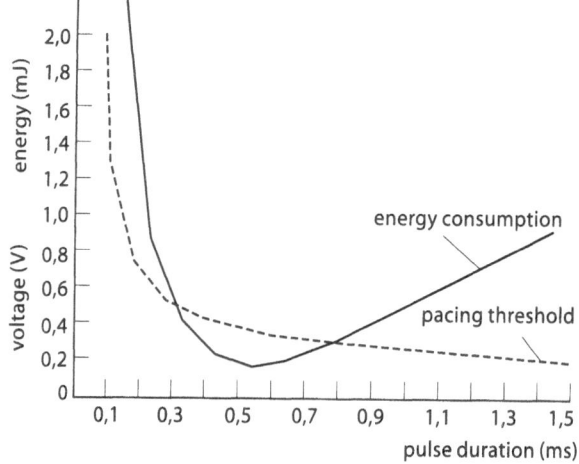

**Fig. 2.7.** The curve of energy consumption has a nadir which coincides with the pulse duration near chronaxie

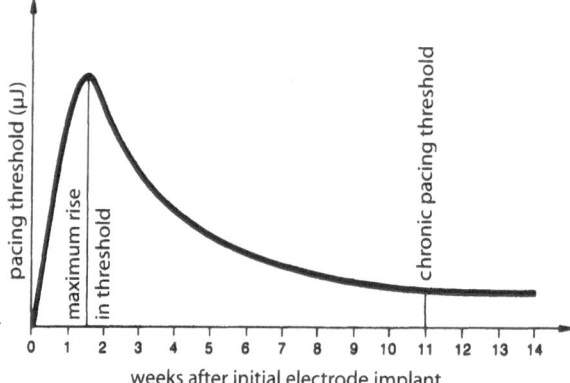

**Fig. 2.8.** In the atrium, the pacing threshold increases during the first weeks, reaching a peak between the 10th and 14th week, and falling to its chronic value after 2 to 3 months. In the ventricle, the peak may be delayed by 1 or 2 months to reach its chronic value at 6 months

antee a 100% safety margin. In contrast, at constant voltage, this safety margin can only be guaranteed by a quadrupled pulse duration (Figs. 2.2, 2.7).

In conclusion, one must program the strength of stimulation with a 100% safety margin by doubling the threshold voltage measured at a pulse duration near the chronaxie. The pacing threshold varies with various factors, including the pacing rate, drugs, metabolic disorders, degree of fibrosis developing in the vicinity of the electrode, electrode configuration, and polarity.

### Influence of Pacing Rate

The pacing threshold decreases with an increase in pacing rate, up to the point where the stimulus falls in the relative refractory period of the preceding cycle. This phenomenon may have important consequences in the case of antitachycardia pacing, when it is customary to use rapid pacing rates.

## Influence of Drugs and Metabolic Disorders

Glucocorticosteroids, epinephrine, ephedrin and isoproterenol decrease the pacing threshold. Spironolactones, propranolol, verapamil, quinidine and amiodarone may raise it, while class IC antiarrhythmic drugs (flecainide and propafenone) raise it predictably. Likewise, hyperkalemia, hypoxia, hypercapnea, hyperglycemia, and metabolic acidosis or alkalosis increase the pacing threshold.

## Influence of Degree of Fibrosis

Over the weeks that immediately follow implantation of the electrode, pacing threshold increases markedly, sometimes to a level twice or three times that measured at implantation, as a result of a foreign body type of inflammatory reaction. The rise in thresholds during the postoperative period is due to the separation of the electrode from the tissues, which increases the virtual radius of the electrode. Consequently, the same layer of inflammatory tissues has more pronounced effects on threshold at the site of a small than a large electrode. The peak of the inflammatory manifestations coincides with the nadir of pacing impedance. This rise in threshold rarely goes beyond the maximal energy able to be delivered by the pulse generator. Later on, threshold falls, however rarely to the level measured at implantation since the fibrosis that has developed increases the distance between the electrode and excitable myocardium. A stable chronic pacing threshold is reached at approximately 3 months after electrode implantation in the atrium, and between 3 and 6 months in the ventricle.

## Influence of Electrode Configuration on Pacing Impedance and Pacing Threshold

Size, shape and electrode materials also modify the pacing threshold. Current density is defined by the quantity of electrical charges which transit by unit of time through a surface perpendicular to the current pathway. As a result, a spherical shape of the electrode is associated with a higher threshold than an annular shape.

The pacing impedance must be as high as possible. It represents the sum of forces opposed to the flow of current in an electric circuit. It is composed of three ohmic-type resistances, including resistance of the conductor, resistance of the tissues, and the heart-electrode interface resistance, and of a capacitive reactance which corresponds to the polarization impedance.

The resistance of the conductor must be as low as possible to minimize energy losses along the lead from heat conversion; the higher the lead resistance, the higher the threshold. Likewise tissue resistance should be as low as possible. In unipolar pacing, this resistance is negligible, while reaching several dozens ohms in bipolar pacing. This partially explains the regularly lower pacing threshold measured with unipolar versus bipolar pacing.

The heart-electrode interface resistance has no effect on the pacing threshold, though it influences the current drain from the pulse generator and, thus, should be as high as possible to reduce the current drain from the pacemaker.

The electrode resistance is inversely and exponentially proportional to the electrode surface which gains from being as small as possible. In addition, a small electrode size minimizes the fibrotic reaction, a determinant of long-term threshold increase.

The phenomenon of polarization opposes the voltage transfer from the electrical environment of the lead to the ionic milieu of the tissues (see Appendix). Consequently, polarization impedance, which is inversely proportional to the electrode surface, must be as low as possible. To maintain a small macroscopic surface, which increases the heart-electrode resistance (and decreases power drain from the pulse generator) while increasing the microscopic surface of the electrode, which decreases polarization (hence, the pacing threshold), porous electrodes have been introduced. Microporous electrodes cause less polarization and are associated with lower pacing thresholds than smooth electrodes. Materials used are also of great importance since biocompatibility decreases the inflammatory reaction and subsequent fibrosis, thus reducing the risk of long-term threshold rise.

### Influence of Polarity

A cathodal electrostimulation is associated with a lower pacing threshold than anodal. A negative stimulation results in a direct drop in the transmembrane potential of the myocytes, whereas a positive one causes cellular hyperpolarization. At the end of the pulse, voltage drops and cells depolarize, creating a situation of hyperexcitability. Moreover, the refractory period is shorter after anodal than cathodal stimulation. Consequently, if a stimulus falls in the vulnerable period of a spontaneous cycle (in the case of sensing failure, for example), the risk of triggering a tachyarrhythmia is higher with anodal than with cathodal stimulation. As a result, anodal stimulation is never advised. Furthermore, bipolar stimulation is theoretically more arrhythmogenic than unipolar if both electrodes (anode and cathode) have the same surface area and the adjacent tissues have the same reactivity. The refractory period after bipolar stimulation is the same as that of anodal stimulation. This is particularly the case in risky situations such as metabolic disorders, hypoxia, ischemia etc. However, modern electrodes minimize this risk considerably since the anodal surface area is ten times larger than the cathodal, lowering the effect of anodal stimulation.

### Influence of the Pacing Stimulus Waveform

The defibrillation threshold is lower with biphasic versus monophasic shocks. It may be important to examine whether the same observations apply to antibradycardia pacing. The rheobase of a monophasic pulse is the same as that of a biphasic one, though the chronaxie of biphasic pulses is shorter. However, given the energies of antibradycardia pacing, depolarization threshold is higher with biphasic pulses, justifying the use of monophasic pulses in cardiac pacing. This should not be confused with the concepts of conditioning or fast recharge pre- and poststimuli, which are distinct from the pulse which depolarizes the myo-cardium.

## Sensing

Sensing defines the ability by the pacemaker of detecting electrical signals of car-diac origin transmitted through the electrode. Just as the strength of stimulation is expressed in volts, the amplitude of the sensed signal is expressed in millivolts (mV).

The pacemaker is equipped with entrance filters which sense P and R waves on the basis of three characteristics: the frequency spectrum (in Hz); the slew rate (in mV/ms); the signal amplitude (in mV).

### The Frequency Spectrum

The frequency of a signal is expressed in hertz (Hz) and is the inverse of its period (Fig. 2.9). Depolarization signals of cardiac origin are mainly contained within a frequency spectrum between 10 and 100 Hz, and are well included within the bandpass of the pacemaker's amplifier. The pacemaker amplifies incoming signals between 30 and 70 Hz (that is the average bandwidth of P and R waves), and its maximal sensitivity is situated in this range of frequency. Sig-nals above and below this range must be of much greater amplitude to be filtered by the pacemaker (Fig. 2.10). Therefore, the chances of sensing ventricular activ-ity by an atrial electrode are relatively slim since the R wave perceived in the atrium is a low frequency signal effectively eliminated by the pacemaker filter. The average frequency of the T wave is in a range below 10 Hz and is also elimi-nated (Fig. 2.10). On the other hand, the frequency spectrum of signals of muscu-lar origin overlap those of P and R waves. Therefore, in a unipolar configuration, the pacing system is vulnerable to interferences of muscular origin (see p. 70 and p. 270).

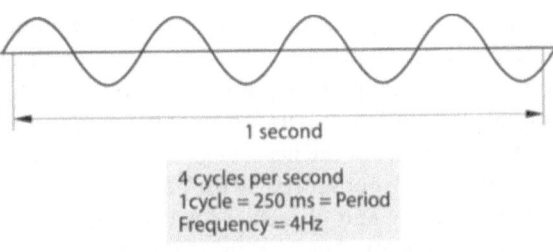

**Fig. 2.9.** Relationship between signal and fre-quency. In this example, 4 cycles occur over 1 sec-ond: the signal has, there-fore, a frequency of 4 Hz. Its period is, thus, 1 s/4, i.e. 250 ms. Hence, the relationship between period and frequency is: Frequency = 1/period, and period = 1/frequency

1 second

4 cycles per second
1 cycle = 250 ms = Period
Frequency = 4Hz

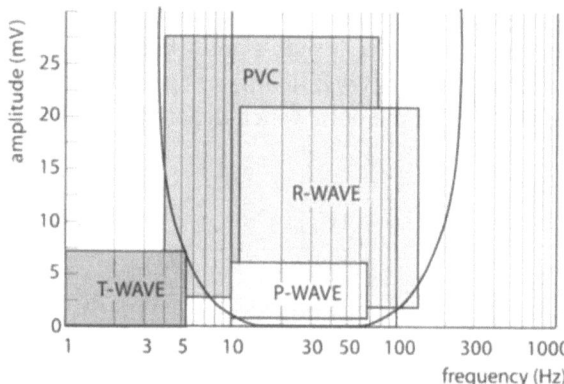

**Fig. 2.10.** Electrical characteristics of the various signals of cardiac origin. T wave: the signal of ventricular repolarization is in a frequency band between 1 and 5 Hz, with an amplitude between 1 and 7 mV. P wave: the atrial depolarization signal is in a frequency band between 10 and 50 Hz, with an amplitude between 11 and 6 mV. R wave: the ventricular depolarization signal in a frequency band between 10 and 70 Hz, and its amplitude is between 5 and 20 mV. PVC: premature ventricular complex is in frequency band between 5 and 40 Hz, and its amplitude ranges between 5 and 25 mV. The system used by pacemakers to sense electrical signals is based on filtration techniques. All devices use amplifiers to detect events whose frequency is comprised between an upper and a lower limit: the bandpass. All signals outside of these boundaries are ignored by the pacemaker. Generally, the bandpass of pacemakers ranges between 25 and 150 Hz, centered around 55 Hz. However, given a sufficiently large amplitude, the T wave may, despite filtering, be sensed as a ventricular depolarization signal

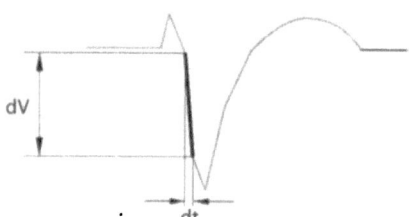

**Fig. 2.11.** The slew rate of an atrial or ventricular electrogram is the ratio of effective amplitude (dV) over time (dt) expressed in mV/ms, and ranges typically between 0.5 and 3 mV/ms

## The Slew Rate

The second main parameter determining sensing of intracardiac electrical signal is the slew rate of the depolarization potential (Fig. 2.11). This parameter describes the change in amplitude of the signal as a function of time (dV/dt in mV/ms)

The T wave is generally not filtered by the pacemaker because of its particularly slow slew rate (Fig. 2.12). On the other hand, some highly fragmented QRS complexes (usually extrasystoles) may not be properly sensed (Fig. 2.13). This may be the source of parasystole, i.e. pacing interferes with the spontaneous electrical activity of the heart (Fig. 2.18). It is generally agreed that a pure signal of a rapid wavefront sensed by the pacemaker has a slew rate of at least 1 mV/ms in the ventricle, and at least 0.5 mV/ms in the atrium. At implantation of the device, the fastest slew rate should be sought to guarantee proper long-term sensing (Figs. 2.14, 2.15).

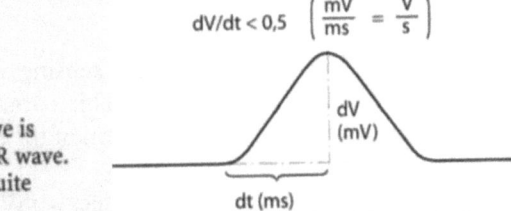

**Fig. 2.12.** The slew rate of the T wave is considerably lower than that of the R wave. Sensing of the T wave is therefore quite unusual

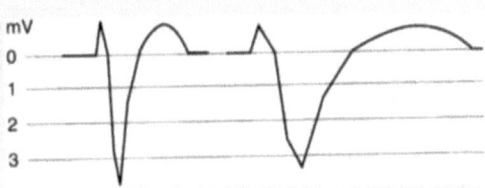

**Fig. 2.13.** In this example, the system sensitivity has been set at 2 mV. The electrogram on the *left* is consistently sensed properly, but not the one on the *right*. This sensing failure is explained by an intrinsic frequency of the signal outside of the bandpass of the filter

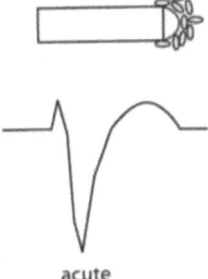

**Fig. 2.14.** Because of the development of fibrosis, the electrogram changes from its initial configuration

acute

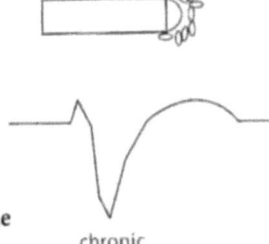

**Fig. 2.15.** The fibrotic layer causes an up to 25% decrease in the signal amplitude

chronic

However, the actual contribution of the slew rate is limited as a result of the different filters utilized by the PSA* and by the implanted pacemaker. Its interpretation is therefore difficult if the implanted device is of a different brand than the PSA, although, even for the same manufacturer, the filters of the pacemaker may be different than those of the PSA. It is important, therefore, to have a recording of the intracardiac electrograms at the time of lead implantation, particularly when the measurements reported by the PSA are borderline.

---

\* Pacer System Analyser

### Signal Amplitude

The third sensing criterion for proper sensing of intracardiac electrograms is the amplitude of the signal (Fig. 2.16). This parameter will be discussed in more details later in this book. Amplification of the signal after it has been filtered is usually programmable.

A sensing threshold of, for example, 4 mV allows sensing of spontaneous potentials of appropriate frequency and slew rate and whose amplitude is at least 4 mV. Smaller signals are left unrecognized by the pacemaker. Consequently, an increase in the programmed sensitivity setting, for example from 4 to 6 mV, means that the sensitivity of the device is decreased, and vice versa. This applies to the threshold measurements made at the time of device implantation, as well as to the chronically implanted pacemaker (Figs. 2.17–2.19).

Ultimately, the accuracy of sensing depends on an optimal combination of these three parameters: signal comprised within the bandpass, in the vicinity of 50 Hz, which means that the electrogram must include a high frequency component, also known as the intrinsic deflection, whose slew rate and amplitude should be as great as possible. In addition, to optimize the stability of a freshly implanted electrode, one should look for an elevation of the signal's ST segment,

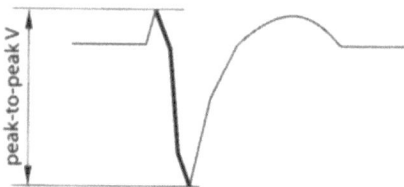

**Fig. 2.16.** The peak amplitude of an electrogram corresponds to the voltage measured between its peak and its nadir. In a depolarization signal, the peak-to-peak amplitude is often irregularly shaped because of the influence of various electrical sources. Sensing by the pacemaker is limited to the intrinsic deflection. After filtering, the signal is rid of some of its components. Thus, peak-to-peak amplitude does not faithfully represents the signal ultimately presented to the pulse generator

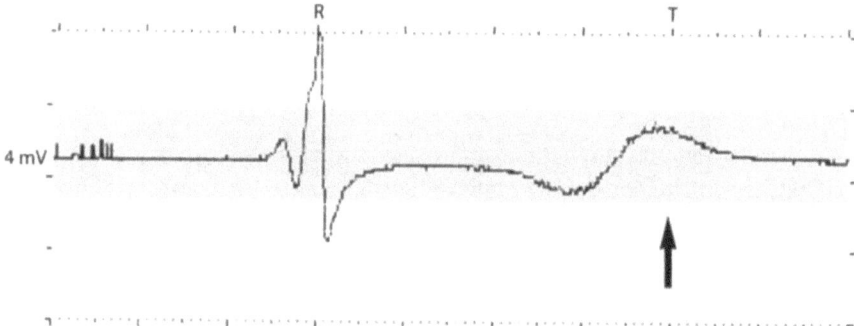

**Fig. 2.17.** Intracardiac ventricular electrogram. The deflections contained within the shaded area are not sensed by the pacemaker since their amplitudes are below the sensitivity programmed at 4 mV. *Arrow:* T wave

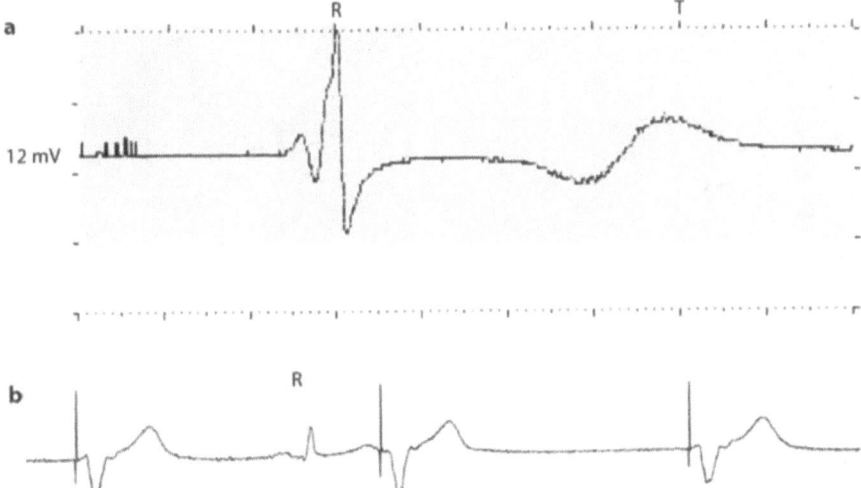

**Fig. 2.18. a** When sensitivity has been programmed at 12 mV, the pacemaker is insensitive, fails to sense all signals of cardiac origin, and paces asynchronously since it is no longer inhibited by spontaneous activity
**b** Failure to sense in the ventricle: a spontaneous complex (*R*) is not sensed by the pacemaker which continues to deliver asynchronous spikes at a fixed rate

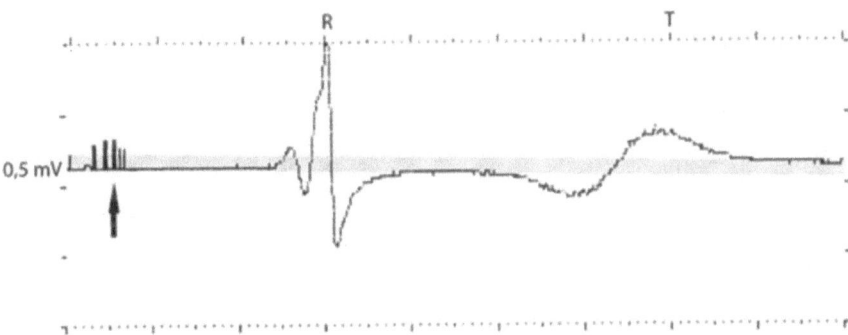

**Fig. 2.19.** The programmed sensitivity is 0.5 mV, such that the pacemaker is highly sensitive. Interferences, e.g. myosignals (*arrow*), are sensed by the pacemaker and improperly interpreted as being of cardiac origin

which indicates the presence of current of injury caused by localized endocardial ischemia. This finding allows to confirm satisfactory pressure of the electrode against the endocardium (Fig. 2.20). Finally, signals originating from other chambers should be as weak as possible to prevent crosstalk as in the case of a ventricular signal sensed by the atrial electrode (Fig. 2.21, see also p. 71–72, 105)

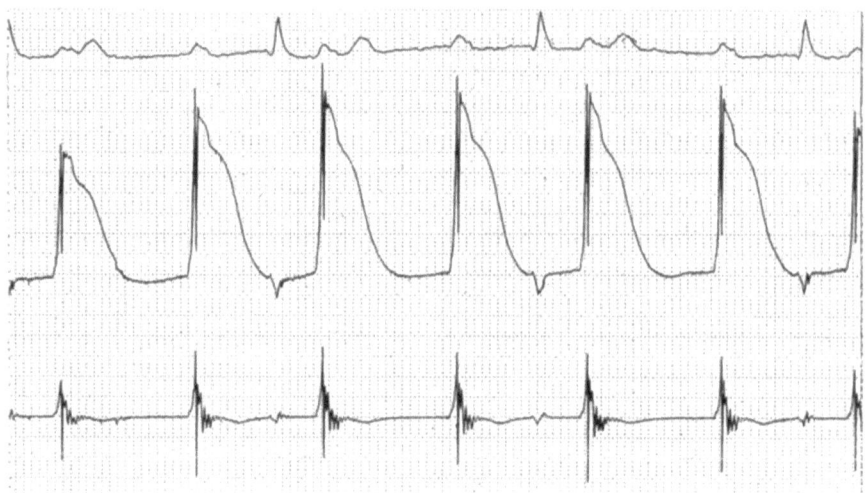

**Fig. 2.20.** Intracardiac atrial signal recorded within minutes of placement of a „screw in" electrode. *Upper trace*: surface ECG; *middle trace*: unfiltered intracardiac atrial electrogram recording (bandpath = 0.05 Hz – 1 kHz); *lower trace*: same signal filtered (bandpath = 30–100 Hz). The unfiltered signal is contaminated by a conspicuous current of injury which artificially increases its peak-to-peak amplitude, but also provides evidence of adequate electrode fixation. Recording speed = 50 mm/s

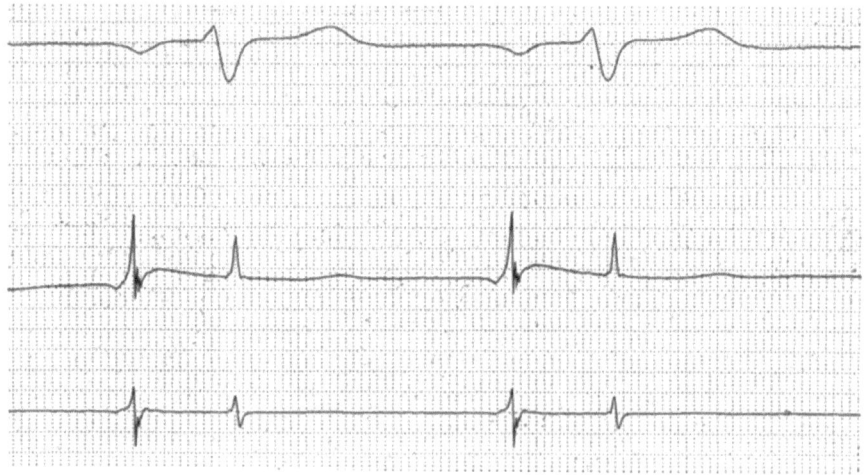

**Fig. 2.21.** The signals recorded are as described in Fig. 2.20. A ventricular electrogram is visible on the atrial channel, making the subsequent development of ventriculo-atrial crosstalk likely. Recording speed = 100 mm/s

Finally, it is important to keep in mind that the intrinsic deflection never occurs in the beginning of the surface ECG QRS complex. This explains the late sensing of the signal sometimes observed in cases of right bundle branch block

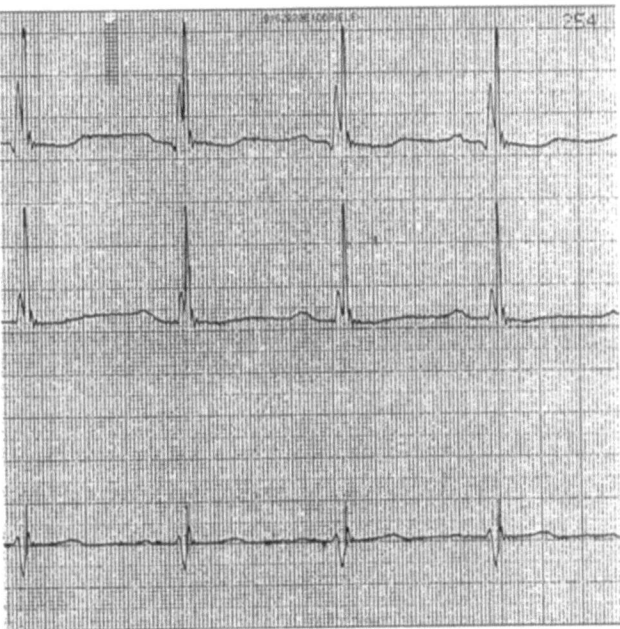

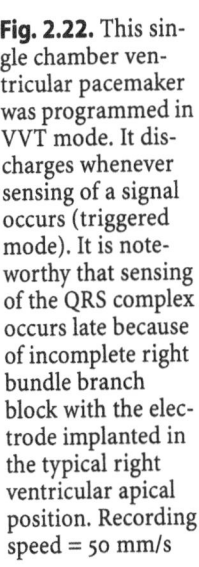

**Fig. 2.22.** This single chamber ventricular pacemaker was programmed in VVT mode. It discharges whenever sensing of a signal occurs (triggered mode). It is noteworthy that sensing of the QRS complex occurs late because of incomplete right bundle branch block with the electrode implanted in the typical right ventricular apical position. Recording speed = 50 mm/s

(Fig. 2.22) since the ventricular lead is implanted in the right ventricle and, thus, senses ventricular activation belatedly.

## 2.2
## The Pulse Generator

### Sources of Pacing Power

Until approximately 1975, the energy used in pacing was provided by a zinc-mercury battery whose main disadvantages were the gas production associated with its decay and a short life span. Nowadays, the iodine-lithium battery does not produce gas allowing its hermetic seal and insulation from the electronic circuitry. Its drawback is a high internal resistance which decreases its output voltage, particularly during high consumption (increase in pacing frequency from dual-chamber or rate responsive pacing).

When the battery nears depletion, its internal resistance increases. The output voltage is 2.8 V for a battery at beginning of life (BOL)*. As it decays, its internal resistance increases from 100 ohms to over 10 kiloohms. This causes a drop in output voltage to the neighborhood of 2.3 V, an indication of approaching end of life (EOL)** and of elective replacement (ERI)***. At 2.1 V, EOL has been reached and the generator is no longer capable of delivering an effective pulse (Fig. 2.23).

---

\* beginning of service (BOS), ** end of service (EOS), *** recommended replacement time (RRT)

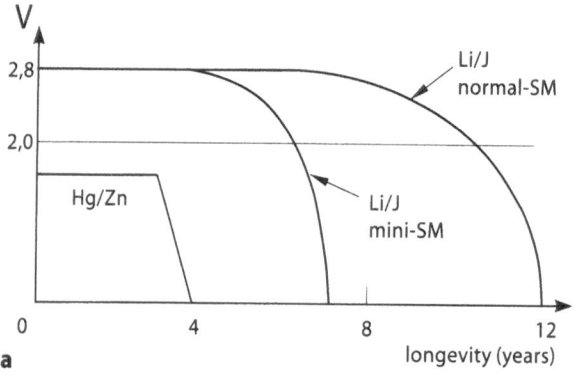

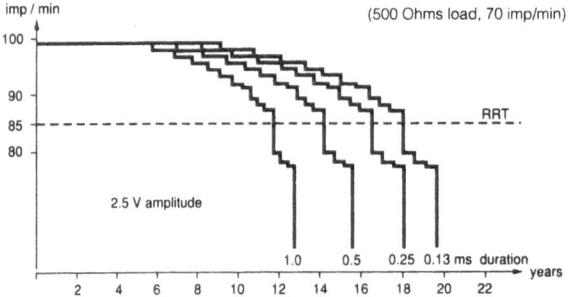

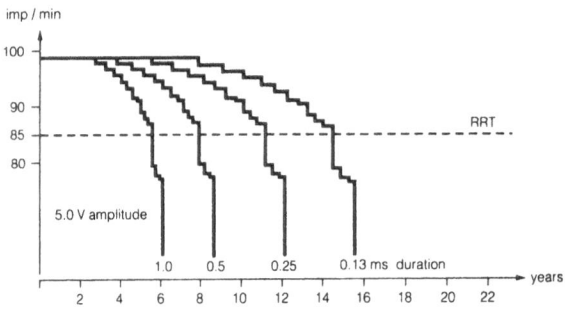

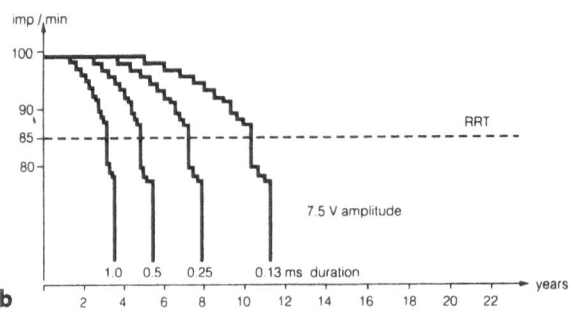

**Fig. 2.23. a** Depletion curves of various types of batteries. The lithium-iodine battery has an initially stable voltage at 2.8 V, followed by a gradual decay until total depletion. Caution is advised with respect to small-sized batteries (Mini-SM) currently offered by manufacturers, since their EOL is reached much more abruptly than with a similar, but larger battery. Zinc-mercury batteries had short lives and sudden EOLs
**b** The speed of decay depends on the programmed amplitude and duration of the pulse. The lifespan may be radically different as a function of these two variables (data from Pacesetter)

**Recommended follow-up intervals after appearance of the "AGEING" message**
(DDD, 60 min⁻¹, 0.4 ms, 100% pacing, 500 Ω).

| Pulse amplitude (V) | 7.5 | 5.0 | 3.8 | 2.5 | 1.2 |
|---|---|---|---|---|---|
| Recommended follow-up interval (months) | 1 | 2 | 3 | 6 | 6 |

months

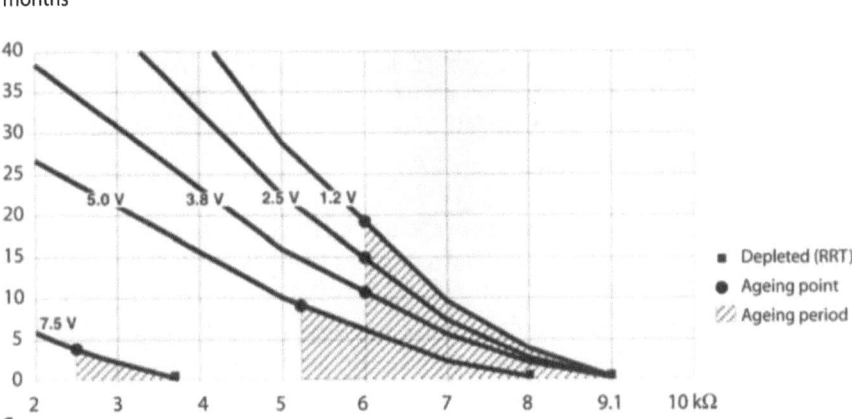

**Fig. 2.23. c** Another way of expressing the status of a battery is to graph its internal resistance as a function of time and programmed voltage. Resistance increases exponentially until the elective replacement indicator (ERI) has been reached. RRT (recommended replacement time) corresponds to ERI (data from Vitatron)
**d** Example of depletion curve of a current pulse generator, retrieved by telemetry. ERI, elective replacement indicator (PM from Ela Medical)

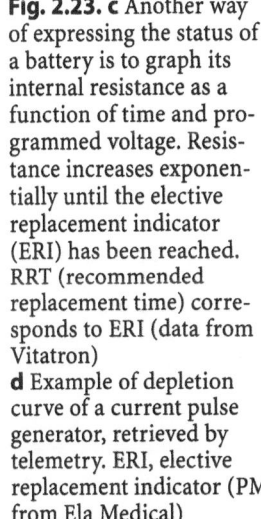

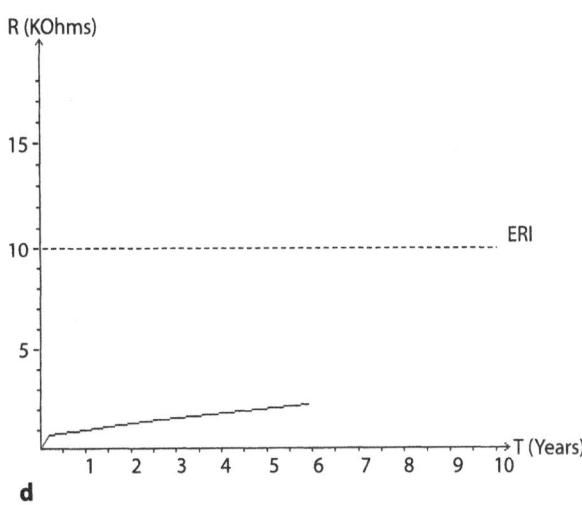

ERI is reached a few weeks before the voltage delivered by the battery reaches such a level resulting in loss of capture. Determination of the ERI is performed in various ways. Monitoring limited to delivered voltage is insufficient since it remains relatively constant, which is less likely to be the case with internal impedance.

The battery delivers a constant voltage at 2.8 V which may not be sufficient to depolarize the myocardium; the pulse generator includes a voltage multiplier to allow the generation of higher voltage. Nuclear batteries, used in the past, had much greater longevity. However, patients were no longer beneficiaries of the rapid evolution of the pacing technology, while not immune from the accidents associated with aging of the electrodes. The reliability of the iodine-lithium battery and other advances in cardiac pacing have lead to the abandonment of nuclear pulse generators.

## The Pacemaker Components

The integration of the basic functions (pacing and sensing), as well as of all complex tasks involved in each separately, requires a computer-like structure (Figs. 2.24, 2.25).

The battery powers the whole of these electronic components, including a microprocessor and associated memories. The circuits consist of a group of complementary C-MOS transistor-based cells which consume very little power.

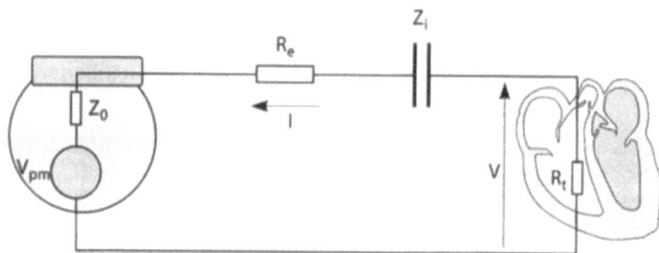

**Fig. 2.24.** The pacing circuit may be schematized as follows: $V_{pm}$ power source; $Z_o$ output impedance of the system; $R_e$ electrode resistance; $Z_i$ heart-electrode interface impedance; $R_t$ tissue resistance. The various impedances and resistances are placed in series. The voltage at the battery's poles is, thus, divided proportionally to the value of each. According to Ohm's law, the following relation applies: $V = I(R_e+Z_i+R_t)$, with I being the current flowing through all elements contained in the circuit

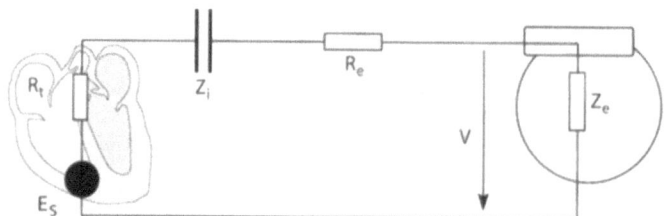

**Fig. 2.25.** The sensing circuit may be schematized as follows: $E_s$ endocavitary signal of myocardial origin; $R_t$ tissue resistance; $Z_i$ heart-electrode interface impedance; $R_e$ electrode resistance; $Z_e$ input impedance of the system. Since the cardiac signal is of very low amplitude, $R_t$, $Z_i$ and $R_e$ must be kept at a minimum. On the other hand, the input impedance into the pulse generator ($Z_e$) must be high (on the order of 15,000 – 20,000 $\Omega$)

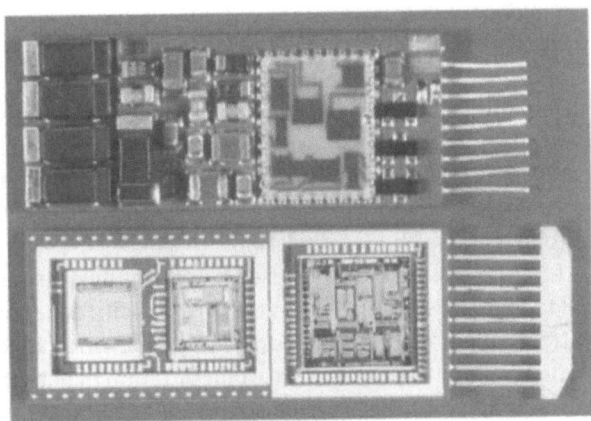

**Fig. 2.26.** Photograph of the electronic circuitry of a dual chamber pacemaker

A single or several integrated circuits constitute the interface between microprocessors, intracardiac electrodes and, when applicable, physiologic sensors. They also maintain communications with the outside world via a bi-directional telemetry system (Fig. 2.26).

The microcomputer consists of hardware and software which contain the programs and databanks. It controls the entire operation of the pacemaker. It is made of a central unit and associated memories. The Read Only Memory (ROM) has a fixed content set at the time of manufacture of the device. The information that it contains cannot be modified subsequently, although some devices do allow certain preprogrammed modifications by special programmers. ROM type memories consume little power. Moreover, their information is preserved even in the midst of powerful electric interference (electric knife, defibrillator, diathermy, etc.).

Random Access Memory (RAM) is an active memory which can be reinscribed. It is typically used to store the programmed pacing parameters, and the results of interim calculations and measurements. It also allows the storage of patient and pacemaker information. The content of RAM can be read and modified via the programmer. In more recent models, it is possible to load not only data, but also complementary programming instructions. This allows to modify, sometimes extensively, the pacemaker function after implantation. Future technology will be profoundly influenced by the development of Megachips, computer micromodules capable of logic functions and containing huge memories.

Microprocessor technology is steadily advancing. In modern devices, the hardware is used as the platform for pacing whose various functions depend on the quality and intelligence of the microprocessor-based software, also known as Central Processing Unit (CPU).

The ROM-RAM dialog is backed by safety measures to eliminate the introduction of erroneous data into RAM. In the unlikely case of memory loss from RAM, the microprocessor switches automatically to a safety mode which paces according to standard parameters.

## Pacemaker Longevity

The longevity of a pacemaker is defined as the time interval between its implantation and the identification of ERI. The longevity of an implanted pacemaker depends on multiple factors: the effective battery capacity, the programming of the pacing parameters and the percentage of time spent pacing, the system impedance, the efficiency of the electronic circuitry, the telemetry functions, and the passive battery depletion.

Lithium-iodine batteries used in pacing devices have a nominal capacity of 0.8 to 2 amperes-hour (Fig. 2.27). This capacity depends mainly on the size of the battery. However, the effective capacity, that which adequately supplies the circuits, is smaller. Indeed, after a certain duration of activity, although there is residual capacity in the battery, the voltage at its poles is no longer sufficient to supply the circuits, such that only the effective capacity can be taken into account, since it guarantees the normal pacemaker function.

The main element which determines longevity is the delivery of pacing pulses and, consequently, its related parameters: the programmed parameters, the percentage of time spent pacing, and the impedance of the system. The higher the pulse amplitude and/or duration, the greater the power consumption, and the shorter the pacemaker longevity. One must, therefore, program the pacing parameters at values high enough to guarantee 100% effective pacing under all circumstances, but low enough to minimize wasting of energy. As a corollary, programming of the device should be such as to minimize the delivery of pacing pulses whenever the hemodynamic and electrophysiologic status permits it.

Hence, a dual chamber rate responsive pacemaker consumes more power than an inhibited single chamber device. Finally, a low pacing impedance increases consumption and vice versa. It is, therefore, important to pay attention to this measurement at the time of implantation and to utilize modern leads with small surface electrodes associated with high pacing impedance. Insulation failure causes a precipitous drop in impedance and causes rapid battery depletion, whereas a non implanted device, thus not connected to a lead, consumes very little energy because pacing impedance is infinite.

Remaining factors entering in the calculation of battery longevity are less important. The consumption by electronic circuit has been considerably reduced with the introduction of C-MOS circuits. That needed for telemetry is virtually negligible. Finally the spontaneous decay of lithium-iodine batteries is minimal (on the order of 5%).

1 Ah = 1 A current for 1 hour
or

1 Ah = 10 mA current for 100 hours
or

1 Ah = 10 μA current for 100 000 hours
     = 10 μA for 11.4 years

Fig. 2.27. Energy sources. A battery with a capacity of 1 ampere hour (*A-h*) can deliver continuously a current of 1 A over 1 h (or a current of 10 mA over 100 h, etc.). Lithium/iodine battery

**Table 2.1.** Influence of a decrease in stimulation amplitude on the energy consumption and thus longevity of a pacemaker. If the impulse amplitude is reduced by half, then current consumption is reduced to 25%, which markedly increases the pacemaker's longevity

| | VVI Mode | | DDD mode | |
|---|---|---|---|---|
| Amplitude | 5 V | 2.5 V | 5 V | 2.5 V |
| Consumption in inhibited mode | 11 A | 11 A | 12 A | |
| Ventricular consumption | 10 A | 2.5 A | 10 A | 2.5 A |
| Atrial consumption | – | – | 10 A | 2.5 A |
| Total consumption | | | | 17 A |
| Longevity (in years) | | | | |
| For a 1.5 A-h battery | 9 | 14 | 6 | 12 |
| For a 1.1 A-h battery | 6.2 | 9.6 | 4.1 | 8 |

**Fig. 2.28.** Current consumption by the pacemaker can be calculated from this formula. By convention, current consumption is estimated at a pacing rate of 70 BPM, an impedance of 500 Ω, a pulse duration of 0.5 ms, an amplitude of 5 V, and a 100% incidence of pacing. In actuality, nowadays,

$$I = I_c + I_n \cdot \frac{F}{70} \cdot \frac{500}{Z} \cdot \frac{t}{0.5} \cdot \frac{V^2}{5^2} \cdot \frac{\% \text{ of } P}{100}$$

it has become more difficult to compare various models because manufacturers, who offer ever smaller batteries, advertise longevity estimates based on pulse durations shorter than 0.5 ms and amplitude lower than 5 V. These longevities are, thus, comparable to previously advertised ones, but based on lesser consumption parameters $F$ frequency of pacing (min$^{-1}$); $t$ pulse duration (ms); $V$ pacing voltage; $Z$ pacing impedance (1/2); $I_c$ current consumption of the electronic circuit in inhibited mode (A); $I_n$ constant; % of $P$ percentage of paced events

From this information, one can predict the longevity of a given device (Table 2.1). Longevity is the ratio between effective battery capacity and current consumption (Fig. 2.28).

One must stress that lithium-iodine batteries do not deplete abruptly as mercury batteries used to do. Warnings from end-of-life indicators allow time for elective scheduling of the pulse generator replacement. However, nowadays, the smaller devices offered by manufacturers contain critically small batteries with reduced effective capacity. The depletion curve of a small battery is much steeper near end-of-life than that of batteries used in devices built during the 1980s. This mandates closer surveillance of the patient implanted with these newer devices to avoid complications due to ineffective pacing or modification of the behavior of a pacemaker near depletion.

It is noteworthy that the incidence of pocket erosion or infection has not changes since the years 1983–1984, despite the continued reduction of the can size; one may, thus, legitimately wonder whether this trend imposed by manufacturers should not be revised in order to guarantee a satisfactory device longevity (on the order of 7 to 8 years for a single chamber device, and 5 to 6 years for a dual chamber and/or rate responsive pacemaker), and, in the same time, enhanced patient safety at the approach of battery depletion.

## 2.3
## Programming and Telemetry

### Programming

The ability to change the pacing parameters non invasively via an external device was viewed as superfluous by some in the beginning. Nowadays, the benefits and the need for programmability are no longer in doubt. This evolution of idea was paralleled by a sharp decline in the number of non programmable devices implanted.

Pacemakers are programmed by placing the programmer head (wand) of the external programmer over the cutaneous surface overlying the pacemaker can, and by sending electromagnetic or radiofrequency signals (Figs. 2.29, 2.30). The coded message contains a safety code that operates as a key on the programming circuit. This safety feature prevents the reprogramming of the device by other external sources („phantom programming"). After having received the message, the device decodes the information and programs its circuits. One must under-line that electromagnetic interferences may occur if another programmer or high energy electrical equipment are located near the patient. Problems may also occur during programming if the patient has been placed on a metallic table (operating or examination table).

Programming is not a technical game, but offers considerable advantages in individual patients, particularly apparent in transient sensing or pacing failures caused by metabolic disorders, for example (see clinical cases, p. 65). Conse-quently, one of the main advantages of temporary reprogramming is to avoid

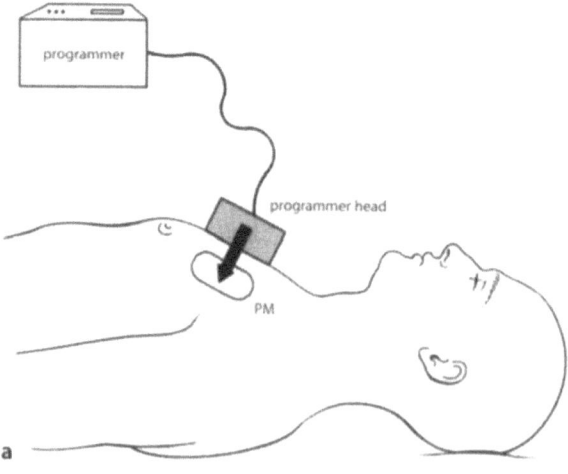

**Fig. 2.29. a** Programming consists of transmitting information from the pro-grammer to the pacemaker

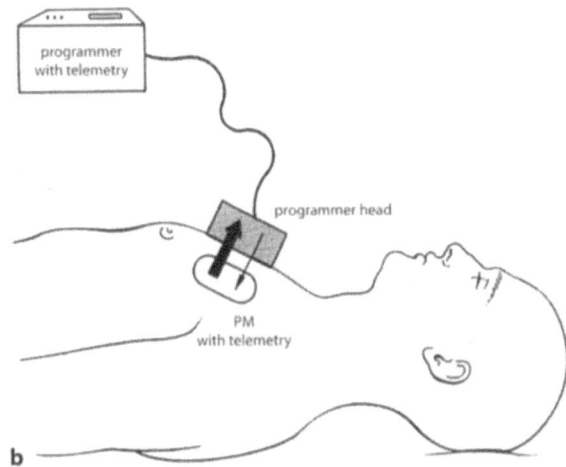

**Fig. 2.29. b** Telemetry is the transmission of information from the pacemaker to the programmer (interrogation)

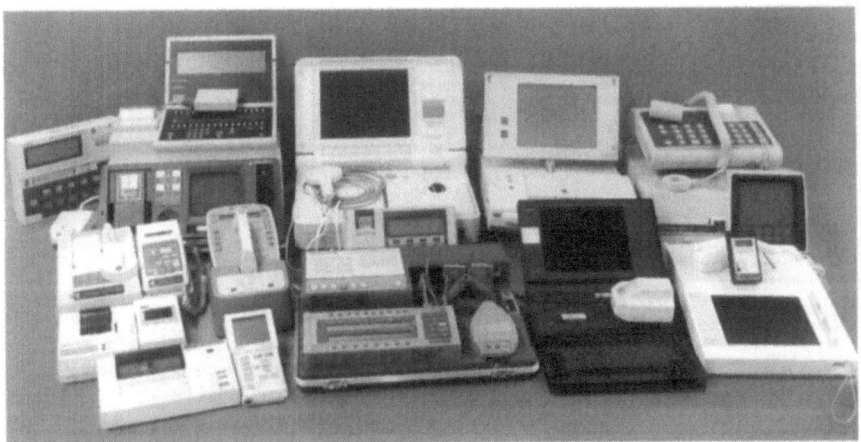

**Fig. 2.30.** A large number of programmers is needed to check and reprogram the many devices marketed by various manufacturers

device replacement for any or all device dysfunctions. One other substantial advantage is the option it confers to decrease the pacing output after implantation according to the chronic pacing threshold (measured 2–3 months after a first implant, or reimplantation of an electrode), which prolongs considerably the device's battery life. Furthermore, an optimal surveillance of a pacemaker, which includes an analysis of pacing and sensing safety margins, cannot be performed without temporary reprogramming of the device.

Besides these important advantages offering enhanced patient safety, cost effectiveness must also be considered. When one takes into consideration the costs involved in a reintervention (new pacing system, hospitalization, surgical costs, loss of work time, and possible complications), and the greater longevity of mul-

```
┌─────────────────────────────┐
│    PROGRAMMED PARAMETERS     │
└─────────────────────────────┘
```

|                                   | INITIAL | PRESENT |        |
|-----------------------------------|---------|---------|--------|
| Mode                              | DDDR    | DDDR    |        |
| Sensor                            | ON      | ON      |        |
| Rate                              | 50→     | 60      | ppm    |
| Hysteresis Escape Rate            | OFF→    | 50      | ppm    |
| Rate Hysteresis Search            | *       | ON      |        |
| A-V Delay                         | 175     | 175     | msec   |
| P-V Delay                         | 125     | 125     | msec   |
| AV/PV Hysteresis w/Search         | *       | 80      | msec   |
| Max Track                         | 135     | 135     | ppm    |
| V. Refractory                     | 250→    | 200     | msec   |
| A. Refractory                     | 275→    | 225     | msec   |
| Blanking                          | 38      | 38      | msec   |
| V. Safety Option                  | DISABLE→| ENABLE  |        |
| Auto Mode Switch                  | OFF→    | DDIR    |        |
| ATech Detect Rate                 | 0→      | 160     | ppm    |
| PVAB                              | 100→    | 150     | msec   |
| PVC Options                       | A PACE ON PMT | A PACE ON PMT |  |
| PMT Options                       | AUTO DETECT | AUTO DETECT |  |
| Rate Resp. A-V Delay              | MEDIUM  | MEDIUM  |        |
| Shortest AV/PV Delay              | 31      | 31      | msec   |
| Magnet                            | TEMPORARY OFF | TEMPORARY OFF | |
| Vent. Pulse Config.               | UNIPOLAR| UNIPOLAR|        |
| V. Pulse Width                    | .8      | .8      | msec   |
| V. Pulse Amplitude                | 2.5→    | 2.0     | Volts  |
| V. Sense Config.                  | BIPOLAR | BIPOLAR |        |
| V. Sensitivity                    | 3.0→    | 4.0     | mVolts |
| Atr. Pulse Config.                | UNIPOLAR| UNIPOLAR|        |
| A. Pulse Width                    | .4      | .4      | msec   |
| A. Pulse Amplitude                | 2.5     | 2.5     | Volts  |
| A. Sense Config.                  | BIPOLAR | BIPOLAR |        |
| A. Sensitivity                    | 1.0→    | .50     | mVolts |
| Maximum Sensor Rate               | 110     | 110     | ppm    |
| Threshold                         | 1.5→    | AUTO (+0.0) |    |
| Measured Average Sensor           | 2.5     | 2.5     |        |
| Slope                             | 8 (Normal) | 8 (Normal) |    |
| Sleep Rate                        | 45→     | 50      | ppm    |
| Reaction Time                     | FAST    | FAST    |        |
| Recovery Time                     | MEDIUM  | MEDIUM  |        |

```
    * Not Applicable
    → INITIAL value differs from PRESENT value
```

```
┌─────────────────────────────┐
│       MEASURED DATA          │
└─────────────────────────────┘
```

| Pacer Rate | 58.7 | ppm |
|------------|------|-----|

Ventricular:
| Pulse Amplitude | 2.0 | Volts    |
|-----------------|-----|----------|
| Pulse Current   | 2.4 | mAmperes |
| Pulse Energy    | 3   | μJoules  |
| Pulse Charge    | 1   | μCoulombs|
| Lead Impedance  | 823 | Ohms     |

Atrial:
| Pulse Amplitude | 2.4 | Volts    |
|-----------------|-----|----------|
| Pulse Current   | 4.2 | mAmperes |
| Pulse Energy    | 4   | μJoules  |
| Pulse Charge    | 2   | μCoulombs|
| Lead Impedance  | 676 | Ohms     |

Battery Data: (W.G. 8788 - NOM. 1.2 AHR)
| Voltage   | 2.78 | Volts    |
|-----------|------|----------|
| Current   | 15   | μAmperes |
| Impedance | <1   | KOhms    |

```
┌─────────────────────────────┐
│        TEST RESULTS          │
└─────────────────────────────┘
```

| R-Wave Amplitude | 8.8     | mVolts |
|------------------|---------|--------|
| Test Polarity    | BIPOLAR |        |
| Safety Margin    | 2.0 : 1 |        |

| P-Wave Amplitude | 3.8     | mVolts |
|------------------|---------|--------|
| Test Polarity    | BIPOLAR |        |
| Safety Margin    | 6.8 : 1 |        |

| Ventricular Capture Threshold | <.5      | Volts |
|-------------------------------|----------|-------|
| Test Pulse Width              | .8       | msec  |
| Test Polarity                 | UNIPOLAR |       |
| Safety Margin                 | >4.0 : 1 |       |

| Atrial Capture Threshold | 1.5      | Volts |
|--------------------------|----------|-------|
| Test Pulse Width         | .4       | msec  |
| Test Polarity            | UNIPOLAR |       |
| Safety Margin            | 1.7 : 1  |       |

**Fig. 2.31.** Complete printout of telemetry interrogation and pacemaker testing. The initial values are those retrieved at first interrogation at the beginning of the test; current values are those currently programmed. Sensing and pacing threshold, along with safety margins with respect to the programmed values, are also printed (Trilogy, Pacesetter)

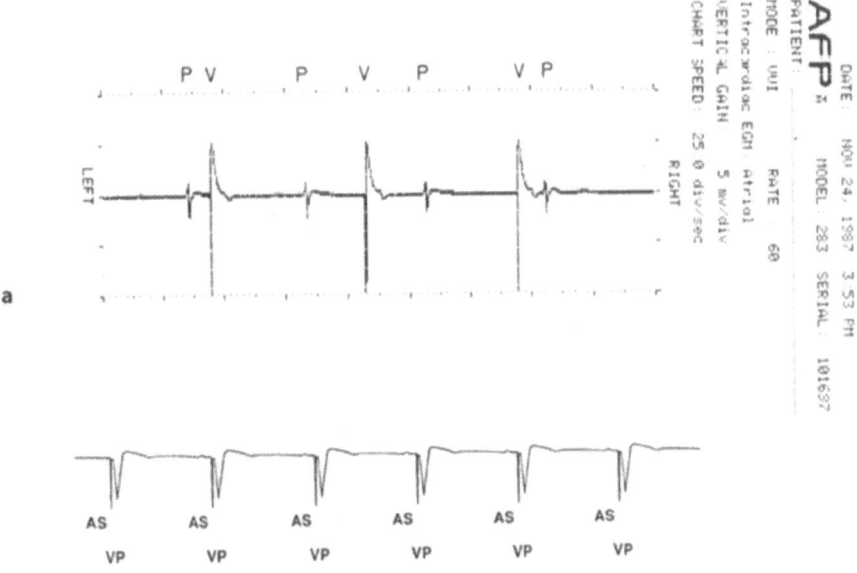

**a**

**b**    DDD, SM-Modell: Symbios 7005

**Fig. 2.32. a** Example of intracardiac atrial electrogram. An atrial electrogram is displayed while the pacemaker is operating in the VVI mode. The high amplitude signals are ventricular pacing spikes, also sensed in the atrium (on the order of 1 V). The lower amplitude signals are atrial depolarizations (on the order of millivolts). This tracing shows that, while it was being obtained, there was no retrograde conduction since the ventriculo-atrial interval (between the ventricular pacing artifact and the P wave) is constantly changing
*P* atrial depolarization; *V* ventricular pacing artifact (spike)
**b** Surface electrocardiogram with simultaneous event markers. Each P wave is sensed (*AS*) and followed by ventricular pacing (*VP*)

tiprogrammable devices from a reduced energy consumption, a cost effectiveness analysis is distinctly in favor of implanting multiprogrammable systems. In view of these various arguments, non programmable pacemakers should no longer be used.

## Telemetry

Telemetry may be viewed as the equivalent of programming with the communication established in the reverse direction, pacemaker–programmer. With the programmer head placed over the pulse generator, the device is interrogated, such that, as opposed to programming, the wand is used as a receiver of messages to be forwarded to the programmer.

The aim of telemetry is to collect essential information pertaining to device function, i.e. the values of the programmed parameters; these depend on the pacemaker model. In most modern pacemakers, one can also retrieve the device's serial number and miscellaneous information relative to battery status, lead integrity (Figs. 2.31, 2.32), and several diagnostic data (see p. 275–308).

## 2.4
## The Pacing Lead

### The Connector

The lead connector makes contact with that of the pacemaker. It is critical to observe a perfect concordance between the two. Otherwise, there is a risk of current leak with rise in pacing and sensing thresholds, and/or alterations in the connectors. Initially connectors sizes were 6 mm and, later, 4.75 mm in diameter. However, the introduction of new connectors standards at 3.2 mm has complicated the situation. The advantage was to reduce the size of the system, especially in the case of bipolar configurations for which a bifurcated lead connector was necessary. However, before coming to the standard type IS-1, which should be universally adopted by manufacturers, the interim use of Medtronic standards, and then of VS-1, has continued to complicate the replacement of devices during this period of transition (Figs. 2.33 – 2.38). It is thus necessary to pay great attention to this concordance before proceeding with replacement of a pulse generator (see p. 373 – 375).

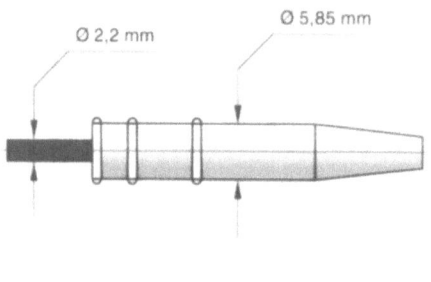

**Fig. 2.33.** In the Cordis standard connection, the silicone plug diameter is 6 mm (5.85 mm) and the diameter of the terminal pin is 2.2 mm. The lead connector is equipped with sealing rings. The 5 mm Medtronic and 6 mm Cordis are not always compatible, depending on the device connector's characteristics (hole diameter, ring dimensions, etc.)

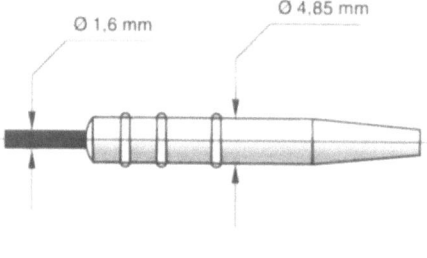

**Fig. 2.34.** In the Medtronic standard connector, the silicone plug is 5 mm (4.85) and the terminal pin diameter is 1.6 mm in diameter. The connector includes sealing rings

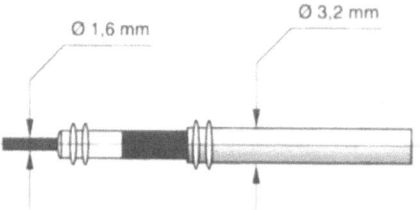

**Fig. 2.35.** The 3.2 mm Cordis connector is distinct from the connector by its longer (9 mm) terminal pin which may interfere with connection (long lead terminal pin, short housing receptacle)

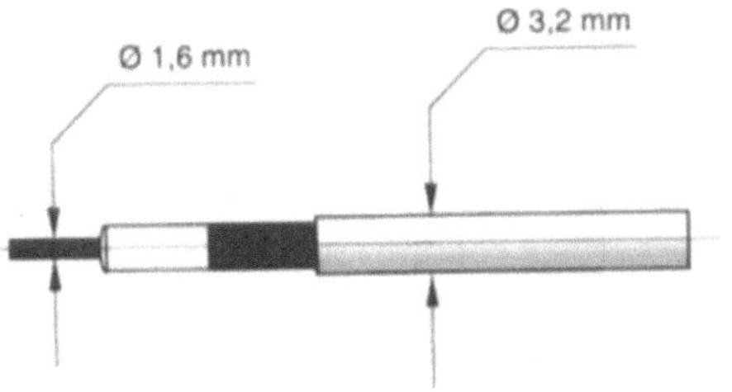

**Fig. 2.36.** The Medtronic VS-1 connector is distinct from other 3.2 mm standards by its long terminal pin and absence of sealing rings. Consequently, the housing receptacle must accommodate long pins and contain seals to guarantee hermeticity

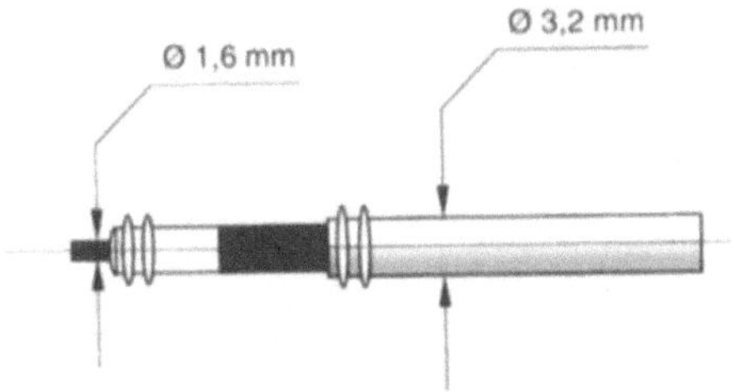

**Fig. 2.37.** The VS-1/IS-1 standard connector is 3.2 mm in diameter at the level of the connector, and its short (5 mm) pin is 1.6 mm in diameter. The sealing rings are on the lead. The housing receptacle may or may not contain sealing rings. The rationale for this normalization attempt by some manufacturers (VS-1) has been revived with a view towards international normalization (IS-1)

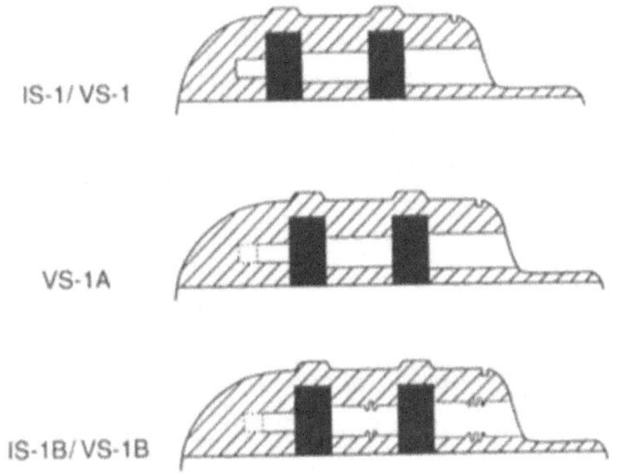

**Fig. 2.38.** Examples of device connectors according to current norms: IS-1/VS-1 connector: no sealing rings, short terminal pin receptacle; VS-1A connector: no sealing rings, long terminal pin receptacle; IS-1B/VS-1B connector: contains sealing rings, long terminal pin receptacle

## The Conductor

The conductor, now helicoidal and multifilar, offers much flexibility and greater mechanical resistance than former monofilar conductors. Stainless steel, abandoned because of its high propensity to corrode, has been replaced by platinum-iridium, carbon or elgyloy (a cobalt, nickel, molybdenum, manganese, chromium and iron alloy) offering higher long-term mechanical resistance. The electrical resistance of modern leads is very low, on the order of 10 $\Omega$.

## The Insulation

The insulation material is of utmost importance. It must be biocompatible, mechanically and chemically perfectly stable over long periods of time, and must not be thrombogenic. It is currently made of silicone rubber or polyurethane. Silicone rubber is highly biocompatible, flexible, and mechanically resistant, but it must be thick (the „high performance" silicone is expected to mitigate this disadvantage) because it tears easily, though can be repaired, and it may become calcified; in addition, its friction coefficient is high. Therefore, two silicone leads introduced in a small peripheral vein may be difficult to manipulate. New surface coatings in development should correct this shortcoming.

Polyurethane 80 A, used in early lead models, has been associated with insulation failure. Cracking of the pellethane insulation resulted from the manufacturing process (uneven cooling of the material) exposing the insulation to various mechanical stresses (further manufacturing, stretching and traumas at the time of implant). In the beginning, microscopic cracks (see Fig. 6.7a) develop in areas of mechanical strain, leading to breakdown of the insulation at points of ligature, between first rib and clavicle, and the bend in the right atrium, and at the interface with the endocardium. Metal-induced oxidation in one another mechanism of insulation failure, due to oxidative degradation of the polyurethane hydrogen peroxide liberated by inflammatory phenomena after the infiltration of fluid inside the lead. As a result, Medtronic 6972, 6990 U and 6991 U leads have had to be systematically replaced. Leads 4004, 4012, 4504, 4512 (Medtronic) and 1010 T (Pacesetter) must be carefully watched. Nowadays, polyurethane 55D is a reliable material, offering high mechanical resistance, low friction coefficient, and small thickness, which allows the construction of smaller leads than silicone rubber. However, it is stiffer and cannot be repaired.

## The Electrode

The electrode is the part of the lead in contact with the endocardium (Fig. 2.39). The influence of size and shape of the electrode on pacing threshold have been discussed (see p. 25–26). Its materials are quite varied. Initially of polished metal, its surface is now porous, which minimizes polarization and improves sensing. The electrode is naturally microporous with carbon, which allows tissular colonization, or is rendered artificially porous, as in the old Laserdish lead, with laser perforated macropores, or encrusted with platinum or elgiloy microspheres, or made of a network of metallic fibers. As a whole, the advantage of a porous electrode are a low polarization, a lesser fibrotic reaction (Fig. 2.40), a better endothelial ingrowth of the electrode, a lower sensing impedance, and a lower pacing threshold.

Medtronic was the first manufacturer to offer electrodes equipped with a central reservoir containing 1 mg of dexamethasone sodium phosphate bound to silicone with passive and continuous diffusion along its concentration gradient (Capsure lead). The diffusion is local, not systemic. Approximately 20% of the drug remains trapped in the reservoir at 4 years. The favorable effects on pacing threshold of glucocorticosteroids administered systemically is attributed to the inhibition of the release of inflammatory mediators by the cells included in the fibrotic tissue. Similarly, steroid eluting electrodes stabilize macrophages, and attenuate myofibrillar disarray and myocyte membrane

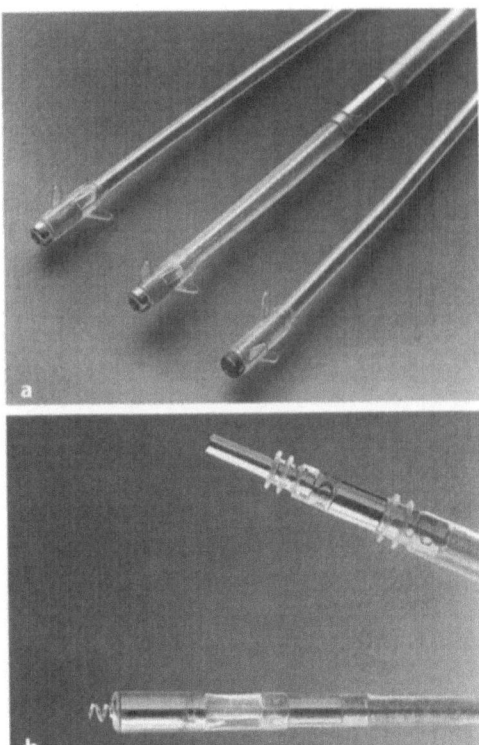

**Fig. 2.39. a** Passive fixation (tined) endocardial pacing electrodes
*Left*: platinum, unipolar
*middle*: platinum, bipolar
*right*: carbon, unipolar (photograph from Ela Medical)
**b** Endocardial pacing electrode with retractable screw

injury. Steroid elution suppresses the slow release of inflammatory mediators, thus preventing the rise in threshold without incurring the risk of systemic effects.

The results of clinical studies have confirmed the validity of this concept by demonstrating a considerable reduction in the amount and duration of the inflammatory process after implantation of the electrode, and a stabilization of the chronic pacing threshold at a lower level than that obtained with similar leads without steroid. Active fixation („screw in") electrodes are now available with steroid, and similar beneficial effects are expected despite greater local injury. Other manufacturers have developed leads with steroid contained in a collar situated at the tip, adjacent to the electrode.

## Fixation Methods

The lead is fixed by various methods (see Fig. 2.40). Initially, in absence of means of fixation, the lead was kept in place at the right ventricular apex by virtue of its rigidity alone, with a considerable rate of dislodgment and myocardial perforation. Then a silicone cone was developed. Nowadays, 2 types of leads are avail-

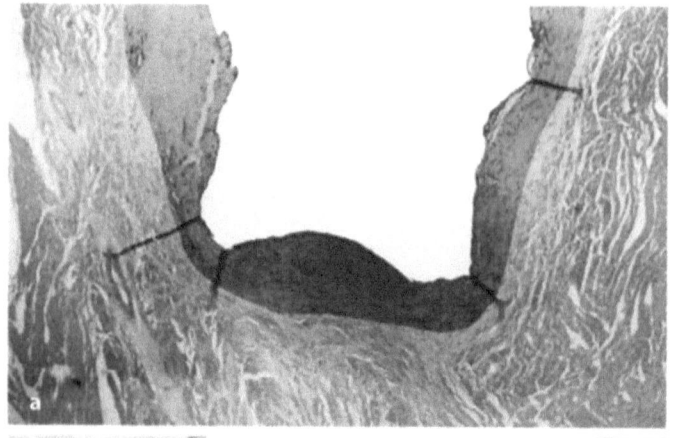

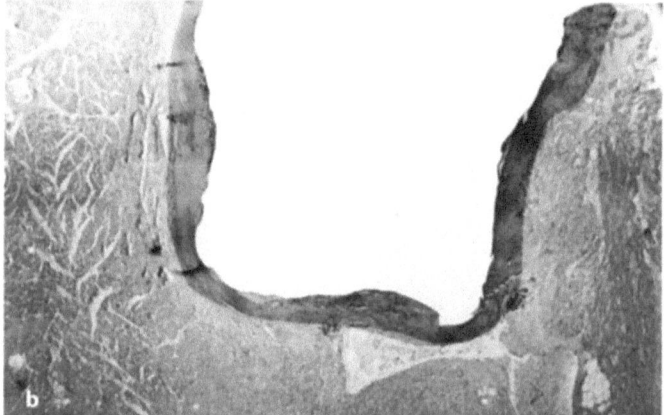

**Fig. 2.40.** More prominent fibrotic reaction caused by a platinum electrode (**a**) as compared to a carbon electrode (**b**) 3 months after implantation in a canine right ventricular apex (data from Ela Medical)

able: passive fixation with outgrowths (tines) of the insulation material near the distal electrode; or active fixation, with a retractable or non retractable screw which may or may not be electrically active. With such devices, the dislodgment rate is less than 1% in experienced hands, at the cost, perhaps, of a slightly higher acute pacing threshold with „screw in" electrodes.

## Unipolarity Versus Bipolarity

Pacing leads are either unipolar or bipolar. With the unipolar type, the electrode is the negative pole (cathode), and the pulse generator can is the positive pole (anode), or „indifferent" pole. In bipolar configuration, the negative pole is located at the very end of the lead, and the positive one is a ring 10 to 25 mm proximal to the negative pole (Fig. 2.41). Both poles of a bipolar lead are thus intracardiac (Fig. 2.42), whereas, in a unipolar system, the electrical field spans from the distal electrode to the pacemaker can, across the thorax and the pectoral muscles (Fig. 2.43).

The disadvantages of the bipolar lead are the following:

- Its caliber is bigger since its has two insulated conductor wires, which explains its greater rigidity and lesser maneuverability than a unipolar lead.
- It cannot be repaired in case of fracture, and it is not advised to convert it into a unipolar lead by abandoning the conductor to the proximal electrode since damage of one of the conductors usually means damage to the entire lead.
- On the surface electrocardiogram, the pacing spike may have a lower amplitude than that of a unipolar lead, which may make it difficult to analyze, even with the use of special filters (Figs. 2.44, 2.45).
- The amplitude of the cardiac signal depends highly on the dipole orientation with respect to the orientation of the depolarization wavefront. Sensing may, theoretically, be hampered if the axis of depolarization of a spontaneous event such as an extrasystole is perpendicular to the lead's sensing dipole (a bipolar signal results from the potential difference sampled by each pole).
- The intensity of the electrical field is distributed between both electrodes of the bipolar lead, and is therefore weaker at each electrode than the intensity of the electrical field in the vicinity of a unipolar lead. In other words, there is a theoretical loss of energy in a bipolar lead. To minimize this energetic loss, the anode must be sizable, and be placed at a considerable distance from the cathode.

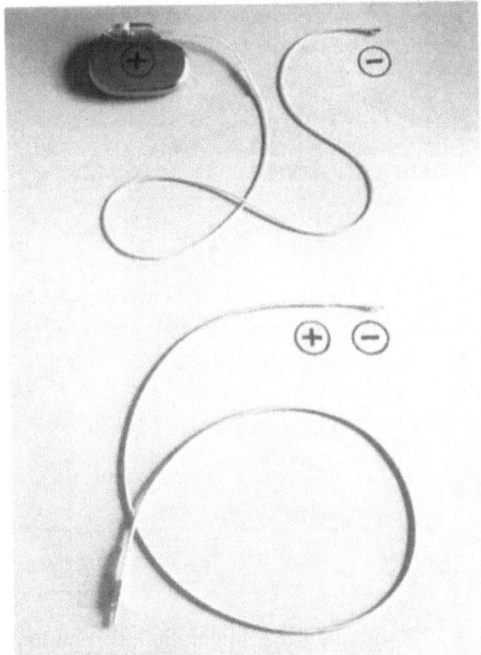

**Fig. 2.41.** A unipolar lead connected to the pulse generator

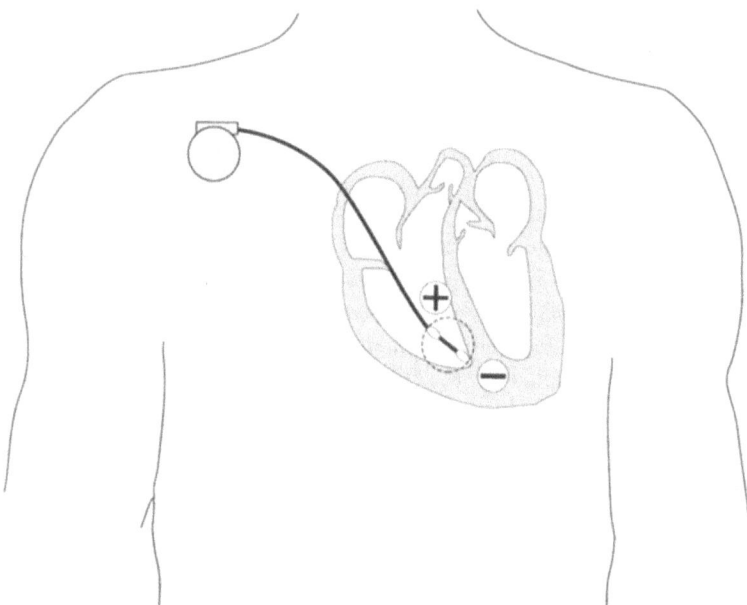

**Fig. 2.42.** In a bipolar configuration, current flows through the lead conductor, reaches the distal electrode, traverses the myocardium, reaches the distal electrode and returns through a second conductor wire to the pacemaker can

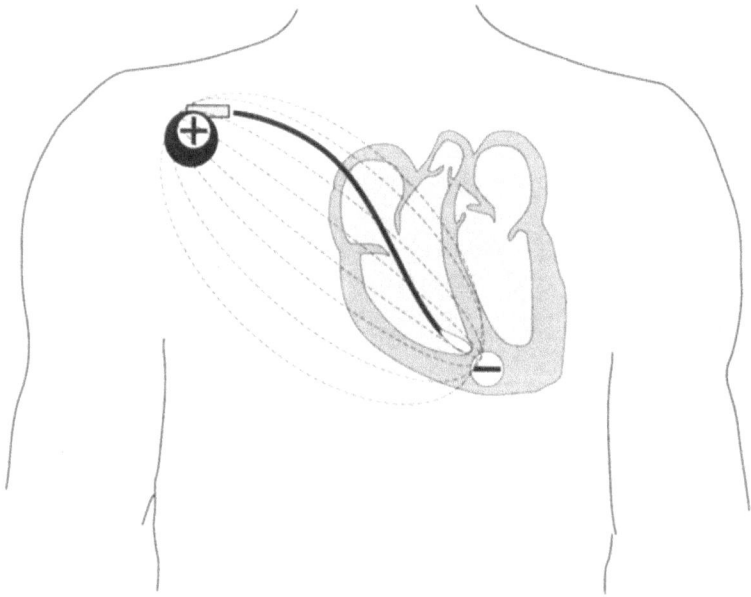

**Fig. 2.43.** In unipolar configuration, current flows through the lead conductor, through the myocardium, and returns to the pacemaker can which constitutes the second electrode

The advantages of the bipolar lead are, however, determinant:

- The electrical field is strictly intracardiac and does not traverse the thorax as in the case of unipolar pacing. Consequently, signals of muscular origin cause virtually no interference with bipolar sensing. The risk of inhibition or triggering of the pacemaker by myosignals is minimized. Likewise, the chances of T wave sensing by a ventricular lead, or R wave by an atrial lead are considerably diminished. Finally, risks of interference by extraneous signals are fewer; this will be more extensively discussed in Chapter 6 (see p. 256 – 262), though the example of adverse interferences by high power, low frequency security systems used in department stores is worth mentioning here.
- Conversely, muscular and diaphragmatic contractions caused by unipolar pacing are practically never encountered with bipolar stimulation.

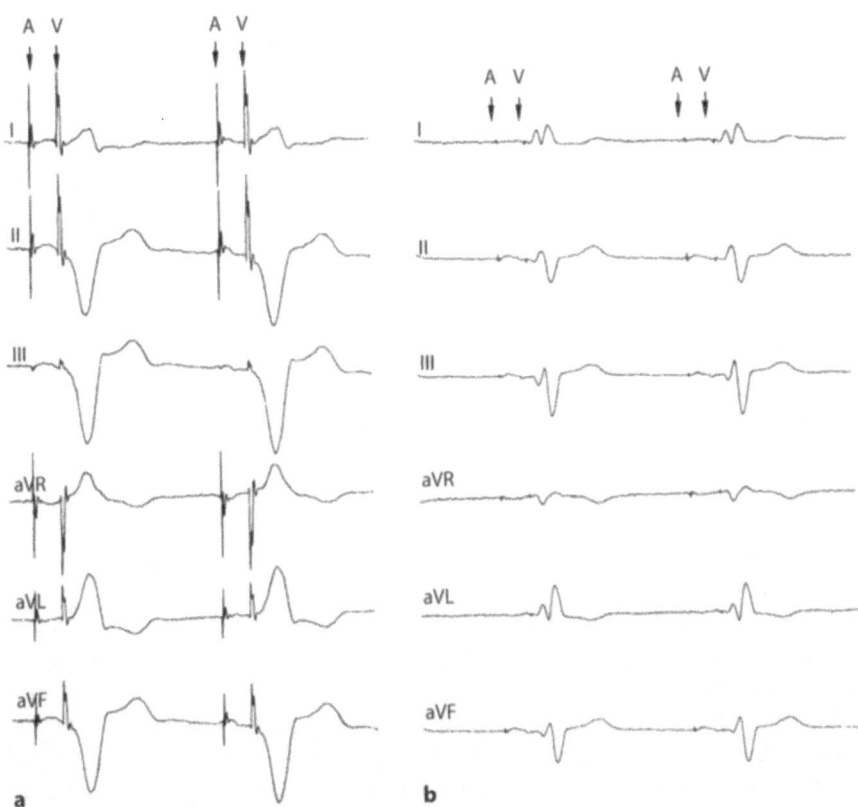

**Fig. 2.44. a** In unipolar configuration, pacing spikes are easy to recognize on the surface electrocardiogram
**b** In bipolar configuration, the spikes are often difficult to identify even after removal of the filters of the electrocardiographic recorder

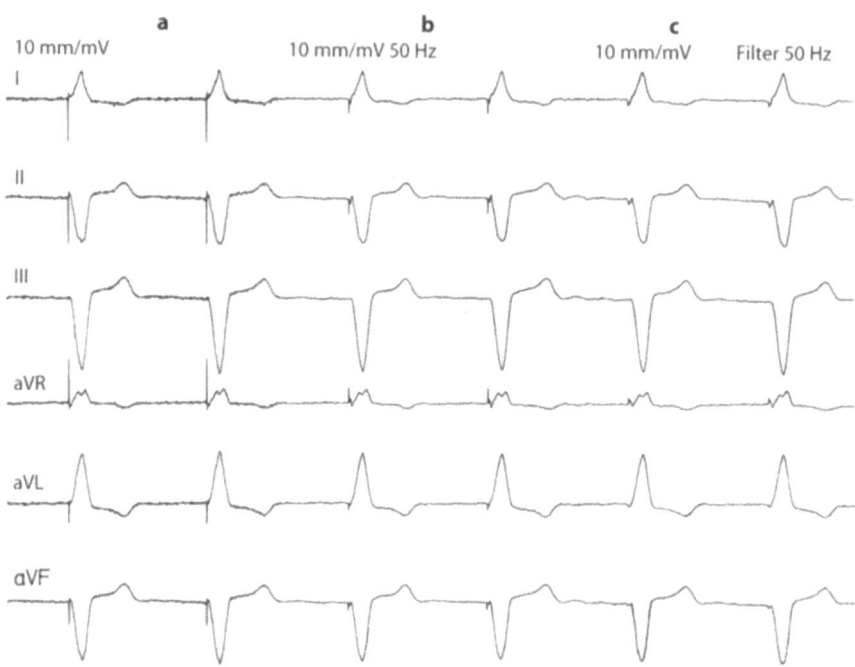

**Fig. 2.45.** The electrocardiographic filters may sometimes render the pacing spikes undetectable in bipolar configuration. The difficult interpretation of the tracing may lead to erroneous conclusions. One can sometimes improve the tracing by changing the filter

**Table 2.2.** The NASPE/BPEG pacemaker lead code (NBL code)

| I | II | III | IV |
|---|---|---|---|
| Electrode configuration | Fixation mechanism | Insulation material | Drug elution |
| U = Unipolar | A = Active | P = Polyurethane | S = Steroid |
| B = Bipolar | P = Passive | S = Silicone rubber | N = Nonsteroid |
| M = Multipolar | 0 = None | D = Dual (P + S) | 0 = None |

In the United States, the preference has been and remains in favor of bipolar leads. In Europe, since the development of 3.2 mm connectors, and the greater flexibility and reliability of bipolar leads, they are being used more and more. Moreover, the selective programming of sensing versus pacing configuration should become widespread. Ideally, pacing should be programmed unipolar (lower consumption of energy, spikes more visible on the surface ECG), and sensing in bipolar configuration (to optimize the reliable function of the pacemaker).

Table 2.2 shows the lead code as proposed by NASPE/BPEG. This classification is not widely used in practice.

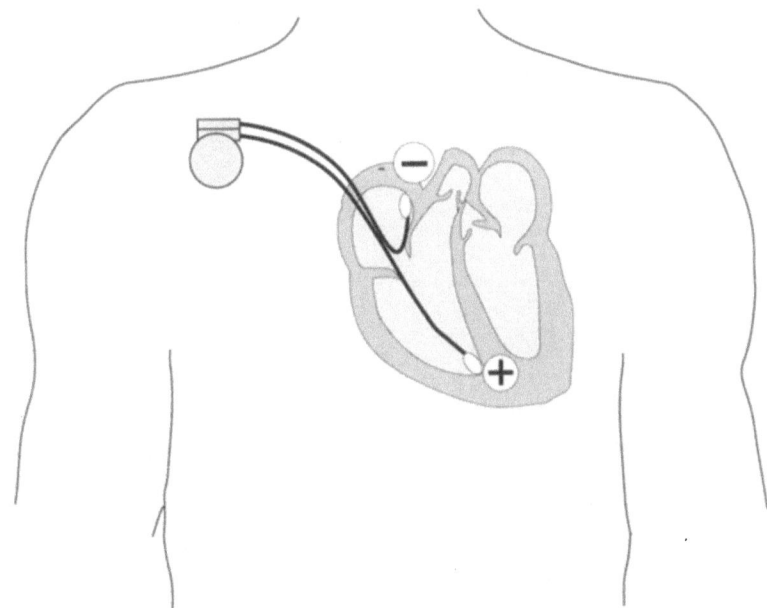

**Fig. 2.46.** During atrial sensing, the atrial unipolar electrode is the cathode and the ventricular electrode is the anode. Although the system is unipolar, the Combipolar configuration reduces the chances of sensing myosignals, thus allowing the programming of a high atrial sensitivity

## Combipolar Concept

Combipolar sensing (Polarity DDDR system, Pacesetter) is intended for atrial sensing, though requires both an atrial and a ventricular lead. The atrial sensing system senses the difference in potential between the atrial and the ventricular electrodes (Fig. 2.46). Both the P wave and the QRS complex are sensed. If the signal represents a P wave (originating from the atrium), the AV delay is initiated. When the atrial amplifier senses a QRS complex, the ventricular amplifier senses it as well. If the ventricular amplifier senses the QRS complex before the atrial amplifier, the signal is identified as a QRS complex and the atrial channel is refractory. However, if atrial and ventricular sensing of a PVC occurs simultaneously, an AV delay is initiated. Consequently, the AV interval should not be programmed „long" when Combipolar is in use.

In general, the risk of myosignal interference is greater in the atrium since the P wave amplitude may be the same or lower than the amplitude of myosignals. In the case of the Combipolar system, the effective field of sensing spans between the atrial and the ventricular lead tips. Compared with the field of a unipolar system, which spans between the lead tip and the pacemaker can, the Combipolar configuration is reduced, resulting in a lower noise amplitude sensed by the pacemaker. Thus, eliminating the pulse generator from the atrial sensing process reduces the risk of sensing interferences.

# CHAPTER 3

# The Pacing Modes

## 3.1
## The International Code[1]

The various pacing modes have been classified according to an international code which allows the immediate understanding of the overall function of a pacemaker. A three letter code was originally used. Technological advances have mandated the addition of a fourth and fifth letter.

- The first letter always indicates the site of stimulation, either the ventricle (V), the atrium (A), both (D), or neither (O) [S also indicates either ventricle or atrium: „single" (single chamber)].
- The second letter indicates the site of sensing, according to the same code.
- The third letter indicates the mode of function: inhibited (I), triggered (T), both (D), or none (neither triggered nor inhibited).
- The fourth letter indicates the programmability, the availability of telemetry, or of rate responsiveness:

  O  Nonprogrammable.
  P  Up to two programmable functions, usually the lower rate and the pulse duration or amplitude.
  M  Multiprogrammable, with three of more functions.
  C  Communication: the availability of telemetry makes the device interactive, with bidirectional exchanges of parameters. It can be interrogated.
  R  Rate responsiveness = rate modulation (increase in pacing rate based on information provided by a sensor which measures an effort-related parameter), now of considerable technological importance.

- A fifth letter is used for antitachycardia pacing function:

  O  None
  P  Pacing (antitachycardia)
  S  Shock
  D  Dual (P+S)

These various pacemaker configurations will be further detailed in upcoming chapters.

---

1 The NBG Code, equivalent to the NASPE/BPEG generic pacemaker code. NASPE, North American Society of Pacing and Electrophysiology; BPEG, British Pacing and Electrophysiology Group (see foldout table)

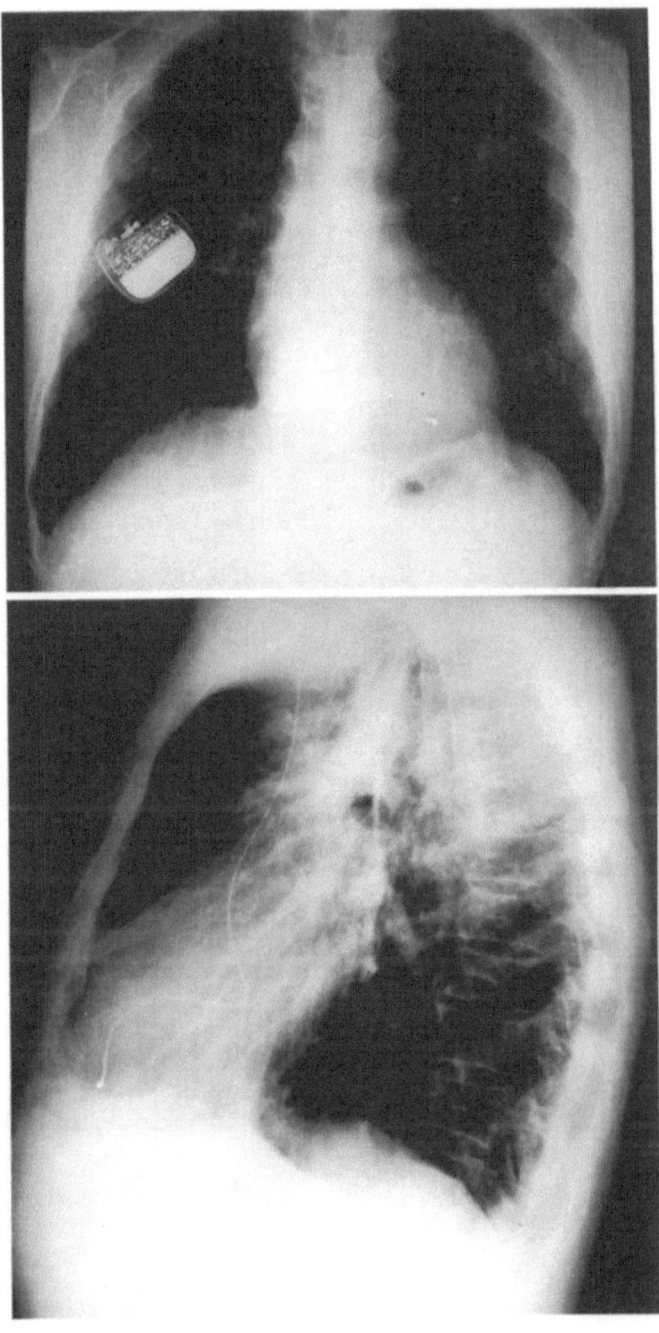

**Fig. 3.1. a** Single chamber pacemaker: the endocardial electrode is in the right ventricle (VVI mode)

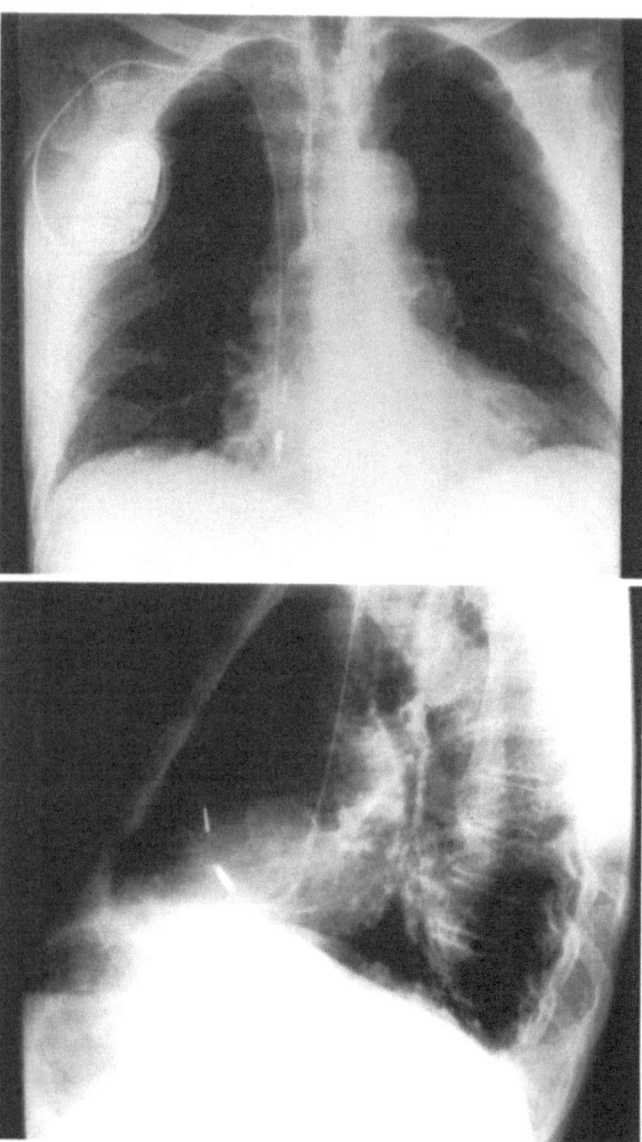

**Fig. 3.1. b**
The lead is in the
right atrium
(AAI mode)

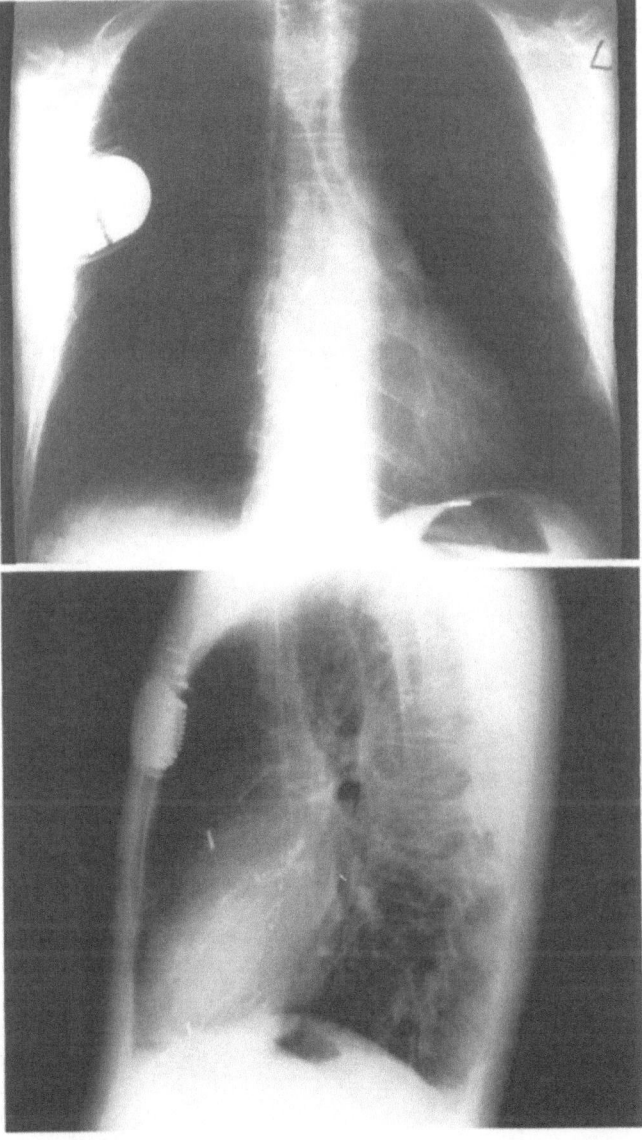

**Fig. 3.1. c** Dual chamber pacemaker: one lead is in the right atrium, the other in the right ventricle

## 3.2
## The Various Types of Pacemakers and Their Programmable Functions

Two main families of pacemakers will be distinguished in the upcoming presentation: single and dual chamber pacemakers. The former are connected to a single right ventricular or atrial lead (Fig. 3.1a,b). The latter are connected to two leads, usually placed in the right atrium and right ventricle (Fig. 3.1c, 3.2). A third

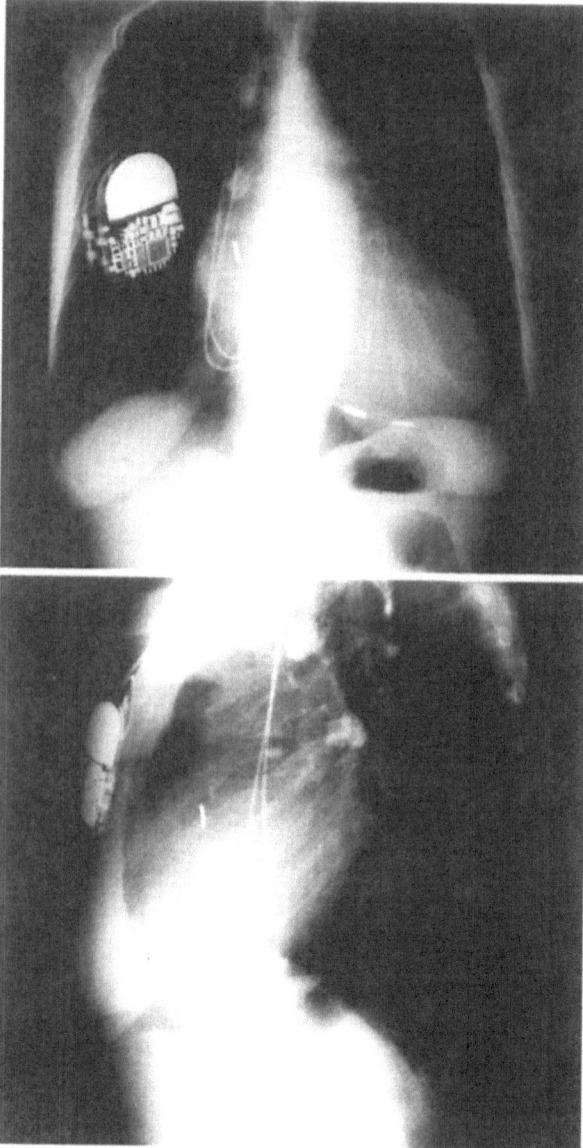

**Fig. 3.2.** Dual chamber pacemaker (Medtronic, Symbios 7008), connected to two bipolar leads. Each lead has two electrodes located inside the cardiac chambers

pacing system has recently been perfected which allows dual chamber pacing with a single lead. Dual chamber pacemakers, the most complex, best reproduce normal physiology.

This chapter will, in order, present single chamber pacing, followed by dual chamber pacing, ending with rate responsive sensors and their integration to single and dual chamber pacing. The programmable parameters will be described, and their value and use explained. Telemetry parameters will be discussed separately (see p. 275 ff.).

## Terminology

### Demand Versus Fixed Rate Pacing

Sensing is an indispensable function of a demand pacemaker. The terms „demand" or „stand by" mean that the pacemaker will only intervene when the spontaneous activity of the heart falls below a precise (programmable) rate (for example 60 BPM). The proper function of the system can be verified by the consistent absence of a pulse below the programmed rate (although the function can be influenced by isolated extrasystoles and resulting pulse deficit). In other words, in contrast to asynchronous, fixed rate pacing, the spontaneous activity of the heart is taken in consideration. The pacemaker abstains from pacing when the intrinsic cardiac rhythm is faster than the programmed lower rate (see Fig. 3.5b).

A distinction is made between *R wave inhibited* (VVI) and *P wave inhibited* (AAI) pacemakers. The former behaves as a pure ventricular demand and the latter as a pure atrial demand pacemaker. Combining the two constitutes a dual chamber system (DDI or, if programmed to track the atrium, DDD).

In asynchronous, fixed rate pacing (Fig. 3.3) sensing is absent: the pacemaker does not take the spontaneous activity of the heart in consideration and, instead, paces steadily at the set rate. This creates a danger of delivery of a stimulus in the vulnerable phase of the spontaneous heart cycle and, under certain conditions, of inducing ventricular tachycardia or fibrillation.

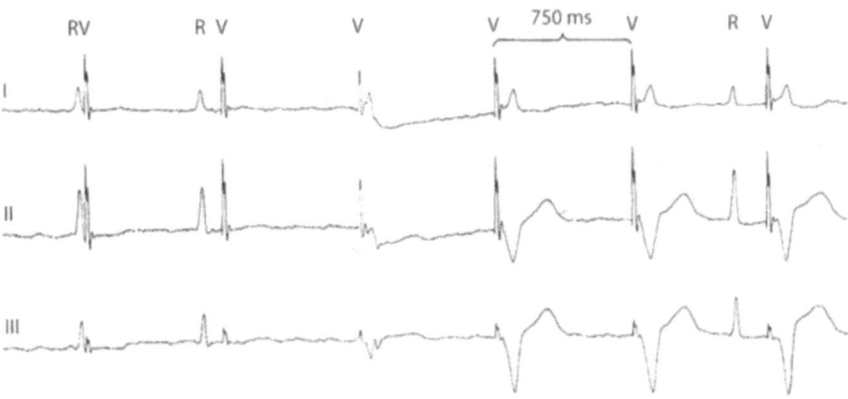

**Fig. 3.3.** Pacing cycle (in asynchronous mode): the interval between spikes measures 750 ms and corresponds to a rate of 80 BPM. In V00 mode, parasystole sets in: ventricular pacing is delivered at a fixed rate without sensing of the spontaneous ventricular rhythm *V* ventricular stimulus; *R* R wave

This pacing mode, nowadays, is used only temporarily during testing of the pacing system, for example by application of a magnet (see p. 78). During magnet application, most pacemaker models will revert to fixed rate pacing (for measurement purpose), usually only while the magnet is being applied. The resulting pacing rate is characteristic of each model and often provides information relative to the device elective replacement time or to the safety margin of the pacing output.

In a few pacemaker models, the effect of the magnet can be turned off by the programmer in order to minimize the risk of external interference by external magnetic fields. This protection, obviously, has its limits in presence of unusually powerful magnetic sources. In other models, sensitivity to magnet can be temporarily turned off while testing of the pacemaker is being performed.

A few pacemakers will deliver a finite number (e.g. three) of asynchronous stimuli at the magnet rate upon magnet application; others will continue to deliver a few more pulses after removal of the magnet. One should also note that, depending on the manufacturer of the programmer, some programmer head contain a permanent magnet, and others not.

The term „non rate responsive" applies to pacing by a regular demand pacemaker (without rate responsive function) which has been set at, for example, a lower rate of 60 or 70 BPM. Under such conditions, the pacing rate cannot increase, unless it has been programmed to a tracking mode (AAT, VVT, DDD), or rate smoothing has been programmed.

For the sake of clarity and consistency, the following definitions are provided of the terms that will be regularly used in forthcoming pages of this book:

- *Asynchronous:* continuous pacing at a set rate irrespective of the spontaneous cardiac activity.
- *Non rate responsive*: the term describes the function of a pulse generator pacing at a demand rate which remains at a programmed value (for example 60 or 70 BPM), in contrast to a rate responsive system which adapts its rate to the level of exercise. This non rate responsive rate, however, is programmable.
- *Fixed rate:* Function of a pacemaker (for instance a stand by device) the pacing rate of which cannot be reprogrammed, and is therefore „fixed". Nowadays such devices are of historic interest only.
- *Programmed lower rate:* slowest rate at which the demand function of the pacemaker has been programmed to escape.
- *Programmed upper rate:* maximal rate at which ventricular pacing is allowed to track atrial activity on a 1 : 1 basis
- *Sensor rate:* Pacing rate determined by the sensor function of a rate responsive system.
- *Maximal sensor rate:* Maximal (programmed) rate at which the sensor is allowed to drive the heart rate.

### Rate Versus Pacing Cycle and Versus Escape Interval

Since 60,000 ms correspond to 1 min, rate (in BPM) and interval (in ms) are calculated as presented in Fig. 3.4 (see foldout table).

The pacing rate (BPM) is often expressed as the so-called pacing cycle, cycle length or pacing interval.

The pacing interval defines the time interval (in ms) between two consecutive pacing pulses delivered during asynchronous pacing (see Fig. 3.3).

The escape interval (of a single chamber system) describes the interval between the last spontaneous cardiac event and the next pacing stimulus (see Figs. 3.5b, 3.7b).

As an example, a programmed lower rate of 60 BPM corresponds to a pacing interval (cycle) of 1000 ms. Upon sensing of an R wave, the pacemaker initiates an escape interval, waiting for a spontaneous cardiac event. Should no spontaneous event occur during that period, the device delivers a pulse at the end of 1000 ms. Conversely, should it sense spontaneous ventricular activity, it will reset its timer and initiate a new escape interval of 1000 ms.

The escape interval applies only to the demand function. In single chamber systems, it corresponds to the pacing interval when no rate hysteresis has been programmed (see Fig. 3.5b).

$$\text{Heart rate (BPM or min}^{-1}) = \frac{60\,000}{\text{cycle (ms)}}$$

$$\text{Cycle (ms)} = \frac{60\,000}{\text{heart rate (BPM or min}^{-1})}$$

**Fig. 3.4.** Conversion formulas to calculate heart rate versus cardiac cycle (interval)

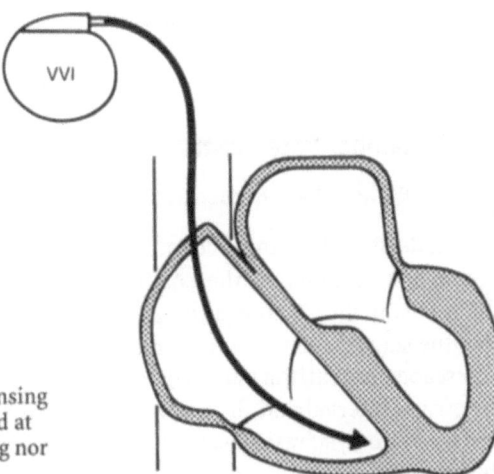

VVI

**Fig. 3.5. a** VVI mode. Pacing and sensing (including of extrasystoles) is limited at the ventricle. There is neither sensing nor pacing in the atrium

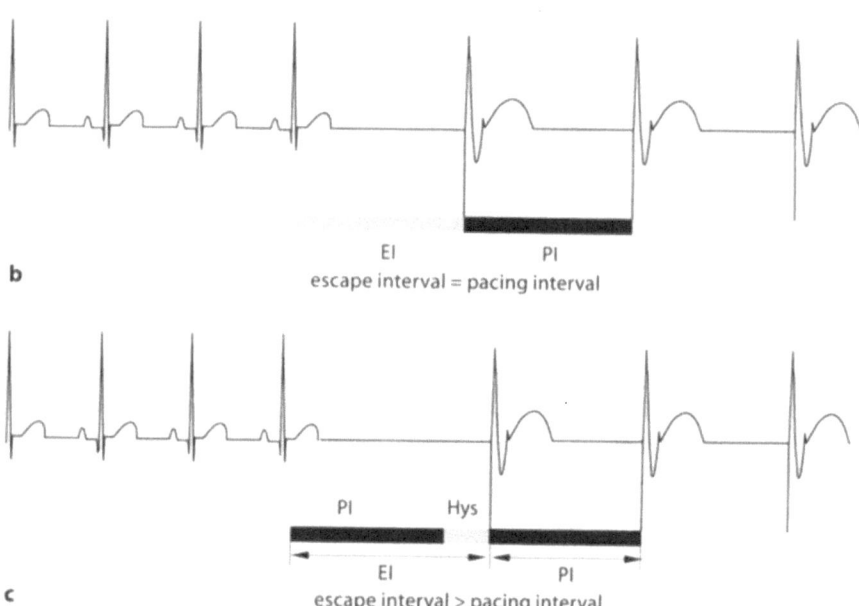

**Fig. 3.5. b** VVI pacemaker function diagram. When sensing ventricular events before the end of its escape interval, the pacemaker is inhibited and resets that interval. In absence of sensed event, the pacemaker delivers a ventricular stimulus at the end of its escape interval. In absence of hysteresis, the escape interval (between a spontaneous event and a paced event) and the pacing interval (between two paced events) are equal
**c** When hysteresis has been programmed, the escape interval is longer than the pacing interval. The difference between the two intervals is equal to the programmed hysteresis

The term „interval" will also be used to calculate the upper pacing rate based on the sum of the refractory period and the AV interval (see p. 89–95) Likewise, hysteresis or indications for pulse generator replacement are defined, with some pacemaker models, as a corresponding prolongation of the escape or the pacing interval (for example 100 ms).

## Single Chamber Pacemakers

### SSI Mode Without Rate Responsiveness

This mode describes single chamber back up pacing. When the pacemaker senses spontaneous activity in the chamber containing the electrode, it is inhibited, which means that it aborts the escape interval that is in progress and resets it from the sensed event. If no spontaneous activity has been sensed by the end of this escape interval, the pacemaker paces the chamber involved (see Figs. 3.5, 3.7). The escape interval and the pacing cycle are identical and equal to the lower rate interval, if no hysteresis has been programmed (Fig. 3.5b and see also p. 74–75). This mode of function applies to the ventricle (VVI) as well as the atrium (AAI).

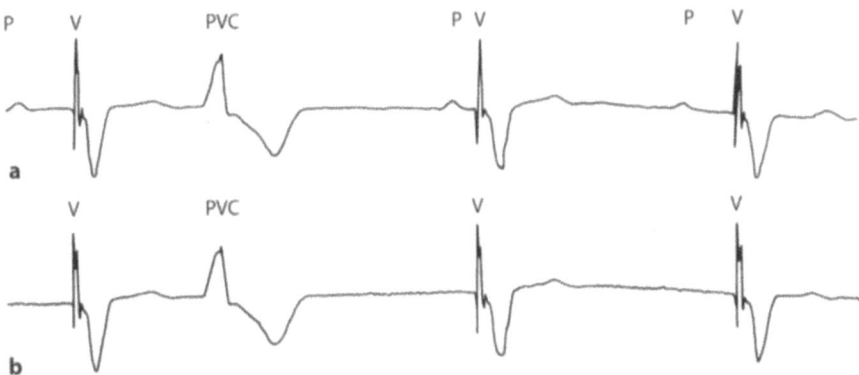

**Fig. 3.6. a** Complete atrioventricular block with persistence of atrial activity. Atria and ventricles are dissociated
**b** Atrial fibrillation with atrioventricular block. In both cases the premature ventricular complex (PVC) is sensed by the pacemaker and resets it

## The VVI Mode

Ventricular pacing, ventricular sensing, inhibited when sensing a ventricular event.

The ventricular pacemaker inhibited by an R wave is the most widely implanted pacemaker in the world. It paces the ventricle, senses the ventricle, and is inhibited by the ventricle (Figs. 3.5, 3.6).

Pacing and sensing are achieved through a lead implanted in the right ventricle, usually transvenously (see Fig. 3.1). On the surface electrocardiogram, a pacing spike is followed by a wide QRS complex, with a left bundle branch block morphology since pacing is performed at the right ventricular apex.

Atrial signals (P wave) are not sensed by a VVI pacemaker. Atrial activity, independent from the ventricles, is thus asynchronous in presence of atrioventricular block (see Fig. 3.8).

## The AAI Mode

Atrial pacing, atrial sensing, inhibited when sensing an atrial event.

This mode is similar to VVI, except that pacing and sensing are performed through a lead implanted in the right atrium, usually transvenously (Figs. 3.7, 3.8, see also Fig. 3.1).

The interval between the atrial pacing spike and the paced P wave, the P wave axis and the P wave morphology, all depend on the location of the electrode(s) within the atrium. Normal atrioventricular conduction is preserved, giving rise, in absence of bundle branch block, to narrow QRS complexes.

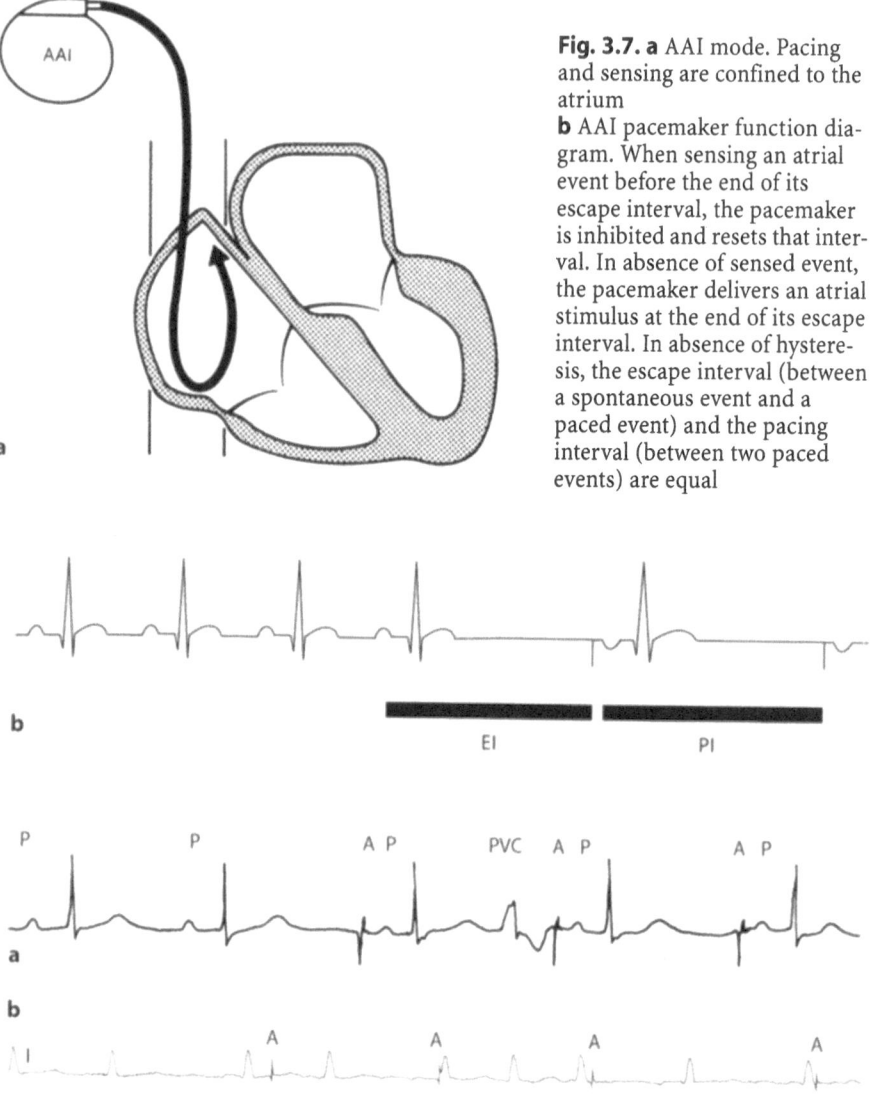

**Fig. 3.7. a** AAI mode. Pacing and sensing are confined to the atrium
**b** AAI pacemaker function diagram. When sensing an atrial event before the end of its escape interval, the pacemaker is inhibited and resets that interval. In absence of sensed event, the pacemaker delivers an atrial stimulus at the end of its escape interval. In absence of hysteresis, the escape interval (between a spontaneous event and a paced event) and the pacing interval (between two paced events) are equal

**Fig. 3.8. a** In AAI mode, a premature ventricular complex (*PVC*) is not sensed
**b** During atrial fibrillation or flutter, the atrial spikes (*A*) have no effect on the atrial rhythm
*P* P wave

## Programmable Parameters in SSI Mode

*Pacing Output*

As discussed in the previous chapter, the control of the pacemaker's power consumption depends on the programming of amplitude and duration of the pacing pulse. The programmability of these two parameters is essential. Post implant, whether the lead was placed de novo or reimplanted, one can expect a rise in pacing threshold due to the inflammatory process occurring at the site of implantation. This acute rise begins two to three weeks after implant in the ventricle, and may start much earlier in the atrium. The chronic threshold is not established before 3 to 6 months (see p. 245). The pacemaker may then be reprogrammed to a more power saving pulse strength to optimize device longevity. Advances in lead technology, particular modifications of their microstructure, have allowed to reduce the pacing threshold (hence, power consumption), and to attenuate the initial rise in threshold. Steroid eluting electrodes appear to lower considerably the pacing threshold, particularly during the first few weeks after implantation of the electrode. During the acute period, other causes of threshold rise, besides the inflammatory process, may be a dislodgment, microdislodgment, or fracture of the lead. At a later stage, endogenous factors, such as myocardial infarction, myocarditis, systemic diseases, or metabolic disorders, may be responsible for a pacing threshold rise.

CASE STUDY

*Example.* A dual chamber pacemaker was implanted in a 62 year old lady with binodal dysfunction (sinoatrial block + atrioventricular block). She had sustained episodes of ventricular asystole and had to be reanimated on several occasions. Two months later, she was rehospitalized for poor control of diabetes (blood glucose = 560 mg/L), associated with atrial sensing failure and rise in atrial and ventricular pacing thresholds (2.5 V at a 0.5 ms pulse duration). Satisfactory capture could be regained by reprogramming the pacing output to 5 V in both chambers. Two days later, after improvement of her metabolic status, adequate sensing and pacing returned; atrial sensing threshold was greater than 2.5 mV, and the ventricular pacing threshold fell to 2.5 V at a duration of 0.06 ms, such that the device could be reprogrammed at a pulse amplitude of 2.5 V and pulse duration of 0.3 ms in both chambers. The patient was no longer pacemaker dependent; a spontaneous rhythm near 70 BPM had reappeared. In the following days, the pacemaker intervened only intermittently, as it used to do before the metabolic derangement.

This example underscores the importance of being able to reprogram the pacemaker, and being able to increase its output up to high values (7.5 – 10 V) when faced with transient health crises.

> Some manufacturers offer devices set at a low nominal pacing output to reduce battery size while guaranteeing an acceptable device longevity. These nominal values are not always high enough to guarantee a sufficient margin of safety with respect to the measured pacing thresholds.

Programmability of the output voltage and pulse duration vary widely from one model to the next. Since pacing threshold may be influenced by several factors, a proper safety margin must be respected when programming the device. After implantation, nominal values of pulse amplitude and duration, as set by the manufacturer, are usually adequate and can be left unchanged. Later on, when pacing threshold has stabilized, programming must be performed again to provide a pacing output at twice threshold and guarantee a wide enough safety margin. In the case of a pacemaker dependent patient, this safety margin should be even wider. As a reminder, power consumption is proportional to the pulse duration, and to the square of the output voltage (see p. 21).

In unipolar configuration, the pacing output must sometimes be reduced because of uncomfortable concomitant stimulation of the pectoral muscle. With atrial stimulation, the lead is often screwed into the lateral wall, which carries a risk of stimulation of the phrenic nerve which courses in the vicinity of the pacing electrode, causing strong contractions of the diaphragm with each pulse delivery from the pacemaker. The same complication may occur with ventricular pacing, particularly when the right ventricle is dilated, by direct stimulation of the left hemidiaphragm. It is, therefore, imperative to perform a test of high output pacing at the time of implant, and to change the electrode placement in case of diaphragmatic stimulation. In clinical practice, a pacing output voltage of 2.5 V and pulse duration between 0.3 and 0.6 ms are usually programmed in both atrium and ventricle once the chronic threshold has been reached.

With recent devices, threshold testing can be performed automatically after device implantation: The pacing output (voltage or duration) is gradually decreased automatically and in a calibrated fashion. Testing is interrupted (by pressing on, or by releasing, a programmer's dedicated key, depending on the model) when loss of capture is noted on the surface ECG continuously recorded during the test. In some old Siemens or Telectronics devices, a „Vario" function can be programmed: the test is magnet activated; by counting on the surface ECG the number of pacing pulses delivered until loss of capture, the pacing threshold may be calculated (Fig. 3.9).

The disadvantage of such methods is that testing is only performed from time to time as part of the device surveillance schedule. In case of unexpected transient rise in pacing threshold, the patient is unprotected and at risk of recurrent symptoms from pacing failure. The ideal system is entirely automatic, included in the device function, and capable of autoprogramming its pacing output by continuously remeasuring the capture threshold (function known as autocapture). This offers obvious advantages: pacing at the lowest possible output, preservation of battery life, uninterrupted safety. This approach was first offered by the Prism model (Cordis), the device tracking the threshold by analyzing the depolarization gradient after ventricular pacing. This system was limited to the ventricle and required a powerful algorithm. Several manufacturers continue to explore this concept. Currently, Microny (Pacesetter) and Eikos (Biotronik) are the only devices which offer autocapture. The Microny continuously analyzes the evoked potential (evoked response, see also Fig. 7.7b), adjusting the pacing output at 0.6 V above the threshold measured every 8 h, and storing the threshold measurements in memory over an 18-week period. In case of failure to sense the evoked potential because of loss of capture after the 13 ms blanking period, a high energy spike is delivered 47 ms after the end of blanking, and a new threshold measurement is initiated to automatically readjust the programmed pacing amplitude. Some other models with autocapture function of various manufacturers are now coming.

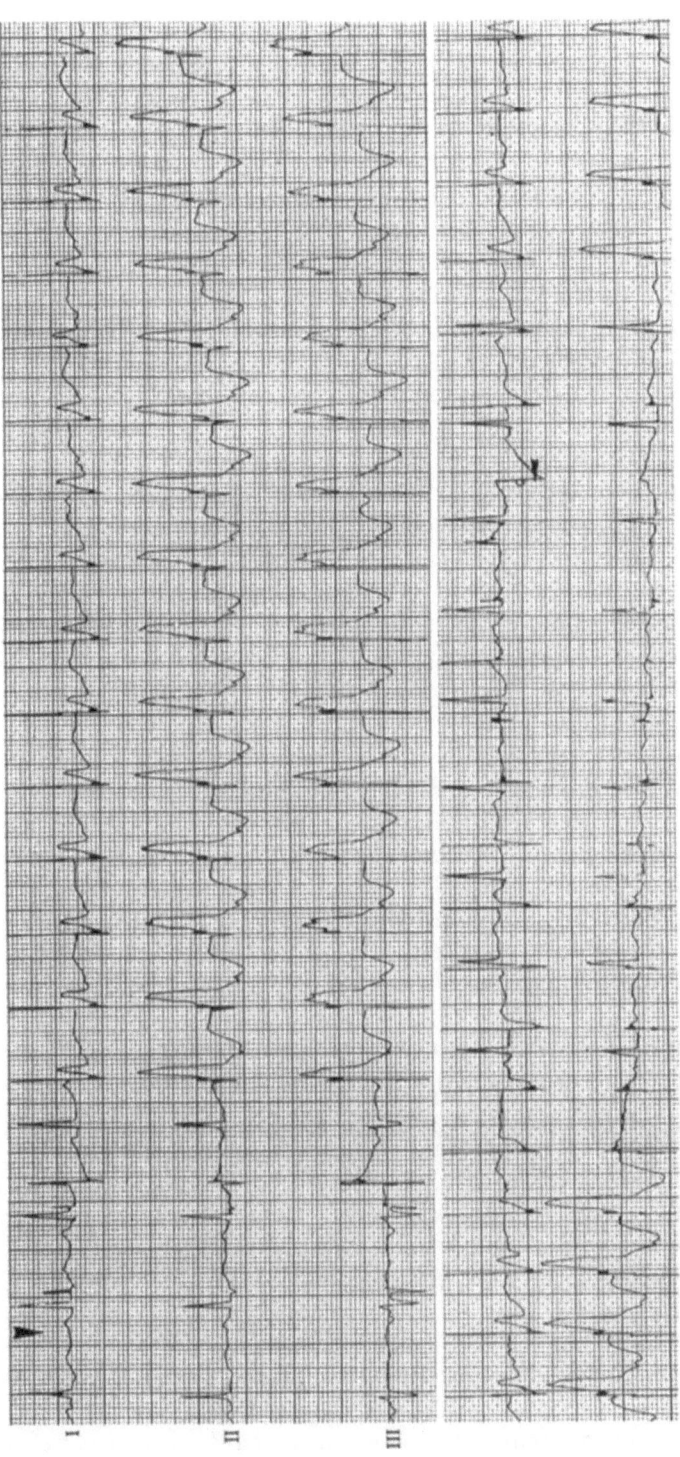

**Fig. 3.9.** Implanted ventricular pacemaker. Activation of Vario testing by magnet (*arrow*), with gradual decrease in pacing amplitude until loss of capture. Paced QRS complexes have a vertical axis because the pacing lead has been placed in the right ventricular outflow tract (*o* and *horizontal arrow*: end of the test)

*Sensitivity*

In unipolar systems, the range of sensitivity programming is between 0.25 and 4.0 mV in the atrium, and 1.0 and 7.0 mV in the ventricle. However, to determine more precisely the sensitivity threshold, wider zones of sensitivity are needed to measure precisely the safety margin offered by a given programmed setting. In Pacesetter systems, for example, the values range up to 14 mV in the ventricle. In absence of such capability, the amplitude of the intracardiac electrogram measured by telemetry may be helpful, although the measured amplitude is often quite different from the effective amplitude of the signal.

In our practice we usually program the sensitivity in the ventricle at 4 or 5 mV, after a study performed in 1987 by Irnich showed that such programming in the unipolar configuration was mostly successful in eliminating sensing of myosignals or other extraneous signals; in the chronic phase, R wave amplitude is mostly above 8 mV, thus offering a wide safety margin.

In the atrium, we use sensitivity settings between 1.5 and 2 mV in the unipolar configuration, according to the size of the atrial electrogram. Failure to sense the P wave occurs in approximately 38% of cases during exercise at such programmed values. One should, thus, underscore the value of a bipolar system if one needs to program a high sensitivity (below 1 mV) to guarantee atrial sensing during effort, while minimizing the risk of unwanted interference. The importance of exercise testing to unmask episodes of sensing failure not apparent at rest is also noteworthy.

In an effort to continuously adapt the sensitivity setting to the various physiologic and pharmacologic conditions which may influence sensing and its safety margin, Intermedics (DDD Cosmos II), developed a self-adaptive tuning of the device's sensitivity, as a function of changes in signal amplitude (autosensing). This principle is now renewed in the model Marathon (Intermedics) (Fig. 3.10).

The ultimate goals of sensitivity programming are to eliminate, as much as possible, the failure to sense cardiac events which need to be sensed (undersensing), and oversensing of events which should not be sensed.

*Undersensing.* When the sensitivity of the sensing system is insufficient (the programmed values are too high), P and R waves are no longer recognized, causing failure to sense also known as „entrance block" (see Fig. 2.18). This phenomenon appears also when the intracardiac signals become so small as to no longer be sensed at a given, stable sensitivity setting. In such case, either lead dislodgment or fibrotic growth around the electrode(s) should be suspected. A back up pacemaker becomes „blind" and behaves as an asynchronous pacemaker: it is no longer inhibited by intracardiac electrograms (Fig. 3.11), and delivers pacing pulses at a fixed rate.

*Oversensing.* When the sensitivity of the sensing system is too high (the programmed values are too low), oversensing may occur (see Fig. 2.19). P and R waves are properly sensed, but other events may be sensed as well, and interpreted as being of cardiac origin, including myosignals (particularly from active

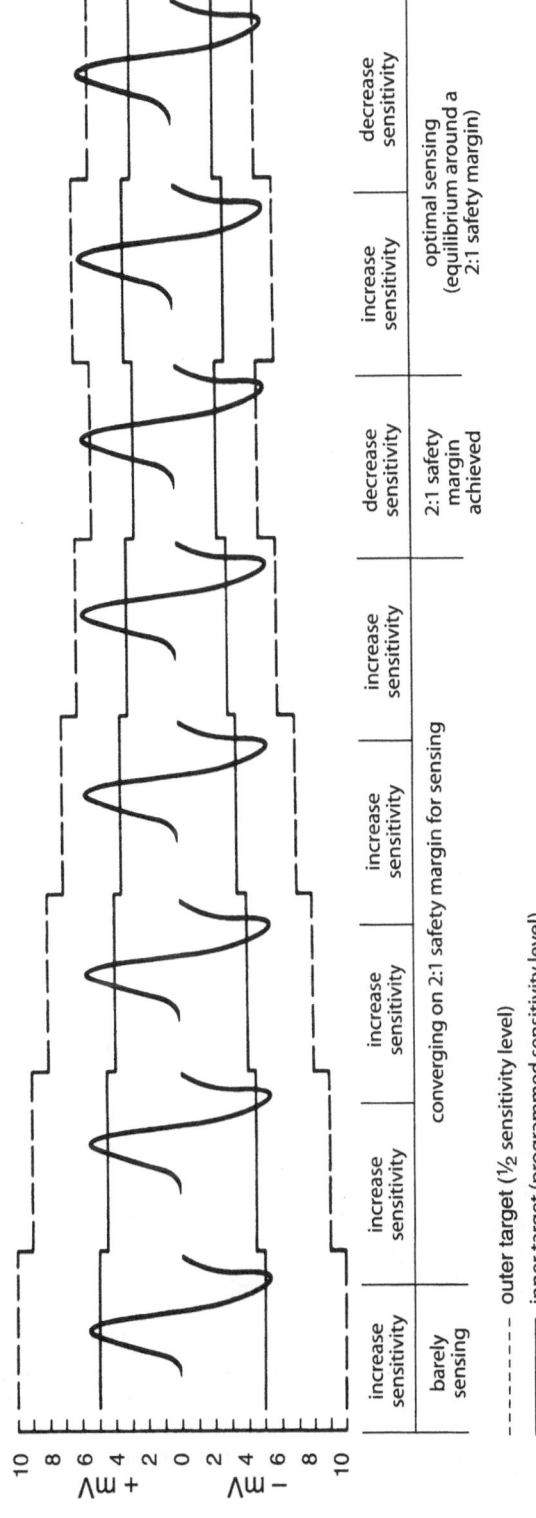

**Fig. 3.10.** Description of the autosensing function used in Intermedics pacemakers (Marathon DR)

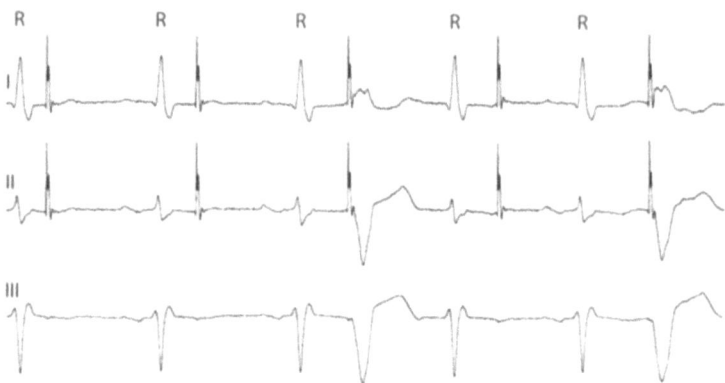

**Fig. 3.11.** The R waves are not sensed by the pacemaker. Pacing is asynchronous at a fixed rate of 70 BPM

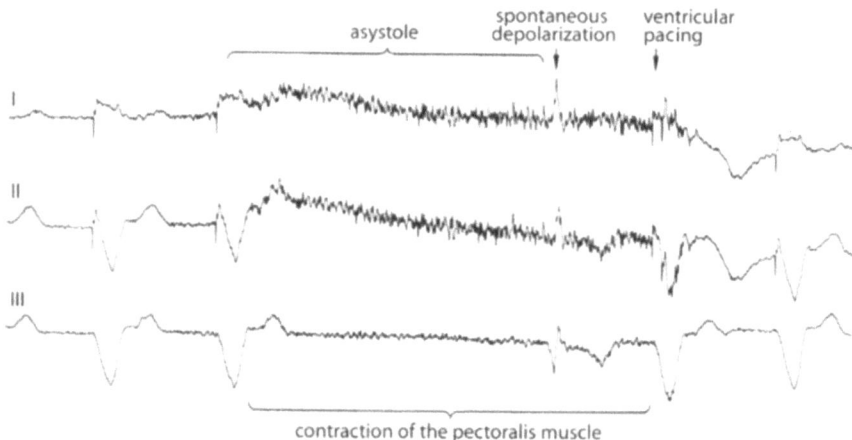

**Fig. 3.12.** Example of a VVI pacemaker inhibition by myosignals, interpreted by the pacemaker as being of cardiac origin, explaining the absence of pacing pulse delivery, resulting in asystole. In this case, the sensitivity of the device was deliberately programmed at a very low value (0.5 mV), causing the device to be highly sensitive

pectoral muscles), T wave, afterpotentials, and exogenous interferences. This may cause inhibition of the pacemaker (Fig. 3.12). This abnormal behavior may cause brief cardiac asystole and, often, symptoms in the form of Stokes-Adams episodes if the patient is pacemaker dependent.

CASE STUDY

*Example.* A completely pacemaker dependent baker (3rd degree atrioventricular block) has recurrent syncopal episodes from sensing of myosignals while he was kneading dough. The symptoms were eliminated by reprogramming the device sensitivity from 2 to 5 mV (decrease in sensitivity = increase in programmed value).

T wave or afterpotential sensing has become rare since the perfection of entrance filters, since the frequency spectrum and the slew rate of the T wave do not overlap those of depolarization signals caused by P and R wave (see also Fig. 2.10 and Fig. 8.29). The same abnormal behavior may be caused by the sensing of extraneous signals, or by signals caused by intermittent contact of the conductor in a fractured lead.

One other instance of oversensing may present from cardiac events occurring outside the chamber which contains the electrode. A particular form of this phenomenon consists of ventriculo-atrial crosstalk: in case of programming of a high sensitivity at the atrial level, the atrial lead may send to the pulse generator a ventricular signal which will be interpreted as an atrial electrogram (far-field R wave sensing) (Fig. 3.13, see also Fig. 3.51).

CASE STUDY

*Example.* An activity driven rate responsive pacemaker was implanted with a bipolar lead in the atrium (see Fig. 3.1b), such that the risk of extraatrial interference was theoretically low. However, while the lower rate was set at 60 BPM, a resting paced rate at 50 BPM was observed. The cause of this discrepancy was elucidated by the electrocardiogram associated with the analysis of the intraatrial event markers (Fig. 3.13). With the sensitivity set at 1.25 mV, the ventricular electrogram (R wave) following atrial pacing was erroneously interpreted as an atrial electrogram by the pacemaker. It was, therefore, intermittently inhibited with a decrease in pacing rate. The problem was corrected by reprogramming the sensitivity at 2.5 mV. The native P waves remained properly sensed, while the R wave amplitude was reduced below the threshold of atrial sensing.

## The Refractory Period

The refractory period is the interval which follows pacing or sensing in a given chamber, and during which the pacemaker, functioning in the inhibited (or triggered) mode, is not reset. If a cardiac event falls during this period, it will be disregarded by the pacemaker which is „blind".

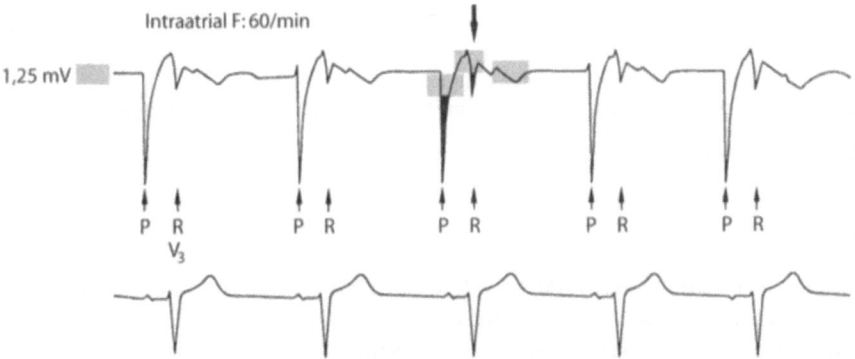

**Fig. 3.13. a** Atrial intracardiac signals recorded from a pacemaker whose sensitivity value has been set very low (hypersensitive pacemaker). The R waves, despite their low amplitude, are sensed by the pacemaker and interpreted as P waves

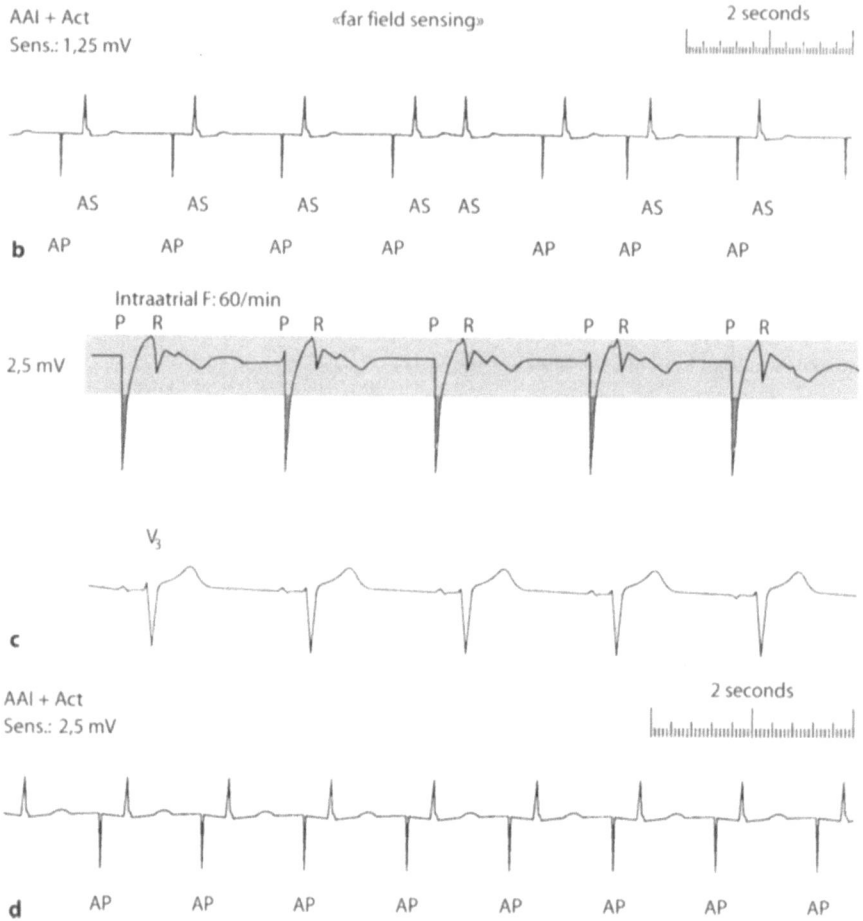

**Fig. 3.13. b** ECG event markers: the atrial signals recorded by an Activitrax (Medtronic) pacemaker implanted in the atrium are, in fact, of ventricular origin. This phenomenon causes a decrease in heart rate during atrial pacing. The pacing cycle is lengthened by the time interval contained between the atrial spike and the R wave
**c** After reprogramming of the sensitivity from 1.25 to 2.5 mV (device rendered less sensitive), only atrial signals are being sensed
**d** When the pacemaker paces the atrium, the heart rate is 70 BPM, precisely the programmed rate
*AS* atrial sensing; *AP* atrial pacing

The refractory period of a pacemaker behaves like the refractory periods of the cardiac conduction system (see p. 9 ff), though it may be reprogrammed.

Refractory periods serve to prevent the inappropriate inhibition of the device e.g. farfield sensing (see above). In VVI mode, the refractory period is usually programmed between 220 and 350 ms. Its aim is to prevent the resetting of the pacemaker by the T wave which would reset the pacing cycle. On the other hand, the programming of an excessively long refractory period carries the risk of

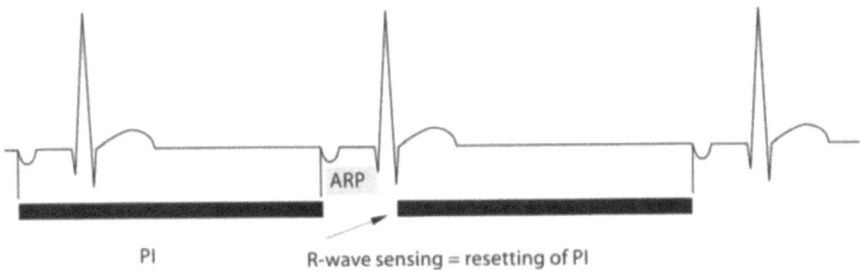

**Fig. 3.14.** The programmed refractory period of an AAI pacemaker must be long enough to avoid its resetting by the R wave sensed in the atrium. In this case the ARP was programmed too short
*ARP* atrial refractory period; *PI* pacing interval

non-sensing of close coupled premature ventricular complexes. In AAI mode, the programming of a refractory period overlapping the R wave is necessary to prevent resetting by ventricular depolarization (Fig. 3.14) (refractory period longer than 400 ms). This risk is theoretically decreased by bipolar sensing but, in clinical practice, this is not always confirmed.

*The Lower Rate*

As discussed earlier in this paragraph, the demand function of a pacemaker implies that the device will pace only when the heart rate falls below a programmed or calculated rate. The pacing rate cannot be slower than the programmed lower rate, except in presence of additional special functions.

The lower rate may be programmed and, for simple (non rate responsive) VVI pacemakers, a rate of 70 BPM is usually set in presence of complete heart block (which is not an ideal indication for VVI mode), a satisfactory heart rate from a hemodynamic standpoint. If, on the other hand, there is persistence of spontaneous atrioventricular conduction, and if the indication for the pacemaker is paroxysmal atrioventricular block, a slow lower rate is preferred to minimize device pacing interference with spontaneous rhythm, to reduce power consumption, and to prevent retrograde conduction, often the source of considerable increase in atrial filling pressures, fall in cardiac output and pacemaker syndrome; this will be further discussed on p. 187, 198. The programming of a relatively slow lower rate is also preferable in case of unstable coronary artery disease, to reduce myocardial oxygen consumption which increases with an increase in heart rate. Furthermore, it has been shown that, at any given heart rate, myocardial oxygen consumption increases with pacing, one additional reason to facilitate the emergence of spontaneous rhythm. Finally the temporary use of very slow lower rates (40 BPM or slower), is particularly helpful when testing device sensitivity; a few devices do allow the programming of temporary 000 mode (Fig. 3.15). Conversely, a faster lower rate may be indicated to suppress premature ventricular complexes, particularly bigeminy (see p. 144f.), or to improve hemodynamics in some cases of cardiac insufficiency. Rapid pacing rates are also necessary in children.

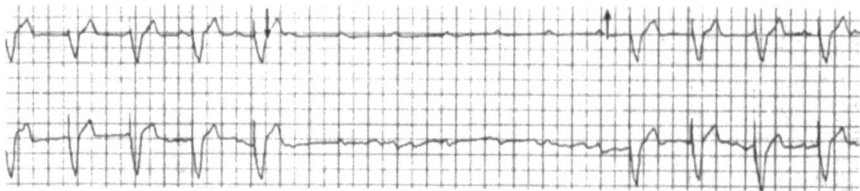

**Fig. 3.15.** Temporary programming of the pacemaker to 000 mode allows to analyze the underlying rhythm in absence of pacing. Interruption of telemetry (by removal of the programmer head) immediately restores the pacemaker's normal functions. Likewise for the temporarily programmed functions. Without such functions, manual programming in search of a pacing threshold carries a nonnegligible risk in pacemaker dependent patients

In fact, nowadays, with several types of pacemakers, the escape rate may be modified by special functions, when the device encounters particular situations. These functions are hysteresis, bradycardic diagnostic functions, rate smoothing, dynamic overdrive, and the sleep rate (see Appendix, p. 393 ff.). Rate responsiveness is yet one other means of modifying the escape rate (see p. 120 ff.).

*Rate Hysteresis*

Hysteresis (from the Greek word „hysterein": that which arrives later) is an interval added to the pacing interval which follows all spontaneous events (Fig. 3.5c, 3.16). Hysteresis is programmable either as a rate value, as an interval, or as a percentage of the lower rate. Consequently, this means that the rate at which the pulse will be delivered will be slower than the programmed lower rate. If hysteresis is programmed at a rate of 50 BPM, while the lower rate has been set at 70 BPM, the pacemaker will begin pacing only if the spontaneous rate falls below 50 BPM. Following this first stimulus (1 beat), the pacemaker returns to the lower rate of 70 BPM. The spontaneous rate must then rise above 70 BPM to inhibit the pacemaker.

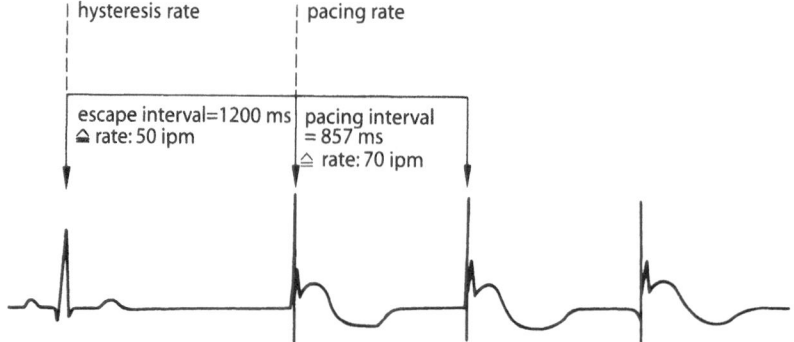

**Fig. 3.16.** When the spontaneous heart rate falls below 50 BPM (which corresponds to an escape interval of 1200 ms), the pacemaker begins pacing at 70 BPM in this particular example (that is a pacing cycle of 857 ms). The hysteresis value is thus 1200 ms – 857 ms = 343 ms

Some devices, such as the Nova II (Intermedics) or Trilogy (Pacesetter) model have a function of „search hysteresis" (see Fig. 8.23). The pacemaker delivers a pulse at the lower rate (70 BPM in our earlier example); then, after 255 pulses delivered at the lower rate, the search function examines the spontaneous rate to determine if it is still below 50 BPM. If it has risen above 50 BPM, the pacemaker is inhibited. If the spontaneous rate has remained below 50 BPM, pacing will restart at the lower rate of 70 BPM for another 255 beats, until the next search pause.

The hysteresis function can be applied in non-pacemaker-dependent patients with infrequent bradycardic episodes (for instance paroxysmal atrioventricular block or carotid sinus syndrome). In VVI mode, hysteresis is meant to preserve spontaneous rhythm (with spontaneous atrioventricular synchrony) as much as possible. Its other objective is a reduction in power consumption by the pulse generator. Nowadays a dual chamber system („DDD + hysteresis", „DDI + hysteresis" or „DDD + special algorithm") would have been preferable, especially in the presence of retrograde conduction.

*Sensor Hysteresis*

Sensor hysteresis is a distinct type of hysteresis which, in some cases, is recommended to be programmed to avoid a competition between paced and spontaneous rhythm in a rate responsive pacing system. It may be applied to atrial or ventricular pacing, as well as to the DDDR or SSIR modes. When a sensor hysteresis has been programmed, rate responsiveness will only be operative when the spontaneous rate remains below a (programmable) value when compared with the rate determined by the sensor. For example, the sensor may be calculating a desired heart rate of 100 BPM. If a sensor hysteresis of 10% has been programmed, rate responsive pacing will only begin when the spontaneous rate falls below 90 BPM, and initiate pacing at 100 BPM.

### Special Functions in Non Rate Responsive SSI Mode that Control the Escape Rate

Other functions which control the lower rate consist of diagnostic algorithms, smoothing functions designed to eliminate sudden decreases in heart rate, dynamic overdrive, which dictates an increase in rate followed by smoothing whenever the pacemaker senses spontaneous activity, and the sleep rate. These various functions are explained in the Appendix on p. 393 f.

### The SST Mode

### The VVT Mode

Ventricular pacing, ventricular sensing, triggered pacing by ventricular sensing.

This mode is rarely used. With each spontaneous event, the pacemaker delivers a pulse which falls in the QRS complex and has, therefore, no effect since it

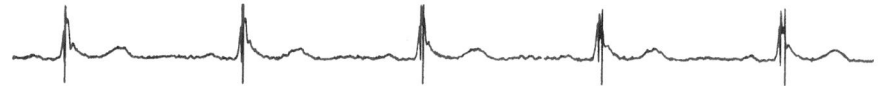

**Fig. 3.17.** In VVT mode, the pacemaker delivers a pulse with each sensed ventricular event. The stimulus is in the QRS and has no effect on ventricular depolarization

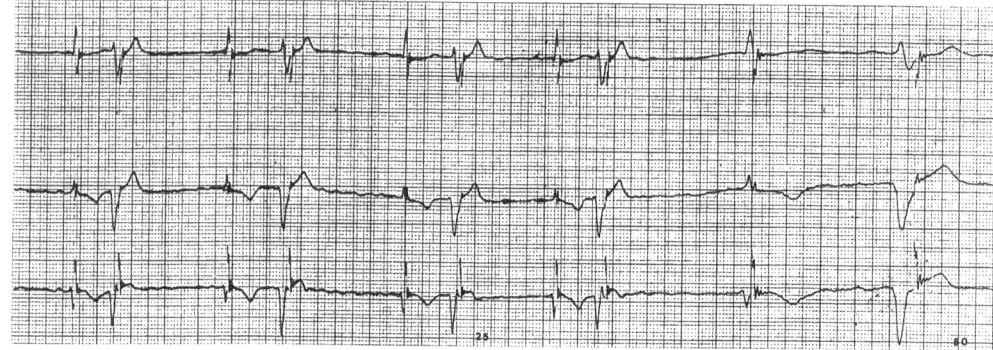

**Fig. 3.18.** The VVT mode allows to determine the timing of QRS sensing. This may be markedly delayed, as in this example of flawless detection of premature ventricular complexes (recording speed at the end of the tracing is 50 mm/s). This phenomenon is not negligible when measuring the apparent duration of the escape interval of a device programmed VVI

occurs during the natural ventricular absolute refractory period (Fig. 3.17). This represents a needless power expenditure. However, it is indicated in patients exposed to powerful external kinds of interference. This prevents the complete inhibition of the pacemaker which, in the VVI mode, would have caused ventricular asystole. Instead, the pulse generator triggers ventricular safety pacing with each interfering signal. Otherwise, its function is no different from the VVI mode. However, because of this peculiarity, it is strongly advised to program a long refractory period, creating an upper pacing rate which will prevent the occurrence of excessively rapid pacing rates (it is, in fact, with an upper triggered rate that this control parameter is offered in the Intermedics Nova II device). With this mode, an external pulse generator is capable of controlling the implanted pacemaker's pacing rate: e.g. in electrophysiologic studies, or antitachycardia pacing.

This mode is particularly helpful during pacemaker checks where the ventricular spike serves as a sensing marker (Fig. 3.18). By varying the programmed sensitivity, one can measure the real sensitivity threshold (see p. 344), as the pacemaker with its filter senses.

### The AAT Mode

Atrial pacing, atrial sensing, triggered pacing by atrial sensing.

This mode is identical to the VVT mode, applied to the atrium. In addition, the atrial triggered mode facilitates the diagnostic of atrial arrhythmias (Fig. 3.19a).

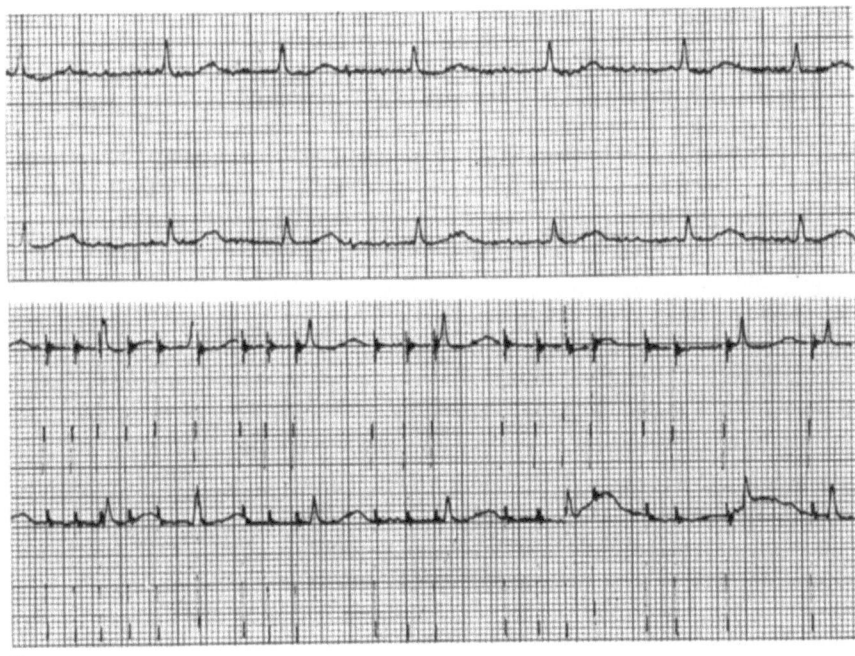

a

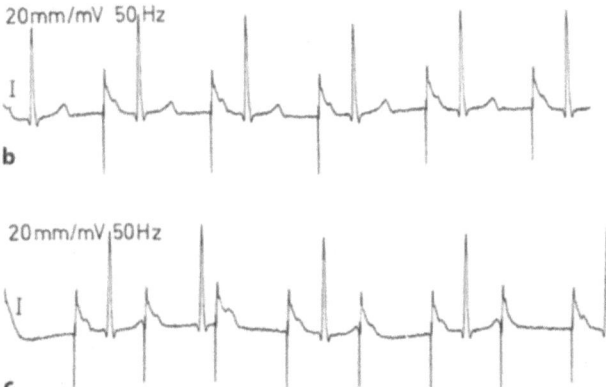

20mm/mV 50 Hz

I

b

20mm/mV 50Hz

I

c

**Fig. 3.19. a** The atrial triggered mode facilitates the diagnostic of atrial arrhythmias as in this example: the device, set in AAI mode at 75 BPM, appears to not function properly with a poorly visible atrial activity (top); once reprogrammed to AAT, flawless sensing of an atrial tachyarrhythmia has become apparent, with appropriate inhibition of the pacemaker (bottom)
**b** Atrial pacing at 60 BPM is associated with 1 : 1 ventricular conduction
**c** 2 : 1 block occurs at a paced atrial rate of 90 BPM, which indicates some junctional dysfunction

Another difference would be with the use of an external pulse generator to measure the anterograde Wenckebach point (Fig. 3.19b,c) during long-term follow up or for antitachycardia pacing. In some models higher rates are programmable in AAT mode in comparison to the AAI mode (see Fig. 3.94).

## The Asynchronous (S00) Mode

Pacing in single chamber, no sensing, asynchronous pacing.

When permanent pacemakers were introduced, pacing was ventricular and performed at a fixed rate (V00 mode). Today, this mode activated by the application of a magnet over the pulse VVI (or VVT) generator (the mode is A00 if the pacemaker is AAI or AAT), is often called the magnet mode. It does not allow sensing of spontaneous events. Consequently, if the patients is not completely pacemaker dependent, a parasystolic rhythm will be observed on the surface ECG, that is the spontaneous rhythm and the paced rhythm will be competing (see p. 59). This may be risky if a stimulus is delivered during the vulnerable period of a spontaneous cycle. This mode is also used to check the battery whose impending depletion will be manifest by a slowing of the so-called magnet rate. But the depletion indicator is not always connected to a slowing of the magnet rate (e.g. Cosmos, Intermedics).

In some pacemaker models it is possible to program „magnet off", either temporarily for testing sensitivity or intrinsic rate or even permanently. In this case there is no asynchronous rate activated by the application of a magnet.

## Dual Chamber Pacemakers

Dual chamber pacemakers, particularly in DDD mode, have been called physiologic. Indeed, harmonious synchrony between atrium and ventricle is guaranteed by an atrial and a ventricular lead (Fig. 3.20). The two leads may be unipolar (see Fig. 3.1c) or bipolar (see Fig. 3.2), like the can which coordinates atrial and ventricular pacing.

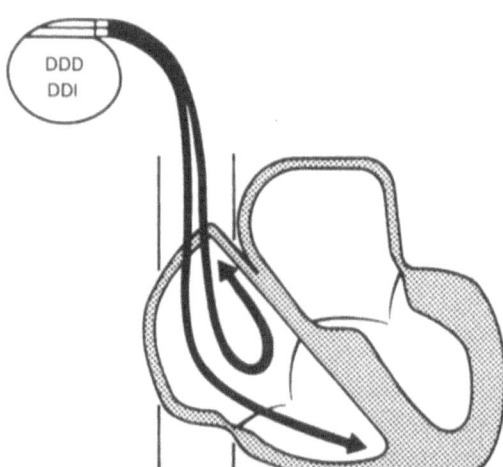

**Fig. 3.20.** Pacing and sensing in atrium and ventricle (DDI), and ventricular triggering by atrial sensing (DDD)

These devices offer a variety of different pacing modes (including single chamber pacing), each with their particular indications. Emphasis will be on DDD, DDI and VDD, the most frequently used modes. The programmable parameters of DDD, which offers the most developed functions of this type of pacing, will be described, though VAT and DVI preceded it historically.

## The DDD Mode

Dual (atrial and ventricular) pacing, dual (atrial and ventricular) sensing, dual (inhibited and triggered) response to sensing.

The principle behind the DDD mode consists of synchronizing ventricular pacing with atrial sensing. Furthermore, if spontaneous atrial activity is present, it inhibits atrial pacing; likewise in the ventricle.

From a few ECGs, it is easy to understand the fundamental behavior of a dual chamber pacemaker:

1. Fig. 3.21: a P wave is sensed in the atrium and an R wave is sensed in the ventricle, with a normal atrioventricular relationship. Atrial and ventricular pacing is inhibited; the surface ECG is normal and shows no pacing intervention.
2. Fig. 3.22: atrioventricular sequential pacing is triggered by the absence of sensing of spontaneous signals in the atrium and in the ventricle.
3. Fig. 3.23: the atrium is paced since no P wave was sensed. In presence of normal atrioventricular conduction, a spontaneous QRS appears during the atrioventricular interval and inhibits ventricular pacing. The function is AAI like.
4. Fig. 3.24 (most important): Ventricular pacing triggered by P wave, atrial pacing inhibited by spontaneous sinus rhythm. The sinus rate increases normally with exercise. Because of underlying atrioventricular block, the pacemaker delivers a stimulus in the ventricle at the end of the atrioventricular delay (programmed here at 150 ms) since no QRS has appeared in the meantime. Ventricular pacing tracks sinus rhythm up to the upper rate (programmed here at 125 BPM).

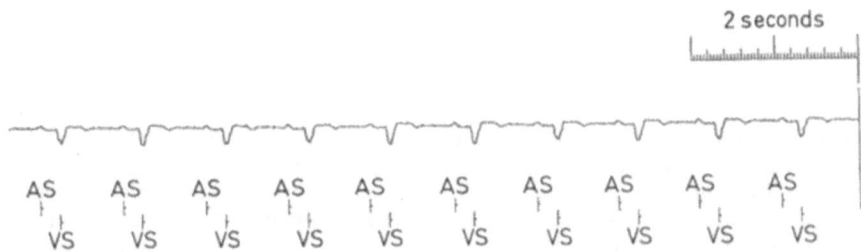

**Fig. 3.21.** Surface ECG with event markers. Atrium and ventricle are sensed by the pacemaker (AS, VS). Atrial and ventricular pacing is inhibited. Normal function

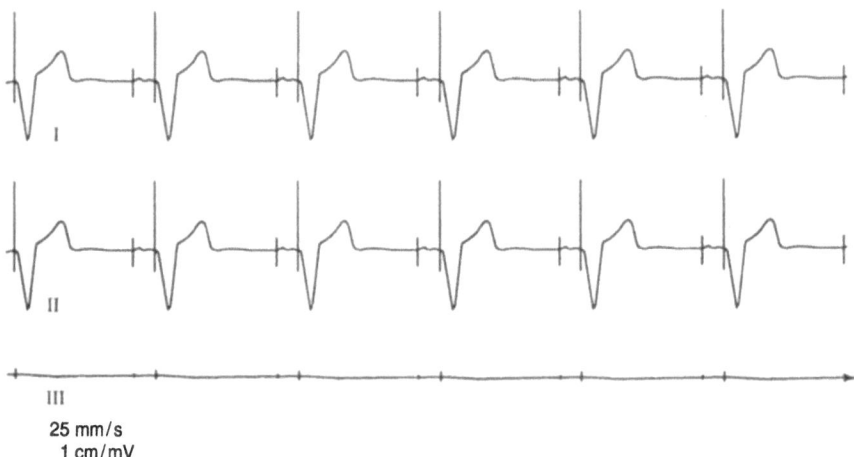

25 mm/s
1 cm/mV

**Fig. 3.22.** No spontaneous signal is sensed by the pacemaker, either in the atrium or the ventricle during the escape interval or the atrioventricular delay, resulting in atrioventricular sequential pacing

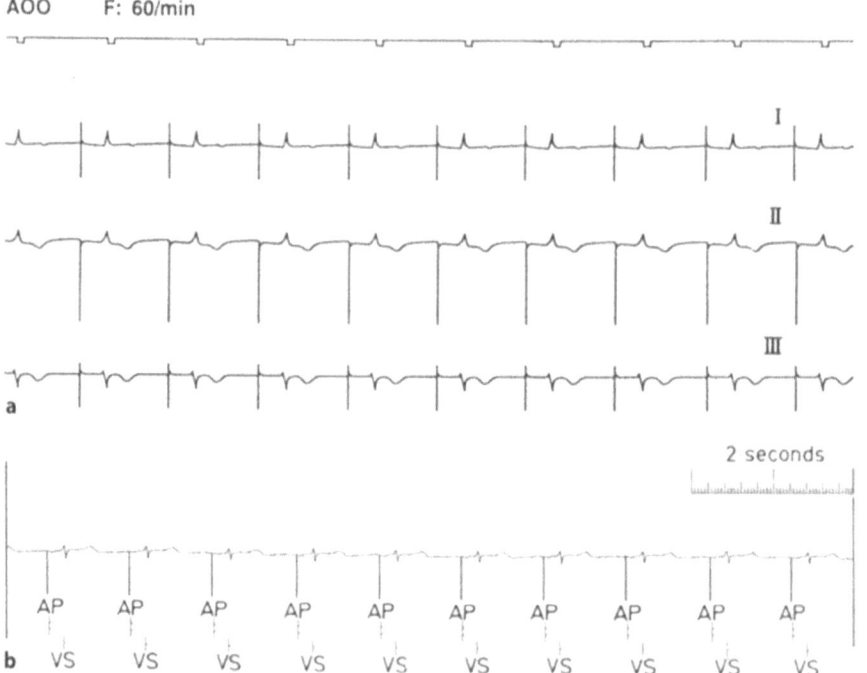

**Fig. 3.23. a** In the atrium no P wave is sensed during the escape interval. Following atrial stimulation, atrioventricular conduction occurs normally and the QRS complex is sensed during the atrioventricular delay, inhibiting ventricular pacing (the PR interval is shorter than the programmed atrioventricular delay).The pacemaker is in DDD mode, but the ECG shows an AAI like behavior
**b** Analysis of the event markers confirms DDD mode function with atrial pacing (AP) and ventricular sensing (VS)

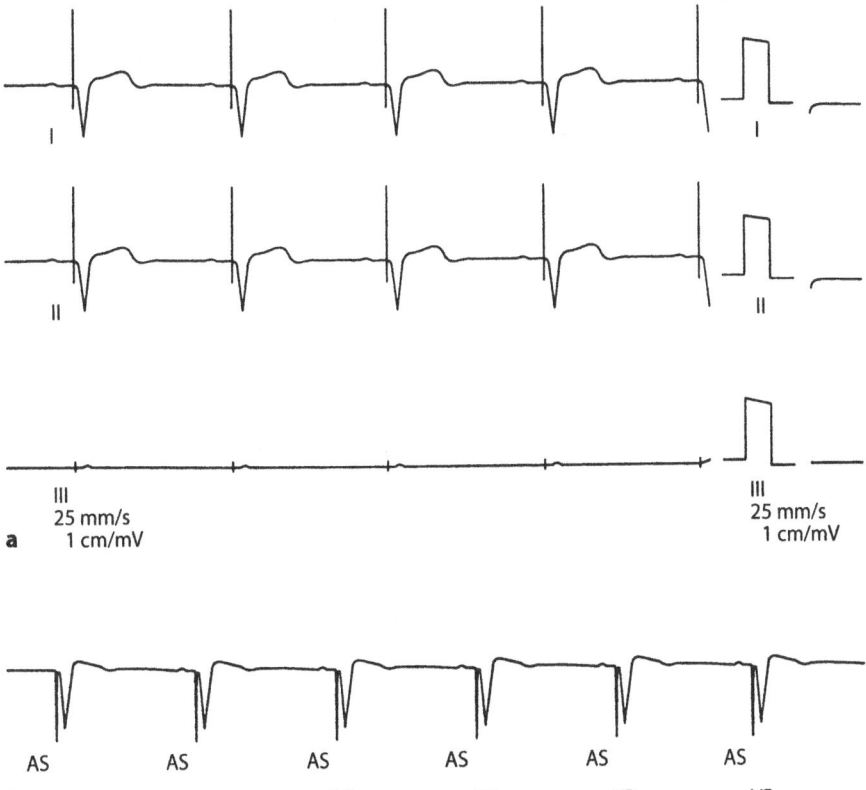

**Fig. 3.24. a** Surface ECG; during exercise, the atrial rate (normal sinus rhythm) increases. Because of underlying atrioventricular block, no spontaneous QRS complex appears during the atrioventricular delay. The pacemaker delivers a ventricular stimulus at the end of that interval (in this case 150 ms), such that the ventricular paced rate is identical to the sinus rate up to the programmed upper rate of 125 BPM (inhibited function in the atrium and triggered in the ventricle)
**b** The event markers confirms this proper function
*AS* atrial sensing; *VP* ventricular pacing

### Standard Programmable Parameters

As with single chamber devices, pulse amplitude and duration, and sensitivity are separately programmable in the atrium and the ventricle by the same procedures. Depending on the model, one can program the pacing and/or sensing polarity, either in both chambers simultaneously, or completely separately. Some pacemakers offer an automatic programming of the polarity according to the lead connected to the device header (Medtronic Kappa). Likewise, lower rate is programmable as in the case of a single chamber device. Conversely, hysteresis and some special functions are not available in all systems. These special functions are detailed in the Appendix (see p. 394 ff).

Other parameters that can be applied in DDD mode must be thoroughly understood if one wants to interpret correctly the ECG tracings generated by these pacemakers. The various periods that correspond to each event of the car-

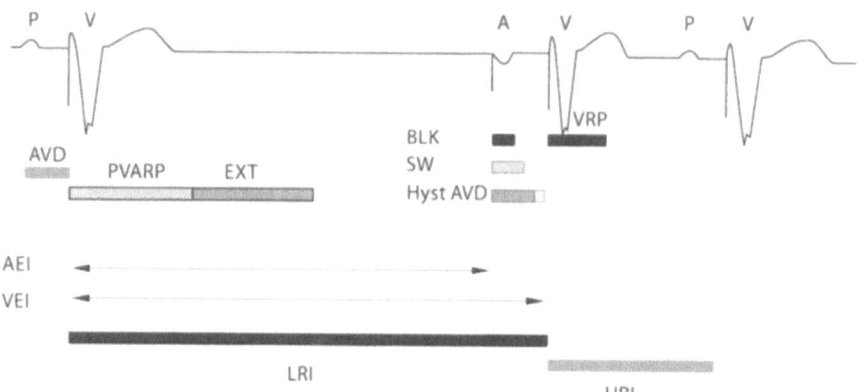

**Fig. 3.25.** Diagram showing the various periods initiated in DDD mode
*P* spontaneous P wave; *A* paced P wave; *V* paced QRS complex; *AVD* atrioventricular delay;
*PVARP* post ventricular atrial refractory period; *EXT* extension of PVARP after premature
ventricular complex; *BLK* postatrial ventricular blanking period; *SW* safety window; *Hyst
AVD* hysteresis of atrioventricular delay; *VRP* ventricular refractory period; *AEI* atrial
escape interval; *VEI* ventricular escape interval; *LRI* lower rate interval; *URI* upper rate
interval

diac cycle will now be reviewed (Fig. 3.25). From an atrial sensed event, an atrioventricular interval is initiated.

### The Atrioventricular Delay

The atrioventricular delay (AVD) is the electronic equivalent of the physiologic PR
interval. In most pacemakers, it represents the interval between atrial and ventricular pacing spikes. In other models, it is the interval contained between a sensed P
wave and the ventricular pacing spike (Figs. 3.25, 3.26). The AVD is an atrial refractory period. If a spontaneous QRS occurs during the AVD, it is interrupted. Values
between 0 and 300 ms can be programmed, depending on which model has been
implanted. The AVD must be programmed such as to offer a satisfactory coordina-
tion of atrial and ventricular contractions, to maintain the highest possible cardiac
output (see p. 189 ff.). At rest, and upon atrial sensing, the optimal range of AVD is
usually between 80 and 120 ms, though interindividual variations are wide. Atrial
pacing initiates other intervals: the AVD from a paced atrial event, distinct from
that from a sensed event, a ventricular blanking period, and a safety window.

### AVD from Paced Versus Sensed P Wave

This function was designed to maintain a stable left mechanical AV interval.
Indeed, left atrial systole is delayed with respect to the paced right atrium: a
delay exists between the pulse delivery and right atrial depolarization, further
lengthening the interatrial delay; these various delays vary according to the electrode position in the right atrium, and from one individual to the other (Figs.

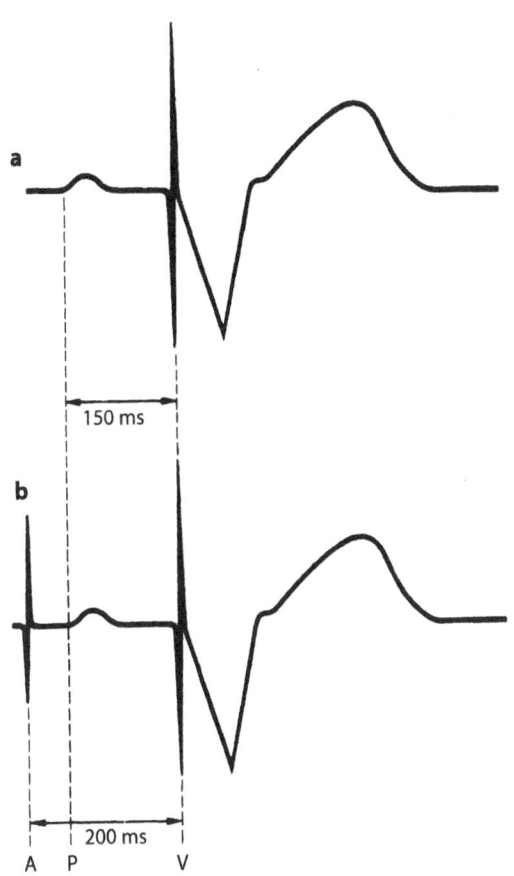

**Fig. 3.26a–c.** Difference between AVD initiated after sensed (**a**) versus paced (**b**) P wave. When the P wave has been paced (**b**), the AVD must be lengthened by an average value of 70 ms. In this example, this difference measures 50 ms **c** A long interval (130 ms) is present between the atrial spike (*A*) and the atrial response (*P*); therefore a long (240 ms) *AVD* (delay between atrial and ventricular spikes) was programmed *A* atrial spike; *V* ventricular spike; *P* paced and spontaneous P wave

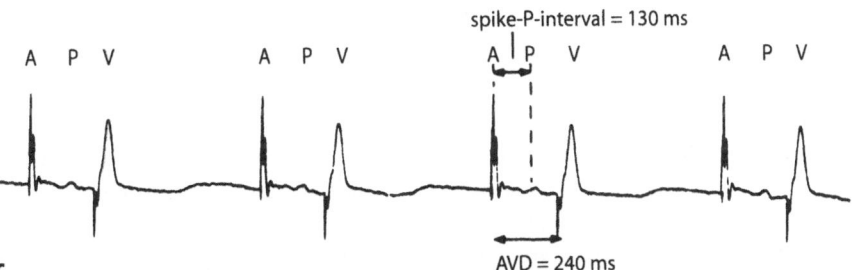

3.25–3.27). Hence, this parameter, AV extension, must be programmable. Only few pacemakers offer this function: fixed values can be found in the Synchrony and the Pacesetter Paragon (25 ms), in the Sorin Living (30 ms), in the Vitatron Diamond (40 ms) and in the Cosmos II (Intermedics) and Relay (50 ms). It is programmable in the ELA Medical Chorus (0 to 94 ms), and in the Chorus II, Chorum and Talent (0 to 156 ms). The greatest programmability is offered by the models Elite, Thera, Kappa (Medtronic), Physios TC 01, Dromos, Eikos and Inos (Biotronik), the Vigor models (CPI), and the Trilogy (Pacesetter), which allow the independent setting of AVD for sensed versus paced P waves. In three sepa-

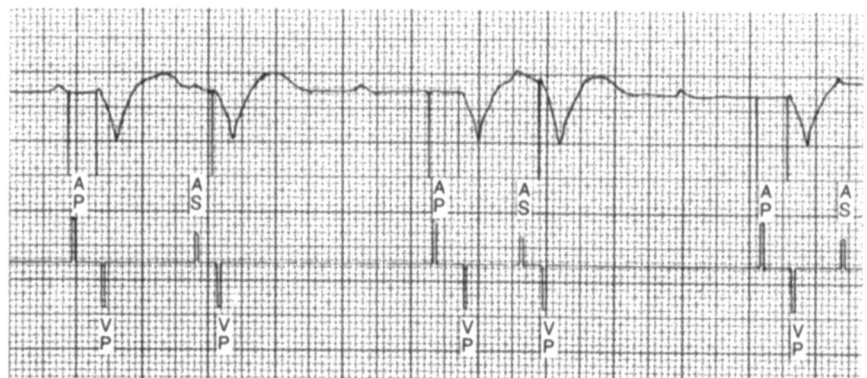

**Fig. 3.27.** The marker channel illustrates the difference in AVD duration depending on whether it has been initiated by an atrial paced event (AP – VP = 180 ms) or an atrial sensed event (AS – VP = 120 ms) The AVD hysteresis is, thus, 180 – 120 = 60 ms. Note, incidentally, the presence of intermittent sensing failure
*AP* atrial pacing; *VP* ventricular pacing; *AS* atrial sensing

rate studies, the average optimal value of the difference paced versus sensed AVD has been 70–75 ms. This function is also valuable by allowing the occurrence of as many narrow QRS complexes as possible, which offers two distinct advantages in presence of preserved of atrioventricular conduction:

1. It decreases power consumption by decreasing the number of paced ventricular events.
2. It maintains a normal sequence of ventricular contraction, since ventricular pacing causes a desynchronization of contraction which is hemodynamically adverse.

With this in mind, the Ruby and Diamond (Vitatron) and the Trilogy (Pacesetter) pacemakers offer a special function called AV delay scanning. It is not an automatic function in search of the optimal difference in AVD as one finds in the Chorus II, Chorum and Talent (Ela Medical) models, but an additional window, added to the AVD, aimed at facilitating spontaneous AV conduction (see p. 397 f.).

In addition to a positive search hysteresis of AVD, the Trilogy pacemaker (Pacesetter) offers a negative AVD search hysteresis function. The AVD is shortened in programmable steps to force ventricular pacing before spontaneous AV conduction occurs. This function is indicated whenever 100% ventricular pacing is needed, as in the case of patients with obstructive hypertrophic cardiomyopathy.

### Adaptation of the AVD to the Atrial Rate[1]

The aim of this algorithm is to reproduce the normal physiologic adaptation of the PR interval with exercise (Fig. 3.28). Its value varies in a linear fashion, here again with wide interindividual variations. The objective is dual:

---

1  rate adaptive AVD

1. To maintain as optimal as possible an AVD over the entire range of sinus rates
2. To shorten the total atrial refractory period, which also raises the 2 : 1 pacemaker AV block rate (which will be extensively covered on p. 88 ff.), in an effort to improve the pacemaker's behavior at peak atrial rates.

The Vitatron Quintech 931 was the first model to offer this function. The hemodynamic value of this feature is discussed in detail in Chap. 4.

### The Ventricular Blanking Period and the Safety Window

The blanking period, a brief interval which follows atrial pacing, is a component of the ventricular refractory period. Its purpose is to prevent the sensing, by the ventricular electrode, of afterpotentials originating from atrial pacing which the pacemaker would erroneously interpret as a signal of ventricular origin. Too short a blanking period may cause atrial pacing, or rather its afterpotentials, to be sensed in the ventricle, a phenomenon known as atrioventricular crosstalk (Fig. 3.29). In presence of crosstalk, prolonged ventricular asystole may occur if the patient has no atrioventricular conduction and is pacemaker dependent (Fig. 3.30). Too long a blanking period may cause failure to sense a ventricular depolarization (for example a premature ventricular complex falling during the blanking period), which may incur the risk of ventricular stimulation at the end of the AVD, in the vulnerable period of the extrasystole (Fig. 3.31).

Ventricular safety pacing is a function complementary to the blanking period. If, after the blanking period, a ventricular event is sensed during the safety window, a ventricular stimulus will be triggered at the end of this window, generally 60 to 100 ms after the atrial stimulus. Two situations are, therefore, possible: if afterpotentials from atrial pacing were sensed at the ventricular level during the safety window period, ventricular pacing is triggered which will prevent ventricular asystole as described in the previous paragraph (Fig. 3.32). If a premature ventricular complex was sensed, ventricular pacing falls during the natural

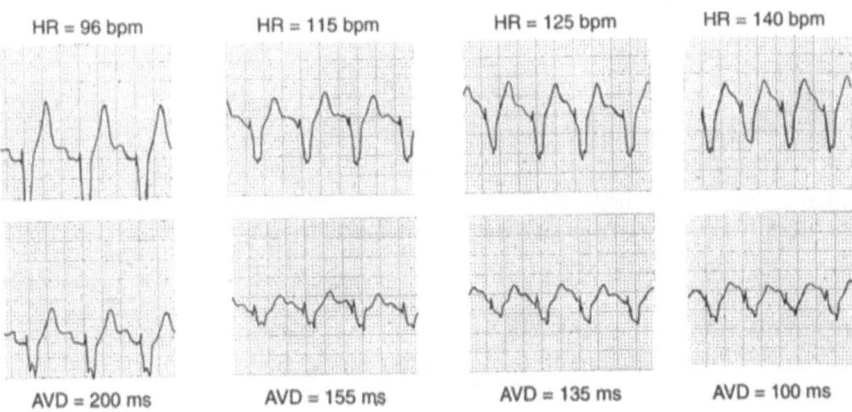

**Fig. 3.28.** Gradual shortening of the AVD with increasing heart rate, reproducing the physiologic response

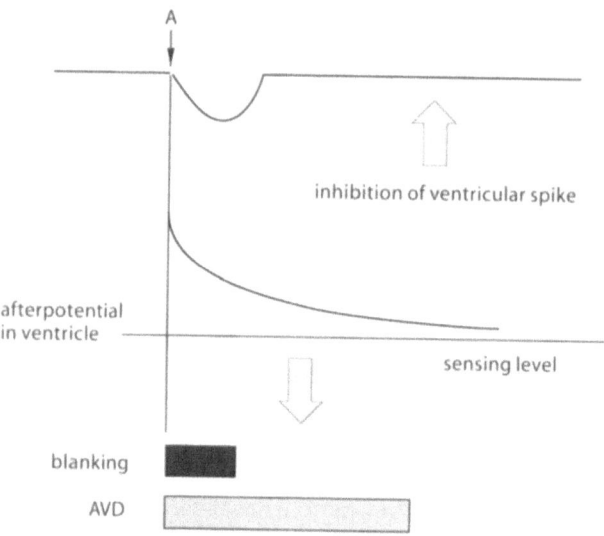

**Fig. 3.29.** When blanking is too short, atrial afterpotentials may be sensed and inhibit ventricular pacing in absence of a safety window
*A* atrial stimulus

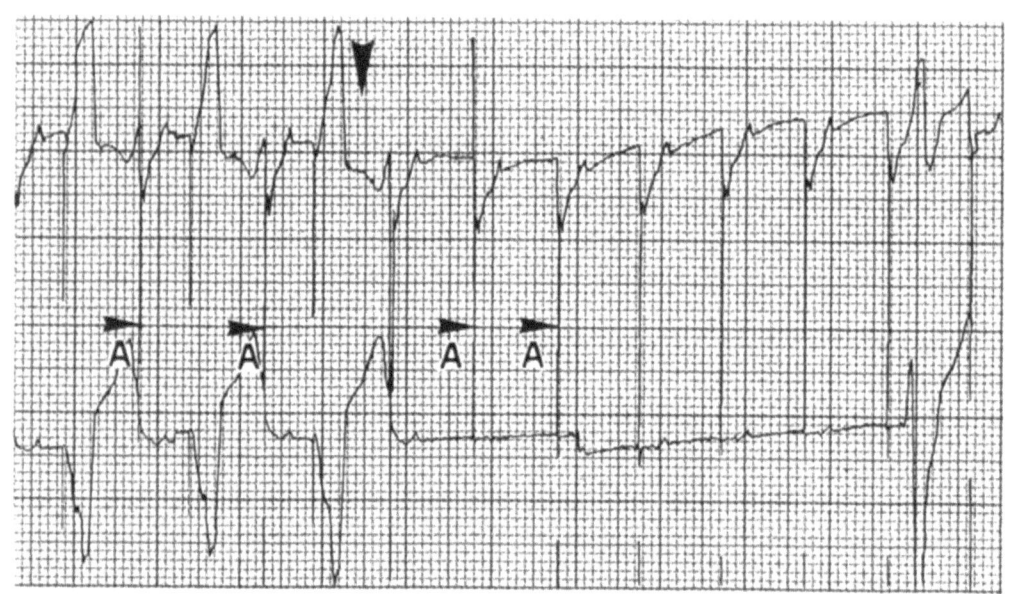

**Fig. 3.30.** In absence of safety window, and in presence of crosstalk, inhibition of ventricular pacing may cause syncope in a patient with complete atrioventricular block

refractory period of the ventricle, and is, therefore, harmless (Fig. 3.33). This function is indispensable in all dual chamber modes which may include atrial pacing. Its recognition is easy since the AVD is set by the safety window.

It is, therefore, important to determine the optimal value of the blanking period: too short, it may cause crosstalk, and the AVD is nonphysiologic, set by

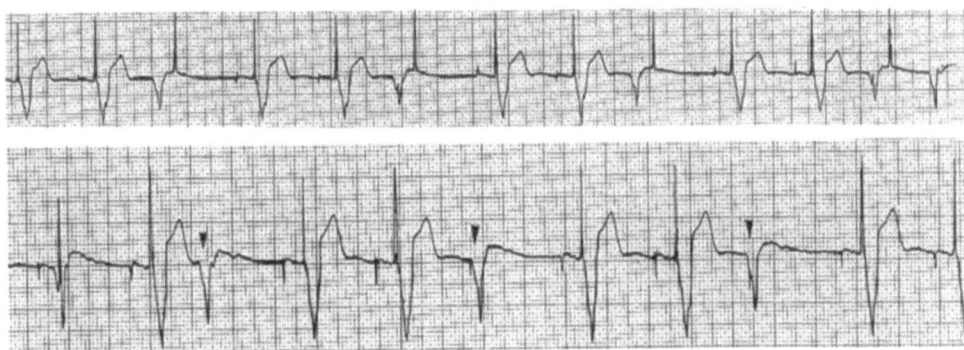

**Fig. 3.31.** Late coupled premature ventricular complexes fall just after the atrial spike, in the blanking period (*upper tracing*). They are not sensed and the pacemaker delivers a ventricular spike at the end of the AVD, during repolarization of the extrasystoles. This situation may be dangerous since it may be arrhythmogenic. After shortening the blanking period (*lower tracing*), the extrasystoles are now sensed and pacing during their recovery has been eliminated

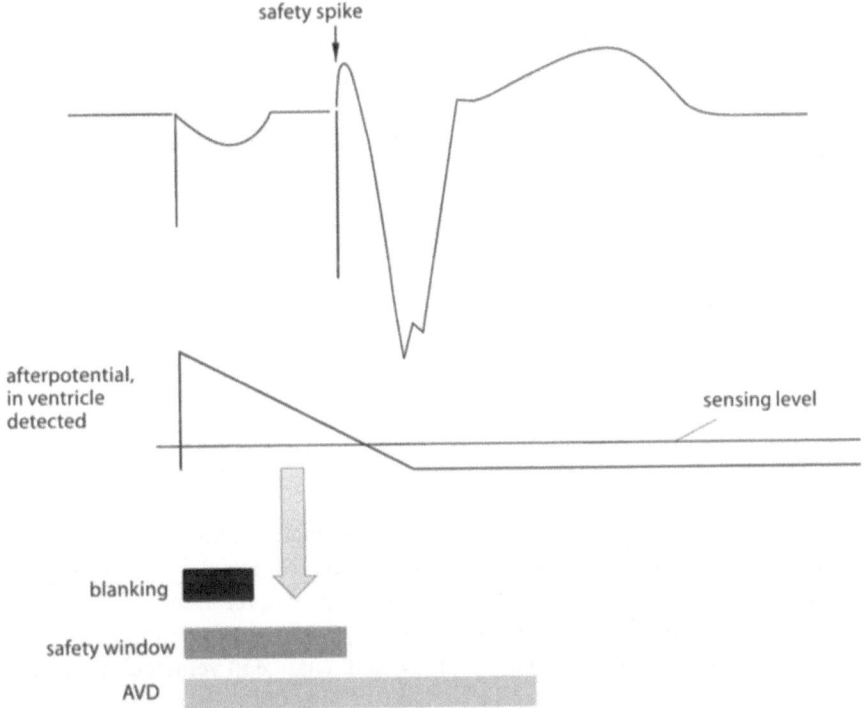

**Fig. 3.32.** Afterpotentials are sensed in the safety window, causing a forced ventricular stimulus delivery at the end of this window (its duration depends on the pacemaker model)

the safety window; too long, it facilitates the non-sensing of premature ventricular complexes. It must also be verified during exercise; indeed, with increasing heart rate, the afterpotentials from atrial pacing and those from the preceding

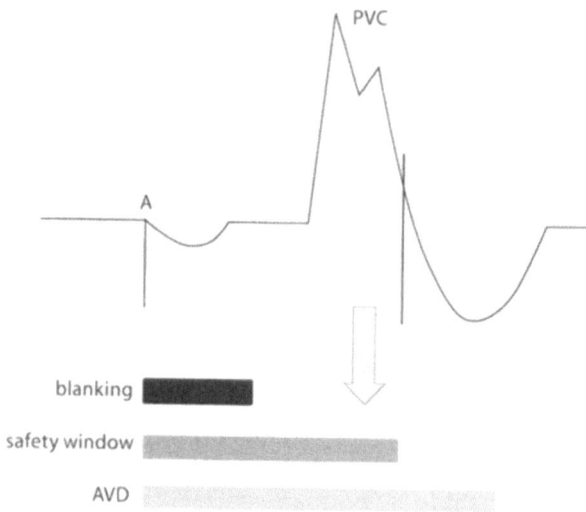

**Fig. 3.33.** A premature ventricular complex (PVC), sensed in the safety window, triggers a premature ventricular spike, however, during the refractory period of the PVC

ventricular pacing may cumulate and facilitate crosstalk, even when the latter was not apparent at rest.

In all cases, the risk of crosstalk is theoretically diminished by programming a bipolar atrial pacing (with low pacing output) and bipolar ventricular sensing configuration. Blanking may then be kept very short, allowing sensing of most late coupled premature ventricular complexes.

### Periods Initiated by Ventricular Events

Whether ventricular depolarization is sensed or paced, it initiates several periods, both ventricular and atrial.

#### The Ventricular Refractory Period

This period has the same purpose than in the single chamber systems: to avoid the resetting of the pacemaker by late potentials from ventricular pacing, or by the T wave. This risk is theoretically minimized by several, more or less associated reprogrammings: polarity switch of either pacing or sensing in the ventricle, lowering of the ventricular pacing output, change in ventricular sensitivity, and lengthening of the refractory period (see Fig. 3.25).

#### The Post Ventricular Atrial Refractory Period and the Total Atrial Refractory Period – the 2 : 1 Pacemaker AV Block Rate

The total atrial refractory period (TARP) is controlled in various ways depending on the manufacturer. Most offer a separate programming of AVD and of the post ventricular atrial refractory period (PVARP). TARP begins at the atrial spike or after atrial sensing, and represents the sum of AVD + PVARP (Fig. 3.34). Others, like Biotronik, offer the programming of a fixed TARP, even if the algorithm of automatic AVD shortening is activated, which means that, for any given increase in heart rate, PVARP increases by a value corresponding to the shortening of AVD.

Whatever the system configuration, a P wave falling during TARP does not initiate an AVD, and is not followed by ventricular pacing. In fact the PVARP of modern pacemakers is composed of two distinct periods: an absolute refractory period, rarely programmable, during which the pacemaker is completely „blind" in the atrium; and, just behind it, a relative refractory period during which atrial sensing may occur and cause very peculiar device behaviors to be discussed further in later sections.

The main purpose of the PVARP is to prevent the sensing of ventriculo-atrial conduction (VAC) which may induce endless-loop tachycardia (ELT). Average values for VAC have been between 220 and 280 ms, such that PVARP must theoretically be set at longer values. Indeed, if a retrograde P wave is sensed outside the refractory periods, it will trigger an AVD followed by ventricular pacing inducing a retrograde P wave, and the cycle starts again. A ELT has been initiated which may become incessant (Fig. 3.35).

TARP determines the maximal atrial rate that the pacemaker can ever sense on a 1 : 1 basis or the 2 : 1 pacemaker AV block rate. Setting of a long AVD at 250 ms and PVARP at 350 ms, for example, the TARP lasts 600 ms, which corresponds to a rate of 100 BPM. The 1 : 1 AV association rate, therefore, cannot be faster than 100 BPM. Beyond that rate, every other P wave falls in PVARP (Fig. 3.36). This means that the ventricular paced rate, in this example, falls from 100 to 50 BPM, a development particularly adverse to the exercise capacity of a patient with complete heart block, possibly leading to collapse. The AV association is 2 : 1.

### The Upper Rate and Wenckebach Behavior

The maximal 1 : 1 AV synchronized rate (upper rate) is the fastest rate at which the pacemaker can pace the ventricle and track a rapid atrial rhythm on a 1 : 1 basis. In other words, the ventricular pacing rate tracks the sinus rate up to a program-

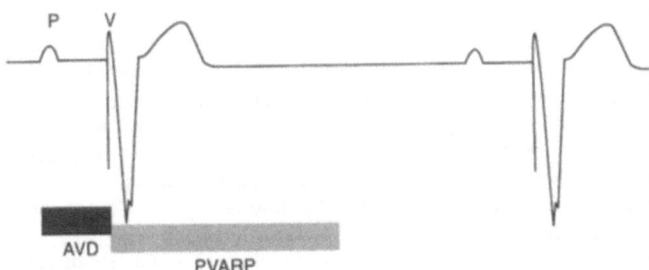

**Fig. 3.34.** All P waves sensed outside the total atrial refractory period (TARP), and whose rate falls between the lower rate and the programmed upper rate, are associated with an AVD as programmed: the atrioventricular association is 1 : 1

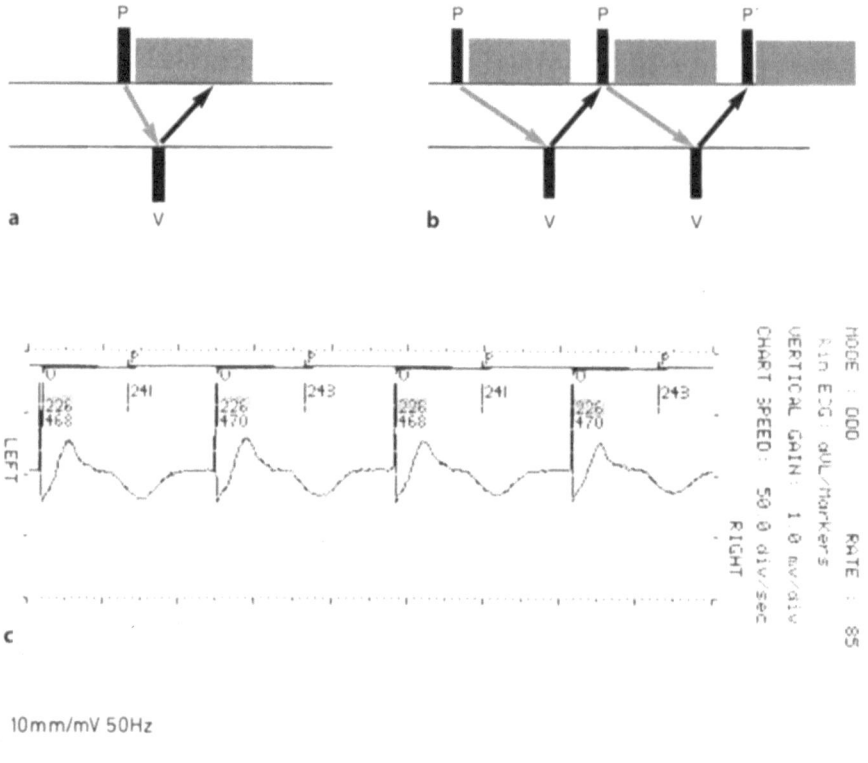

**Fig. 3.35. a** When AVD is programmed within normal limits (not too long), it is unlikely for retrograde (ventriculo-atrial) conduction to reach the atria before the end of the natural refractory periods of the conduction system or atria (*shaded areas*)

**b** To initiate an endless-loop tachycardia, a long enough AVD is needed to allow a long enough recovery time for the nodo-hisian and atrial tissue to be depolarized retrogradely after the end of their natural refractory periods (shaded areas)

**c** The event markers and the surface ECG are simultaneous. A P wave is sensed 226 ms after the ventricular stimulus because of retrograde conduction

**d** In the same patient, a pacemaker induced tachycardia at a rate of 130 BPM is initiated because the PVARP is shorter than 226 ms. The pacemaker senses the retrograde P waves and perpetuates 1 : 1 synchronized ventricular pacing

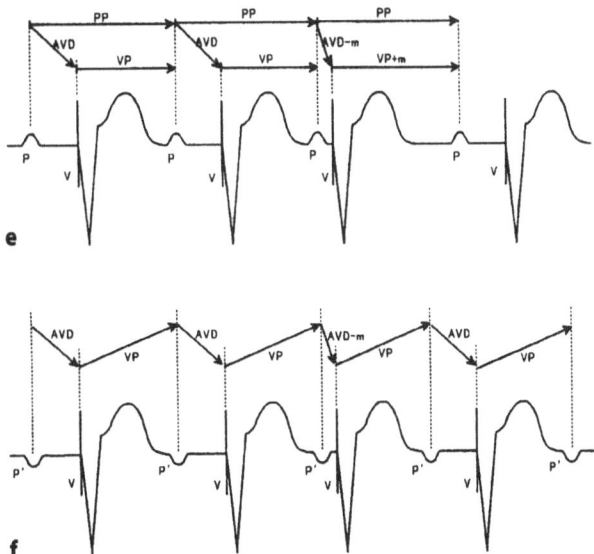

**Fig. 3.35. e** Permanent sinus rhythm tracking ventricular pacing. After the third P wave, AVD is shortened (AVD minus m); Since it is sinus rhythm, the PP cycles have the same duration. The shortening in the AVD results in a lengthening of the following VP interval that becomes equal to the measured VP interval during the previous cycles plus m
**f** Endless-loop tachycardia. Each ventricular pacing is followed by a retrograde wave (P') after a constant VP' interval. After the AVD modulation (shortening in the AVD minus m), the VP' time remains constant since the P wave depends on the previous ventricular pacing. The ELT diagnosis is actually possible since the retrograde conduction time remains constant, even though there is an AVD modulation
*P* spontaneous P wave; *V* ventricular pacing; *P'* retrograde P wave

mable limit. However, the upper rate is conditioned by the maximal atrial sensing rate, or 2 : 1 pacemaker AV block rate, itself dependent on TARP, which is equal to AVD+PVARP. The upper rate is usually programmed within a zone ranging between 100 and 180 BPM. One should not confuse the upper rate with the limit of ventricular run a way, which applies to all modes, and is not programmable. The latter very dangerous dysfunction is usually due to a technical failure which, fortunately, has become quite rare.

Spontaneous atrioventricular conduction is not affected by programming of the upper rate. Consequently, supraventricular tachycardias with spontaneous AV conduction, and ventricular tachycardias, both independent from pacing, may go on at a rate faster than the upper programmed rate without intervention from the pacemaker, which is inhibited by spontaneous events as long as they do not fall in its refractory periods.

What happens to a pacemaker-dependent patient with complete atrioventricular block?

If the atrial rate goes beyond the programmed upper rate, but stays below the 2 : 1 pacemaker AV block rate, a Wenckebach-like behavior takes place. Since the ventricular pacing rate is limited by the programmed upper rate, any accelera-

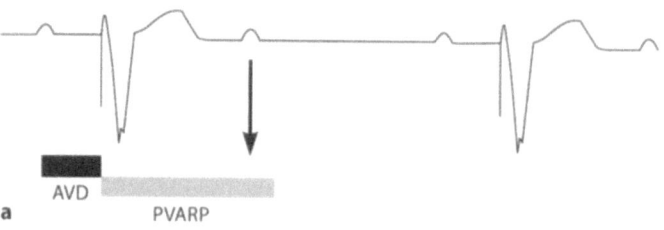

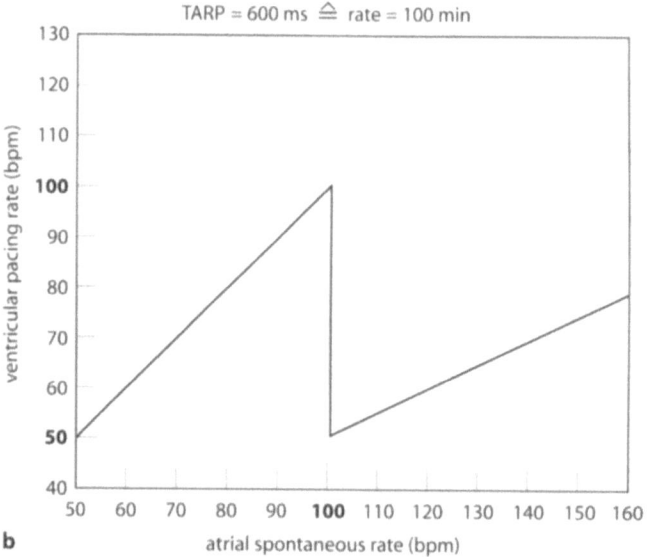

**Fig. 3.36. a** When the atrial rate crosses the 2 : 1 pacemaker AV block rate, the first P wave is normally conducted to the ventricles with the programmed AVD. The next P wave is blocked in the PVARP and initiates no AVD. The association is 2 : 1

**b** If the spontaneous atrial rate goes beyond the 2 : 1 pacemaker AV block rate (in this case 100 BPM, TARP = 600 ms), in a patient with complete AV block, the ventricular rate falls abruptly to a rate equal to one half the atrial rate, i.e. 50 BPM. or to the programmed lower rate, if the latter is faster than 50 BPM

tion of the atrial rate beyond this limit results in an extension of the AVD, cycle after cycle. After a few 1 : 1 ventricular paced cycles, a P wave ends up falling in PVARP and is not followed by ventricular pacing (Fig. 3.37). The latter resumes with the following P wave, and so on. The end result is that, as the atrial rate increases beyond the programmed upper rate and approaches the 2 : 1 pacemaker AV block rate, the average ventricular rate decreases because of a growing proportion of blocked P waves (falling in PVARP), until it reaches a value equal to the 2 : 1 pacemaker AV block rate divided by 2, as the atrial rate has reached the 2 : 1 pacemaker AV block rate (Fig. 3.38). Consequently, it is important to remember that, if the atrial rate goes beyond the programmed upper rate, and one wishes to maintain a level of ventricular pacing near that upper

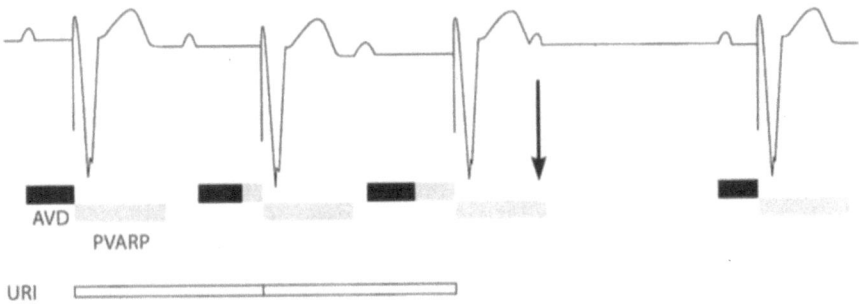

**Fig. 3.37.** The Wenckebach function is characterized by ventricular pacing at the programmed upper rate, interrupted by longer cycles due to P waves blocked in PVARP *URI* upper rate interval; *AVD* AV delay

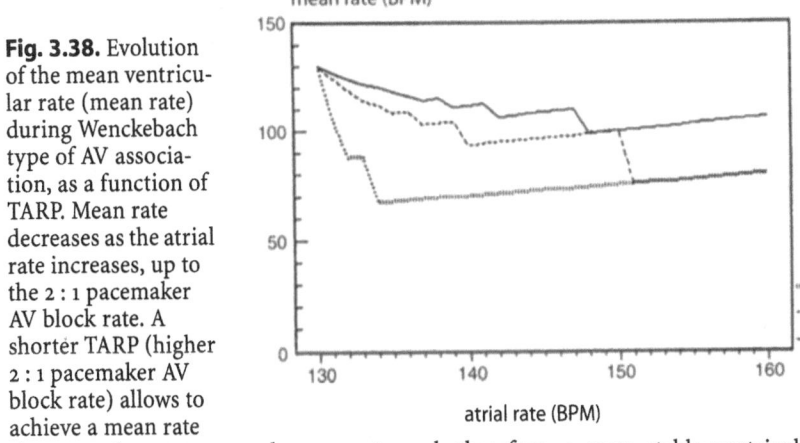

**Fig. 3.38.** Evolution of the mean ventricular rate (mean rate) during Wenckebach type of AV association, as a function of TARP. Mean rate decreases as the atrial rate increases, up to the 2 : 1 pacemaker AV block rate. A shorter TARP (higher 2 : 1 pacemaker AV block rate) allows to achieve a mean rate closer to the programmed upper rate and, therefore, a more stable ventricular rate response

rate, it is mandatory to program a high 2 : 1 pacemaker AV block rate, which means short AVD and PVARP (Fig. 3.39). This objective is partially fulfilled by the algorithm of AVD shortening with increasing atrial rate (see p. 84). On the other hand, the programming of a short PVARP exposes to the sensing of retrograde P waves and consequent risk of pacemaker induced tachycardia. In such cases, the use of protections, to be described in the next chapter, is necessary. Programming a high 2 : 1 pacemaker AV block rate allows also to increase the value of the upper rate, especially if the patient is young and physically active, and to avoid the switch to the Wenckebach mode which is detrimental to exercise capacity.

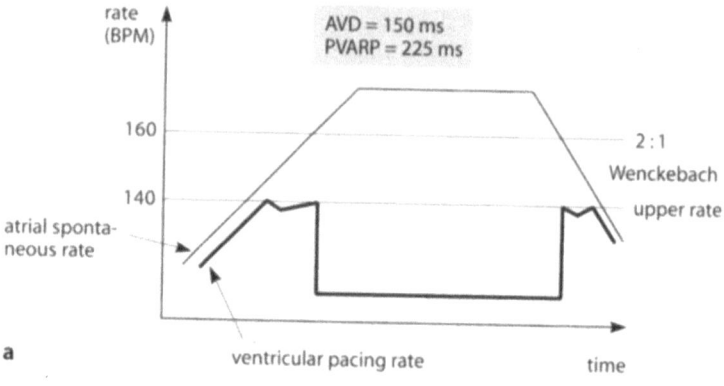

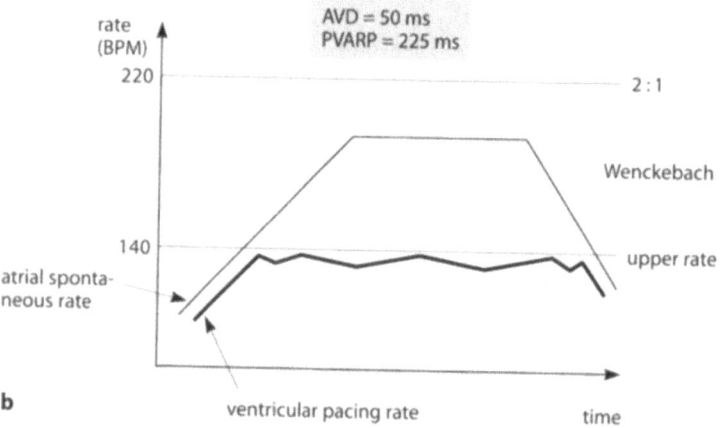

**Fig. 3.39. a** Consequences of a low 2 : 1 pacemaker AV block rate (160 BPM) relative to the programmed upper rate (140 BPM) on the Wenckebach type association. When the atrial rate goes beyond 160 BPM, the ventricular pacing rate falls abruptly to 80 BPM (synchronized on the atrial activity sensed on a 2 : 1 basis by the pacemaker)
**b** When the 2 : 1 pacemaker AV block rate has been programmed at 220 BPM, relative to the same upper rate of 140 BPM, the Wenckebach zone is widened: the duration of Wenckebach function is lengthened, and the fall in ventricular paced rate would be attenuated should the atrial rate cross the 2 : 1 pacemaker AV block rate

CASE STUDY

*Example.* A 35 year old patient with third degree AV block has received a DDD pacemaker and complains of reduced exercise capacity when bicycling. An exercise ECG is performed. The programmed upper rate is 130 BPM. During exercise, the patient's spontaneous atrial rate rose to 135 BPM. Because of Wenckebach behavior (with gradual lengthening of the AVD and loss of ventricular pacing, in this case after the 4th P wave), the patient experiences a sudden loss of energy. After reprogramming of the upper rate to 150 BPM, the patient recovered his usual exercise capacity (Fig. 3.40).

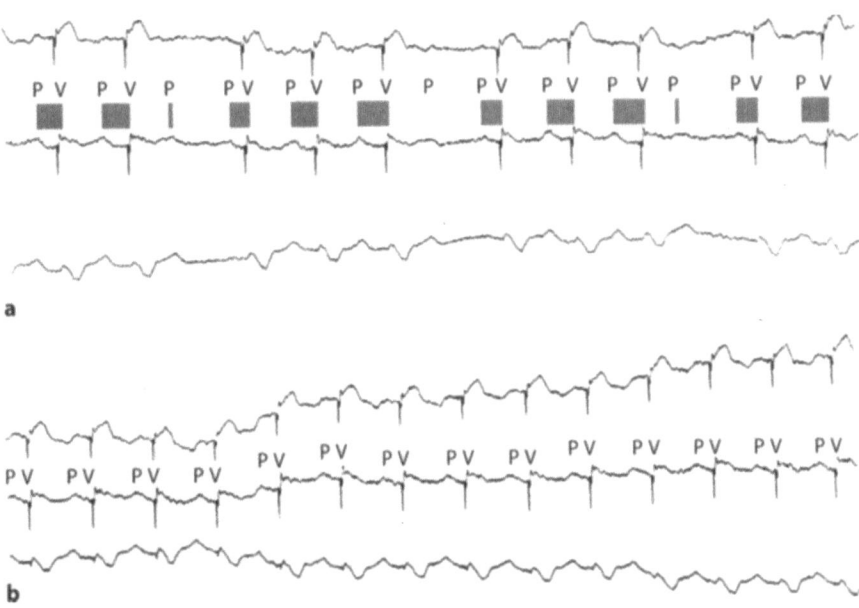

**Fig. 3.40. a** The upper rate has been programmed at 130 BPM. During exercise, as the atrial rate has reached 135 BPM, the pacemaker switches to Wenckebach mode. The AVD increases from cycle to cycle as a result of the upper rate set at 130 BPM, until a P wave falls in PVARP. No ventricular pulse is delivered, causing a ventricular pause until the next P wave. The patient develops symptoms
**b** After reprogramming of the upper rate to 150 BPM, an increase in atrial rate to 145 BPM is accompanied by 1 : 1 AV association and elimination of symptoms
*P* P wave; *V* ventricular pacing

This example is in support of a recent study which confirmed the important hemodynamic alterations that are induced by Wenckebach periodicity compared to 1 : 1 synchronization during exercise, with fall in systolic arterial pressure due to the decrease in ventricular rate, and wide cyclic variations in blood pressure related to the irregularity of the ventricular rhythm.

Consequently, our recommendation is to offer the greatest possible 1 : 1 AV association during exercise by programming a short TARP and a high upper rate. This implies compromising with various programmable parameters, including AVD and PVARP, and a thorough knowledge of several clinical characteristics such as patient age, overall exercise capacity, underlying heart disease, presence of retrograde conduction, etc.

## Protection Algorithms Against Endless-Loop Tachycardia

The term pacemaker mediated tachycardia (PMT) includes two types of pacemaker related tachyarrhythmias:

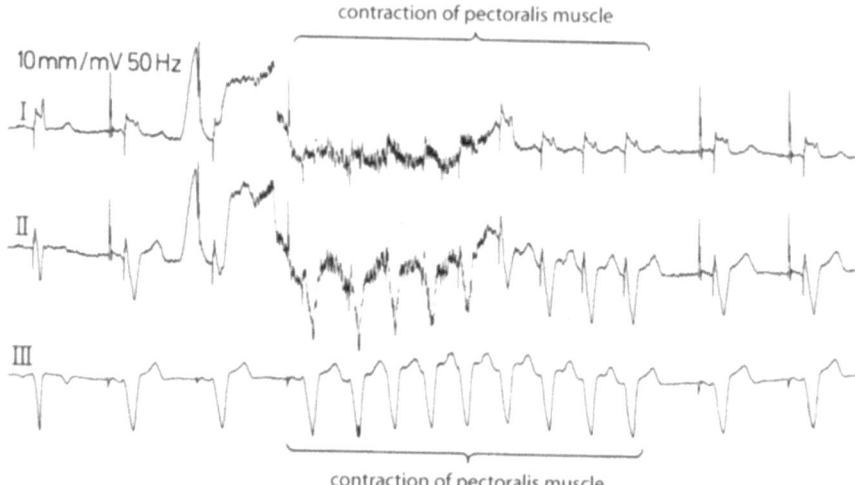

contraction of pectoralis muscle

10 mm/mV 50 Hz

I

II

III

contraction of pectoralis muscle

**Fig. 3.41.** Example of ventricular acceleration induced by DDD pacemaker tracking myosignals at the atrial level at a rate of approximately 140 BPM, the programmed upper rate being 150 BPM. This type of behavior belongs to the family of tachycardias mediated by dual chamber pacemakers (PMT)

1. Those due to tracking of atrial arrhythmias or extracardiac interferences sensed by the pacemaker atrial channel, and expressed as an acceleration of the ventricular pacing rate (Fig. 3.41)
2. „Endless-loop" tachycardia (ELT), a form of reentrant tachycardia mediated by the pacemaker

ELT will be discussed in this chapter. The term PMT, which is more encompassing, is often used instead of ELT, but not the reverse.

The onset of an ELT implies preserved retrograde conduction from ventricular depolarization. If the latter has been synchronized to a spontaneous P wave, retrograde conduction is blocked since the AV conduction system is refractory at the time of ventricular activation. However, if AV desynchronization occurs, retrograde conduction may take place. It is noteworthy that retrograde conduction may be preserved in cases of complete anterograde block. The average prevalence of preserved retrograde conduction in an overall population of pacemaker patients is 40%. During exercise, retrograde conduction may appear when it was not present at rest, such that the overall prevalence may reach 75%. This means that protective measures are essential, and that it is futile to look for it at the time of device implantation. Instead, it seems preferable to assume that it may develop in all patients, particularly during sympathetic activation.

The various phenomena that may induce retrograde conduction, and potentially trigger ELT are the following:

- Too long a programmed AVD
- Isolated premature ventricular complexes (Fig. 3.42a)

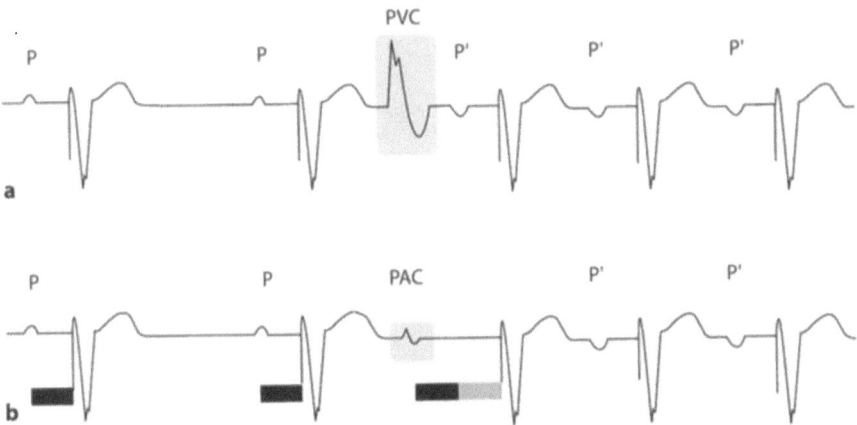

**Fig. 3.42. a** The premature ventricular complex (PVC), timed well after the last spontaneous P wave, retrogradely depolarizes the atria via the conduction system which has recovered its excitability, thus initiating ELT

**b** The atrial extrasystole (PAC: premature atrial complex) is conducted to the ventricles with an obligatory lengthening of the programmed AVD (observance of the upper rate limit). As a result of this phenomenon, the conduction system becomes open to retrograde conduction (*shaded area*), and initiation of ELT

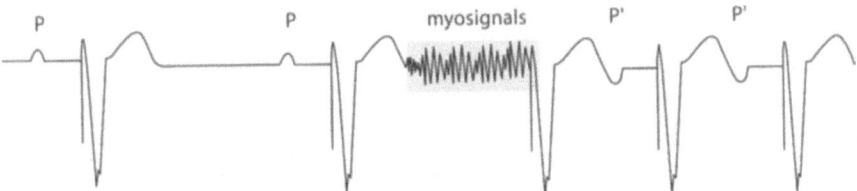

**Fig. 3.43.** The myosignals sensed by the atrial electrode trigger ventricular pacing. Retrograde activation of the atrium is possible since it is outside its refractory period

- Very early premature atrial complex (Fig. 3.42b)
- Sensed artifact at the atrial level such as outside interference
- Myosignals (Fig. 3.43)
- Failure of atrial sensing or pacing (Fig. 3.44)
- Absence of PVARP extension after magnet removal (Fig. 3.45) or at the time of 1 : 1 AV reassociation after fall-back or mode switch.

The rate of ELT depends on the relative values of the retrograde conduction time, of the programmed upper rate, and of the ongoing AVD. If the sum of retrograde conduction time + AVD (at the upper rate) is less than the interval corresponding to the upper rate (60,000/upper rate), the rate of ELT will be equal to the upper rate, and the AVD is lengthened to comply with the programmed upper rate (Fig. 3.46a).

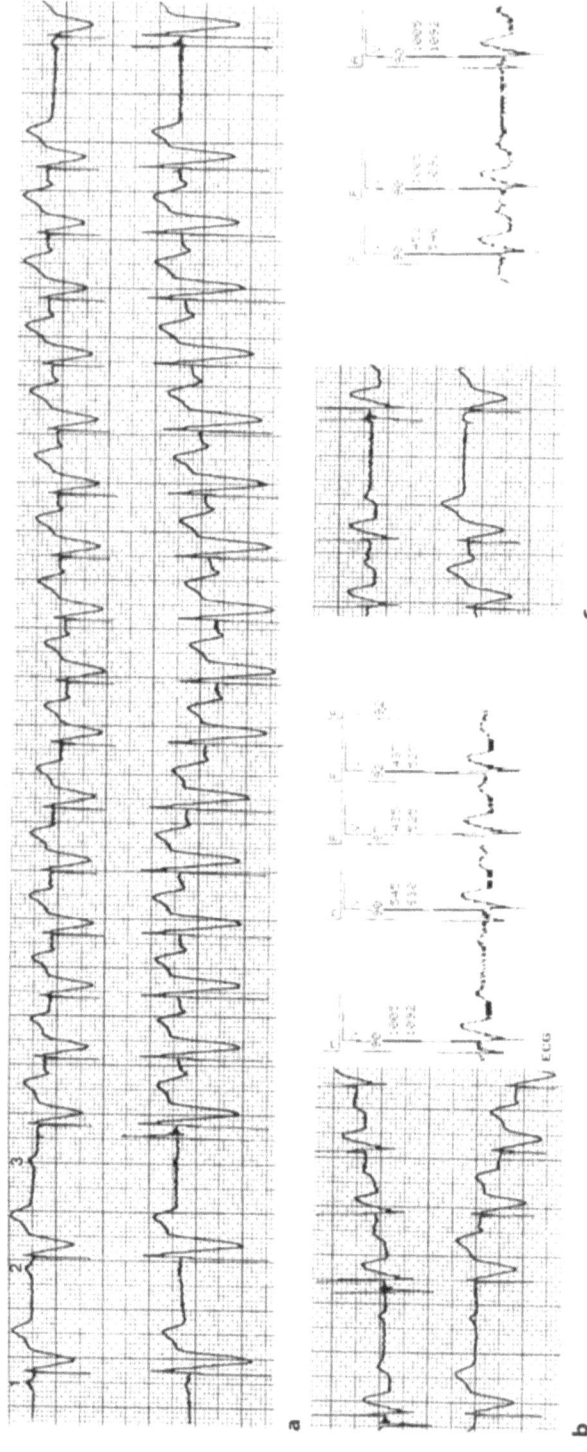

**Fig. 3.44a–b.** DDD mode, 55/122 BPM, AVD = 90 ms, PVARP = 400 ms, atrial sensitivity = 2 mV

**a** Failure of atrial sensing (P3) with atrial pacing in the atrial refractory period, retrograde conduction from ventricular pacing and initiation of ELT which ends spontaneously by block in the retrograde direction

**b** The event markers reveal the presence of a retrograde conduction time of 525 ms and

**c** the spontaneous termination of ELT

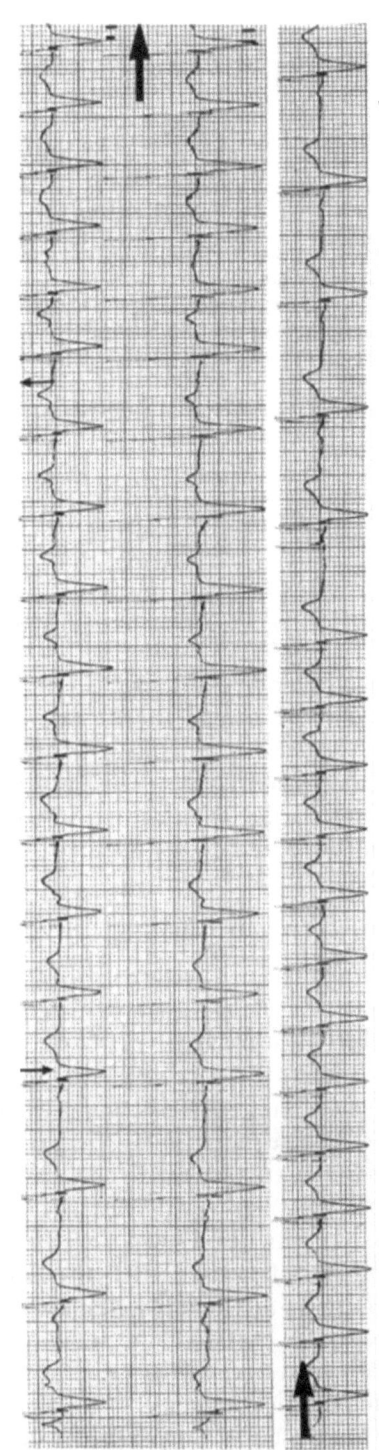

**Fig. 3.45.** DDD mode, 60/120 BPM, AVD = 160 ms, PVARP = 280 ms, magnet test. Onset of ELT upon magnet removal from a pacemaker converted to D00 mode during magnet application (*small downward arrow*), allowing retrograde conduction because of absence of automatic increase in PVARP at the time of magnet removal (*small upward arrow*)

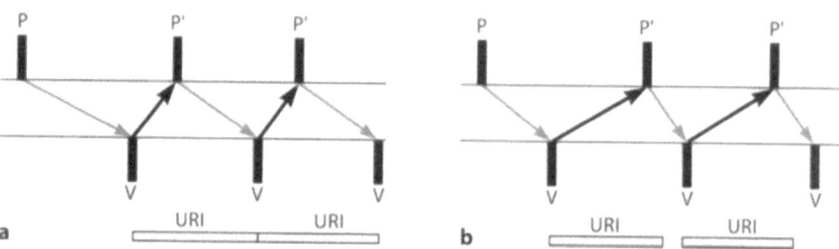

**Fig. 3.46. a** The sum of retrograde conduction time + AVD (ongoing PV delay at the upper rate) is shorter than the upper rate interval (*URI*). The AVD is therefore lengthened so that the ventricular paced interval complies with this upper rate interval
**b** The sum of retrograde conduction time + AVD (PV delay at the ongoing rate) is longer than the upper rate interval. The rate of ELT is, consequently, slower than the programmed upper rate
*P* spontaneous P wave; *V* ventricular pacing; *P'* retrograde P wave; *URI* upper rate interval

CASE STUDY

> *Example.* Upper rate = 150 BPM (400 ms), retrograde conduction time = 220 ms, AVD = 100 ms. The sum of the time intervals = 320 ms, less than the upper rate interval (400 ms). The rate of ELT will be equal to the upper rate with lengthening of AVD after each retrograde P wave to observe the shortest paced cycle length.

If the sum of the AVD (at the ELT rate) + retrograde conduction time is longer than 60,000/upper rate, the ELT rate will be slower than the upper rate (Fig. 3.46b) and equal to 60,000/(AVD + retrograde conduction time).

If the retrograde conduction time is 350 ms, and AVD is 100 ms, their sum is 450 ms, and the rate of ELT is slower than the programmed upper rate. The average incidence of ELT slower than the programmed upper rate is 35%.

### The Classic Prevention of ELT Onset

Theoretically the retrograde conduction time should be measured, and PVARP should be set at a longer value to maintain a safety margin and total protection. This will avoid the induction of ELT since the retrograde P wave can only fall during this refractory period. However, this way of programming is not without consequences on the exercise capacity of the paced patient.

In the example shown in Fig. 3.35c, retrograde conduction, that is the interval between the ventricular pacing spike and the following P wave can be measured at 226 ms on the marker channels. The PVARP was programmed at 325 ms. Nevertheless, the patient did suffer from a few episodes of reentrant tachycardia. It is only after extending the PVARP to 400 ms that all episodes of ELT were eliminated. However, this imposes a limitation of the upper rate since TARP is equal, in this particular example, to 400 ms + AVD (150 ms) = 550 ms. The programmed upper rate, therefore, cannot be set above 109 BPM, too slow a heart rate for a young individual. The main objective is indeed to protect the patient against ELT, but also to preserve an intact exercise capacity. To that effect, one has to rely on the various protective mechanisms against the consequences of an active retrograde conduction, and try to program a short TARP. One option is to activate the algorithm of automatic shortening of the AVD, which will shorten TARP by the amount of AVD shortening.

However, the best way to shorten TARP remains to shorten PVARP, particularly since it is not always desirable to use the algorithm of automatic AVD reduction. One has, then, to rely on the various methods of ELT onset prevention.

### The Modern Prevention of ELT Onset

Factors facilitating the development of ELT may be eliminated by choosing a bipolar configuration of sensing, which, as opposed to unipolar, minimizes the risk of extracardiac interference, or by programming a short rather than long AVD, since a long interval allows the AV nodal tissue to recover its excitability before being exposed to the retrograde wavefront coming from the right ventricle. Following premature ventricular complexes, magnet application, the end of fall-back or mode switch, noise reversion, or a programming session, protection is accomplished by the programmable or fixed extension of PVARP to „cover" the retrograde conduction time (Fig. 3.47, 3.48). Atrial pacing synchronous with premature ventricular complexes may be triggered to prevent retrograde conduction (Fig. 3.49).

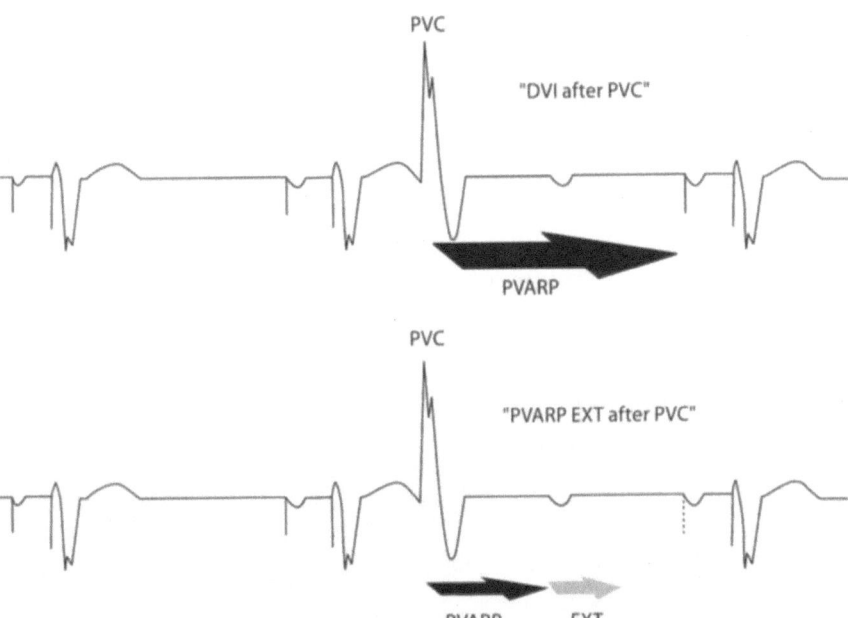

**Fig. 3.47.** To prevent any triggering of ELT after a sensed premature ventricular complex, some pacemakers extend the PVARP over the entire atrial escape interval („DVI after PVC", *top tracing*), while others extend the PVARP over some of the VA interval („PVARPext after PVC", *bottom tracing*) to allow the return of proper atrial sensing toward the end of the atrial escape interval
*PVC* premature ventricular complex

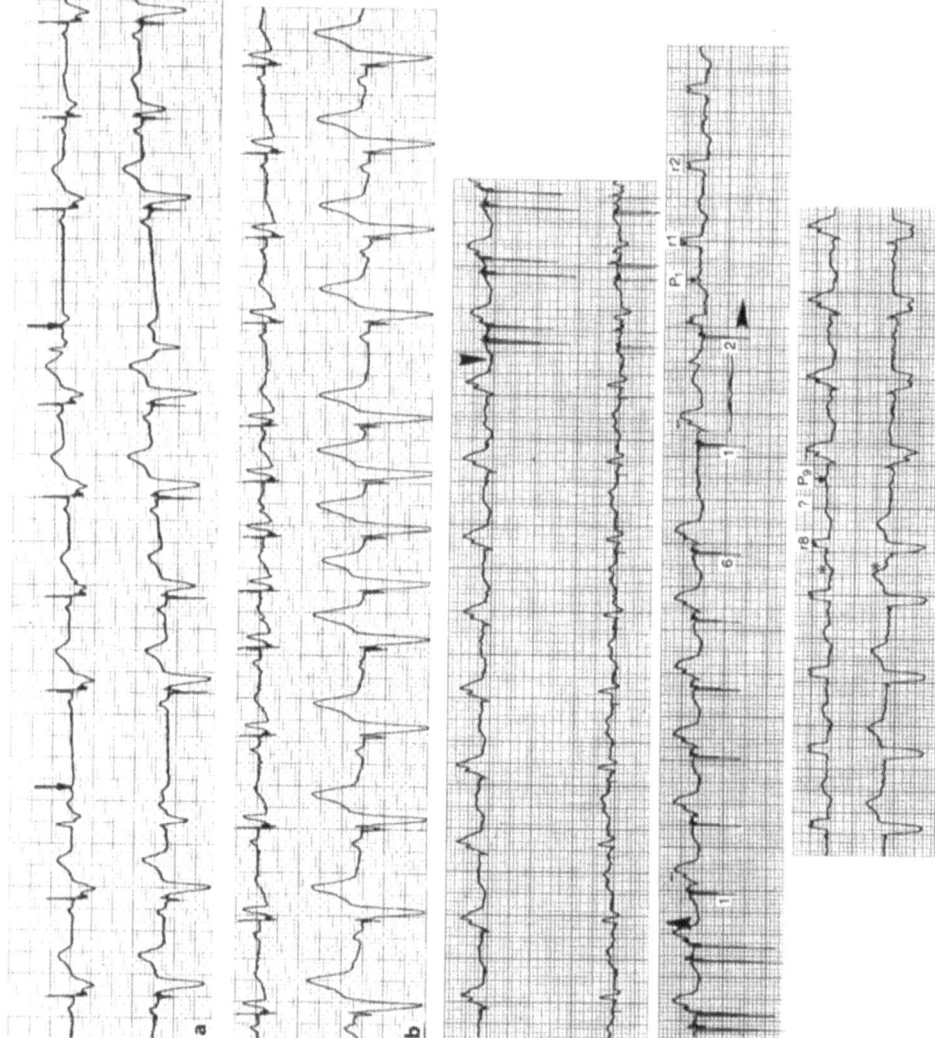

**Fig. 3.48.** VDD mode, 51/120 BPM, AVD, 156 ms, PVARP, 125 ms

**a** Two premature ventricular complexes are followed by P waves unsensed by the pacemaker (*arrows*). This is normal function since, with the Sorin Physiocor 300 model, PVARP is extended to 406 ms after sensing of a premature ventricular complex

**b** After sensing of two P consecutive waves separated by an interval shorter than the minimal interval corresponding to the programmed upper rate (500 ms for a rate of 120 BPM), the pacemaker switches to the VVI mode, pacing at the upper rate for four beats. Atrial sensing is then reestablished

**c** DDD mode, 60 BPM, AVD = 156 ms, PVARP = 297 ms. Indication for pacing: syncope, first degree AV block and left bundle branch block (LBBB). Example of dysfunction related to the protection against the onset ELT of by lengthening of PVARP upon magnet removal. This pacemaker, upon magnet application (downward arrow), functions in D00 mode at 96 BPM with its programmed AVD. Upon removal of the magnet (*upward arrow*) 6 atrioventricular paced beats are delivered at a rate of 96 BPM, followed by 2 beats at the lower rate of 60 BPM. At that moment (*horizontal arrow*), the PVARP is extended to 453 ms. This causes the second asynchronous QRS, at the lower rate, to be followed by a PVARP of 453 ms, which overlaps the following P wave (*P1*) with return of spontaneous rhythm (first degree AV block and left bundle branch block), disappearance of the ventricular spikes, all QRSs being interpreted as premature ventricular complexes (from *r1* to *r8*). This causes a lengthening of PVARP with each cycle and perpetuation of the phenomenon. This will be interrupted after the premature atrial complex (*), which shifts the following P wave (*P9*) and brings it out of PVARP. The programmed AV synchrony has been restored

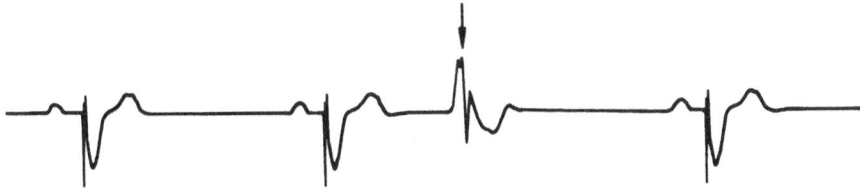

**Fig. 3.49.** Other method of protection against ELT (Vitatron). An atrial stimulus is delivered when a premature ventricular complex is sensed to block retrograde conduction

Methods of prevention of ELT include the following:

- Programming a PVARP longer than the retrograde conduction time
- Use of bipolar sensing to minimize the risk of ELT induction by myosignals
- Programming a short AVD
- Automatic lengthening of PVARP after premature ventricular complexes
- Atrial pacing synchronous with premature ventricular complexes
- DVI mode after premature ventricular complexes
- Use of some fall-back or mode switch algorithms

These methods, though effective, remain insufficient. Indeed, nothing may prevent a premature atrial complex, which can prolong AVD, or an artifact or extracardiac interference sensed as P wave, to cause AV asynchrony, the basis for the initiation of ELT. Consequently, the pacemaker must be equipped with a system to recognize and terminate ELT.

*ELT Termination*

All available methods are effective to variable degrees. Most are based on the recognition, by the pacemaker of ventricular pacing synchronous with atrial activity occurring at the same rate, over a fixed or programmable number of cycles, at a rate equal to the programmed upper rate. In general, after 6 or 16 cycles (Cosmos II, Relay, Marathon), the pacemaker omits synchronous ventricular pacing to break ELT. However, as discussed earlier, the rate of ELT is not uncommonly below the programmed upper rate.

To offer maximum protection against ELT at rates below the programmed upper rate, the Paragon and Synchrony pacemakers allow the programming of a rate different than the upper rate, from which at the 10th and every 127th cycle, the pacemaker does not initiate an AVD or ventricular pacing, to interrupt a possible tachycardia. This system, however, lacks specificity.

Completely automatic functions are found in the Chorus series which makes a diagnosis of ELT on the basis of a fixed retrograde conduction time after a variation on the AVD (Fig. 3.50, see also Fig. 3.35e, f). This completely automatic system reprograms its AVD and PVARP in case of frequent episodes of ELT. This information can be retrieved by interrogation of the device's statistics. Clinical experience with this system has shown it to offer the best remedy to this complication.

The Diamond (Vitatron), Trilogy (Pacesetter) and Phymos (Medico) models use the same analysis of the retrograde conduction time to diagnose ELT.

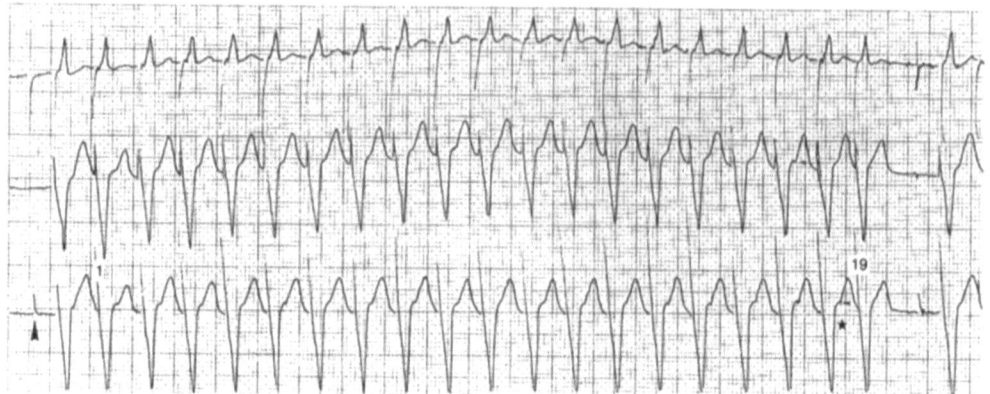

**Fig. 3.50.** ELT induced by failure of atrial pacing (*arrow*). The rate of the tachycardia is equal to the programmed upper rate (DDD mode, 70/150BPM, AVD = 140 ms, PVARP = 141 ms). The tachycardia is interrupted after modulation of the AVD, shortened by 47 ms (*). The VV interval (*19*) is shortened. Retrograde conduction is blocked since the nodo-hisian conduction system is refractory when the last ventricular spike is delivered

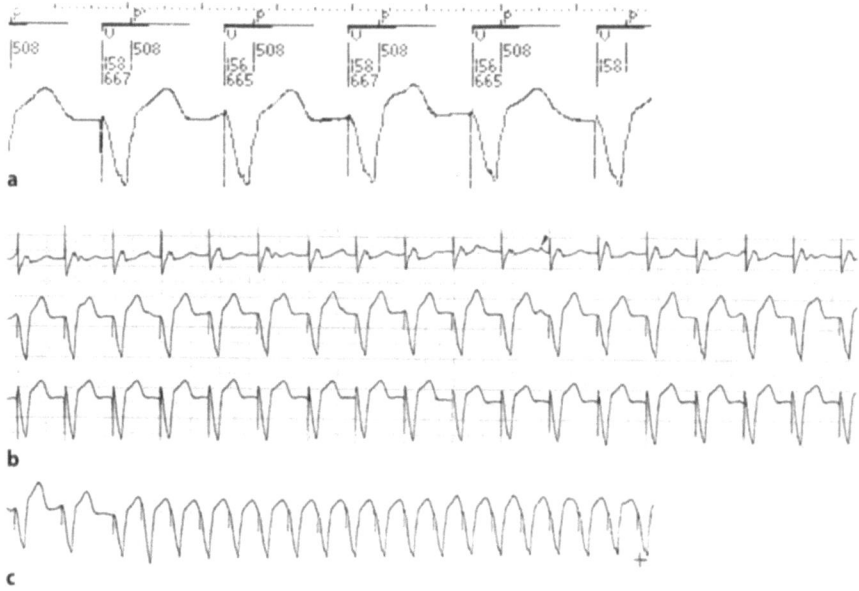

**Fig. 3.51.** Example of ventriculo-atrial crosstalk
**a** from sensing of paced ventricular complex at the atrial level after the end of PVARP whose value is very short (approximately 156 ms). This phenomenon explains
**b** the AV dissociation, and **c** the sudden acceleration of ventricular pacing when the upper rate is reprogrammed from 90 to 150 BPM (Fig. 3.51 d, e see p. 105)

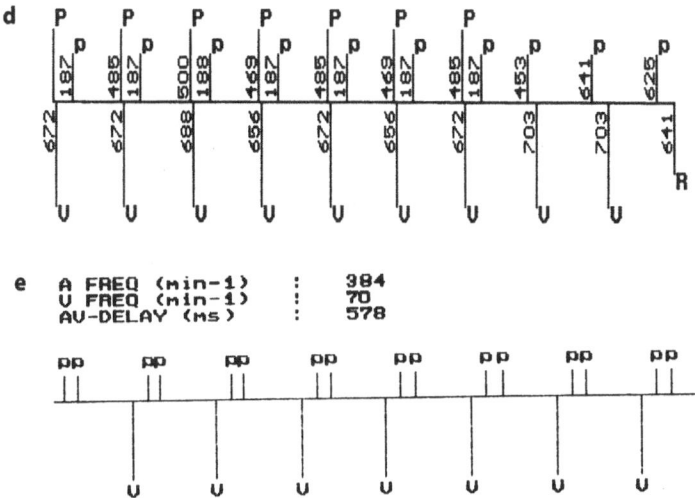

**Fig. 3.51. d** VA crosstalk recognized in a special Holter function with markers of the Chorum pacemaker, Ela Medical: 187 ms after the first (regular) P wave a second one appears. This P wave, caused by far-field R wave after ventricular pacing, is detected by the atrial channel due to a very short absolute atrial refractory period (blanking) and as P-wave misinterpreted by the pacemaker. Additionally there is to see the beginning of fallback (mode switch) function
**e** VA crosstalk identified by a special function with event markers in the Chorum pacemaker (ELA Medical). The pacemaker is programmed in VDD and there is sinus dysfunction: each ventricular pacing is followed by a first P wave corresponding to the far-field R wave sensed just after the atrial blanking; then a second P wave appears which corresponds to a retrograde P wave

## VA Cross-Talk

The PVARP of modern pacemakers is divided in two intervals: 1/ a short absolute refractory period; it is rarely programmable (50 – 300 ms) and, depending on the pacemaker model, is set at 100 to 150 ms; and 2/ a relative refractory period. Atrial sensing during this second period neither initiates an AVD nor triggers ventricular pacing. It is, however, logged in the pacemaker's diagnostic memory as a premature atrial event. VA crosstalk is due to a sensing of the far-field R wave by the pacemaker's atrial channel, after the end of the absolute PVARP, during its relative second period. The systematic sensing of a far-field R wave (usually a paced R wave since pacing delays the propagation of ventricular depolarization) causes double counting in the atrium: the sinus or paced P wave, and the far-field R wave. This results in erroneous diagnoses of atrial arrhythmias, and in the inappropriate trigger of mode switch according to the particular algorithm assigned to each pacemaker model.

The Vitatron system offers an automatic, permanent extension of post-ventricular atrial blanking if the retrograde conduction time is found to be very short (< 150 ms), to suppress what the pacemakers considers to be crosstalk (Fig. 3.51).

### Automatic Mode Switch AAI/DDD

This mode is proper to the Chorus II, Chorum and Talent (ELA Medical) models. As long as AV conduction is preserved, the pacemaker functions in AAI mode with refractory periods confined to the atrium, although it continues to monitor the occurrence of a QRS after each non-premature P wave (ADI mode).

When AV conduction fails (no QRS at the end of AVD + a monitoring window of 31 ms), the pacemaker switches automatically to DDD mode, including all protective functions (anti ELT, mode switch), followed, when appropriate, by return to AAI mode and return of spontaneous AV conduction (Fig. 3.52).

This mode, like the AV delay scanning function of Vitatron and Pacesetter (see p. 397 f.) is meant to limit the power consuming ventricular pacing, and facilitate the synchronization of ventricular contraction. These particular modes apply to situations when ventricular pacing is rarely used, as in the carotid sinus syndrome, vaso-vagal syncope, sino-atrial block, or paroxysmal AV block.

### The DDI Mode

> Atrial and ventricular (dual) pacing, atrial and ventricular (dual) sensing, inhibition by atrial and ventricular events.

This is a distinct form of dual chamber pacing. Pacing and sensing are activated in both chambers. The pacemaker takes charge of atrioventricular syn-

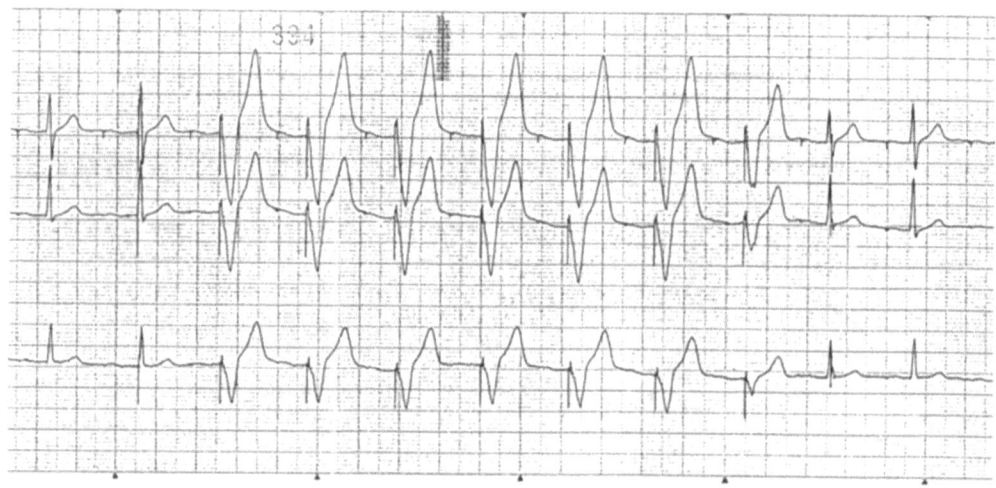

**Fig. 3.52.** Automatic mode switch of the Chorus II (ELA Medical). In the beginning of the tracing, the rhythm consists of atrial pacing and ventricular sensing. The AR interval is long (260 ms). Upon carotid massage, the pacemaker switches to DDD mode, at an atrial pacing rate near that present before. The mode remains DDD until spontaneous complexes return to inhibit ventricular pacing. The pseudo-AAI mode has been restored

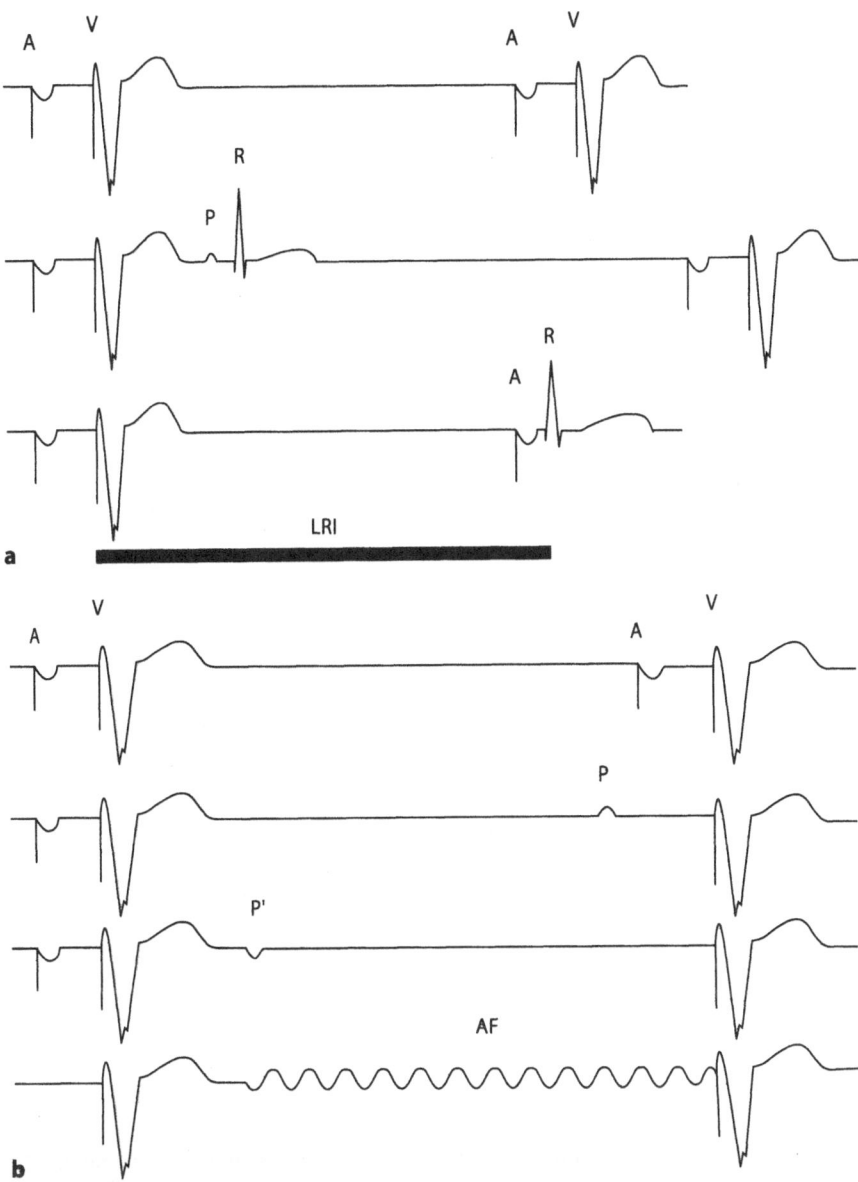

**Fig. 3.53. a–d** Examples of normal DDI function
**a** Resetting of the pacemaker from R wave sensing
**b** Absence of synchronization with isolated atrial activity. This offers the advantage of avoiding a sudden acceleration of the ventricular rate from sensing an atrial tachyarrhythmia (*bottom tracing*)

chrony only when atrial and ventricular rates are both below the lower rate, that is only during periods of sinus bradycardia (Fig. 3.53). When the pacemaker senses spontaneous atrial or ventricular signals at a rate above the programmed lower rate, pacing is inhibited. However, as opposed to the DDD mode, sponta-

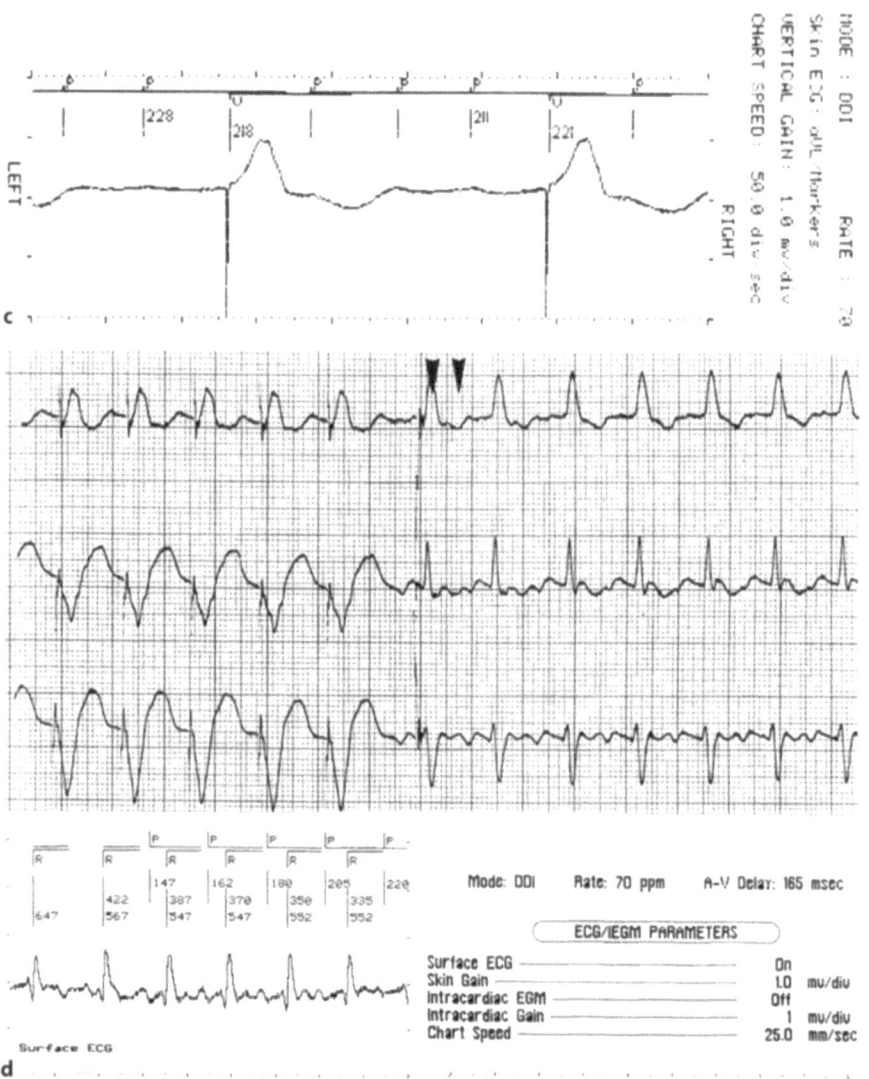

**Fig. 3.53. c** Simultaneous recording of surface ECG and event markers in DDI mode. The atrial rate is 270 BPM, the ventricular rate is 70 BPM. As opposed to the DDD mode, the atrial activity does not cause ventricular pacing to accelerate
**d** switch from rapid tracking in DDD mode to completely inhibited DDI mode and intrinsic rhythm (*arrows*). The event markers (*bottom left*) confirm the proper inhibition of the pacemaker at both the atrial and ventricular levels in DDI mode switching, see p. 402 ff.
*AF* atrial fibrillation; *LRI* lower rate interval; *P* P wave; *V* ventricular pacing stimulus

neous atrial activity initiates neither an AVD nor ventricular pacing, such that, in the event of an atrial tachycardia, ventricular pacing rate does not increase in presence of atrioventricular block (Fig. 3.53), and the device's behavior is VVI

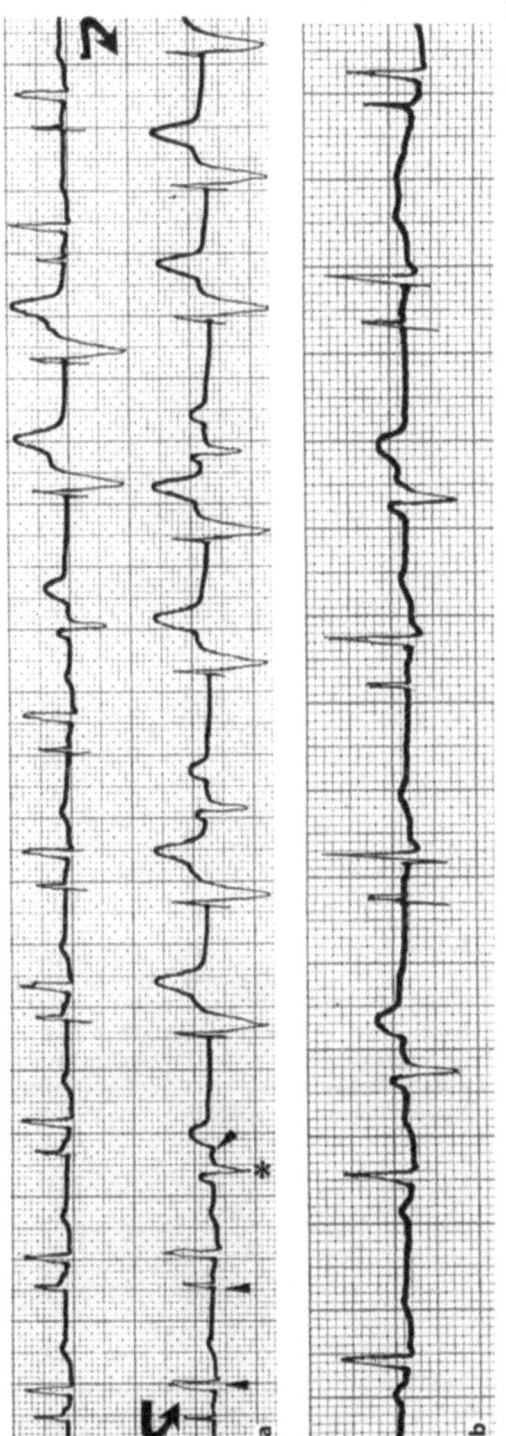

**Fig. 3.54. a** DDI mode, 70 BPM, AVD = 200 ms, atrial sensitivity = 2 mV. Premature ventricular complexes (*) are followed by retrograde P waves (*oblique arrow*) sensed by the DDI pacemaker, resulting in inhibition of atrial pacing. At the end of the escape interval, and in absence of a sinus P wave, the pacemaker paces only the ventricle, causing further retrograde atrial activation **b** by lengthening PVARP to 280 ms, the retrograde P waves are no longer sensed by the device with improvement in AV synchrony

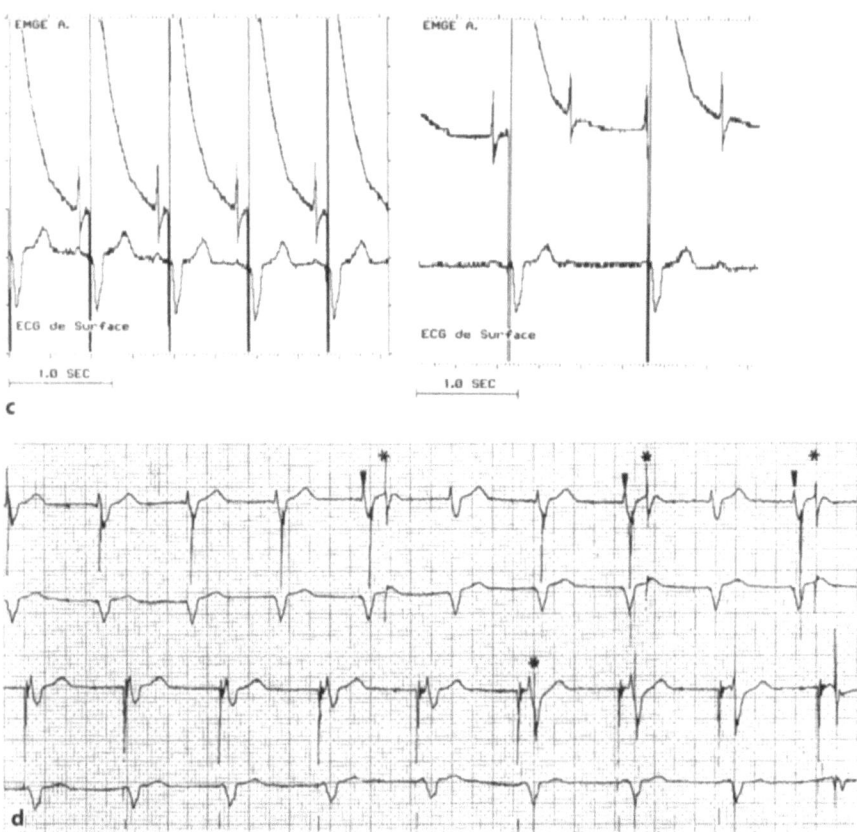

**Fig. 3.54. c** *Upper trace*: atrial electrogram; *lower trace*: surface ECG; *left*: in DDD mode, each P wave triggers a ventricular paced complex at the end of the programmed AVD; *right*: the device has been reprogrammed to DDI. Atrial sensing inhibits atrial pacing. The behavior is pseudo VVI with AV asynchrony. Complete AV block is a contraindication to DDI
**d** DDI mode, 60 BPM, AVD = 165 ms, PVARP = 325 ms, pulse amplitude = 4 V/0.5 ms in both chambers, sensitivity = 1 mV in atrium and 2 mV in ventricle, blanking period = 13 ms. Accelerated junctional rhythm is sustained. Atrial pacing is delivered at the end of the AV interval within sensed R waves (pseudo-pseudofusions). The R waves marked by arrows are not sensed because of their timing within the blanking period, resulting in ventricular pacing on the T wave, after completion of the AVD. Possible solutions: increase the lower rate, shorten the AVD to eliminate ventricular pacing on the T wave, program a short blanking period (as was done in this example)

like. This implies that the DDI mode is contraindicated in presence of AV block or junctional rhythm at a rate above the lower rate (Fig. 3.54), unless the patient has known atrial arrhythmias and the pacemaker does not have an automatic mode switch function.

Since this mode offers AV synchrony only at the lower rate, or at the smoothing rate (if rate smoothing has been programmed), the risk of tracking an atrial tachyarrhythmia by the pacemaker is none. In this mode, the programmable

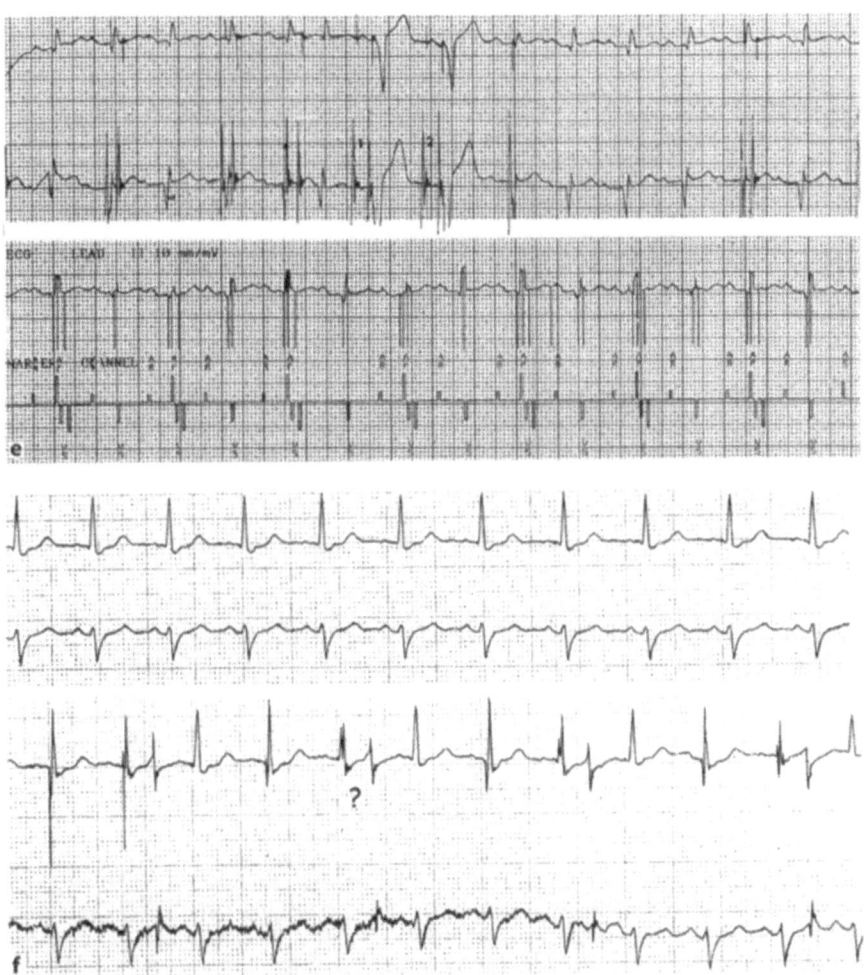

**Fig. 3.54. e** DDI mode, 90 BPM, AVD = 150 ms, PVARP = 300 ms, atrial sensitivity = 0.5 ms, ventricular safety pacing: on. The P waves are sensed during the refractory period. The pacemaker delivers atrial spikes in the beginning of the QRS and senses the R wave. It delivers ventricular spikes at the end of the safety window (120 ms), in the ST segment
**f** DDI mode, 75 BPM, AVD = 240 ms, PVARP = 475 ms, atrial sensitivity = 0.6 ms, blanking period = 38 ms. An exercise test allows to uncover a system dysfunction not observed at rest during which the pacemaker was inhibited by the intrinsic rhythm. During exercise, P waves are no longer systematically sensed because of a long PVARP. Atrial pacing is delivered in the QRS which is not sensed because of its timing within the blanking period. This causes ventricular pacing to occur on the peak of the T wave

parameters are: pulse amplitude and duration, sensitivity, blanking period and safety window, AVD, ventricular refractory period, and PVARP. The upper rate needs to be programmed only if rate smoothing has been turned on, to indicate the maximal rate at which rate smoothing needs to become active.

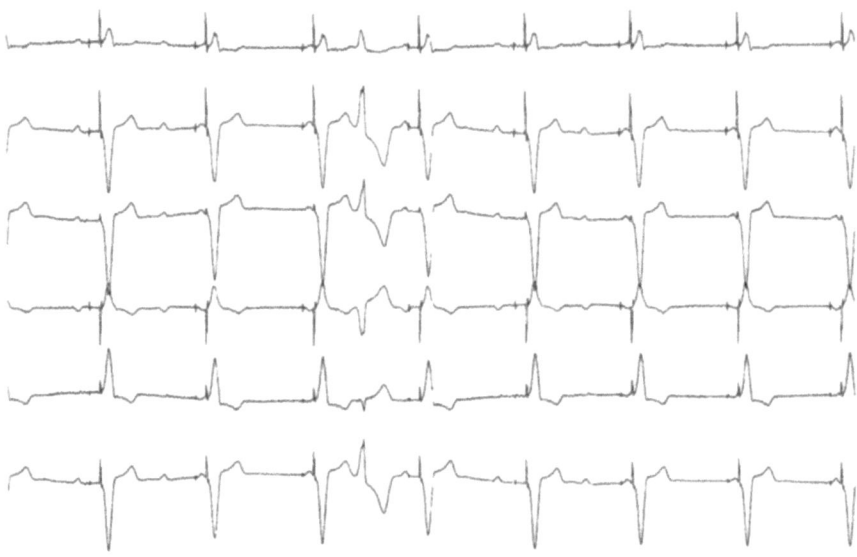

**Fig. 3.55.** In D00 mode, the atrioventricular pacing rate is fixed. Intrinsic atrial and ventricular complexes are not sensed (including extrasystoles)

### The D00 Mode

Asynchronous atrioventricular sequential pacing.

Upon application of a magnet over the pulse generator can during testing sessions, the device switches to D00 mode, except for the Quadra (Telectronics) which switches from DDD to V00), with fixed rate atrioventricular pacing without regard to the underlying intrinsic rhythm (Fig. 3.55).

### Other Modes of Dual Chamber Pacing

### The VDD Mode

Ventricular pacing, atrial and ventricular (dual) sensing, ventricular pacing triggered by P wave, ventricular inhibition by ventricular events.

In this mode, atrial pacing is inexistent. Otherwise, the device behavior is identical to the DDD mode (Fig. 3.56). The same parameters are present, except amplitude and duration of atrial pulses, blanking period and safety pacing window, all related to atrial pacing. This mode is valuable in presence of single lead, dual chamber systems (see VDDR, p. 116).

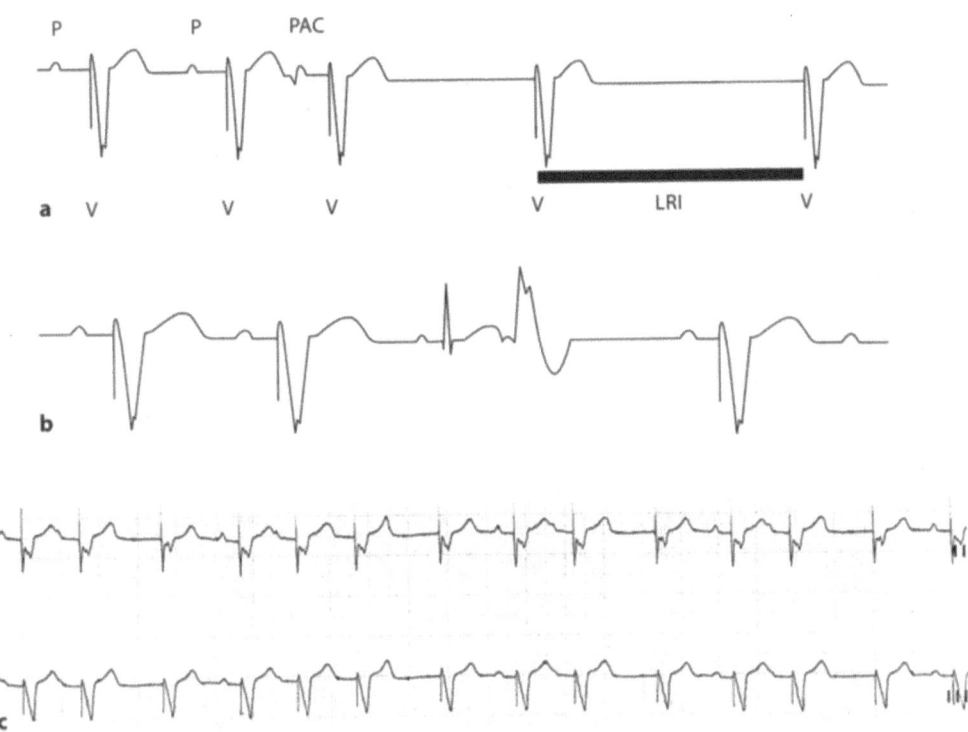

**Fig. 3.56. a** In absence of atrial and ventricular activity, pacing is confined to the ventricle
**b** Spontaneous ventricular events inhibit the VDD pacemaker whose main function is to guarantee atrioventricular synchrony by tracking of the P wave
**c** The VDD mode allows the acceleration of ventricular pacing up to the upper rate, with Wenckebach like behavior occurring when the sinus rate rises above the programmed upper rate. However, after a P wave falling in PVARP, the pacemaker delivers an asynchronous pulse if no P wave has been sensed during the escape interval (3rd, 7th, 10th and 12th paced QRS complex)
*LRI* lower rate interval

## The VAT Mode

Ventricular pacing, atrial sensing, ventricular pacing triggered by P wave.

Now obsolete, this was the first available dual chamber mode. The atrium cannot be paced and, in particular, the ventricle is not sensed. It is, therefore a ventricular pacing mode triggered by any atrial sensing. The absence of ventricular sensing implies a lack of premature ventricular complex sensing, which is potentially dangerous.

### The DAT Mode

Atrial and ventricular (dual) pacing, atrial sensing, ventricular pacing triggered by P wave.

Similar comments apply to this mode, available in the Quadra (Telectronics) and Physios (Biotronik) models, and which offers atrial pacing capability. It is valuable only in cases where ventricular pacing inhibition by myosignals cannot be corrected in a pacemaker dependent patient. Though not the most satisfactory, this mode may be helpful until exchange of the lead for a bipolar system.

### The DDT Mode

Same as DDD plus pacing for all sensed events in a given chamber.

This mode, available in the Physios (Biotronik), Chorum (Ela Medical) and Phymos (Medico) models is used to suppress inhibition of the pacemaker by myosignals, or as a test mode.

### The DVI Mode

Atrial and ventricular (dual) pacing, ventricular sensing, inhibition by ventricular events.

In DVI, the pacemaker is inhibited by signals of ventricular origin. Its behavior is, then, VVI like. Atrial pacing occurs in conjunction with ventricular pacing. It is, therefore, a form of AV sequential pacing which does not pay attention to the spontaneous atrial activity (Fig. 3.57). Several types of DVI mode have been developed along with the evolution of technology: committed, noncommitted, semi-committed. All modern devices offer the semi-committed ventricular pacing mode.

- The committed mode (historical): all atrial paced events are systematically followed by ventricular pacing, regardless of intervening spontaneous ventricular events (R wave).
- Noncommitted mode: a ventricular blanking period is initiated after atrial pacing. If the pacemaker senses a ventricular event after the end of the blanking period, ventricular pacing is inhibited (Fig. 3.58).
- Semi committed mode: the pacemaker includes a safety pacing window in addition to the blanking period.

This dual chamber mode of pacing is no longer used except as a rescue mode pending revision of the system.

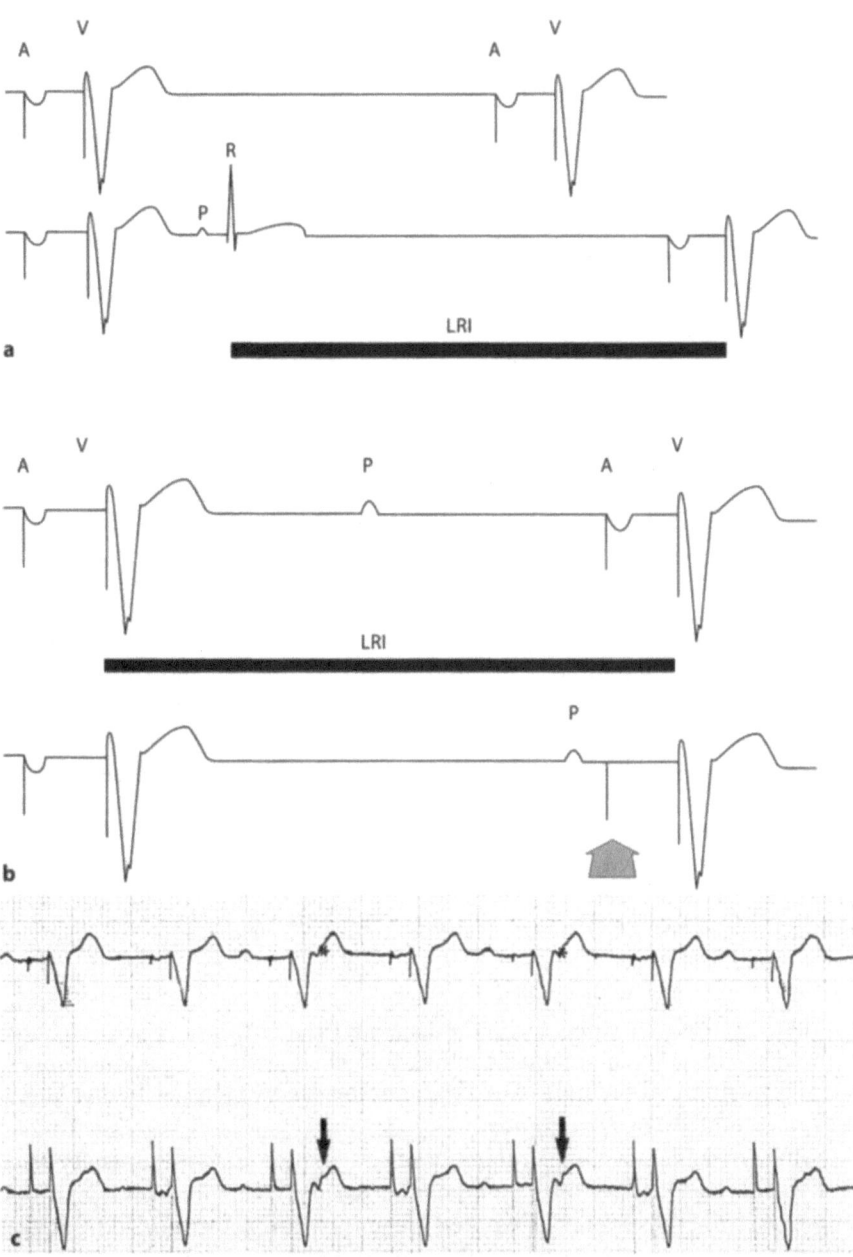

**Fig. 3.57. a** The DVI mode guarantees AV synchrony at the lower rate in absence of spontaneous ventricular activity

**b** The occurrence of intrinsic P waves has no effect on the pacemaker which can be reset only by spontaneous QRS complexes

**c** Spontaneous P waves do not modify the behavior of the pacemaker. Absence of intrinsic ventricular activity accounts for the AV sequential pacing at the lower rate. Some of the atrial spikes fall in the natural atrial refractory period, which explains the appearance of retrograde atrial activation behind the paced QRSs (*arrows*)

*LRI* lower rate interval

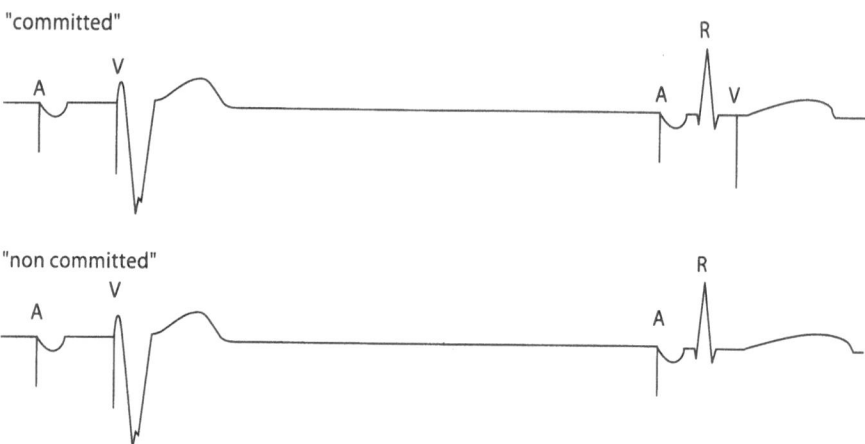

**Fig. 3.58.** In the committed DVI mode, all atrial paced events are systematically followed by ventricular pacing. In the noncommitted DVI mode, sensing of a ventricular event after the atrial spike, before the end of the AVD, inhibits ventricular pacing

## The VDD(R) Mode

The single lead VDD(R) systems were originally offered, and continue to be developed, by Italian investigators (Antonioli 1979). Most manufacturers are building such systems, using a single pacing lead. Atrial sensing is performed via two or more electrodes floating in the right atrium. The single catheter lead has a distal unipolar or bipolar ventricular electrode and, 11 to 15 cm proximally, two atrial electrodes in variable configurations, depending on the system: either annular, separated by 0.5 to 3 cm, or orthogonal, partially circumferential and placed at 180° from each other, at the same level on the body of the lead, or distant from each other, in a diagonal configuration (Fig. 3.59a). The atrial electrogram amplitude recorded varies with the dipole configuration within the atrium and its relationship with the atrial wall, and also with respiratory and cardiac motion. Electrodes in contact with the atrial wall seem to produce a larger amplitude signal, however, more unstable than those that are floating in the center of the right atrium. This requires the programming of very high sensitivity, such as 0.07 mV in the Biotronik Dromos.

Some systems (Biotronik Dromos, Medico Phymos, Intermedics Unity, Vitatron Saphir and Vitesse) offer a *differential sensing*: the bipolar electrogram is generated from the difference between the unipolar signals recorded from each electrode in reference to the pacemaker can (pseudo bipolar sensing at the atrial level). Its advantage is an excellent rejection of the extracardiac interferences and of the ventricular electrograms, allowing a high sensitivity setting. Far field signals such as myosignals or R wave reach the electrodes nearly simultaneously and with similar amplitudes. Therefore, the difference in electrogram amplitude originating from each electrode is minimal, resulting in absence of detection of such signals by the atrial amplifier. Conversely, signals whose source is near the electrode and with favorable vector orientation do not reach each electrode

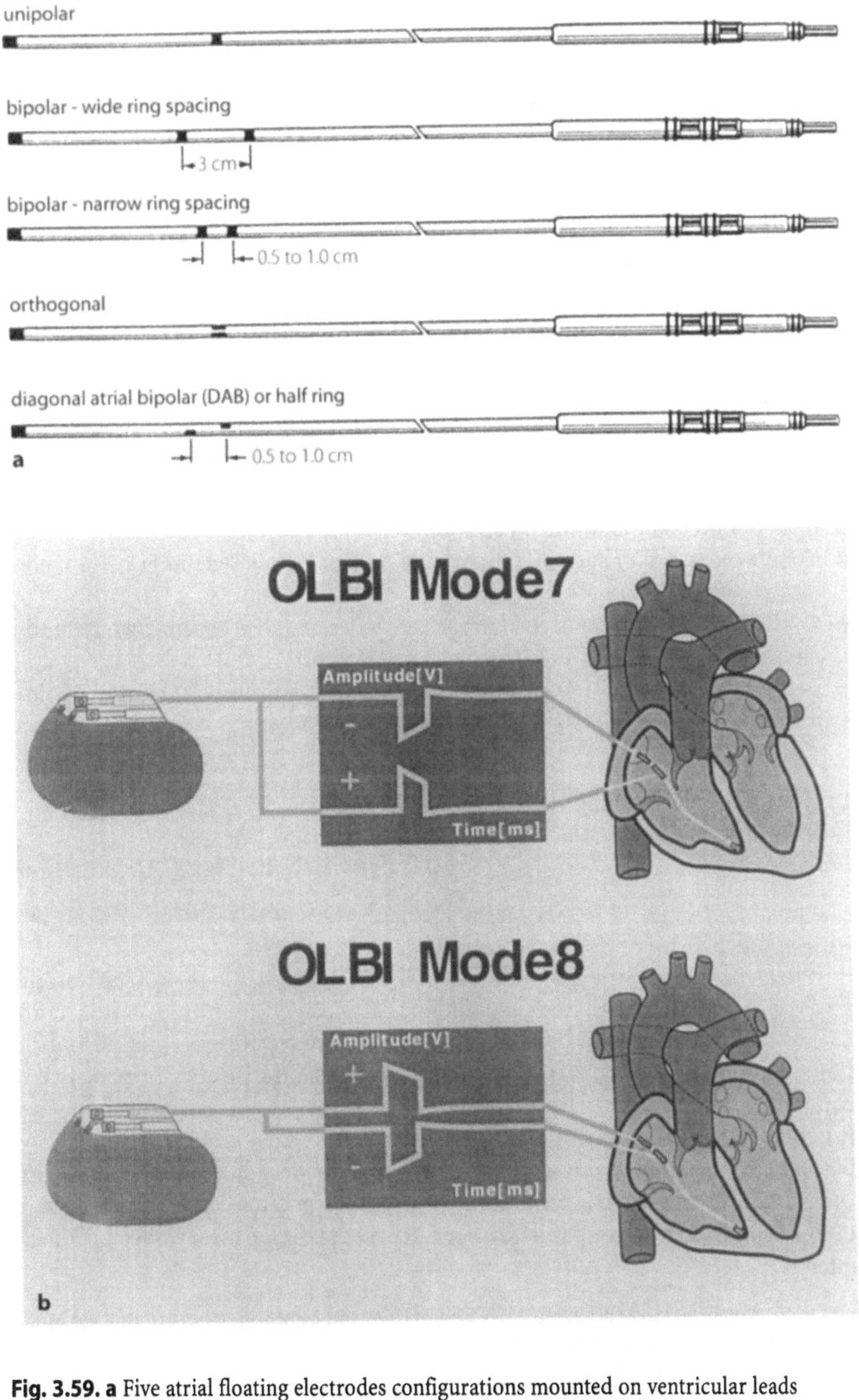

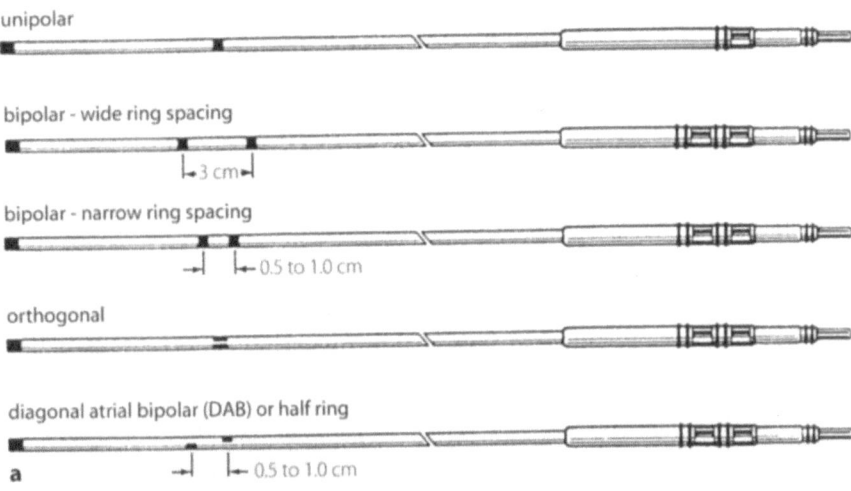

unipolar

bipolar - wide ring spacing
3 cm

bipolar - narrow ring spacing
0.5 to 1.0 cm

orthogonal

diagonal atrial bipolar (DAB) or half ring

**a**    0.5 to 1.0 cm

## OLBI Mode7

Amplitude[V]

Time[ms]

## OLBI Mode8

Amplitude[V]

Time[ms]

**b**

**Fig. 3.59. a** Five atrial floating electrodes configurations mounted on ventricular leads
**b** The OLBI concept is used with a single lead VDD to allow atrial pacing. The system triggers
two simultaneous pulses of inverted polarity on each atrial electrode of the single lead VDD

simultaneously. This causes the amplifier to emit two distinct signals. In other words, if electrogram A is exactly like electrogram B, the amplifier does not emit a signal; but if they are different, they are not canceled and can be amplified to allow sensing of a P wave. Thus, the goal of the differential amplifier is to improve sensing specificity, particularly since single lead VDD(R) systems call for high sensitivity levels.

### Advantages of the Single Lead VDD(R) Systems

- Compared to the standard implantation of a dual chamber system, the implantation of single lead simplifies and shortens the operative technique. However, special attention must be paid to the position of the atrial dipole.
- The amount of indwelling material implanted is less, which facilitates the subsequent addition of new leads if necessary. It is also a logical choice in patients who already have defective leads that have been abandoned.
- The development of fibrosis along the lead is probably less than with the two leads of a standard dual chamber system.
- It causes no trauma to the atrial wall.
- Compared to a VVI system, physiologic pacing is possible under certain conditions (see below).
- A VDD system can be used temporarily in emergency to improve hemodynamics (AV block with preserved sinus function)
- Certain features of VDD pacing systems, such as differential amplification, may also be of help in standard dual chamber pacing.

### Disadvantages of the Single Lead VDD(R) Systems

*Problems Related to the Absence of Atrial Pacing and Reliability of Atrial Sensing*

The reliability of atrial sensing is suboptimal, particularly during exercise and with changes in posture.

When considering the implantation of a VDD system, the presence of proper sinus node function must be verified, that is absence of sinus bradycardia, chronotropic incompetence, or bradycardia – tachycardia syndrome, and the indication should consist of an atrioventricular conduction disorder. In presence of complete AV block, it may be difficult to exclude the presence of sinus node dysfunction on the basis of traditional methods such as exercise testing (not always feasible in a patient with complete AV block), or ambulatory monitoring (because of poorly visible P waves). The presence of sinus node dysfunction is often recognized after implantation of the pacemaker, or it may develop subsequently.

- During bradycardic episodes, a VDD(R) system can only operate in a VVI(R), or more precisely in a VDI(R) mode since it continues to monitor atrial activity, with all its drawbacks: loss of AV synchrony, risk of pacemaker syndrome, and increased risk of atrial arrhythmias (see p. 198).

- If retrograde conduction is present, ELT may be induced. Protection algorithms may correct this drawback. However, several of these algorithms are followed by atrial pacing, for instance after PVARP extension, and are not available in a VDD(R) system. This may cause repetitive ELT, or alternans of ELT and switches to VVIR mode, or the persistence of VVIR function as long as the sinus rate does not rise above the ventricular lower rate or if the pacemaker is not equipped with a special hysteresis function.
- In the event of atrial tachyarrhythmias (bradycardia-tachycardia syndrome or post AV node ablation for atrial arrhythmias) antiarrhythmic drug therapy is often needed. Sinus bradycardia precipitated by these treatments often leads to undesirable AV asynchrony.
- Similar effects can be expected from atrial sensing failure which occurs more often due to the floating characteristics of the electrodes.

### Choice of Electrodes

The right heart chambers dimensions must be properly measured before implantation to choose the optimal lead model with the proper distance between distal electrode and atrial rings. If this evaluation is not performed correctly, the electrode must be exchanged, which is expensive. Two distinct situations may present: either the right ventricular or atrial dimensions are too large, causing the atrial electrodes to placed near the tricuspid valve, with poor atrial sensing; or unsatisfactory pacing thresholds at the right ventricular apex require implantation in the inflow chamber, placing the atrial poles in the superior vena cava, or causing recoiling of the lead into the right atrium as one tries to advance it to optimize atrial sensing.

Cardiac dimensions may change after implantation, leading to complete loss of function: chamber dilatation from progression of the underlying heart disease, or reduction in cavity size as a result of the hemodynamic improvement from AV synchrony.

Nowadays, the argument of cost saving by VDD systems compared to other dual chamber systems is no longer valid.

### The OLBI Concept

Atrial pacing was not possible until Medico developed a pacing system capable of pacing the right atrium from the floating dipole in a conventional bipolar pacing mode. 95% of cases atrial capture was observed, however at high pacing output only, and in 19% of cases diaphragmatic pacing was noted at atrial capture threshold. Nowadays, Biotronik offers the OverLapping Biphasic Impulse (OLBI) system which generates simultaneous pulses of opposite polarity from each floating atrial electrode (Fig. 3.59b). OLBI reduces atrial pacing threshold significantly compared to conventional uni- or bipolar configurations on floating atrial electrodes. However, pacing thresholds recorded with OLBI are higher than those obtained with conventional tined or active fixation leads. This system is also associated with a wider separation between atrial capture and diaphragmatic stimulation thresholds.

### Indications for VDD(R) Systems

- As a temporary mode of pacing, it is more effective than the VVI mode to improve a patient's hemodynamic status in emergency.
- It should be considered for a young individual in whom the system is being implanted for a life time, reserving a dual lead system in case of subsequent lead failure, or of development of sinus node dysfunction. The indication, here, consists, of AV block and preserved sinus node function.
- It may also be considered in the event of a difficult catheterization because of fibrosis around previously implanted electrodes.
- In elderly patients without sinus node dysfunction, to maintain AV synchrony as much as possible and shorten the implant procedure.

To conclude, VDD(R) systems, quite interesting from a scientific standpoint, need further developments. From a clinical standpoint, despite their superiority over VVI pacing, VDD(R) pacemakers (as the technology stands now) should be reserved for exceptional situations. As a matter of principle, the most effective mode of pacing must be offered, which usually does no allow to omit atrial pacing.

## Rate Responsive Pacemakers

Rate responsive pacemakers may be viewed, in a broad sense, as physiologic pacemakers, although the various sensors incorporated in these devices do not reproduce exactly the physiologic response of sinus node acceleration.

While single chamber pacemakers without rate responsiveness pace at a fixed rate (usually programmed between 50 and 70 BPM) whether the patient is at work or asleep, rate responsive pacemakers adjust the pacing rate to various types of activity. Consequently, they are generally utilized in patients whose spontaneous heart rate is no longer capable of an appropriate increase with exercise (sinus node dysfunction or severe sinus bradycardia without proper increase in sinus rate with effort: sinus node chronotropic incompetence). Rate responsiveness is also applied to dual chamber systems when AV synchrony is to be preserved in presence of chronotropic incompetence.

Thus, the goal is to restore a near physiologic adaptation of the heart rate by means of as specific as possible a sensor of metabolic demand. Sensors are there to replace the normal control by the sino-atrial node and act as artificial modulators of heart rate.

The following are criteria of sensor quality:

- The information provided must be of metabolic nature or in direct relation with the sympathetic system.

- This information must be in direct linear relationship with the level of exercise.
- The sensitivity of the system must be optimal to reduce the system's response time.
- The variation measured must be wide enough as to be specific.
- The information must be reproducible.
- An interface must be devised to transfer the information to the pacemaker.
- The sensor must be miniaturized to allow its inclusion in the device can, and its power consumption must be minimal.

Several types of sensors have been developed and are included in commercially available systems. Their strengths are variable, and their advantages and disadvantages will be discussed.

### The Various Sensors

### Sinus Rhythm

The very best sensor of physical exercise is the atrial signal sensed by the atrial electrode since the atrial rate is under direct influence of circulating catecholamines and of the autonomic nervous system. This type of rate responsiveness is that utilized in all dual chamber models with ventricular pacing after atrial sensing (VDD, DDD, DAT, VAT, DAD, DDT). The advantages are obvious, while the disadvantages consist mainly of difficulty in atrial implantation, complications related to dual chamber pacing, and particularly of the subsequent development of atrial arrhythmias.

### Activity

Systems based on this concept are currently the most commonly used in the world. The sensor is a piezoelectric element applied to the inside of the pacemaker can (Fig. 3.60). Deformation of this element by vibrations is converted into electrical energy sensed and quantified by the pacemaker. The signals sensed must be above the programmed threshold, which determines the upper and lower sensitivity boundaries; any signal crossing these boundaries triggers a rate responsive algorithm (Fig. 3.61). In addition a so-called rate-responsive slope must be programmed.

Certain advantages are unarguable: simplicity, use of traditional pacing leads, excellent sensitivity at the onset of effort, and good correlation between physical performance and heart rate modulation under condition of walk testing or daily life effort. On the other hand, limitations exist: the information is not physiologic, causing the pacemaker to accelerate unnecessarily for extraneous vibrations such as street traffic, poor road conditions when riding a car, bicycle or motorcycle, vibrations in airplane, from dental procedures, prolonged pressure on pacemaker can, etc.; in addition, as opposed to other sensors, heart rate is not influenced by fever or emotional stress. When the muscles activated by effort are

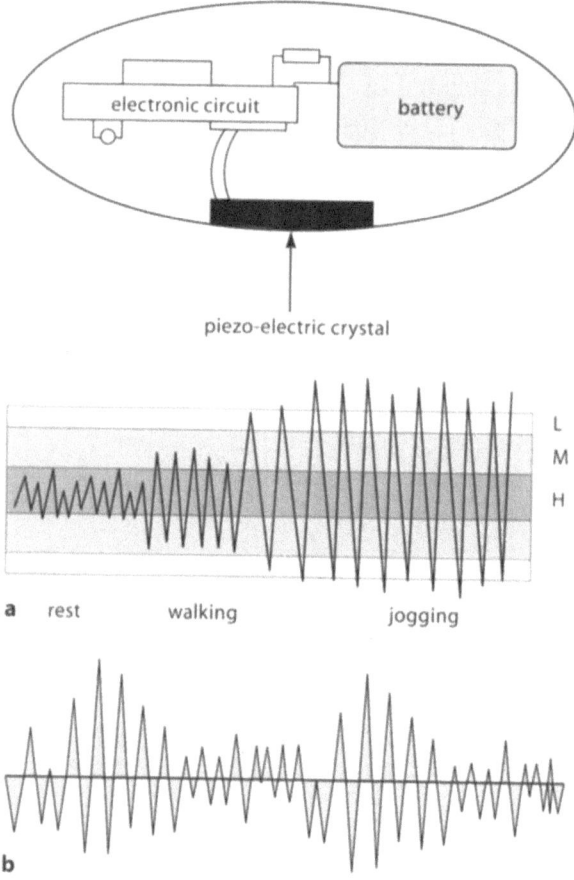

**Fig. 3.60.** The common sensor of all systems based on activity is a piezoelectric element affixed to the inner surface of the pacemaker can. It is a mechanical sensor: body movements deform the sensor which transforms this mechanical energy into an electrical signal

**Fig. 3.61. a** Activitrax type pacemakers (Medtronic) function in an „all or none" manner, unable to modulate the rate responsiveness according to the work load. If the sensitivity is low and the work load increases gradually, the maximal heart rate is never reached; conversely it is reached very rapidly is the sensitivity has been set high

**b** In a Sensolog type pacemaker (Siemens), the signals are integrated: global energy is computed by the rate responsive algorithm, along with frequency and amplitude. The pacing rate can be gradually modulated according to the work load

remote from the device implantation site (as in the case of riding a bicycle), the sensor response is attenuated.

Despite its imperfections, the overall performance of this system is satisfactory.

## Acceleration

To remedy some of these shortcomings, the accelerometers have been developed. The principle behind these sensors is based on changes in acceleration currently measured in the antero-posterior plane. The advantages are the same as those of activity sensors, while the drawbacks are less bothersome, particularly because of a lesser influence of external vibratory interferences (Fig. 3.62). In addition, the resulting acceleration seems better related to the level of effort, although it

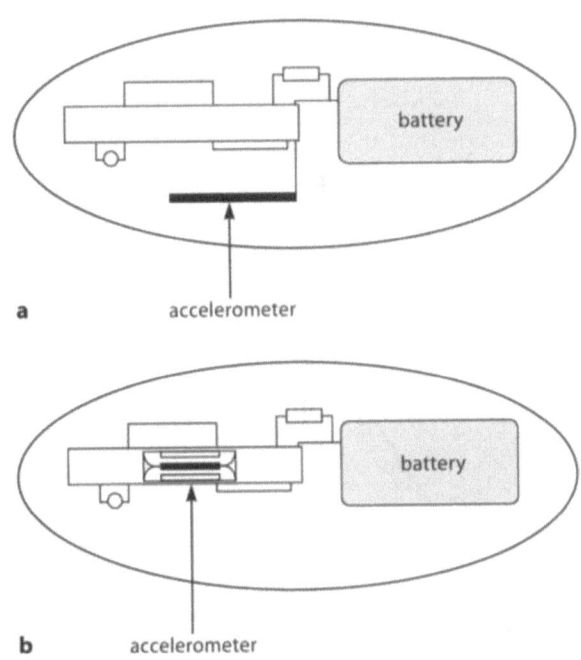

**Fig. 3.62. a** Piezoelectric accelerometers use an elastic mass to generate a force proportional to the frequency of vibrations. Piezoresistive strain gauges are solid silicate resistant circuits which convert mechanical strain into electricity
**b** The variable capacity accelerometer is composed of a single element mounted on a silicate plate. It is a sensor capable of responding linearly to accelerations, sufficiently robust, stable and relatively less susceptible to external interference

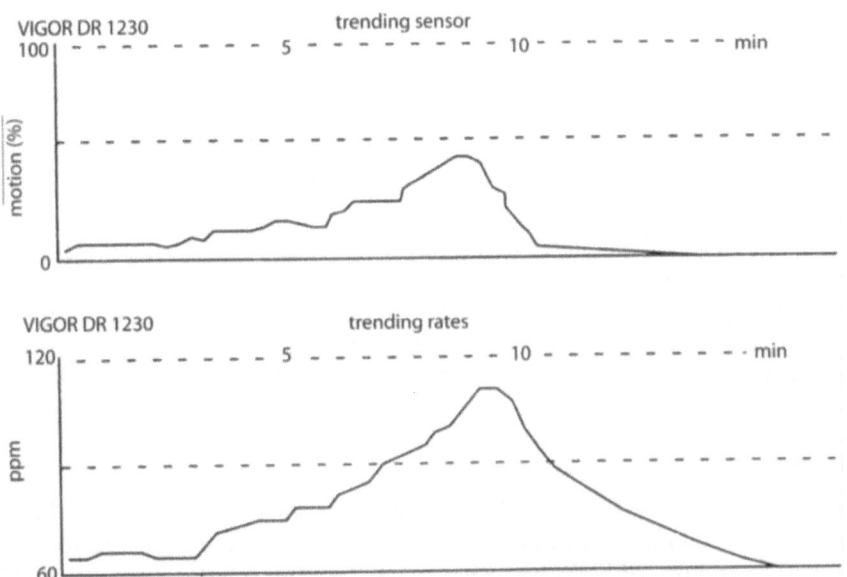

**Fig. 3.63.** Information retrieved by telemetry from a Vigor (DR) CPI pacemaker. An acceleration signal curve is displayed top, along with the calculated sensor rate bottom (data from CPI)

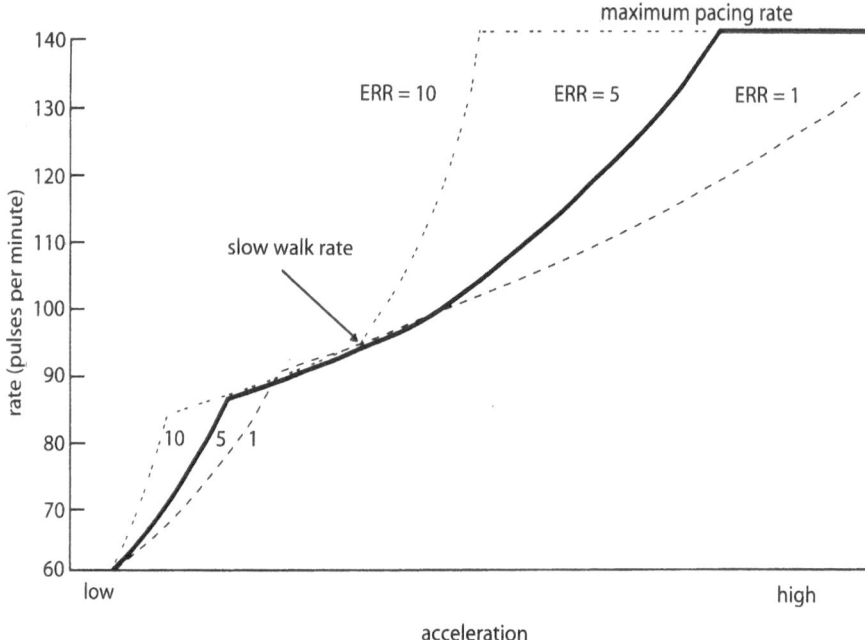

**Fig. 3.64.** Rate responsive algorithm of the Intermedics pacemakers. An initial slope of rate acceleration brings the heart rate to the level of slow walking, programmed on the basis of sensor information calibrated during a test performed after device implantation. The second slope corresponds to the rate response to moderate to vigorous exercise (data from Intermedics, Marathon DR)

tends to be of an „on/off" type. Consequently, with the CPI Vigor, ELA Medical Opus G, and Biotronik Dromos models, the algorithm requires a satisfactory rate smoothing function to offer the proper progression of pacing acceleration (Fig. 3.63). With the Intermedics models (Dash, Relay), the algorithm offers an intermediate, so-called „slow walking" rate, sometimes separately programmable. Only when the effort is vigorous does the pacemaker increase its rate significantly, and quite rapidly (Fig. 3.64). The Intermedics systems include a simulation function which allows the fine tuning of the rate responsive function (see Fig. 7.11b).

### Gravity

The gravimeter included in the Swing and Living pacemakers (Sorin) collects information from a drop of mercury which changes shape from gravity and establishes contact within a cage (Fig. 3.65). This information, of an „on/off" type, is modulated by a powerful algorithm which integrates the duration of contact by the mercury, and the number of contacts with respect to the cardiac cycle. Clinical reports on the use of this system are encouraging.

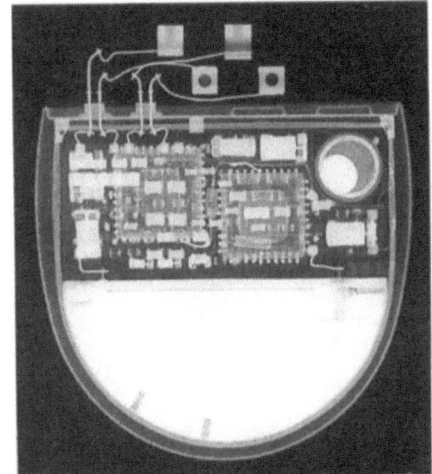

**Fig. 3.65.** The Swing (Sorin) pacemakers use as an activity sensor the acceleration of a droplet of mercury inside a casing visible in the upper right corner of this identification radiograph (photograph by Sorin)

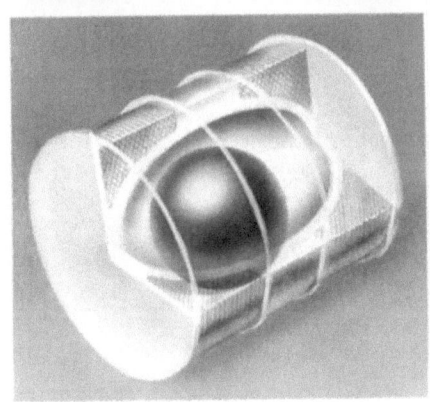

**Fig. 3.66.** The Sensorithm (Siemens) include a ball which moves freely in an elliptical cavity surrounded by a double coil of copper wire. The variations in magnetic field caused by the ball's movements create an electrical field inside the coil (photograph by Pacesetter)

### New Concept in Activity Sensor

Included in the Siemens-Pacesetter Sensorithm 2045 model, this sensor consists of a magnetic ball which moves freely within an elliptic cavity surrounded by a double coil of copper wire (Fig. 3.66). When the patient is active, the ball oscillates, and the variations that it causes in the magnetic field create a current inside the coil. The signal is integrated to provide the surface of the curvature. This total surface as a function of time is the parameter used to determine the heart rate. This sensor consumes no power, and the risk of heart rate acceleration by pressure is eliminated.

### Ventilation

The first device utilizing this concept was based on a measurement of the respiratory rate. The principle consists of measuring the variations in impedance corresponding to the changes in respiratory volume. The system injects a current of known intensity and samples the resulting current at a second electrode. Rossi

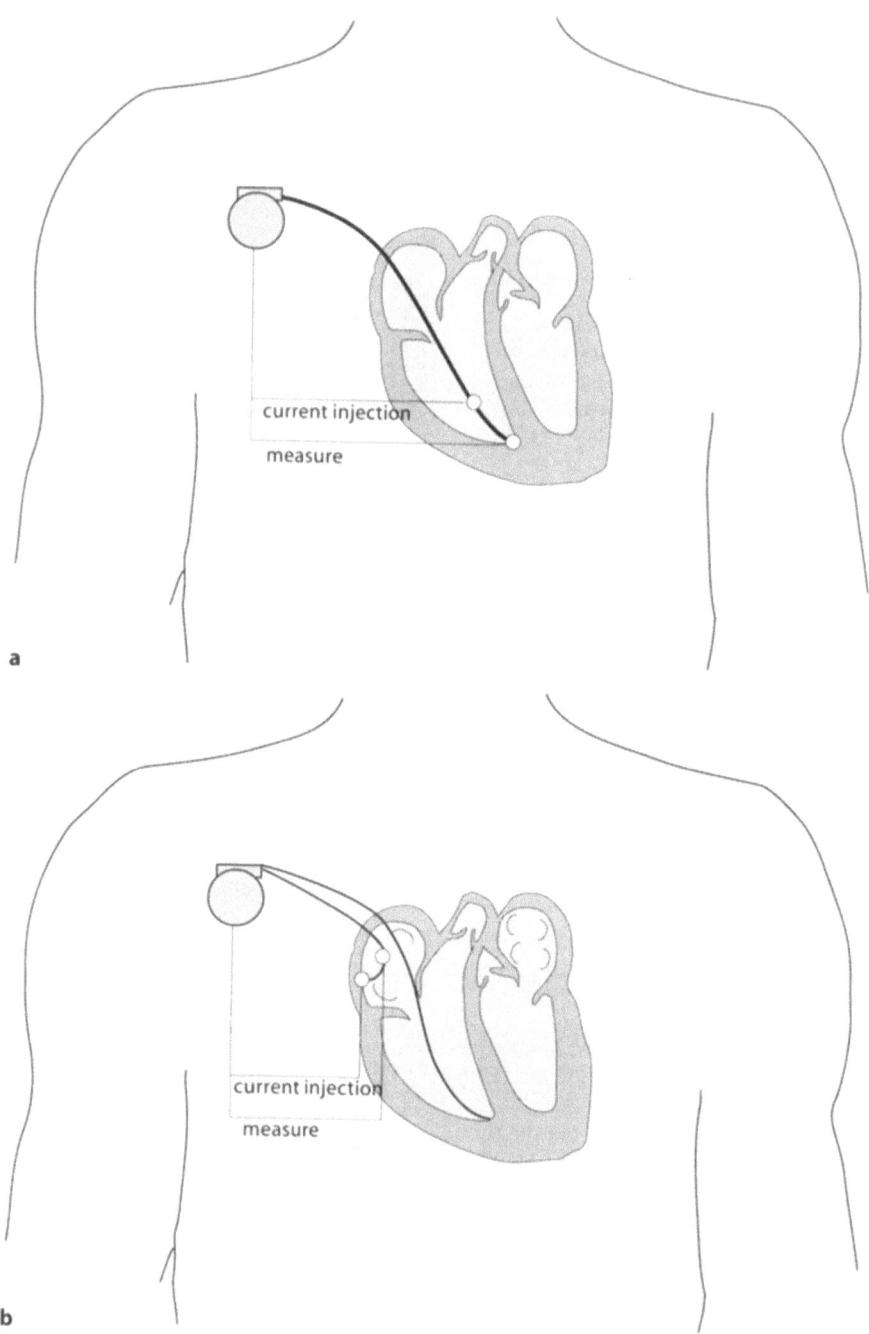

**Fig. 3.67. a** Minute ventilation is the product of tidal volume and respiratory rate. This highly physiologic parameter, which correlates well with heart rate ($r = 0.90$) and with oxygen consumption, is derived from the measurement of intrathoracic impedance. With the Meta MV (Telectronics), current is injected at the proximal electrode of a bipolar lead implanted in

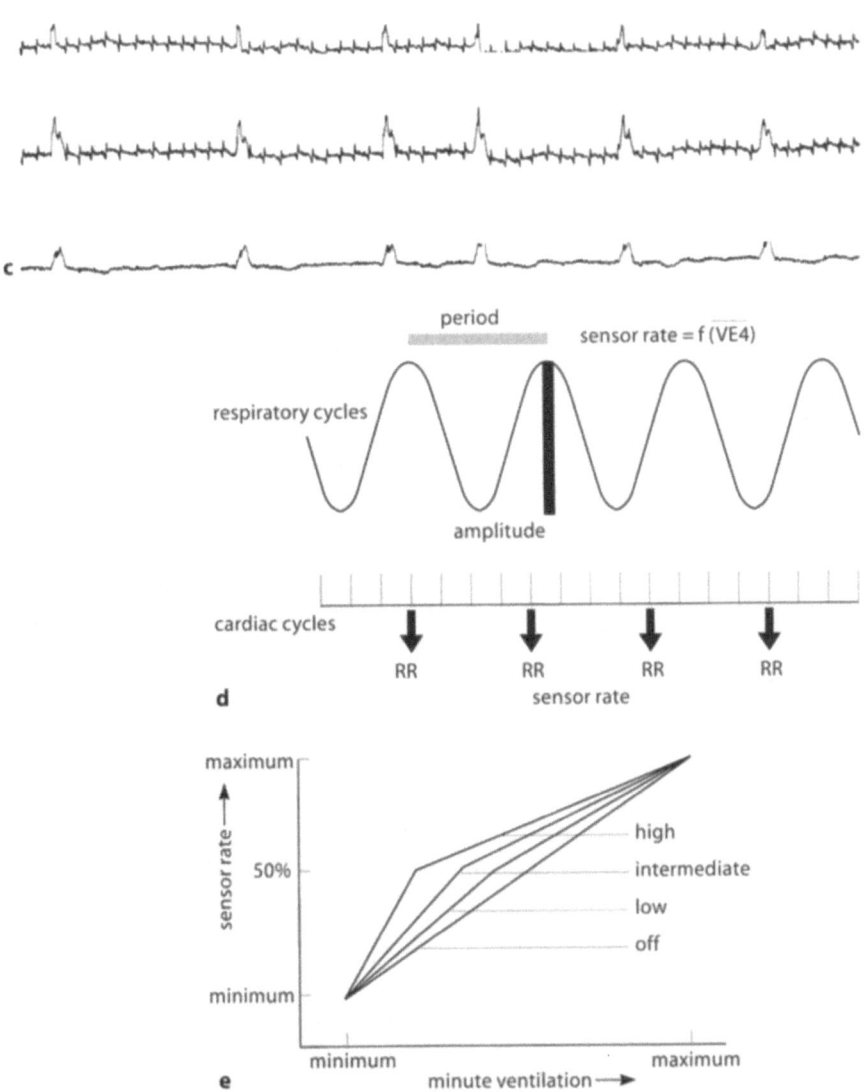

the right ventricle, and impedance is measured between the distal electrode and the pacemaker can

**b** With the Chorus RM, current is injected either at the distal electrode of an atrial bipolar lead, with sampling performed at the proximal electrode, or at a unipolar ventricular electrode or distal bipolar, with sampling at a unipolar or distal bipolar atrial electrode

**c** The current injection causes micropotentials which may be recorded on the surface ECG

**d** The filtered signal allows the sensing of respiratory rate between six and 45 cycles per minute. Ventilation is calculated from the ratio amplitude/ period. The sensor rate (sensor escape interval) is a function of the average of four respiratory cycles (VE4 – ELA Medical). A new sensor rate is calculated every four cardiac cycles to respond rapidly to exercise

**e** The relationship heart rate – minute ventilation is not linear. To reproduce normal physiology, Telectronics introduced a relationship composed of two distinct slopes (data from Telectronics)

has shown an excellent correlation between heart rate, respiratory rate, and oxygen consumption during vigorous exercise. The original principle relied on the measurement of changes in transthoracic impedance from an additional subcutaneous electrode (Biotec). The clinical results were satisfactory; however, the need for an additional electrode with its own complications was a limitation of the method. This was improved by the introduction of a single endocardial bipolar electrode providing the measurements between an intracardiac pole and the pacemaker can.

Several studies have shown a better correlation between heart rate and respiratory parameters by using minute ventilation. This is particularly apparent at the onset of exercise since respiratory rate increases only after several seconds, whereas minute ventilation increases immediately by an adaptation of tidal volume. Moreover, by placing the site of measurement on the pacing lead itself inside the thorax (standard bipolar lead), sensing is more precise, the quality of the information is optimized, and the system suffers from fewer limitations (Fig. 3.67a). In addition, better function is obtained when the lead is implanted in the atrium instead of the ventricle. It is also possible to use this concepts in dual chamber unipolar pacing by injecting the current in the ventricle and sampling in the atrium (Fig. 3.67b). Finally, a single parameter, the slope of rate responsiveness, requires programming. These qualities make this type of sensors probably the best that is currently available.

A few disadvantages must be pointed out: depending on the algorithm applied, the response time at the onset of exercise may be slightly delayed; the pacing rate may remain rapid after the cessation of brief bursts of intense physical activity because of the persistence of a high minute ventilation following this type of exercise; an increase in pacing rate may be caused by rotating movements of the shoulder on the side of the implant, or even by certain truncular movements since muscle activity may modify the measurement of impedance. However, these imperfections remain minor in clinical practice. The main contraindication for the use of this type of sensors is restrictive pulmonary disease characterized by an inordinate increase in respiratory rate with the least effort. The systems currently developed are the Meta III and DDDR (Telectronics), the Legend plus and Kappa (Medtronic) which combines ventilation and activity, and the Chorus RM, Chorum and Talent (minute ventilation and acceleration) (ELA Medical). In contrast to the formers, which have a somewhat delayed response time (improved in the last version of the Meta MV III), the ELA models have a short response time, on the order of 15 seconds or less, underscoring the importance of the algorithm governing this type of sensor to yield a physiologic response. The ELA series also has an autocalibration and simulation system which allows to define rapidly the optimal parameter values to program (see Fig. 7.11c). Physiologically, the heart rate – minute ventilation relationship is linear only at the onset of exercise and the slope changes beyond the anaerobic threshold. The Meta III is currently the only device which differentiates the slope of heart rate -ventilation according to the level of exercise (Fig. 3.67d).

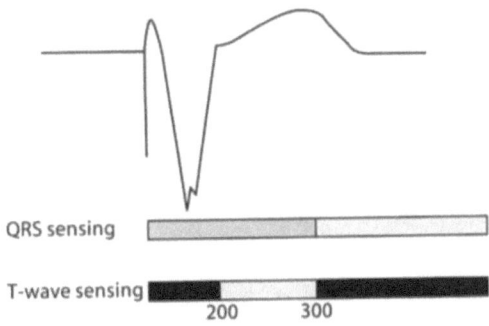

**Fig. 3.68.** The QT interval on the surface ECG coincides to ventricular depolarization – repolarization. The rate responsiveness sensor measures the interval between the ventricular pacing spike and the corresponding intracavitary T wave. The QT interval shortens with exercise and increasing heart rate under the influence of the autonomic nervous system and release of catecholamines. The sensor measures the T wave during exercise within a window of 200 to 300 ms after the spike. The pacing rate is a function of the measurement of the interval between stimulus and T wave

## QT Interval

The algorithm is based on the recognition that the QT interval shortens with exercise and that this relationship is directly dependent on the amount of circulating catecholamines. The intracardiac QRS complex is sampled, and the QT interval is measured within an interval of 200 to 300 ms (Fig. 3.68). In actuality, the relationship between QT interval and heart rate is not linear, which may cause aberrant pacemaker behavior. This has, however, become less frequent with recent pacemakers as a result of modifications of the algorithms. Nevertheless, it remains that a certain number of patients do not have changes in the QT interval with exercise, that the response of the system is slow because of a delay between onset of exercise and changes in QT interval, that cardioactive drugs, metabolic disorders and ischemia may profoundly modify this parameter's behavior during exercise, that there are spontaneous circadian variations, and that such pacemakers can only be used in the ventricle. The Vitatron models are the most original by their self adaptation of the slope of rate responsiveness which avoids multiple exercise tests. This sensor parameter is best combined with more responsive ones, such as activity, as is offered in the Vitatron models.

## Temperature

During physical exercise, considerable heat is generated by muscular activity. At the very onset of exercise, the sudden increase in venous return causes an initial drop in central venous temperature, on average 0.25°C for 1 to 3 min, followed by a rise if exercise continues. On average, the increase in central venous temperature increases by 1.5°C during exercise (Fig. 3. 69). In presence of congestive heart failure, this change takes place more slowly, which suggests that this system may not be the most appropriate in such cases. The sensor's behavior is physiologic since a hot bath or the postprandial period do increase the pacing rate, whereas the consumption of hot drinks does not. However, the response of the system is slow because of the initial drop in temperature, especially with moderate physical activity. This decrease in temperature is registered by the algo-

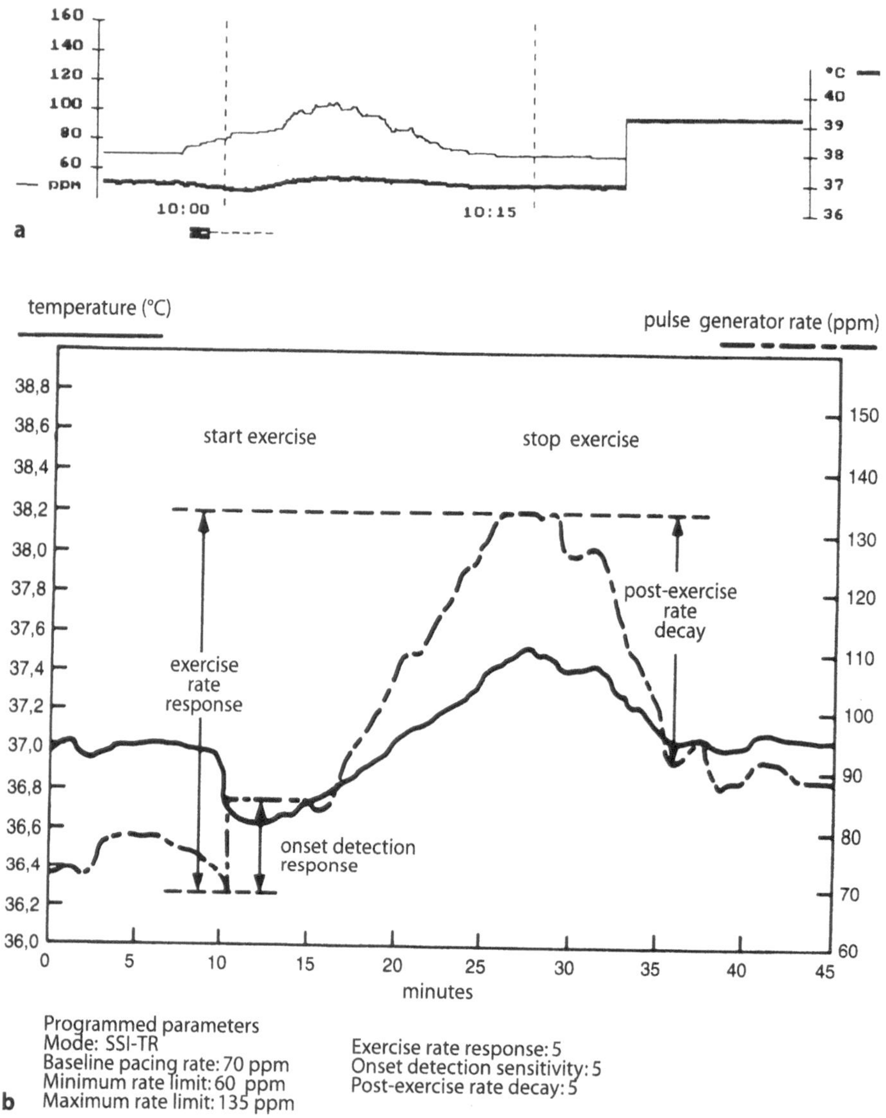

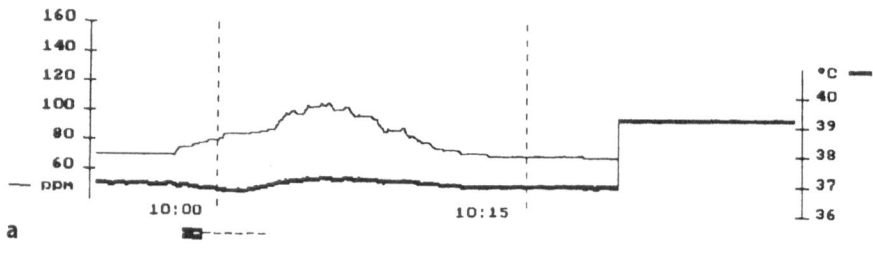

**Fig. 3.69. a** Information provided by the screen of the Thermos pacemaker programmer. The appropriate recognition of an initial temperature drop is noteworthy (data from Biotronik)
**b** Algorithm of the Nova MR pacemaker responsive to the central venous temperature (data from Intermedics)

rithm and causes a temporary increase in pacing rate. This slow response also explains the persistence of a rapid heart rate, for several dozens of seconds after vigorous effort. Finally, the lead is sensor specific and cannot be implanted in the atrium.

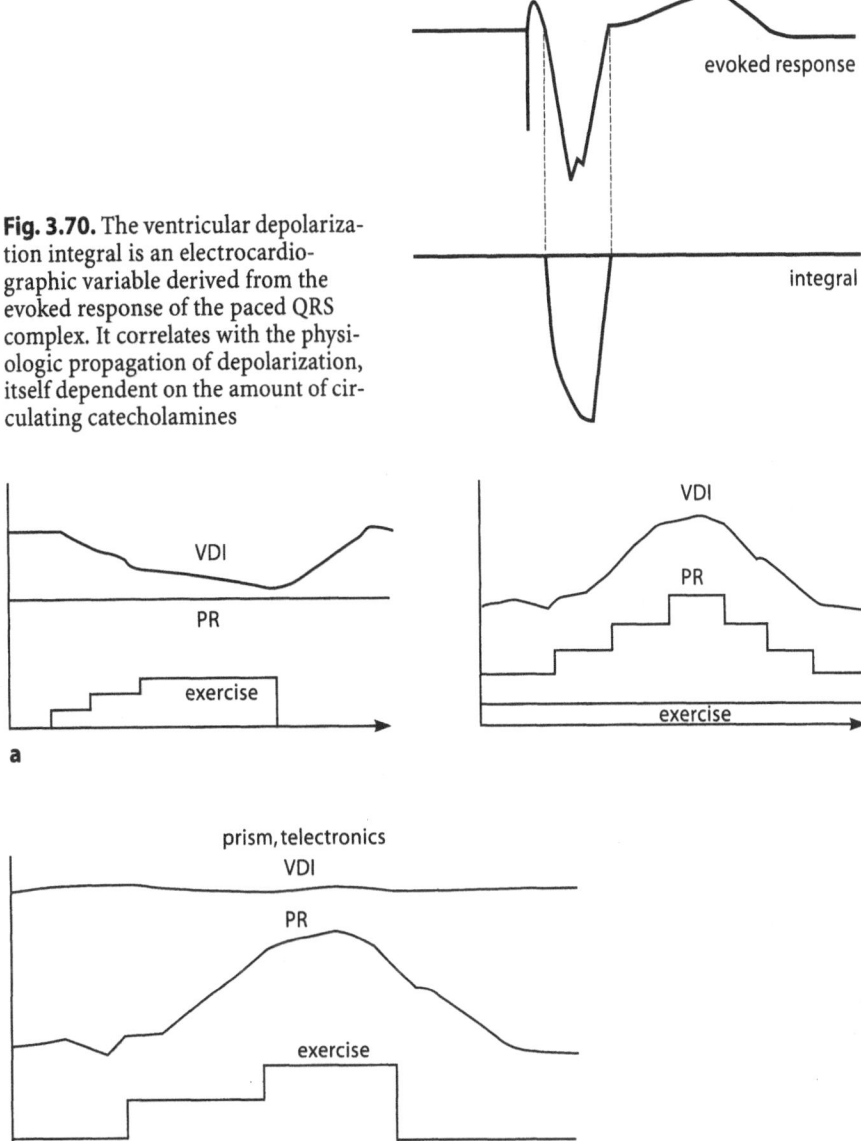

**Fig. 3.70.** The ventricular depolarization integral is an electrocardiographic variable derived from the evoked response of the paced QRS complex. It correlates with the physiologic propagation of depolarization, itself dependent on the amount of circulating catecholamines

**Fig. 3.71. a** The integral of the QRS area decreases during physical activity or mental stress. *Left*: The ventricular depolarization integral (VDI) decreases during exercise at a fixed pacing rate. *Right*: It increases during incremental ventricular pacing performed at rest

**b** The rate responsive algorithm operates as follows: when the ventricular depolarization integral *(VDI)* decreases, the pacing rate increases until the gradient returns to its reference value; when it increases, the pacing rate slows

*PR* pacing rate

### Ventricular Depolarization Integral

The ventricular depolarization integral is also named ventricular depolarization gradient in the literature. This measurement decreases significantly with exercise, as a direct function of the amount of circulating catecholamines. It is less influenced by cardioactive medications than the QT interval, and can be performed with a standard pacing lead. On the other hand, effective pacing is necessary for this measurement, which mandates an artificial increase in the pacing rate in presence of spontaneous rhythm. Finally, this sensor can only be used in the ventricle. Nevertheless, its concept is interesting since the sensor operates under constant feed-back with a so-called closed-loop algorithm. It measures the evoked response, that is the R wave following the pacing stimulus, and adjusts the pacing rate accordingly. The ventricular endocavitary signal resulting from pacing is sampled by the ventricular electrode, and the information is converted into the corresponding pacing rate (Figs. 3.70, 3.71). Furthermore, with the Microny (Pacesetter) model and the Inos 2 DR (Biotronik), the pacemaker is able to verify automatically the presence of effective pacing. In the event of exit block (see p. 253), the pacemaker responds by delivering the maximal output (known as high output pacing), and adjusts the permanent pacing output according to the measurements made, maintaining a safety margin based on its

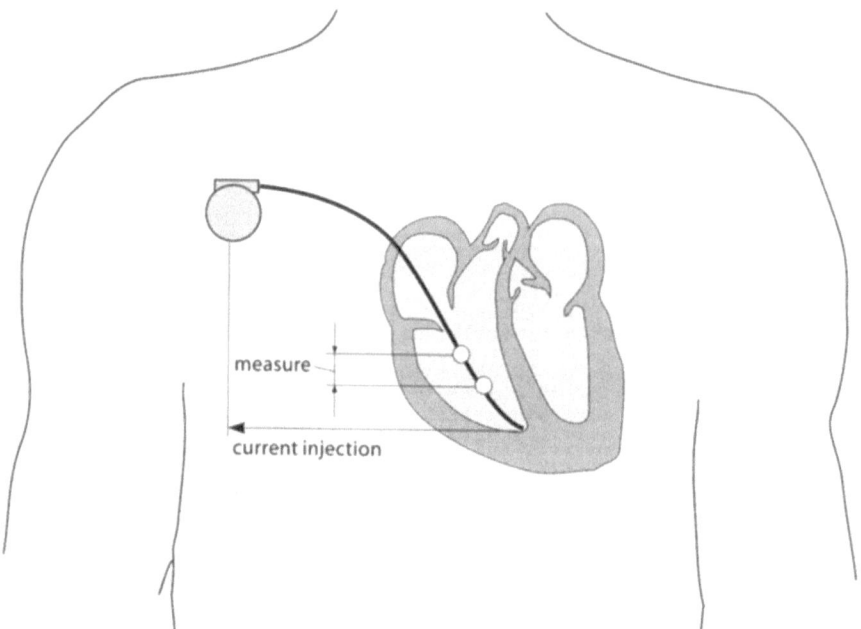

**Fig. 3.72.** Sensing of changes in systolic volume and/or preejection period is performed by measuring the electrical resistance of the right ventricular blood volume between two intracardiac electrodes. The measurement of the relative changes in the signal are compared to a baseline value instead of an absolute value

assessment of the pacing threshold. To allow a rapid and accurate analysis of the evoked response after the pacing spike, a system of triphasic stimulation was developed which requires a powerful algorithm. In the Talent pacemaker (ELA), this concept is utilized to measure the pacing margin of safety which remains programmed at 100%. The system tests the pacing threshold from time to time. In case of a rise in threshold and deviation from the 100% safety margin, the pacemaker reprograms its pacing output to recover the safety margin.

### Preejection Period and Intraventricular Volume

Several experimental studies have shown a remarkably linear relationship, without direct influence of the ventricular rate, between the preejection period and exercise. This interval includes the electromechanical delay and the phase of isovolumetric contraction, which seems to be the most important of the two components of preejection. The information is derived from impedance changes measured by a multipolar electrode, according to the same principles as minute

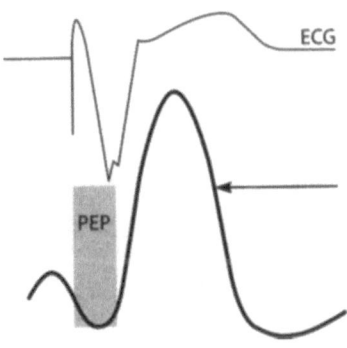

**Fig. 3.73. a** The preejection period extends from the onset of the QRS complex to the onset of the rise in systolic pressure. In hemodynamic terms, it corresponds to the isovolumetric contraction which immediately precedes systolic ejection. It depends on the state of the autonomic nervous system and reflects myocardial contractility
**b** Impedance variation signal correlates with changes in right ventricular volume, recorded by the Precept pacemaker (data from CPI)
*PEP* preejection period; *SV* systolic volume

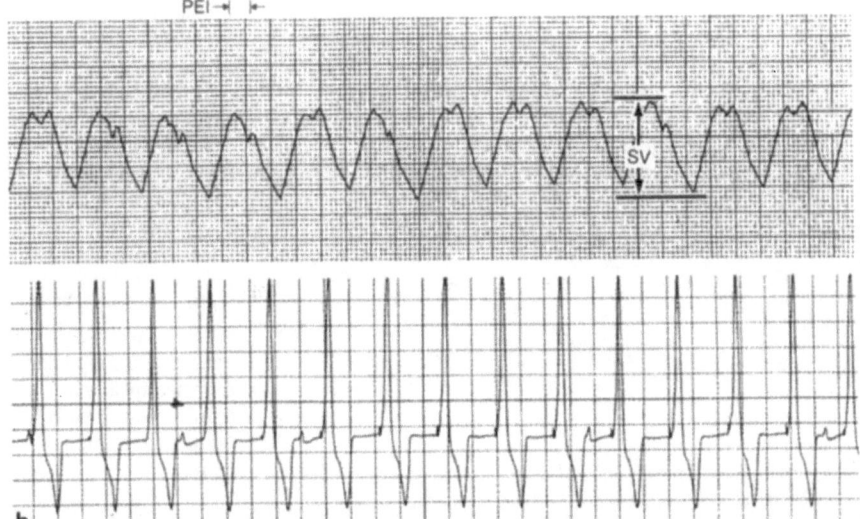

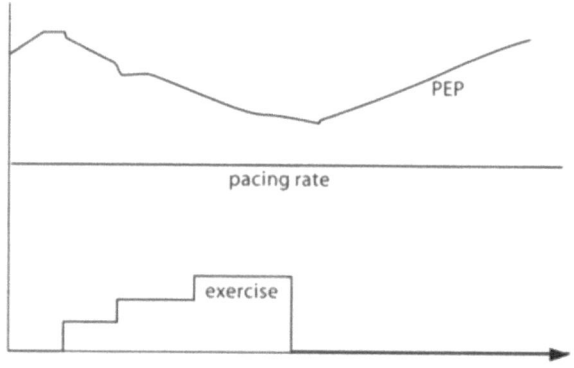

**Fig. 3.74.** During exercise, the preejection period (PEP) decreases and systolic volume increases. When the preejection period decreases, pacing rate increases

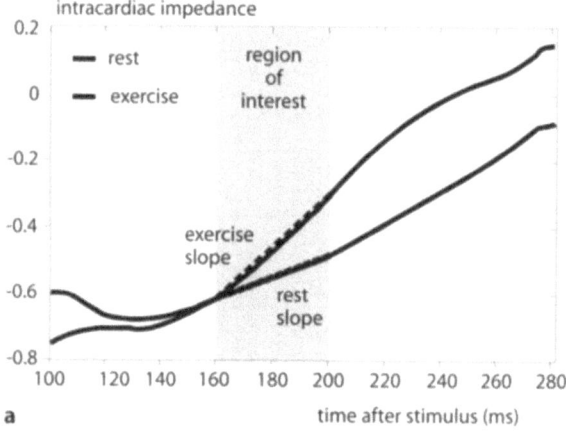

a

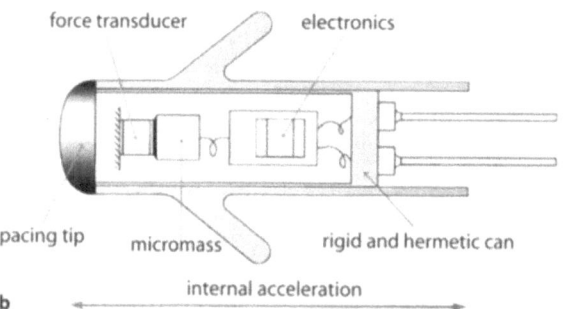

b

**Fig. 3.75. a** Evaluation of the impedance signal. The morphology of the intracardiac impedance waveform during the isovolumetric and early ejection phase is dependent on the patient's physical activity or emotional status. Upon calibration, a patient-specific interval is selected (*Region Of Interest*, ROI) in which the slope, a so-called ventricular inotropic parameter (VIP) is calculated as a measure of contraction velocity and, thereby, of the contractile state of the myocardium. The VIP is the sensor signal **b** Illustration of the distal segment of the BEST lead. A sealed, rigid cylinder, located behind the pacing electrode, contains an accelerometer which generates a signal conditioned by an electronic circuit before being sent to the pulse generator

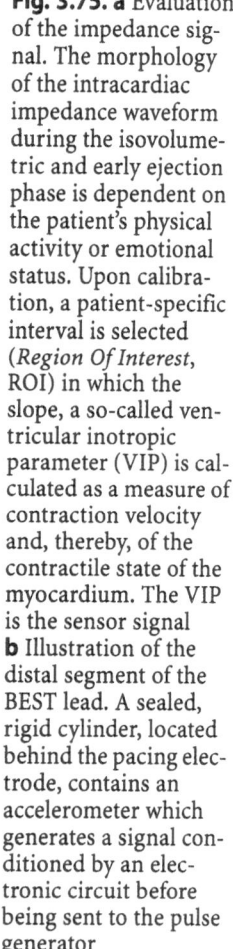

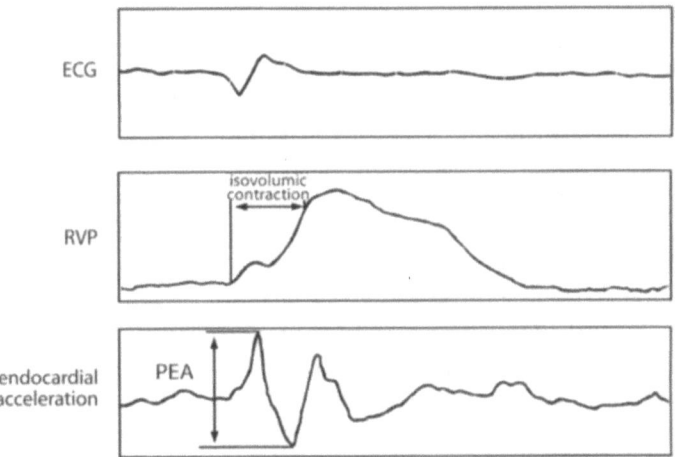

**Fig. 3.75. c** High speed recording. *Top*: surface ECG; *middle*: right ventricular pressure; *bottom*: peak endocardial acceleration (PEA) signal. PEA occurs just after the QRS, at the onset of rise in ventricular pressure. It is synchronous with the first heart sound and results from the forces generated by the onset of tension of the myocardial mass in the very beginning of ventricular contraction

ventilation, but at a faster sampling rate (Figs. 3.72–3.74). Its rapid response time makes this concept theoretically attractive; however, it may be difficult to determine precisely the end of the preejection period, and data are still lacking regarding its performance in various pathological situations. Offered in the Precept (CPI) model, the sensor is not regularly available commercially because of instability of the signal under various conditions, notably variations in body posture. This technique could also be used to verify proper ventricular capture. Some manufacturers are currently pursuing this concept.

### Intracardiac Impedance

Biotronik utilizes the first derivative of the change in impedance measured in the right ventricle. The fastest variation corresponds to ventricular ejection. Consequently, the system is capable of modulating the heart rate which correlates well physiologically with the degree of contractility (Fig. 3.75a). The system incorporated in the Inos DR uses a standard ventricular lead and can operate only when ventricles are paced. However, contractility measurements limited to the right ventricle may differ, in particular circumstances, from that of the left ventricle. Nevertheless, preliminary results have been encouraging.

## Peak Endocardial Acceleration

Introduced by Sorin (BEST Living), an accelerometer is imbedded at the distal end of the pacing lead and monitors cardiac motion. Acceleration measurements are filtered and amplified by the electronic components contained in a sealed, rigid cylinder behind the pacing/sensing ventricular electrode (Fig. 3.75b). The sensor is therefore, sheltered from the influence of volume changes or degree of nearby fibrosis. The signal occurs immediately after the QRS, at the very onset of the rise in intraventricular pressure, and is synchronous with the first heart sound (Fig. 3.75c). The pacing rate does not influence the signal which correlates with the degree of myocardial contractility. The peak of endocardial acceleration (PEA) correlates with changes in left ventricular dP/dt. Inferior vena occlusion decreases PEA and left ventricular dP/dt simultaneously. Occlusion of the pulmonary artery increases right ventricular dP/dt, and the fall in left ventricular dP/dt results in a corresponding fall in PEA. Myocardial ischemia, which decreases dP/dt, causes a concomitant decrease in PEA. PEA increases proportionally with increasingly larger bolus injections of inotropic agents, with level of exercise or mental stress, and with increasingly faster normal sinus rhythm. It decreases with beta adrenergic blockade. This system is currently being evaluated and may find many applications in cardiac pacing, for instance autocapture, and in other areas of cardiology: monitoring of transplant patients, of ventricular function, and of the effects of cardioactive drugs. The pacemaker also has a second sensor (gravity).

## Oxygen Saturation

In theory, this measurement is a good indicator of level of exercise. During exercise, oxygen extraction by muscles causes an increase in arteriovenous saturation difference. The method used for the measurement consists of hemoreflectometry, which is a measure of blood reflectivity after emission of infrared light from a diode, and sampling by phototransitors (Fig. 3.76). The lead has to be dedicated. Several technical problems remain to be solved, including alteration of long-term lead function by fibrin deposits, and sensing disturbances by lead motion from ventricular contraction. Much remains to be tested with this sensor included in the OxyElite (Medtronic) model and in the Synchrony $O_2$ and Solus $O_2$ (Pacesetter); the last 2 models are dual sensor devices monitoring $O_2$ and activity, and are in clinical testing.

## Right Ventricular Pressure

The increase in circulating catecholamines with exercise causes an increase in ventricular myocardial contractility which can be assessed by measuring dP/dt via a piezoelectric element implanted in the right ventricle. This system, therefore, requires dedicated instrumentation. A linear relationship exists between heart rate and dP/dt during exercise. It is noteworthy, however, that a mere increase in heart rate, without exercise, increases dP/dt. As a result, the rate

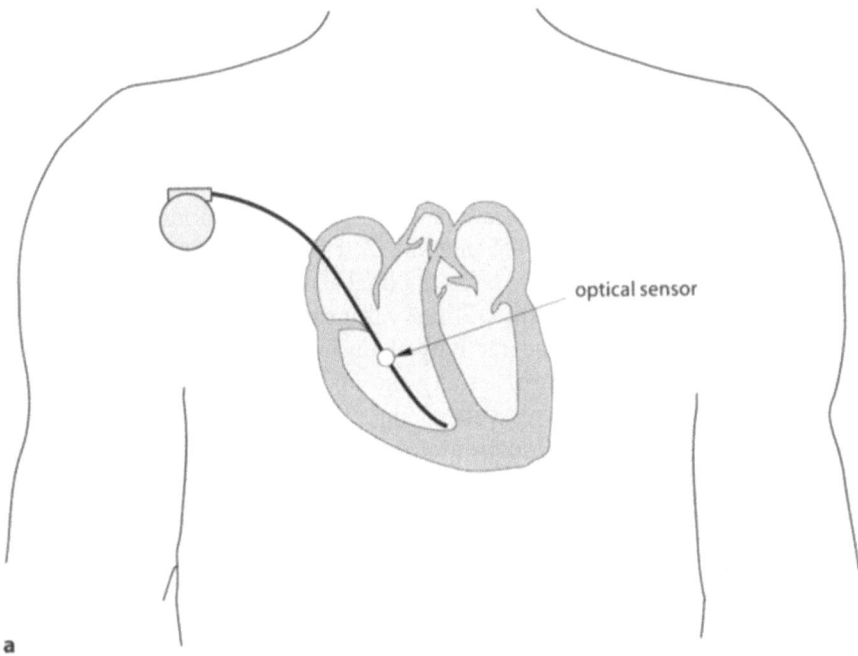

a

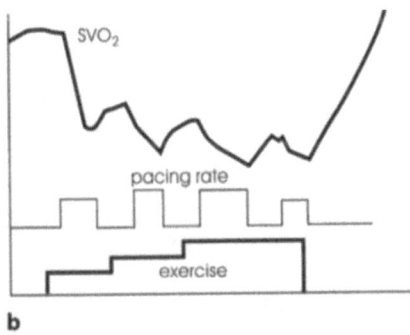

b

**Fig. 3.76. a** Changes in metabolic demand during exercise can be sensed by a special intracardiac lead which carries an optical sensor for oxygen saturation measurement
**b** During exercise, oxygen extraction by active muscles increases gradually. Venous blood returns to the right heart depleted in oxygen („blue" blood). This color change can be measured by an optical sensor mounted on a special right ventricular electrode (hemoreflectometry). This is a rapidly changing parameter, comparable in its dynamics to the sino-atrial node

responsive algorithm is complex, and its clinical performance remains uncertain in patients suffering from heart failure, atrial fibrillation, or treated with cardioactive medications. Initially tested clinically by Medtronic (Deltatrax), this sensor is not currently available commercially.

This list could not possibly be comprehensive, since the near future will undoubtedly give birth to further developments.

### Dual Sensor Pacemakers

Another line of research has sought to use two or more sensors in a single pace-maker; the mutual supplementation of some parameters could probably increase the wealth of information pertaining to metabolic demand, and screen out arti-facts from one sensor by the functions of another. The best association seems to be that of a sensor with a short response time, such as activity, accelerometer or oxygen saturation (which is also a metabolic sensor), and a metabolic sensor, such as minute ventilation, the QT interval, or temperature. Currently, Vitatron is the first manufacturer to have offered a dual sensor (Topaz, Saphir and Dia-mond), combining activity with QT interval measurement, with encouraging results (Fig. 3.77). In case of hyperactivity of one of the 2 sensors, while the other does not confirm the presence of activity, the comparison of information forces the hyperactive sensor to decrease its pacing rate (Figs. 3.78, 3.79). The Legend Plus and Kappa pacemakers (Medtronic) are other examples of dual sensor sys-tem, combining minute ventilation and activity, and the Talent (ELA) combines body acceleration and minute ventilation. The living (Sorin) combines peak endocardial acceleration and gravity.

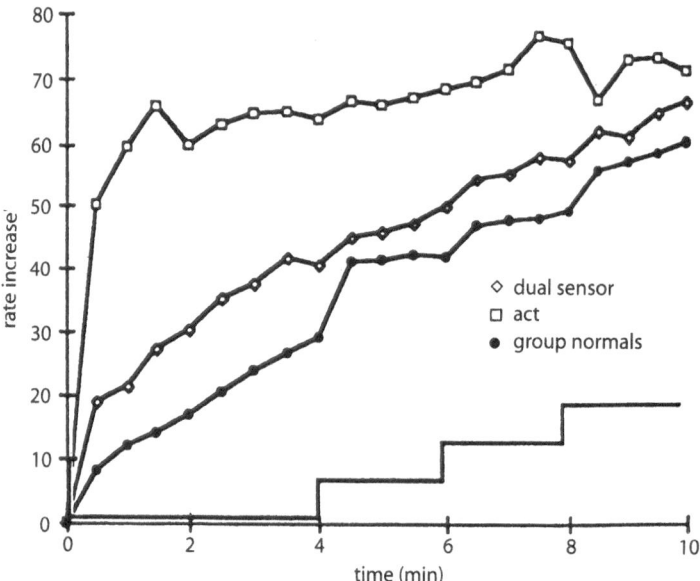

**Fig. 3.77.** Advantage of the dual rate responsive sensor combination (QT + activity). While the activity sensor generates an excessive response, the combination of both sen-sors brings the rate acceleration curve back toward that of the normal subjects (data from Vitatron)

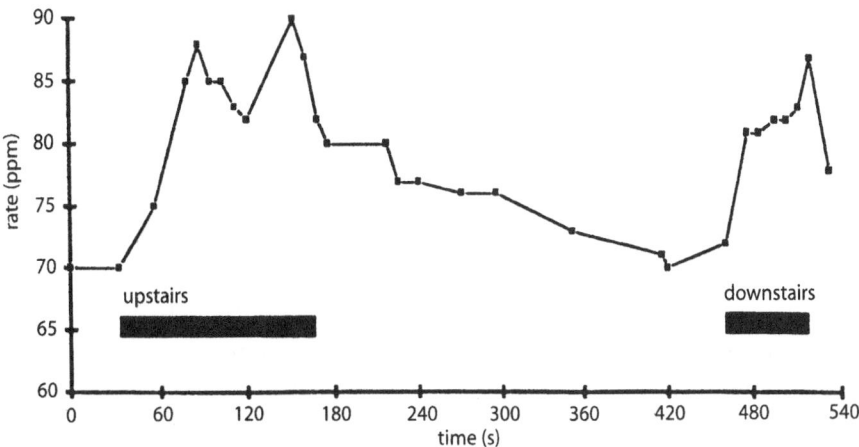

**Fig. 3.78.** Attenuation of the adverse effects of an activity sensor by a QT interval sensor: usually, the activity sensor causes a marked acceleration of the pacing rate upon going downstairs which, in this case, has been successfully attenuated

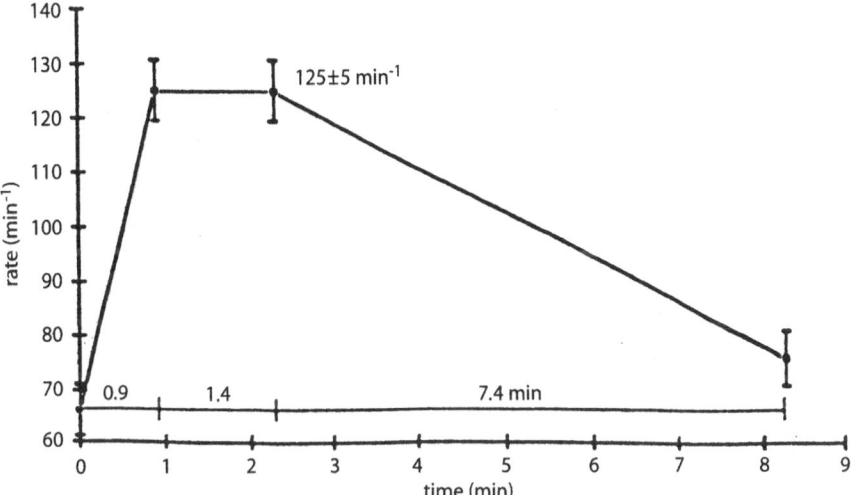

**Fig. 3.79.** Tapping on the pacemaker can causes an increase in the paced rate based on the activity sensor. This information is not confirmed by the QT interval sensor, which forces a return to the lower rate (data from Vitatron)

## Integration of Rate Responsiveness in Single and Dual Chamber Pacemakers

### In Single Chamber Pacing (SSIR Mode)

Rate responsiveness controls the pacemaker's escape interval. Its basic operation is otherwise unchanged, and the device remains in stand-by with all currently available functions except for rate smoothing, which is unnecessary since one of the sensor's role is precisely to smooth the rate during recovery from exercise.

## In Dual Chamber Pacing

*The DDDR Mode*

Atrial and ventricular (dual) pacing, atrial and ventricular (dual) sensing, inhibited and triggered (dual) response to sensing, rate responsive pacing.

In this mode, the basic functions of the pacemaker are the same as that of a DDD system. On the other hand, at high rates, the operation of the device is largely influenced by the rate responsive function. The 2 : 1 and Wenckebach operations remain in effect in DDDR pacing, since the basic operating mode is DDD. From the standpoint of atrial electrical stability, it may be risky to not recognize these functions, to not understand the indications for this pacing mode, and to improperly program the pacing parameters.

A clear understanding of the DDDR mode requires to keep in mind that rate responsiveness controls the pacemaker's escape interval which varies according to the information provided by the sensor. When the sensor signals exercise, the pacemaker gradually shortens its escape interval between the programmed lower rate and the maximal sensor rate. This corresponds to an acceleration of the lower rate, and means that if the sinus rate is slower than the rate responsive rate, the DDDR function takes charge of pacing altogether, at least in the atrium. If, conversely, the sinus rate is faster than the rate responsive rate, ventricular pacing will depend on the sinus rate between the programmed lower rate and the programmed maximal synchronous rate.

With some of the commercially available DDDR pacemakers, it is possible to distinguish two upper rates: one upper rate that can be considered typical, synchronous with the P wave, corresponding to that usually found in typical DDD pacing, and one other upper atrioventricular pacing rate linked to the rate responsive function (maximal sensor rate). Users need to know when to program a maximal sensor rate below, at or above that of the P wave synchronous rate, and understand the meaning of these various choices. The behavior of the DDDR pacemaker as a result of these different options is described in the Appendix (p. 399 ff.).

In DDD mode, the programming of a high 2 : 1 pacemaker AV block rate, that is of as short as possible a PVARP and short AVD at rapid rates (TARP = AVD + PVARP), optimizes the pacemaker's behavior at rapid atrial rates. The benefits are important: ability to program a high upper rate, optimization of the mode switch functions from proper sensing of pathologically rapid atrial rates, longer Wenckebach periods when the sinus rate crosses the upper rate, prevention of a 2 : 1 AV association. Some authors have described as an advantage the use of rate responsiveness of DDDR pacemakers to mitigate the abrupt drop in ventricular pacing rate as the sinus rate crosses the 2 : 1 pacemaker AV block rate. Indeed, during vigorous effort, the rate response shortens the escape interval, such that when the sinus rate crosses the 2 : 1 pacemaker AV block rate, the drop in ventricular pacing rate is considerably attenuated. The rate response is used, in such case, as a parachute for the ventricular rate. What about the atrium? A certain

number of spontaneous P waves are not sensed by the pacemaker since, by defi-
nition, they fall in PVARP during 2 : 1 function. No AVD is initiated from these P
waves. Therefore, they must wait for the end of the atrial escape interval, which
began with the P wave preceding the blocked P wave and is controlled by the rate
response, to deliver an atrial stimulus. During exercise, this escape interval is
short, such that it is quite likely for that stimulus to fall during the natural atrial
refractory period, or in the vulnerable period. There again, while resolving the
problem of the drop in ventricular pacing rate linked to the 2 : 1 pacemaker AV
block rate, a risk is incurred to cause an atrial arrhythmia. However, more recent
pacemakers such as the Thera (Medtronic) or Diamond (Vitatron) allow atrial
pacing only after a minimal delay after the preceding P wave, unless it was sensed
(outside the post-ventricular atrial blanking period).

Another problem pertaining to the 2 : 1 pacemaker AV block rate in DDDR
mode is that, in all likelihood, pacing is occurring in the atrium, and that, consequently, the 2 : 1 pacemaker AV block rate is equal to 60,000/AVD set for atrial
pacing (longer than for atrial sensing) + PVARP. Even if some DDDR pacemakers force atrial pacing during PVARP to reach the maximal sensor rate, there is
no more room for atrial sensing. This confirms the need to program a short
AVD during exercise, and, thus, to have available an algorithm of automatic
shortening of the AVD with faster atrial rates, as well as a short PVARP with a
protection algorithm against ELT. Of course, keeping the PVARP long would
avoid such problems, but would also prevent the pacemaker from diagnosing
atrial arrhythmias; moreover, atrial pacing would be unnecessarily energy consuming.

*The DDIR Mode*

Atrial and ventricular (dual) pacing, atrial and ventricular (dual) sensing, inhibition by
atrial and ventricular events, rate responsive pacing.

The DDIR mode functions like the DDI mode. The only consequence of the rate
response is the control of the escape interval which shortens with exercise.
Several risks exist:

- If the rate response is faster than the acceleration in sinus rate, and if, for
  example, a premature ventricular complex with retrograde conduction is
  sensed outside of PVARP, ventricular pacing will be associated with 1 : 1 retrograde conduction during exercise, thus behaving as a VVIR pacemaker (Fig.
  3.80).
- If the sinus rate is faster than the rate response and if, in presence of AV block,
  AV asynchrony occurs, the mode will be VVIR. Moreover, as a result of AV
  asynchrony, some of the P waves fall in PVARP and remain undetected such
  that, here again, premature, ineffective atrial pacing, or arrhythmogenic pacing in the atrial vulnerable period, may occur (Figs. 3.81, 3.82).

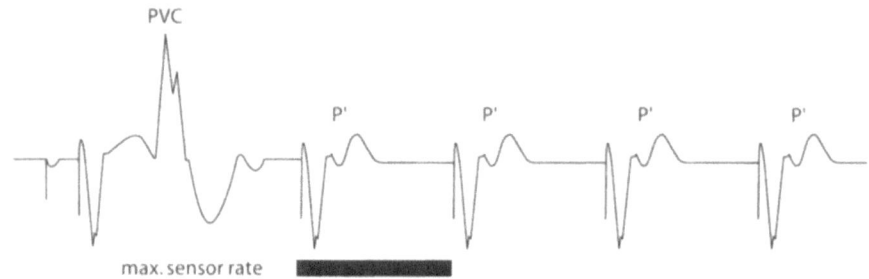

**Fig. 3.80.** In DDIR mode, and in the event of a premature ventricular complex with retrograde conduction, ventricular pacing risks inducing 1 : 1 retrograde conduction and VVIR pacemaker syndrome
*P'* retrograde conduction; *MSR* maximal sensor rate

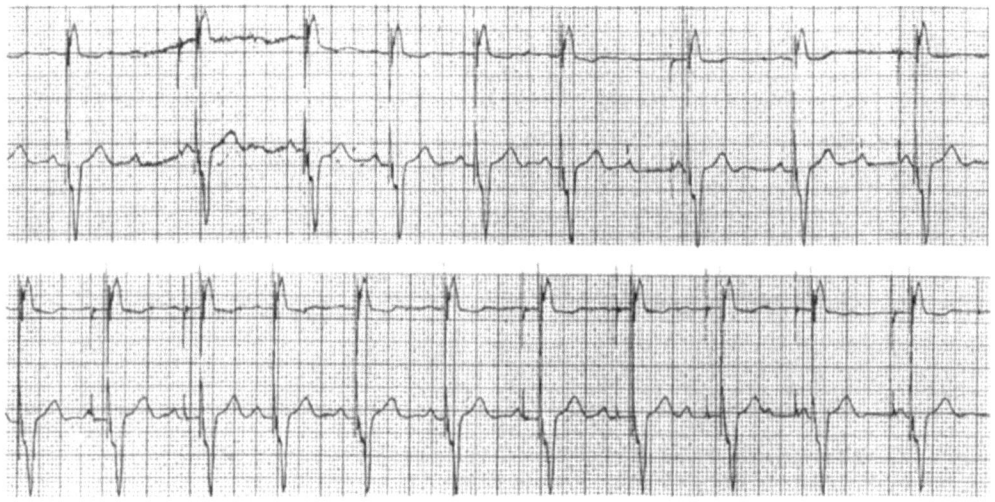

**Fig. 3.81. a** DDD mode, 50/125 BPM, AVD = 150 ms, atrial sensitivity = 0.5 mV (highest for this device). Atrial sensing failure occurs causing prolongation in the ventricular pacing cycles particularly bothersome during exercise
**b** DDDR mode, 50/125 BPM, maximal atrial sensitivity. With moderate effort, and despite intermittent atrial sensing failure, AV sequential rhythm remains stable. Programming of rate responsiveness has allowed to avoid ventricular pauses, but cannot correct AV asynchrony

The only true indication for the DDIR mode is the bradycardia-tachycardia syndrome with very frequent arrhythmic episodes in a patient who has received a pacemaker without a satisfactory mode switch algorithm and/or poorly protected against ELT.

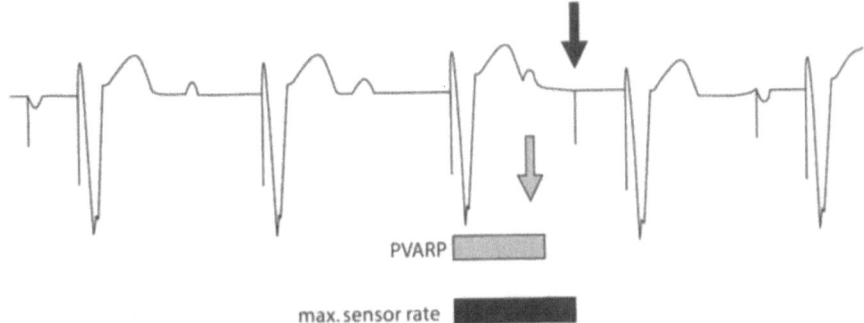

**Fig. 3.82.** In DDIR mode, when the sinus rate is faster than the rate responsive rate, and in presence of AV block, AV asynchrony sets in, which is equivalent to VVIR pacing. In addition, some P waves fall in PVARP and the interval following the blocked P wave ends with an atrial pacing stimulus which is likely to be too early, ineffective or arrhythmogenic

*The VDDR Mode*

> Ventricular pacing, atrial and ventricular (dual) sensing, atrioventricular (dual) synchronous pacing, rate responsive ventricular pacing.

The VDDR pacemakers currently available are the Unity (Intermedics), the AddVent (Pacesetter), the Dromos and Inos2 DR (Biotronik), the Thera VDD (Medtronic), the Swing VDR (Sorin), and the Saphir (Vitatron) which uses two sensors (activity and QT interval). This mode creates competition between the spontaneous atrial rate (VDD) and that calculated by the sensor (VDIR = VVIR with continuous analysis of the atrial signals). With respect to the spontaneous atrial rhythm, the pacemaker functions in VDD or VVIR mode.

If the slope of rate responsiveness is steeper than the acceleration of the atrial rate, the rate responsive function induces only ventricular pacing and AV asynchrony sets in, or even retrograde AV conduction which may trigger ELT.

The algorithms of sensor hysteresis, included in the Saphir (Vitatron) and Unity (Intermedics) represent an improvement: if the sinus rate falls just below the rate response, it becomes possible to resume AV synchrony and to avoid the continuation of VVIR pacing. The other algorithm currently available is the automatic mode switch from VDD(R) to VVIR, or more precisely VDIR. The rate responsive sensor takes charge of ventricular pacing in the event of an atrial arrhythmia (see p. 151ff.). Finally, in case of atrial sensing failure during sinus rhythm or atrial fibrillation, the pacemaker functions in VVIR mode, remaining in VDD mode as long as the atrial signals are properly sensed.

In conclusion, the typical VDD mode is incapable of atrial pacing. One relies strictly on spontaneous P waves to accelerate the ventricular rate during exercise. As a result, the risk of ELT or other pacemaker mediated tachyarrhythmias is high. The VDDR mode is not of great value because of the persistence of the above mentioned problems, and the likelihood of a VVIR behavior during exercise. This mode, in fact, is a form of automatic mode switch from VDD to VVIR in case of loss of atrial sensing from alteration of the intracardiac signal or from development of an atrial rhythm disturbance. Its value is mostly confined to the use of single atrioventricular leads (see p. 116 – 120).

## Antitachycardia Pacing

### Atrial Tachyarrhythmias Prevention

The protective effect of pacing against bradycardia dependent ventricular arrhythmias has been recognized since the 1960s. Later on, this technique has been used to treat torsades de pointe by pacing the ventricle at a rate between 80 and 100 BPM. This same method has been used in the long QT syndrome with, as a result, a shortening of refractory periods. Its preventive effect against atrial arrhythmias has been recognized much later, at the end of the 1970s, when atrial leads and dual chamber systems became available. The meta-analysis by Kenny and Sutton published in 1986 showed a benefit of this type of pacing in patients suffering from sinus node dysfunction. It also showed a reduction in thrombo-embolic complications secondary to arrhythmias, and in mortality, compared to ventricular pacing. These results were later confirmed by Danish investigators in a prospective study.

These observations spurred the development of algorithms such as dynamic overdrive and rate smoothing, as well as the use of rate responsiveness. In fact, it appears that many patients are controlled solely by atrial pacing. Indeed, since implantable Holter functions have become available, it is not rare to identify rhythm disturbances that the patient may not have perceived, and which reveal (despite the observation of sinus rhythm at routine visits, and the absence of symptoms) that this prevention is only partial. This demonstrates that background pharmacologic antiarrhythmic therapy remain often necessary, though not completely effective.

Other preventive methods are within the realm of modern pacing and represent an interesting line of research, even after many years of exploration. Data management capabilities and algorithms offered by microprocessors open new perspectives which should not be stifled because of unsuccessful past experiences. It is, for instance, possible to load in the Chorus II, RM and Talent (ELA Medical), and soon in the Vitatron DDDR models, RAM dedicated software aimed at suppressing the compensatory pauses of ventricular or premature atrial complexes. The goal consists of eliminating bigeminy, which may be poorly tolerated hemodynamically, and of reducing the number of episodes of sustained arrhythmias. The preliminary results have shown inconsistent reliability of such programs, though individual results have been spectacular (Fig. 3.83).

One other method applied to the prevention of atypical flutter with interatrial conduction delay facilitating its onset, originally described by Daubert, consists of resynchronizing the atria with one electrode placed in the usual right atrial position and another one placed in the coronary sinus to pace the left atrium. These leads need to be connected to an AAT pacemaker if AV conduction is pre-

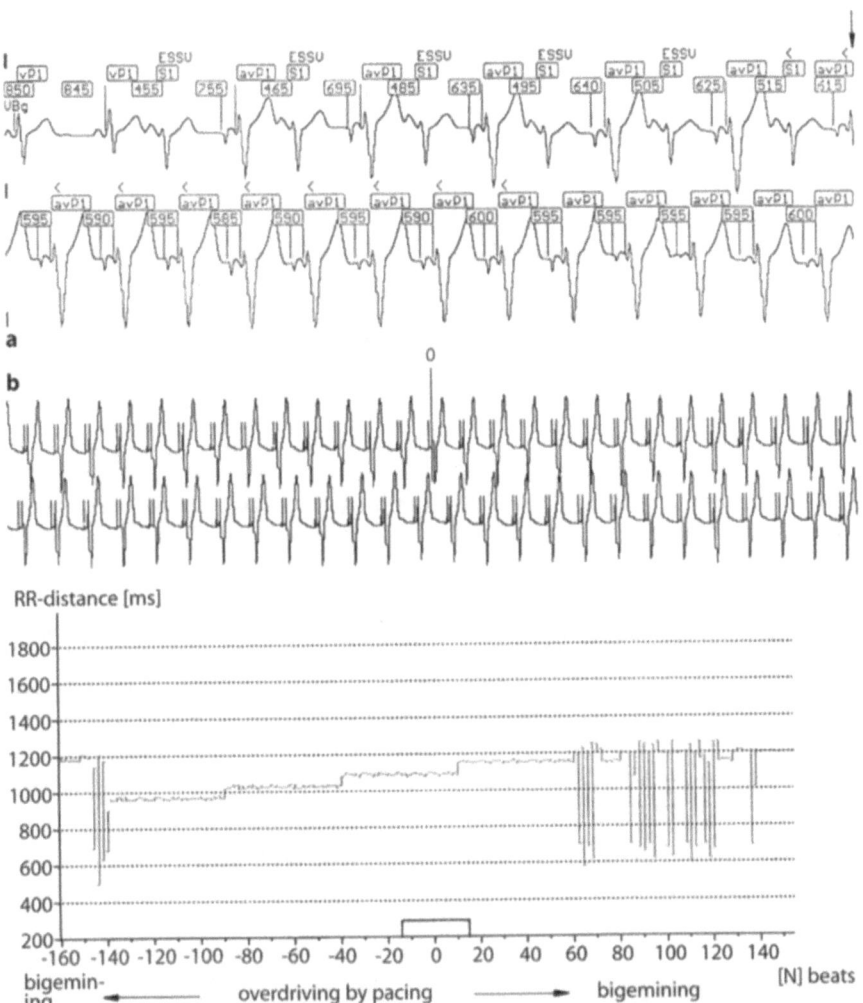

**Fig. 3.83. a** Atrial bigeminy, sensed by the pacemaker, increases the atrial pacing rate which completely suppresses the emergence of further extrasystoles
**b** In the beginning of the tracing, atrial bigeminy has induced an increase in the pacing rate which has eliminated all extrasystoles (overdriving). Every 50 cycles, the pacemaker decreases its pacing rate. When the rate has slowed, bigeminy reappears (data from ELA Medical)

served, or an atrial triggered dual chamber device (by loading a special function in RAM) if AV conduction is disturbed. Preliminary results are promising.

Another approach has been described by Saksena who implants a high right atrial lead, and a low right atrial lead in the coronary sinus ostium. Others have explored the option of stimulating the right atrial septum. The aim of all three approaches is to eliminate defects of right atrial, or of interatrial conduction, which are known to facilitate the onset of atrial arrhythmias. These avenues of research, combined with the prevention of atrial arrhythmias by atrial or dual chamber pacing, will perhaps improve the prevention of sustained atrial arrhythmias.

## Protection Against Sustained Atrial Tachyarrhythmias

### Protection Against Atrial Arrhythmias is Necessary

If it is timed outside the pacemaker's refractory periods, any abnormal P wave, (that is with a short coupling interval), will trigger synchronized ventricular pacing following an AVD. If the atrial rhythm is abnormal, the risk of a sustained accelerated ventricular rate is high, which may have serious hemodynamic consequences, particularly in presence of underlying heart disease, as illustrated in this clinical case:

CASE STUDY

*Example.* A 55 year old patient presents with hypertrophic cardiomyopathy and severe diastolic dysfunction diagnosed at echocardiography. Following a syncopal episode due to AV block, a dual chamber pacemaker is implanted without complications. Four years later, the patient presents in the emergency room in congestive heart failure, and a pacemaker driven heart rate of 140 BPM, noticed by the patient since its abrupt onset, 3 weeks earlier (the upper rate had been programmed at 150 BPM). Following magnet application, which brought the ventricular rate to the programmed lower rate, it became apparent that the patient was in flutter at an atrial rate of 280 BPM, sensed by the pacemaker in a 2 : 1 fashion, thus resulting in a ventricular pacing rate of 140 BPM. The pacemaker was reprogrammed to VVI mode at a rate of 70 BPM and the symptoms of heart failure resolved.

This example illustrates the need of protection against atrial arrhythmias. The various algorithms are described on p. 150 and p. 402, after the description of other pacing modes and of rate responsive sensors.

Two conditions are necessary to increase the pacing rate in presence of atrial tachyarrhythmias:

- The abnormal atrial signals must be of large enough amplitude to be sensed. Indeed, the amplitude of pathologic atrial electrograms is often reduced, below the programmed sensitivity, even if maximal. This is frequently the case with atrial fibrillation.
- The second condition is the ability to sense abnormal rapid atrial rates, which depends on the relative ongoing atrial rate, and that of the maximal sensing rate (2 : 1 pacemaker AV block rate).

This may place the physician before two distinct situations:

- *The amplitude of abnormal atrial signals is below the programmed sensitivity.* The pacemaker does not sense in the atrium. In presence of AV block, the behavior is DVI (see p. 114), with atrioventricular pacing at the back up or rate responsive rate (Fig. 3.84). Atrial pacing is useless and power consuming. In absence of AV block, spontaneous QRS complexes inhibit the pacemaker when the ventricular rate is above the ongoing pacemaker escape rate. In this case, the patient is protected since the ventricular rate does not increase. This may be an argument to program atrial sensitivity at a value low enough to sense normal sinus P waves but not abnormal atrial activity. This may pose two problems: on one hand, the sinus P wave amplitude often decreases with exercise, causing loss of atrial sensing and absence of ventricular pacing acceleration with exercise; on the other hand, the pacemaker is incapable of memorizing the atrial arrhythmia episodes, which precludes a retrospective diagnosis.

- *The pacemaker senses abnormal P waves.* Several situations may be encountered. In presence of AV block, if each P wave falls outside the pacemaker's refractory periods, and if the rate of the arrhythmia is between the lower rate and the programmed upper rate, the paced rhythm is 1 : 1 associated. If the

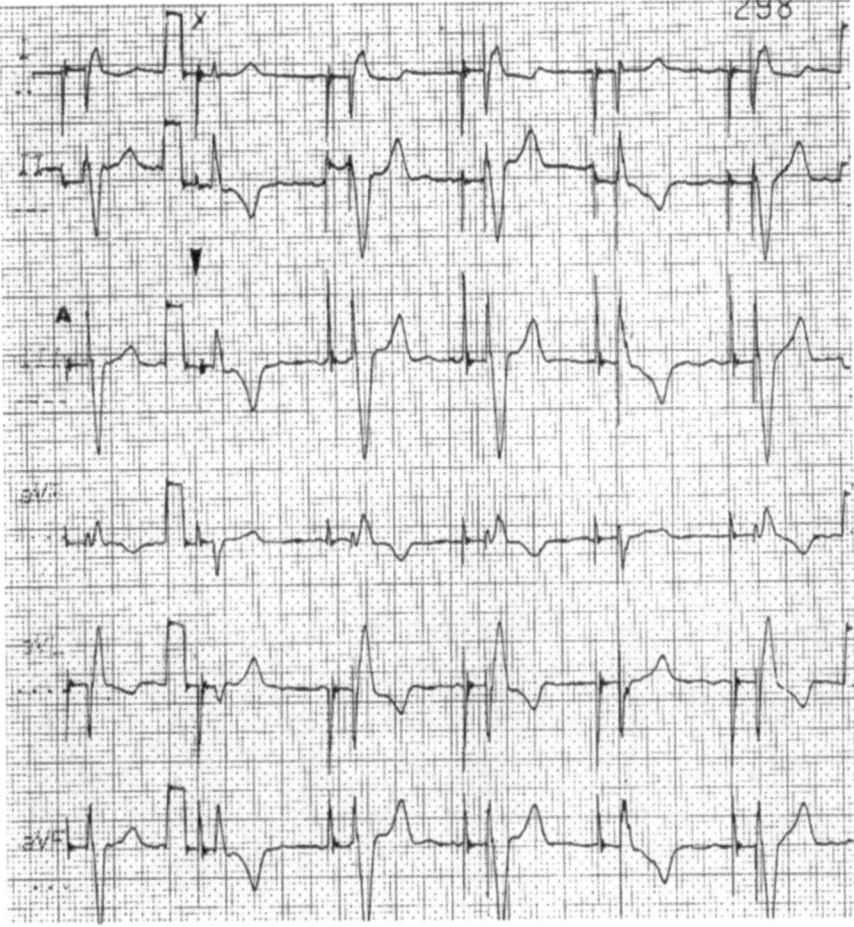

**Fig. 3.84.** DDD mode, 60/100 BPM, AVD = 170 ms, PVARP = 275 ms, atrial sensitivity = 0.5 mV. DVI-like pacing in a patient with atrial fibrillation not sensed by the pacemaker

atrial rate is above the upper rate, but below the maximal atrial sensing rate (2 : 1 pacemaker AV block rate), the AV association will be of a Wenckebach type (Fig. 3.85). If the atrial rate is above the maximal atrial sensing rate, two types of AV association may occur: if the atrial rate is less than twice the maximal atrial sensing rate, the association is 2 : 1 (Fig. 3.86); if the atrial rate is faster than twice the maximal atrial sensing rate, the association is of a Wenckebach type.

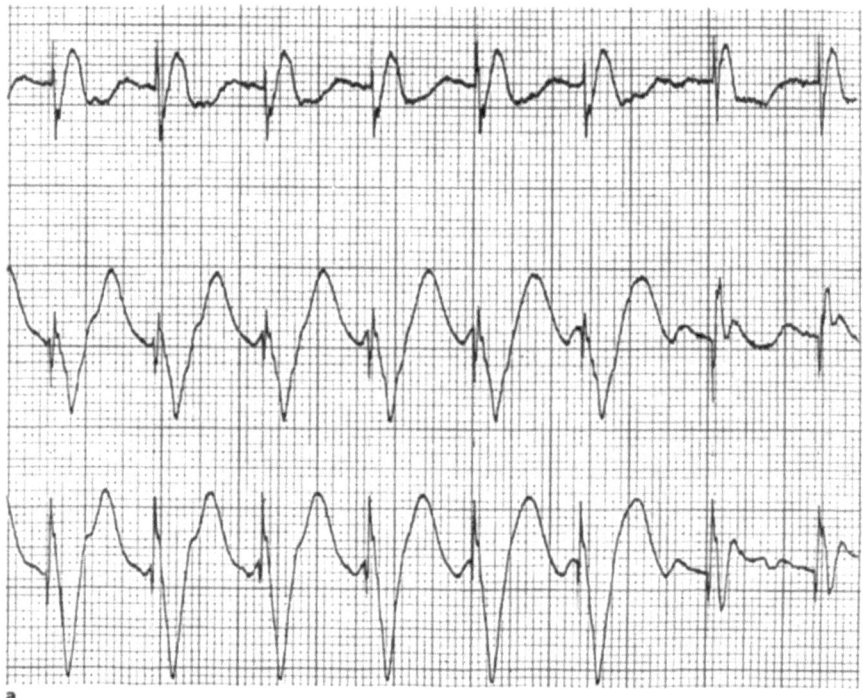

a

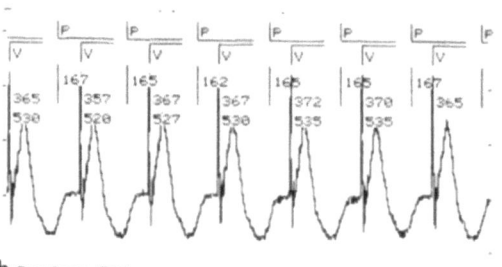

b Surface ECG

**Fig. 3.85a–b.** DDD mode, 60/130 BPM, AVD = 165 ms, PVARP = 250 ms, atrial sensitivity = 1.2 mV
**a** Atrial flutter detected on a 2 : 1 basis by the DDD pacemaker
**b** Event markers in DDD. Every other P wave is sensed with 2 : 1 AV synchrony

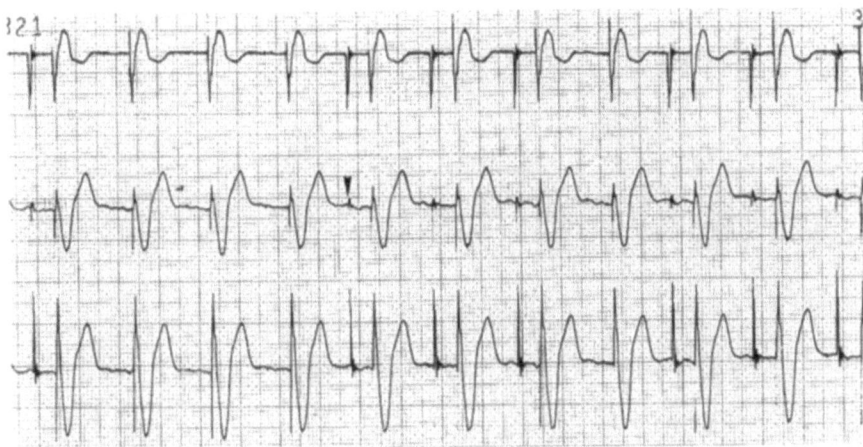

**Fig. 3.86.** DDD mode, 70/100 BPM, AVD = 230 ms, PVARP = 475 ms. The 3 tracings are simultaneous. In the beginning of the recording, the ventricle only is paced, confirming proper sensing of the atrium. AV synchrony cannot go beyond 85 BPM given the programmed pacing parameters. Upon magnet application (*arrow*), D00 mode is induced, with confirmation of the underlying atrial arrhythmia

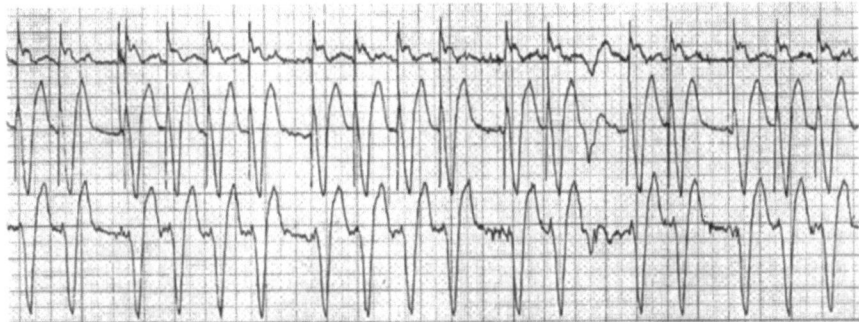

**Fig. 3.87.** DDD mode, 60/110 BPM, AVD = 90 ms, PVARP = 325 ms, atrial sensitivity = 0.8 mV. Inconsistent sensing of atrial fibrillation accounting for an irregular pattern of the paced ventricular rhythm

### Atrial Sensing is Inconsistent

The ECG interpretation is difficult and the ventricular rate is erratic (Figs. 3.87, 3.88). In absence of AV block, the spontaneous QRS complexes inhibit the pacemaker.

Without specific protective algorithm, the various means of protection, which remain rudimentary, are:

- The DVI mode, obsolete nowadays since incapable of atrial sensing (see p. 114).
- The DDI mode with its limitations such as VVI like behavior in presence AV block (see p. 107).

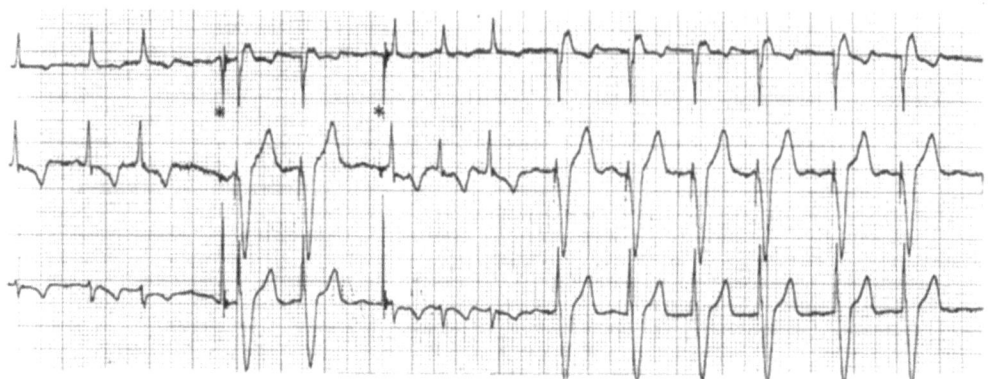

**Fig. 3.88.** DDD mode, 70/1200 BPM, AVD = 140 ms, PVARP = 350 ms, atrial sensitivity = 1 mV. Atrial sensing is inconsistent with delivery of atrial spikes (*) and persistence of a dissociated ventricular rhythm

- Limitation of the upper rate with risk of Wenckebach periodicity during exercise.
- Differentiated programming of the upper rate in rate responsive mode (see p. 399 ff.).
- The VVI mode is the last resort if other measures do not restore proper pacing functions.

The best approach, however, consists of using a dedicated protective algorithm, when available, and when the atrial arrhythmia is sensed by the pacemaker.

### Protection Algorithms Against Atrial Arrhythmias in DDD/DDDR, or Automatic Mode Switch

Automatic mode switch and protection algorithms against atrial arrhythmias are at the forefront of development in cardiac pacing. All manufacturers have a technical solution to offer. With respect to automatic mode switch, the switch from AAI(R) to DDD(R) that takes place in the Chorus II, Chorum and Talent (ELA Medical) models, developed to improve hemodynamics (Fig. 3.52), should not be confused with automatic switches aimed at preventing run-away ventricular pacing from tracking an atrial tachyarrhythmia DDD(R) VDI(R) or DDI(R). Each model has its own, specific algorithm (see p. 402 ff.).

*Algorithm Response*

It is either immediate from one cycle to the next, or delayed by a preliminary analysis of the atrial rhythm.

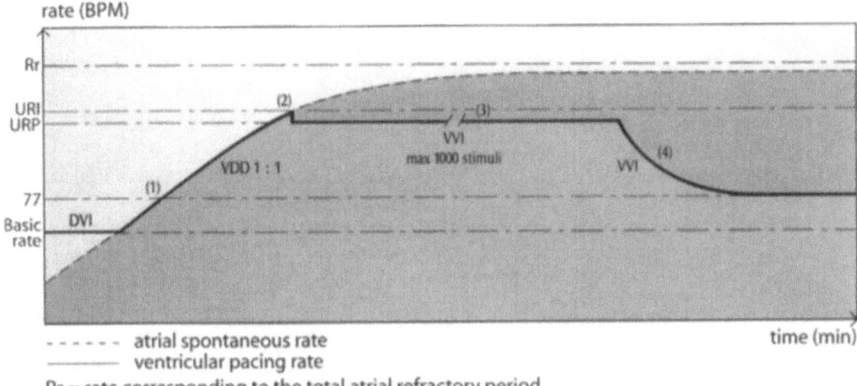

**Fig. 3.89.** Peculiarity of the Sorin Physiocor pacemaker. Wenckebach association is not present and, instead, is replaced by a VVI mode with a cycle equal to the shortest programmed cycle + 100 ms. After 1000 cycles, the pacemaker switches to fall-back

### Discrimination Between Sinus and Abnormal Rhythm

This is the cornerstone of each system. The differential diagnosis hinges on one or more of the following findings:

- The maximal programmed ventricular rate in so-called fall-back systems after a certain number (which may be programmable) of Wenckebach cycles (Fig. 3.89)
- Sensing of an atrial event in the refractory period (dual demand system), with a given prematurity compared to the ambient sinus or rate responsive rhythm
- Sensing of „n" short or premature, consecutive or not consecutive atrial cycles (Fig. 3.90), or of a mean calculated atrial rate above a rate set in the pacemaker's memory

### Methods of Protection

The response may consist of the following:

- A switch from VDD(R) to DVI(R) (dual demand), or to VDI(R), or to DDI(R)
- A change in the maximal ventricular rate
- A change in AV association (n:1)

### AV Reassociation

AV reassociation takes place from one cycle to the next after analysis of a few atrial cycles

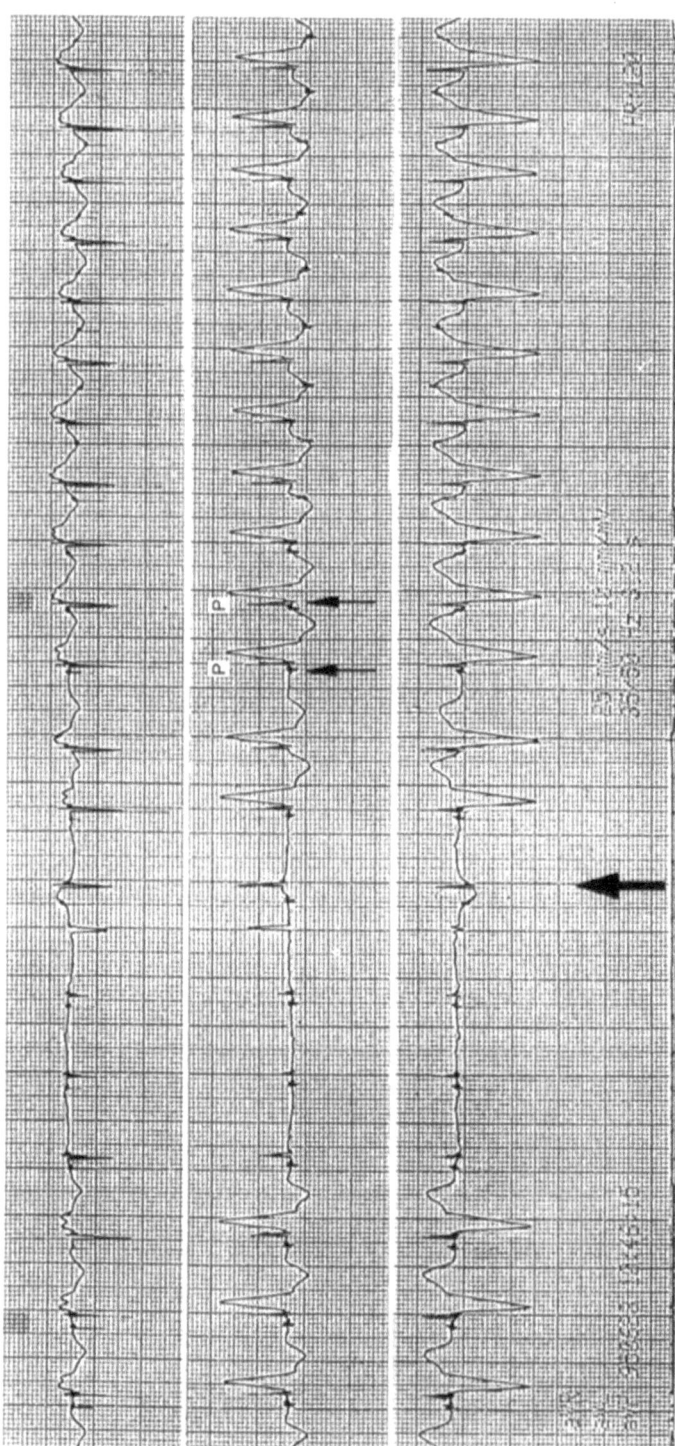

**Fig. 3.90. a** Fall-back algorithm of the Chorus RM (ELA Medical). The programmed upper rate is 120 BPM. A special algorithm, loaded in RAM, causes the delivery of an atrial spike with each sensed event in the DDD or DDDR mode. These atrial sensing markers disappear when the pacemaker converts to the VDIR mode at the time of automatic mode switch imposed by the fall-back function for atrial arrhythmia. At the end of a ventricular threshold test (*large arrow*), an atrial tachycardia develops. The pacemaker paces at the upper rate in Wenckebach mode (from the *two small arrows* on).

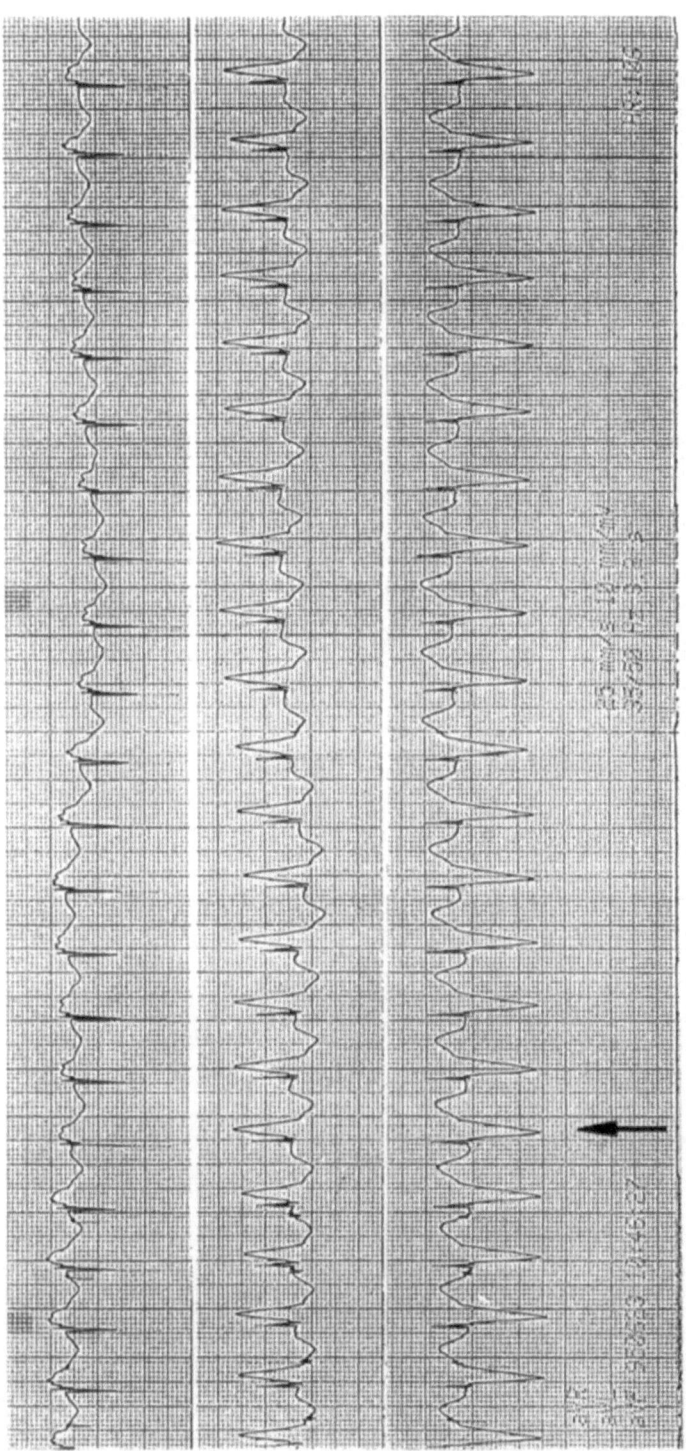

**Fig. 3.90. b** After 16 cycles, fall-back starts with a switch to the VDIR mode (*arrow*). The atrial sensing spikes disappear. The pacing rate slows down to that dictated by the rate responsive sensor.

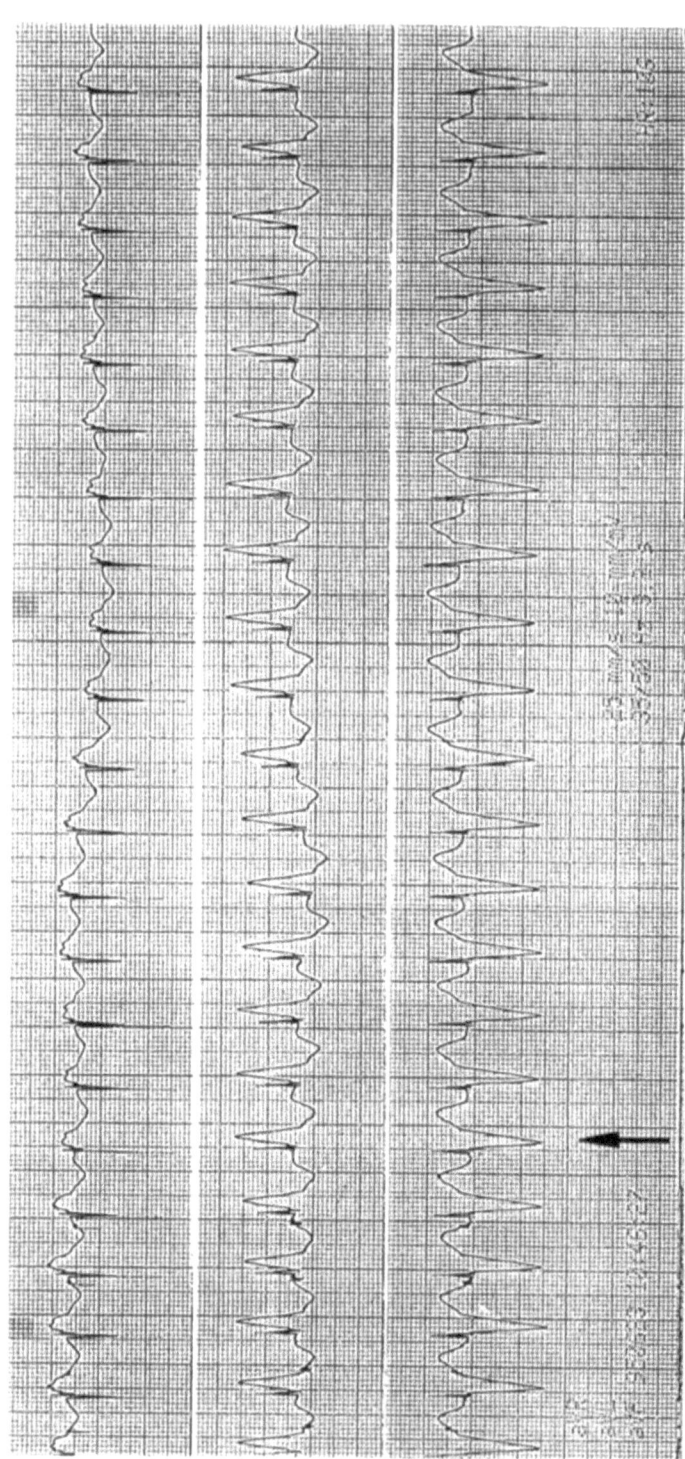

**Fig. 3.90. c** The rate responsive heart rate has been reached

*Diagnostics*

The various systems may or may not provide information regarding the atrial arrhythmias that were sensed and which caused a mode switch. The analysis is retrospective upon interrogation of the device. The data are either mere statistics (tally of the number of algorithm activations, date, duration of the episodes), or more complex, in the form of histograms, diagrams, electrograms, or markers.

These systems are effective only when atrial sensing is reliable during sustained arrhythmia since proper sensing of all abnormal cycles is required. This explains the recent development of pacemakers which diagnose arrhythmias based on probability. The diagnosis hinges on a complex and continuous analysis of the atrial rhythm to enhance sensitivity in the event of intermittent undersensing of abnormal atrial signals.

The best mode of protection may depend on the patient's clinical characteristics. More information is provided in the Appendix (p. 402 ff.) regarding the methods available in individual models.

### Multimode Switch

This mode is specific to Chorum and Talent pacemakers (ELA Medical). A real time mode adjustment to the patient's rhythm and conduction is achieved. In presence of normal AV conduction without atrial rhythm disorders, the mode is AAI (AAIR, if chronotropic incompetence is present). If AV conduction is pathological, the pacemaker operates in the DDD(R) mode. If an atrial tachyarrhythmia occurs, the pacemaker switches from AAI(R) or DDD(R) to the DDI(R) mode.

### Role of Antitachycardia Pacing in Permanent Cardiac Pacing

#### Automatic Antitachycardia Functions

The value of antitachycardia pacing by implantable pacemakers has evolved considerably in recent years. At the atrial level, the advent of new therapeutic modalities has virtually eliminated the indications for the implant of a permanent antitachycardia pacemaker. Bypass mediated or other forms of reentrant tachycar-

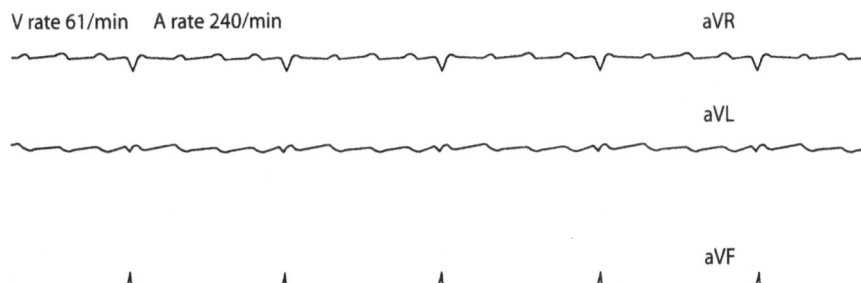

**Fig. 3.91. a** Surface ECG before burst pacing. The atrial rate is 240 BPM and the ventricular rate 61 BPM

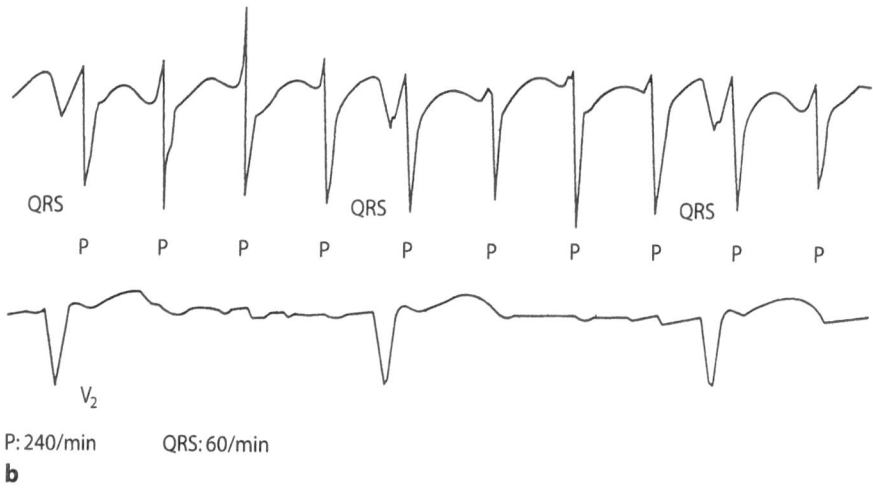

QRS                    QRS                    QRS

P      P      P      P      P      P      P      P      P      P

$V_2$

P: 240/min      QRS: 60/min

**b**

burst pacing at 1100 pulses/min

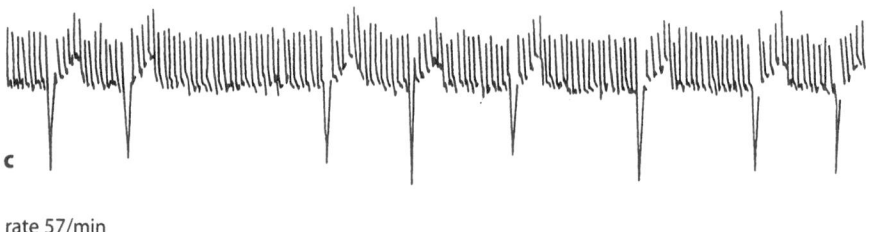

**c**

rate 57/min

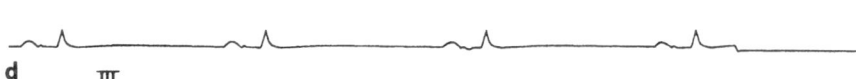

I

II

**d**   III

**Fig. 3.91. b** Same ECG with intracardiac atrial electrograms
**c** Following unsuccessful overdrive and underdrive pacing efforts, burst stimulation at 1100 BPM is delivered
**d** Return to sinus rhythm.

dias are now best definitively cured by ablation procedures. Possible remaining indications are pure, drug resistant, atrial tachyarrhythmias; these must be regular, flutter-like for example, without associated episodes of atrial fibrillation, and responsive to antitachycardia pacing. These several conditions limit considerably the indications for this treatment, particularly since ablation techniques

atrial electrogram rate: 60/min

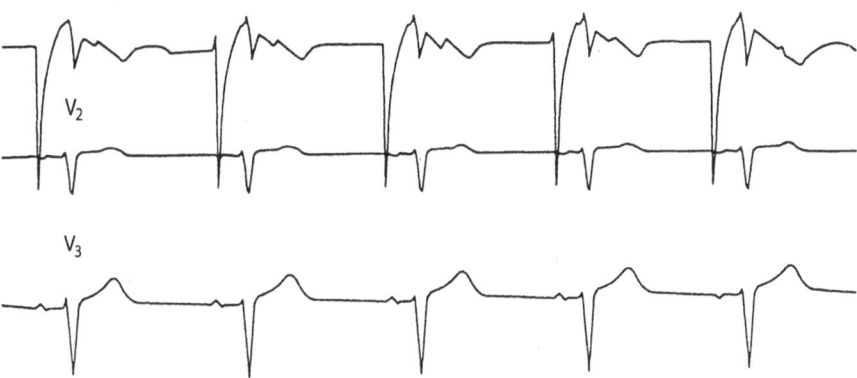

**Fig. 3.91. e** Same ECG as in d with intracardiac atrial electrograms. Sinus rhythm remains stable

may also be applied as a treatment of choice to interrupt an area of slow conduction of a reentrant mechanism (instead of ablating the AV node/His bundle region and implant a permanent VVIR or DDDR pacemaker).

It may be desirable, nevertheless, to have a simple function included in standard pacemakers to automatically burst terminate a regular atrial tachycardia after its diagnosis has been firmly established (Figs. 3.91, 3.92). This function exists currently only in the Intertach II (Intermedics).

At the ventricular level, antitachycardia pacing has been abandoned as a single therapy. Indeed, in 5% – 15% of cases, attempts to pace terminate ventricular tachycardia is complicated by its acceleration, or transformation to ventricular fibrillation, requiring immediate cardioversion or defibrillation. Therefore, safe ventricular antitachycardia pacing should be limited to devices which, in their most recent versions, combine it with cardioversion, defibrillation and antibradycardia pacing.

### Activation of Temporary Antitachycardia Functions

Some pacemakers do allow attempts at high rate atrial pacing. The pacemaker must be either in the A00 mode with control of the pacing rate (Fig. 3.93) or, depending on which chamber needs to be paced, in AAT or VVT mode to be driven by an external stimulator connected to the patient's thorax (Fig. 3.94), and programmed to a special mode allowing high rate stimulation. Esophageal stimulation can also be attempted. However, when using these easily activated techniques, their objectives, risks and necessary precautions must be clearly kept in mind (Fig. 3.95). Others have proposed a programmer-based electrophysiologic testing function to allow the induction or termination of supraventricular or ventricular tachycardias (Fig. 3.96). These modes are only temporary, activated and controlled by the programmer with a physician in attendance. Such systems allow the noninvasive management of sustained tachyarrhythmias via previously implanted pacemakers.

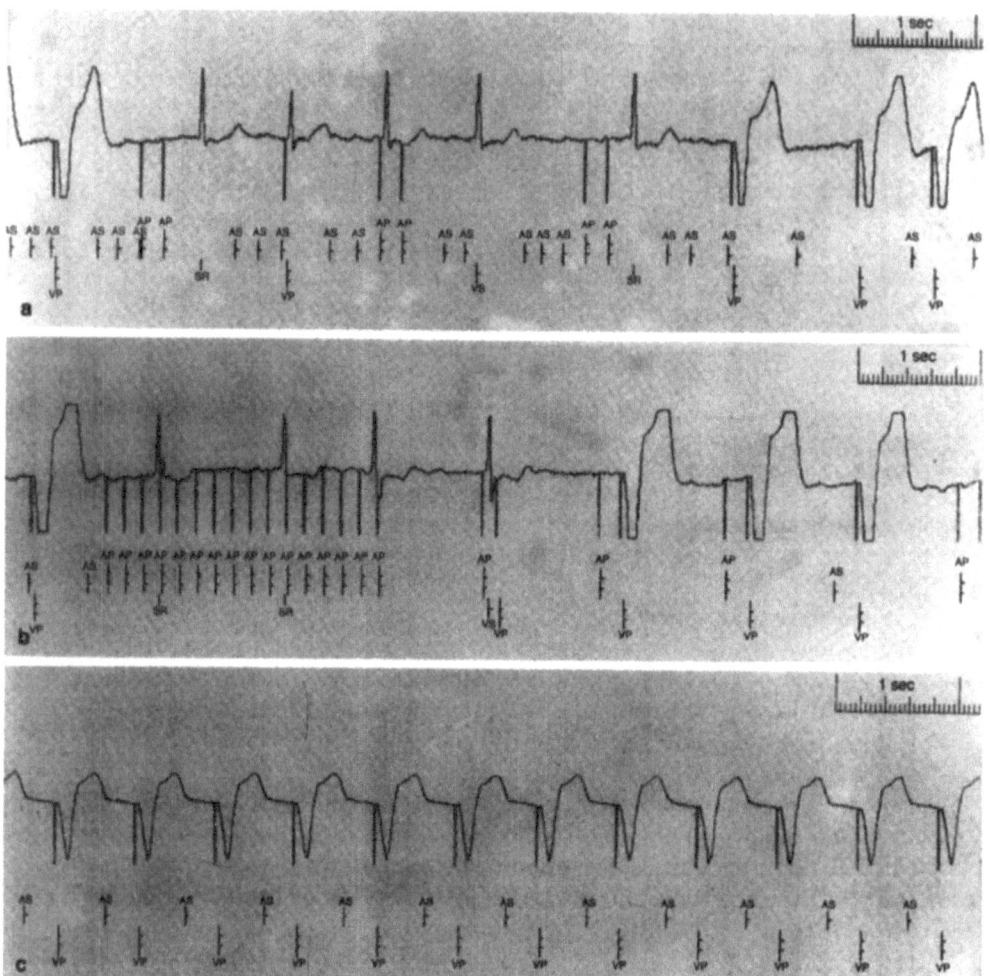

**Fig. 3.92a–c.** Several methods of termination of supraventricular tachycardia. DDD mode with atrial burst. Various bursts (from two to 16 stimuli per burst) at various cycle lengths, are tested
**a** Two stimuli per burst
**b** Sixteen stimuli per burst
**c** Return to sinus rhythm
*AS* atrial sensing; *AP* atrial pacing; *VP* ventricular pacing

In conclusion, permanent antitachycardia pacing is rarely indicated and no longer used as the only treatment modality. Nonpharmacologic treatment of tachyarrhythmias is now discussed in textbooks primarily dedicated to implantable cardioverter-defibrillators or ablation procedures. This topic, although derived from methods applied to cardiac pacing, has become too vast to be covered, even briefly, in a textbook dedicated to antibradycardia pacing.

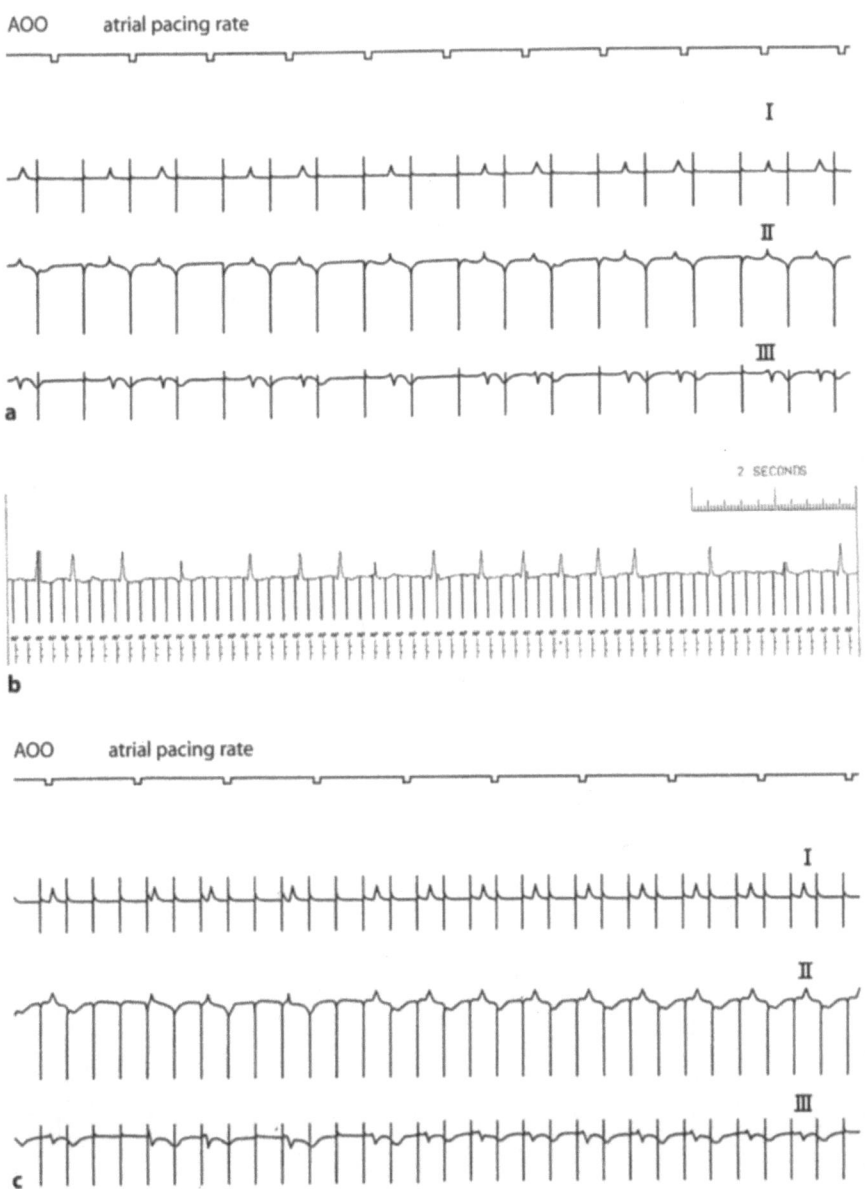

**Fig. 3.93. a–c** An old Symbios 7005 (Medtronic) pacemaker is used to deliver temporary rapid atrial pacing in A00 mode, either to perform simple electrophysiologic testing, or to terminate an atrial tachycardia

**a** At a pacing rate of 100 BPM, Wenckebach periodicity appears

**b** Attempt to terminate flutter by A00 pacing at 400 BPM. Markers are displayed by the programmer

**c** Flutter has been converted and the pacing rate is now programmed at 200 BPM

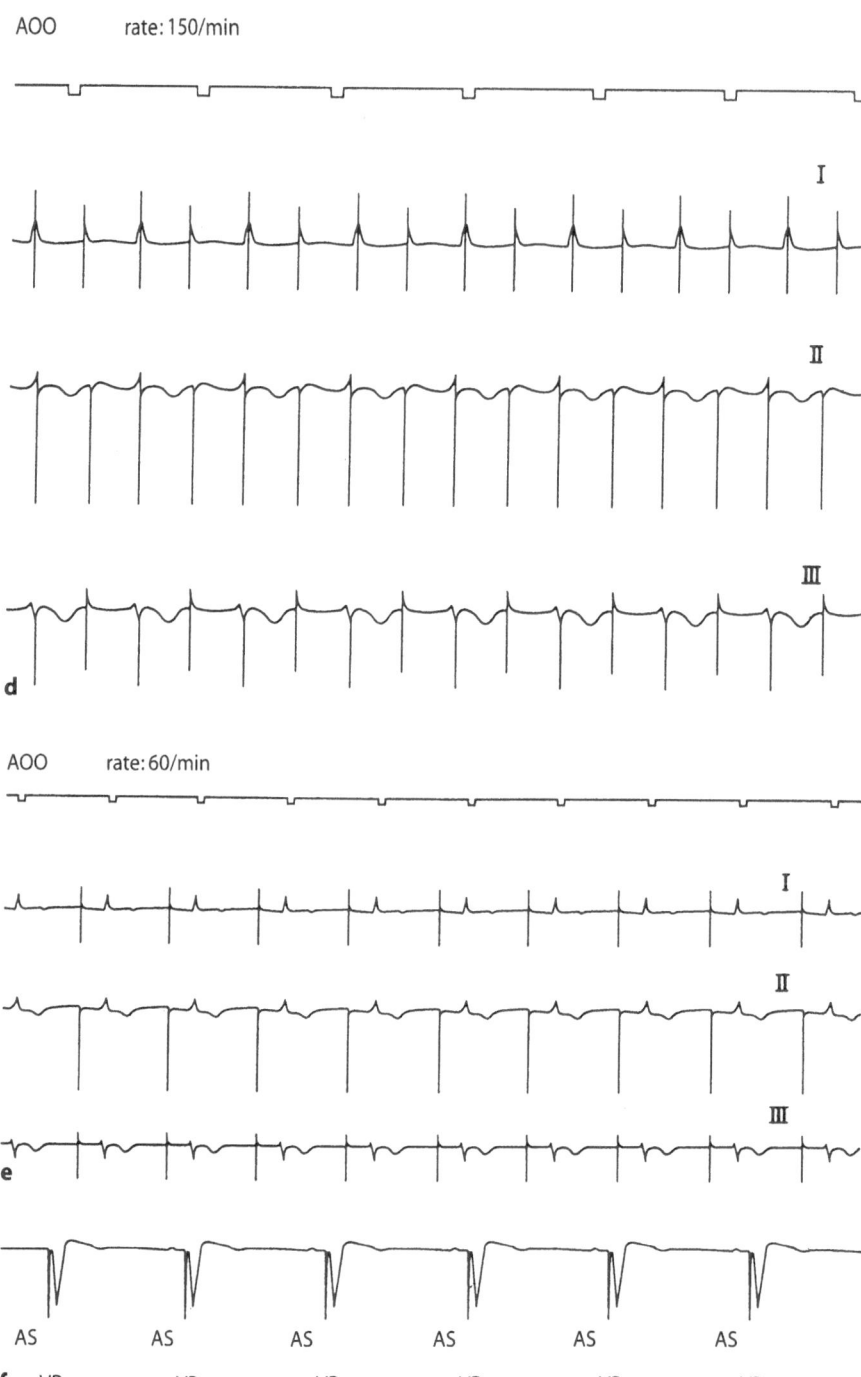

**Fig. 3.93. d–f** An old Symbios 7005 (Medtronic) pacemaker is used to deliver temporary
**d** At a rate of 150 BPM, 2 : 1 block is noted
**e** At 60 BPM, the patient is continuously paced in A00 mode with 1 : 1 conduction
**f** DDD mode with event markers
*AP* atrial pacing; *AS* atrial sensing; *VP* ventricular pacing

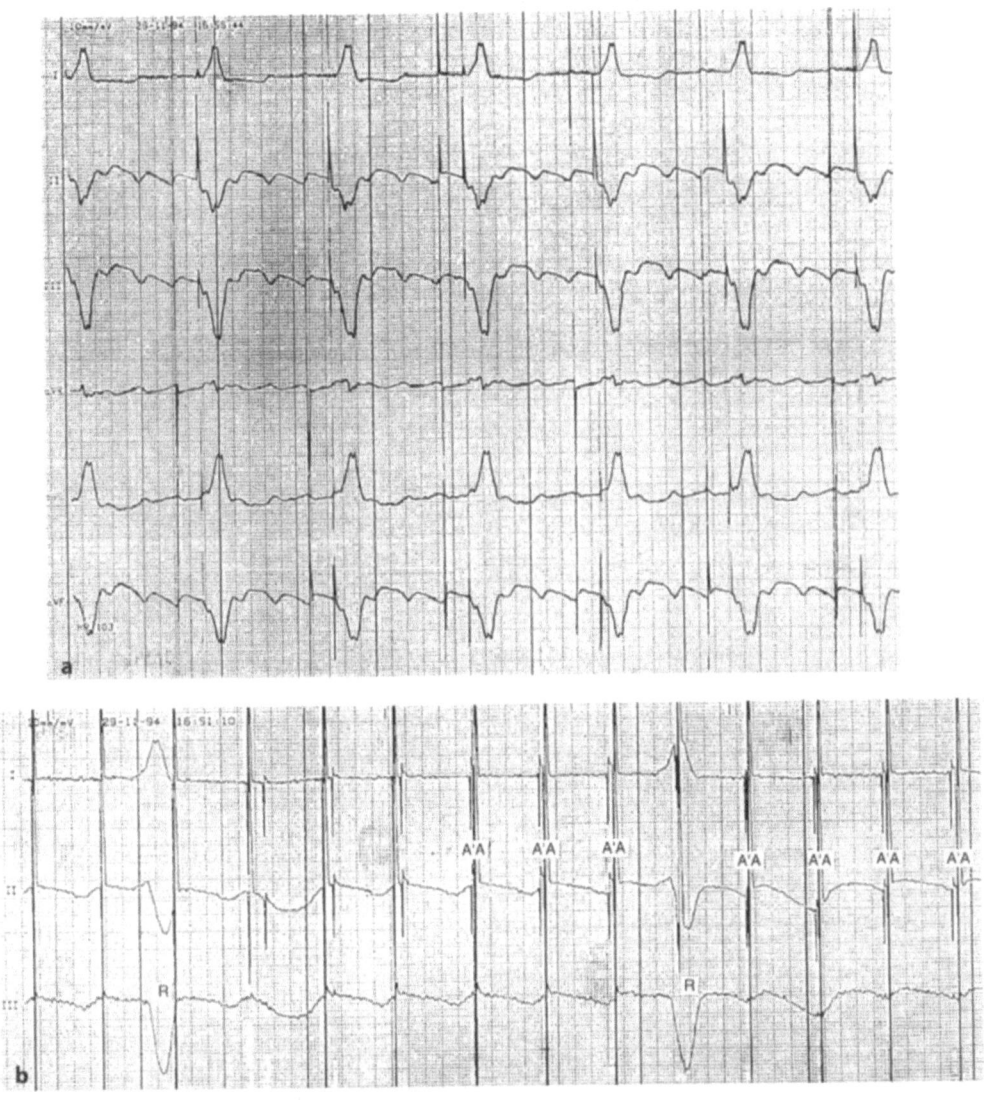

**Fig. 3.94. a** Atrial flutter with atrial rate at 270 BPM on surface ECG
**b** Flutter was terminated by external stimulation driving a Chorus 6034 (ELA Medical) implanted pacemaker in AAT mode with unipolar atrial sensitivity programmed at 0.4 mV. Two electrodes were placed on the patient's thorax (positive near the pacemaker can, negative over the distal atrial electrode). Ten cycles of high output pacing at a rate of 300 BPM were applied while the heart rate limitation suppression function was temporarily activated. Stimulus artifacts from the external device (*A'*) and spikes from the permanent pacemaker (*A*) are visible

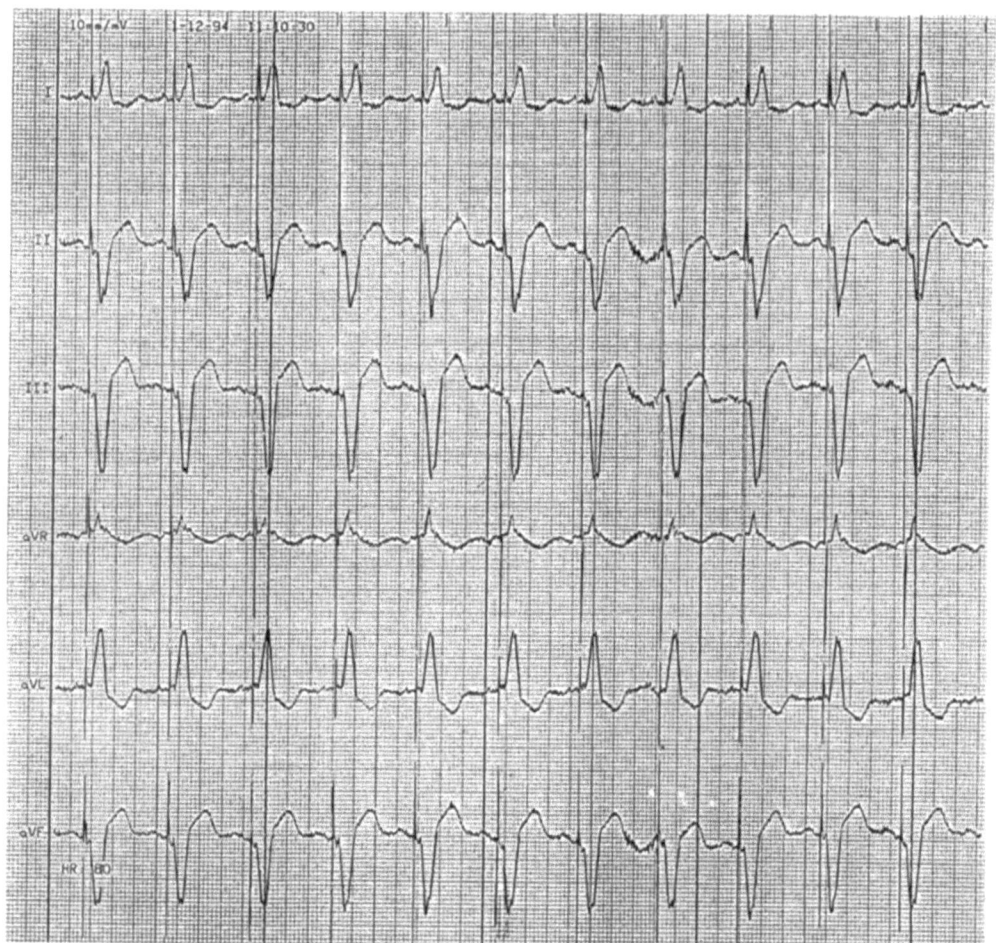

**Fig. 3.94. c** This maneuver restored sinus rhythm

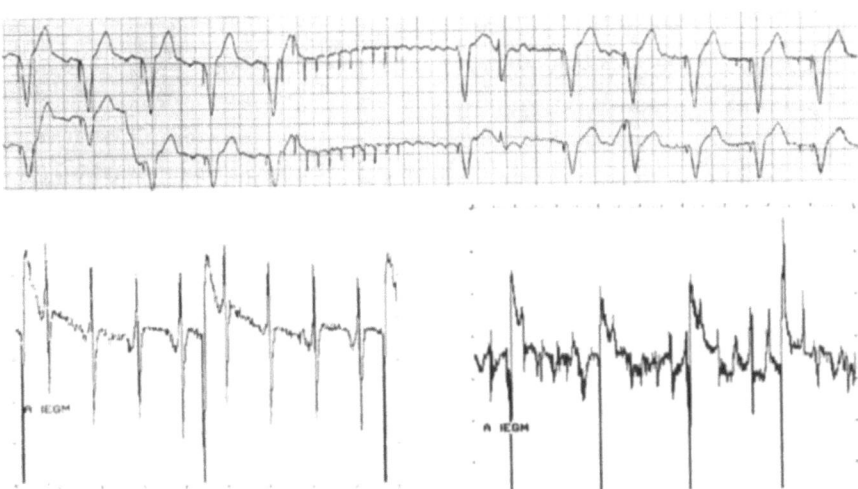

**Fig. 3.95.** Attempts to terminate a tachyarrhythmia in a patient with a pacemaker implanted for complete AV block must be made with great caution. In this example, esophageal pacing to convert atrial flutter causes inhibition of the pacemaker. Note that atrial flutter was converted to atrial fibrillation

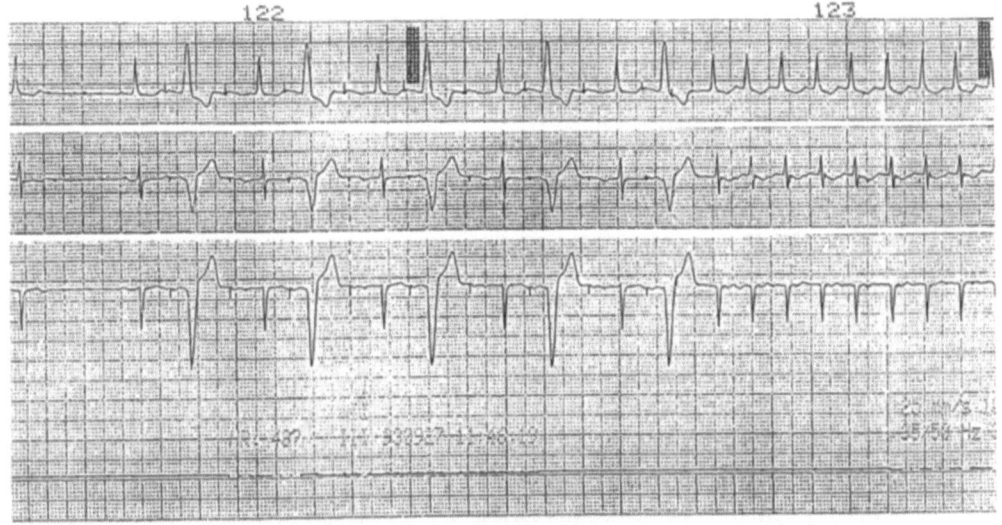

**Fig. 3.96. a** Example of utilization of an implanted pacemaker as an electrophysiologic device (Chorus II, ELA Medical). An atrial extrastimulus during paced rhythm at a cycle length of 600 ms induces AV junctional reentrant tachycardia. Recording speed = 25 mm/s

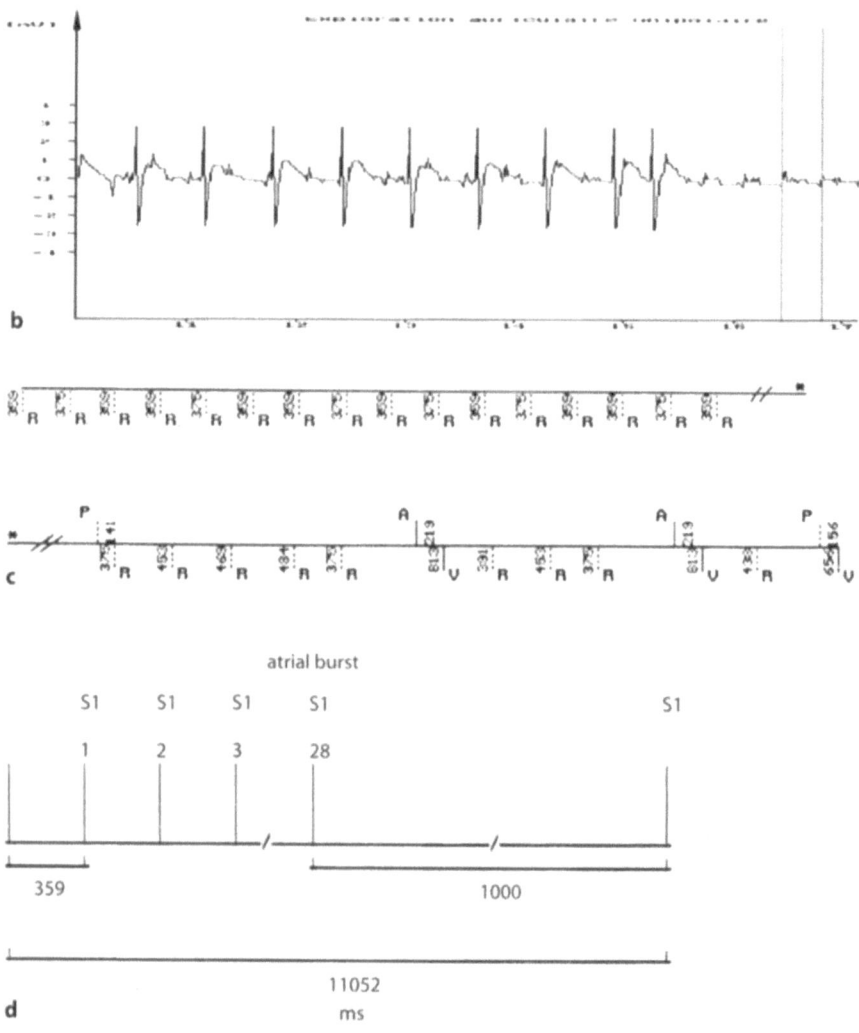

**Fig. 3.96. b** Examination of the intracardiac electrograms: the tachycardia induced has a cycle length of 375 ms

**c** The memory-based marker channel has recorded a ventricular cycle length of 360 to 375 ms. Due to the induced AV junctional reentrant tachycardia, P waves falling in the absolute refractory period are not sensed (no corresponding atrial marker)

**d** Programming of stimulation protocol on programmer screen: 28 cycles delivered at a cycle length of 359 ms

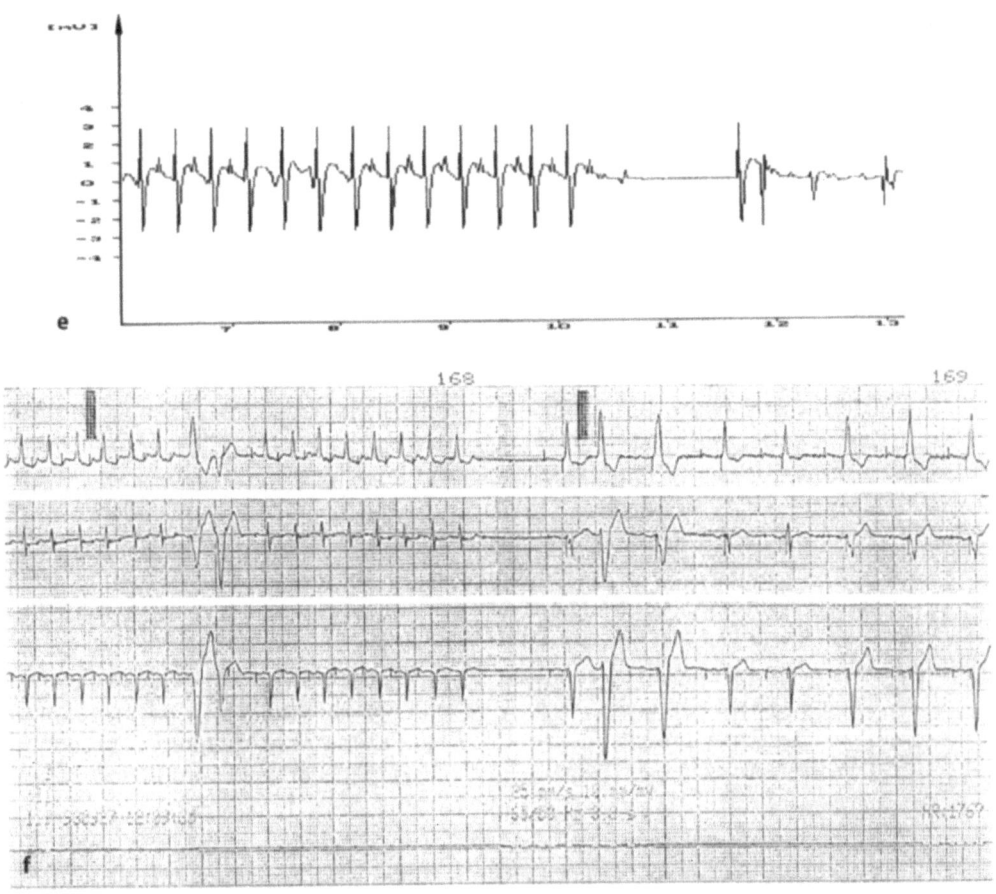

**Fig. 3.96. e** Examination of intracardiac electrocardiogram: tachycardia termination
**f** Surface ECG recording during programmed stimulation procedure
*A* atrial pacing; *P* P wave sensing; *V* ventricular pacing; *R* ventricular sensing

# Chapter 4

# Indications for Permanent Pacing and Choice of Pacemaker

The indications for the implantation of a permanent pacemaker should be clear cut. A poor indication, or the choice of an inappropriate system may have disastrous consequences (see p. 187, pacemaker syndrome), and discredit the treatment. When considered for a patient suffering from an incurable illness, each case must be evaluated individually, including the patient, family and referring physician in the decision making process.

When the decision of implanting a permanent pacemaker has been made for a specific indication, the optimal pacing system needs to be chosen. Old age, or various underlying illnesses, are not, a priori, contraindications to the implant of a sophisticated pacemaker. Elderly patients may benefit greatly from such systems which may provide them with a better exercise capacity, more autonomy, and greater well-being. The main goal of cardiac pacing is to prevent death from cardiac standstill, though control of circulatory and neurologic symptoms due to bradycardia is an important aim as well. Nowadays, besides the classic electrocardiologic diagnoses, new, primarily hemodynamic indications for pacing have emerged.

The diagnosis and the choice of a pacemaker hinge on a thorough knowledge of the patient's medical history and a few tests:

- Physical examination
- Resting electrocardiogram, including during carotid sinus massage
- Chest radiograph

Then, according to the serial results of the tests, the following should be carried out:

- 24 h ambulatory electrocardiogram
- Atropin test
- Echocardiogram
- Upright tilt-table test
- Electrophysiologic study

# 4.1
# History and Investigation

## Clinical History

This is the most important diagnostic element. A classic history consists of Stokes-Adams attacks, i.e. sudden loss of consciousness, without prodrome, often with injury, sometimes associated with urinary incontinence and seizure, of short duration and followed by a rapid return of full consciousness without post-ictal state. Other cardinal symptoms consist of near syncope or lightheadedness, particularly when paroxysmal. On the other hand, a confused mental status would only be attributable to bradycardia if it is corrected by temporary pacing or clears up during periods of normal rhythm.

A slow pulse measured during or just after syncope must be interpreted with caution since it may be secondary to a vaso-vagal reaction, or incessant bigeminy, or even to a post tachycardia bradycardia. Conversely, bradycardia may precipitate the occurrence of atrial or ventricular arrhythmias which may cause palpitation, thromboembolic complications or transient ischemic events. However, the diagnosis of bradycardia-induced tachycardia can only be made after several episodes have been documented. In many individuals (not just trained athletes) a predominant vagal tone may cause resting, asymptomatic bradycardia as slow as 40 BPM, and does not represent an indication for pacing. In contrast, rates below 40 BPM usually cause symptoms. Athletes must be considered separately (particularly those engaged in endurance sports), whose bradycardia does not interfere with physical performance, but who may develop symptoms as in the following example.

CASE STUDY

*Example.* An athlete has suddenly interrupted his routine training, consisting of 200 km/week of cross country jogging, to build a house. He began to experience brief syncopal spells with alarming bradycardia while driving his automobile. A pacemaker would not have been helpful in his case since the symptoms were not only due to bradycardia, but also to some degree of autonomic dysregulation. The gradual resumption of his physical training resulted in the disappearance of symptoms.

A further example illustrates the occurrence of unusual symptoms, of a psychiatric nature, due to bradycardia.

CASE STUDY

*Example.* A 35 year old, depressed woman has been under psychiatric care for 6 months. She, until then, had mentioned neither syncope nor lightheadedness. A resting electrocardiogram, obtained by her family physician showed third degree atrioventricular block with a ventricular escape rhythm at a rate of 40 BPM. The etiology of this block remained unclear despite a complete evaluation. Following implantation of permanent dual chamber pacemaker, all psychiatric symptoms resolved and the patient returned to her usual activities.

Congestive heart failure is rarely attributable to bradycardia, except when it occurs in the context of a diseased heart and precipitates cardiac decompensation. Likewise, chronotropic incompetence is an indication for permanent pacing only in presence of typical symptoms.

Certain types of bradycardia are only temporary and do not require permanent pacing:

- Digitalis intoxication, particularly if combined with hypokalemia
- Intoxication with other antiarrhythmic drugs of any class
- Intoxication with psychotropic medications such as lithium, tricyclics and benzodiazepins. Some medications are administered in unusual formulations which may have important systemic effects, such as ophtalmic preparations which may contain a beta adrenergic blocker
- Metabolic or endocrine disorders

Sleep apnea may cause conduction disturbances which may have to be treated if persistent despite treatment of the sleep disorder.

## Physical Examination

The physical examination looks for signs of cardiac decompensation secondary to bradycardia, underlying heart disease, or an extracardiac source of conduction abnormality.

### Resting and Ambulatory Electrocardiogram

The surface electrocardiogram is key in the diagnosis of the arrhythmia and orients toward further diagnostic steps. Holter monitoring over 24 h is an important electrocardiographic complement. Transesophageal recordings may be useful to diagnose unusual rhythm disturbances and for a simple assessment of sinus and AV nodal functions.

### Exercise Testing

Exercise testing is useful to identify chronotropic incompetence (which would prompt the choice of a rate responsive pacemaker), as well as exercise-induced paroxysmal arrhythmias such as atrioventricular block, sino-atrial block during recovery, or miscellaneous tachyarrhythmias.

### Atropin Test

An insufficient increase in sinus rate after the injection of atropin, 1 mg i.v., can assist in the diagnosis of sinus node dysfunction. The test is in support of a sick sinus node if the resulting rate increases by less than 25% of the baseline rate, or does not go beyond 90 BPM within 5 min after the injection (Blöhmer 1975). The usual contraindications to the use of atropin such as glaucoma or prostatic hypertrophy must be observed.

## Carotid Sinus Massage

Carotid sinus massage is important, particularly in absence of a precise diagnosis. At first, brisk head movements are prompted while an electrocardiogram is recorded. If symptoms occur that reproduce the spontaneous symptoms, the diagnosis is firmly supported. Otherwise carotid sinus massage should be carried out with caution since there is a risk of embolic complication from the break off of an atheromatous plaque. It is advised to regularly perform a doppler sonographic study of the carotid bifurcations, and to withhold the test if stenotic or ulcerated lesions are found. Moderate pressure should be applied for 5 s while continuously recording the electrocardiogram and the arterial pressure noninvasively during and after massage (Fig. 4.1). The test should be performed while the patient is supine and upright, and should be repeated at various times of the day given the well known variability of baroreflex responses.

## Upright Tilt-Table Testing

Upright tilt-table testing serves to provoke a vaso-vagal reaction. Arterial pressure and electrocardiogram should be continuously monitored while the patient rests supine on a tilt-table test for at least 20 min. The table is then tilted in the upright position (usually to a 60° angle) with the patient securely fastened to the table. Vaso-vagal reactions often appear within 25 and up to 45 min of the tilt, which should closely reproduce the patient's spontaneous symptomatology. Some clinicians perform the procedure with the addition of isoproterenol to increase the test's sensitivity, which is likely to be highest shortly after a spontaneous event.

## Invasive Testing

Invasive tests are indicated only when the tests described earlier have remained inconclusive. They should be preceded by a chest radiograph. Electrophysiologic studies of the sino-atrial node and of atrioventricular conduction involves the introduction of endovenous catheters under local anesthesia. The diagnostic information gathered by this type of testing has been briefly discussed on p. 11.

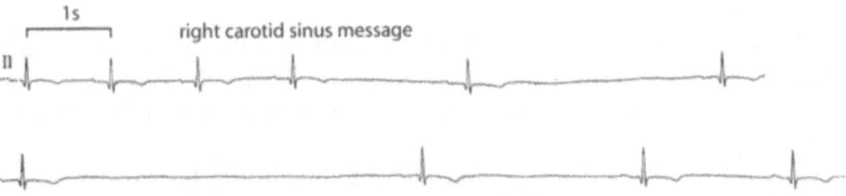

**Fig. 4.1.** Carotid massage causing asystole for several seconds

## 4.2
## Temporary Cardiac Pacing

Before scheduling the implant of a permanent pacemaker it is essential to establish that the conduction disturbance is not caused by an acute, reversible process which would only require temporary pacing.

## Indications

During the acute phase of myocardial infarction, various conduction disturbances may occur. Sino-atrial conduction abnormalities develop most often after occlusion of the right coronary artery; pacing is only needed in presence of symptoms, or if aggravation of the bradycardia is expected from the initiation of treatment with negatively chronotropic medications. Nonresponse of the bradycardia to atropin may be another criterion justifying the placement of a temporary pacing lead.

All forms of atrioventricular block may be encountered. In inferior infarction, conduction disturbances, usually gradual in their development, are often associated with narrow QRS escape rhythms at rates between 50 and 60/min of nodal or hisian origin. In such cases, temporary pacing is only justified in presence of poor hemodynamic tolerance of the slow ventricular rhythm. Conversely, if the atrioventricular conduction disturbance (type I or II second degree, or third degree AV block) is associated with wide QRS complexes, temporary pacing is indicated because of the risk of sudden hemodynamic deterioration.

Finally, in all cases of atrioventricular conduction disorders associated with infarction of the right ventricle, dual chamber (or VDD if sinus node function is preserved) pacing has the best chance of improving hemodynamics. In anterior infarction, atrioventricular block develops often suddenly, and temporary dual chamber pacing is usually needed for hemodynamic reasons. The development of left bundle branch, or of bi- or trifascicular block may signal the need for prophylactic temporary pacing. In critical cases, consideration should be given to emergency revascularization.

In the postoperative phase of cardiac surgery, temporary pacing, often useful, is performed via epicardial electrodes left in place at the time of operation.

In infective endocarditis, particularly that involving the noncoronary aortic cusp (since it is closest to the nodo-hisian conduction system), the occurrence of first degree atrioventricular, or of left bundle branch, block dictates temporary pacing. Likewise in acute myocarditis which often masquerades acute myocardial infarction.

Neck tumors involving the carotid sinus, or surgery of the carotid bifurcation, can cause temporary conduction disturbances, as well as the local effects of some treatments such as radiation therapy, all representing legitimate indications for temporary pacing.

Lyme's disease is a chronic systemic illness caused by tick bites received several weeks or months earlier. It causes a pathognomonic skin rash, followed, in various combinations, by joint and neurologic involvement, myocarditis or myo-pericarditis. In presence of the latter complication, a right ventricular biopsy allows the recovery of spirochetes and, in up to 85% of cases, various degrees of atrioventricular conduction abnormalities appear. Serologic tests may be of help in the diagnosis. The treatment of Lyme's disease consists of tetracyclin, doxy-cyclin or amoxicillin; the conduction abnormalities are transient and require temporary pacing only.

Some have recommended the placement of a temporary pacemaker lead dur-ing right heart catheterization in patients with preexistent left bundle branch block, in the event of additional, traumatically induced, right bundle branch block. Conversely, in case of left heart catheterization in a patient with preexis-tent right bundle branch block, the risk of inducing complete heart block is neg-ligible. Following injection of contrast material into the right coronary artery, brief cardiac standstill is not unusual which does not justify prophylactic tempo-rary pacing. This risk is slightly higher during coronary angioplasty procedures and should be anticipated.

To undergo general anesthesia, prophylactic temporary pacing is rarely justi-fied, even in the case of first degree AV block combined with bifascicular block. On the other hand, previous unexplained syncope associated with obvious con-duction abnormalities may be a reason to consider intraoperative prophylactic temporary pacing.

Some chemical agents with negative chronotropic properties (particularly anti-arrhythmic drugs), or metabolic disorders are typical reasons to offer temporary pacing while waiting for the resolution of secondary conduction abnormalities.

Temporary cardiac pacing is also used to prevent, not a cardiac arrest, but major bradycardia-dependent tachyarrhythmias. A typical example consists of torsades de pointe, in which one of the most effective preventive measures is often rapid (> 100 BPM) pacing. This tachyarrhythmia, which is often of toxic or iatrogenic origin, is due to abnormally long refractory periods resulting in a marked prolongation of the QT interval.

*Temporary pacing may be indicated:*

- During the acute phase of myocardial infarction; a watch – and – wait approach may rather be assumed with AV blocks associated with a posterior wall infarc-tion, whereas with an anterior wall infarction a complete AV block (with a poor prognosis) can occur relatively abruptly without corresponding warning signs
- As a precautionary measure in the postoperative phase of heart surgery
- In complicated cases of bacterial endocarditis or acute myocarditis involving the conduction system
- In the presence of neck tumors or neck surgery
- In the presence of local irritations in the carotid body following radiation therapy
- Because of AV conduction disturbances associated with Lyme disease, in which only temporary blocks will usually occur
- As a result of interventional procedures such as percutaneous transluminal coronary angioplasty (PTCA) of the right coronary artery

- Because of intoxication, side defects, or overdose of negative chronotropic medications
- In the presence of electrolyte imbalance
- During resuscitation
- As a temporary measure in the presence of symptomatic bradyarrhythmias until a permanent pacemaker system is implanted
- Because of pacing system malfunctions and complications such as pacemaker sepsis requiring removal of the system
- For performing overdrive pacing in the presence of recurrent ventricular tachycardias, like in the treatment of torsade de pointe
- Previous unexplained syncope associated with obvious conduction abnormalities
- To prevent, not a cardiac arrest, but major bradycardia-dependent tachyarrhythmias
- Temporary stimulation involving the atrium (DVI, DDD.) is preferable for patients with heart failure. A temporary single lead VDD system is suitable for transient AV conduction disturbances

## Techniques of Temporary Pacing

Several techniques are available to perform temporary pacing, which have evolved considerably and benefited from the techniques used in cardiac electrophysiologic studies and in permanent pacing. Only the techniques used in cardiac pacing with the goal of correcting symptoms due to bradycardia, or of limiting the risk of sudden death by stimulation of the heart will be discussed. These techniques are, without saying, associated with other methods of cardiac massage and emergency ventilation.

### Mechanical Stimulation

Chest thump and cough can both interrupt prolonged cardiac standstill. Chest thump, which consists of vigorously hitting the patient's sternum with closed fist, is effective if applied soon after the onset of cardiac arrest. Cough, also able to cause powerful mechanical stimulation, can only be used during the first seconds of the cardiac arrest. This method, implemented by the conscious patient himself, is familiar to coronary angiographers who use it when the injection of iodine contrast material into the coronary artery causes a prolonged cardiac pause.

### Transcutaneous Electrical Stimulation

An external pacing device is connected to patch electrodes placed on the thorax after cleaning of the skin. The stimulator delivers pulses of 20 to 25 ms duration to reduce the pacing energy and, thereby, the chances of striated muscle stimulation. On average, the current needed to achieve effective 1 : 1 cardiac pacing is 20 to 80 mA. The electrodes have a wide surface coated with a high conductivity gel which reduces the pulse strength necessary to achieve satisfactory capture. The cathode is placed anteriorly between the left nipple and the sternum, and the posterior anode is placed between the spine and the scapula. The electrodes may have to be repositioned to obtain the lowest pacing threshold by avoiding the interposition of bony structures. The stimulation mode is V00 or VVI. The heart is paced approximately 40 ms after delivery of the pulse, and the hemodynamic results are close to those obtained with endocavitary right ventricular pacing. This technique can be implemented very rapidly, does not interfere with closed chest massage and is safe from the standpoint of the rescuers.

Striated muscle stimulation is an adverse effect usually acceptable to the patient for a few hours, sometimes longer, never for days as has been reported. This technique does not cause a rise in cardiac enzymes, nor any other serious complication, including arrhythmias even in presence of acute infarction or cardiomyopathy.

Causes of high pacing thresholds include

- Just-ended cardiac surgery because of residual air left in the pericardium or mediastinum
- Emphysema
- Positive end-expiratory pressure
- Pericardial effusion
- Hypoxia, and
- Acute myocardial ischemia or
- Infarction
  Despite these obstacles, transcutaneous stimulation can be successfully accomplished in 90% of cases.

### Transesophageal Stimulation

Some authors have described the use of this simple pacing method in emergency, while waiting for a more reliable and more subjectively tolerable technique.

### Endocardial Stimulation

The temporary pacing technique of choice remains the placement of a transvenous temporary lead connected to an external pacing device. This requires an experienced operator prepared to face complications. The equipment used depends on the chamber that needs to be paced. Bipolar, platinum electrodes (J shaped or „screw-in" for the right atrium) are mounted on 5 or 6 Fr leads that must be rigid enough to be maneuverable through the cardiac chambers. Placement of the electrode is accomplished in the electrophysiology laboratory or the operating room, under local anesthesia, with fluoroscopic guidance, and by Seldinger's technique (described on p. 208). Table 4.1 summarizes the advantages and drawbacks of the various venous accesses.

The pacing threshold should be less than 1 mA or 1 V, and the sensing threshold should be 5 mV or higher in the ventricle, and 1 mV or higher in the atrium.

**Table 4.1.** Temporary endocardial pacing: venous access

| | Means of venous access | | | | |
| | Basilic | External jugular | Internal jugular | Subclavian | Femoral |
|---|---|---|---|---|---|
| **Advantages** | | | | | |
| 1 | Reduced risk of infection | Stability | Stability | Stability | Ease of placement |
| 2 | No risk of venous puncture | Low risk of venous puncture | Low TE risk | Patient comfort | |
| 3 | | Low TE risk | | Reduced risk of infection | |
| **Disadvantages** | | | | | |
| 1 | Catheterization may be difficult | Catheterization may be difficult | Risk of carotid puncture | Risk of pneumothorax | Risk of arterial puncture |
| 2 | Instability | Discomfort | Discomfort | Risk of femoral puncture | Risk of nerve lesion |
| 3 | | | | Requires trained operator | Instabililty |
| 4 | | | | | High TE risk |

A single ventricular lead is usually sufficient, though in cases of acute infarction (particularly of the right ventricle), of hypertrophic or dilated cardiomyopathy, or postoperatively, dual chamber or single lead VDD pacing may yield remarkable hemodynamic results.

Complications are common, particularly lead dislodgment, and include atrial and ventricular arrhythmias, threshold rise, local and systemic infection, and rare myocardial perforation with tamponnade.

Mention will also be made of transcoronary pacing which, in emergent situations, may be life-saving by pacing the ventricle through an intracoronary guiding sheath.

### Transthoracic Pacing

The last resort consists of epicardial pacing via transthoracic electrodes. This technique, which requires considerable experience, has been largely replaced by transcutaneous and endocardial pacing, except in the cardiac postoperative period, when it is accomplished via electrodes placed during the operation.

# 4.3
# Permanent Cardiac Pacing

The indications have been listed in a few publications which summarize the recommendations from various task forces: the American College of Cardiology and American Heart Association, published in 1984 and revised in 1991, the French Cardiac Pacing Group in 1986, the British Pacing and Electrophysiology Group in 1991, and the Working Group in Cardiac Pacing from the German Cardiology Society in 1991 and 1996. When the indication is unequivocal, it is ranked as class 1; when it is typical, but debatable on the basis of individual characteristics (patient's general condition, limited prognosis, opposition by the patient or the family, etc.) it is ranked as class 2. Class 3 denotes the absence of indications by consensus.

## Pacing Indications Based on Abnormal Electrocardiogram

### Sino-Atrial Dysfunction

Sino-atrial dysfunction may take several forms, including

- Isolated sinus node dysfunction
- Sino-atrial block
- Alternans of bradycardia and tachycardia (bradycardia-tachycardia syndrome) often associated with post tachycardia pauses, and
- Chronotropic incompetence (see p. 11)

The indication for implantation rests mainly on the surface ECG, particularly serial Holter recordings, rarely on the results of invasive electrophysiologic studies. In cases of chronotropic incompetence, the amount of sinus node acceleration, and the impact of the incompetence during exercise have to be measured. In the case of sinus node dysfunction, survival is not lengthened by cardiac pacing, but the clinical situation is improved.

Class 1    The implantation of a permanent pacemaker is indicated when sino-atrial dysfunction causes cardiac or cerebral symptoms consisting of lightheadedness, syncope, cardiac insufficiency, angina pectoris, palpitation, as well as changes in brain functions in the form of decrease in concentration or thought process, memory loss, or even a cerebral vascular accident. Sinus bradycardia or sino-atrial block at a rate below 40 BPM, or intermittent sinus pauses are considered class 1 indications if clearly associated with symptoms.

Class 2    A permanent pacemaker may be indicated in cases of moderate sinus node dysfunction associated with chronotropic incompetence during exercise (the cause of exertional dyspnea), or symptomatic sinus bradycardia due to drug therapy that cannot be withhold. For example, in the bradycardia-tachycardia syndrome, periods of atrial tachyarrhythmia must be suppressed with antiarrhythmic drugs which can only be given after a permanent pacemaker has been implanted.

Class 3    Asymptomatic sinus bradycardia, or all instances in which symptoms cannot be related to sinus node dysfunction are not indications for permanent pacing. As already mentioned, sinus pauses up to 3 s can be present in normal individuals as well as marked sinus bradycardia, particularly in trained athletes.

### Atrioventricular Block

Atrioventricular conduction disturbances are divided into

- First degree AV block
- Mobitz type I (Wenckebach) second degree AV block (progressive prolongation of the PR interval until a block occurs)
- Mobitz type II second degree AV block (single P waves that are not conducted with constant PR intervals occurring before and after the block)
- 2 : 1 and higher grade AV block
- Third degree (complete heart block) AV block

Permanent cardiac pacing for atrioventricular block does no only improve quality of life, but also long-term prognosis. Atrioventricular conduction disturbances include fixed or intermittent atrioventricular block at the level of the atrioventricular node, the His bundle, or below the His bundle. Conduction blocks below the His bundle are less well tolerated than more proximal ones. The QRS complex is larger since the site of subsidiary impulse formation is more distal (see p. 15) with a bundle branch block morphology. This distortion of depolarization is accompanied by an alteration of ventricular contraction synchrony and its known detrimental hemodynamic effect which is independent of the bradycardia. Consideration for pacing hinges on symptoms as well as on the nature of the electrophysiologic disorder.

Isolated first degree AV block or Mobitz I second degree AV block at rest with narrow QRS complex are a priori manifestations of mild alterations of AV nodal conduction. In absence of symptoms, these abnormalities have no prognostic significance. In the event of symptoms and/or in case of associated bundle branch block, intracardiac electrophysiologic investigations are warranted.

In contrast, the Mobitz type II second degree AV block and the acquired third degree AV block with a broad QRS complex are usually situated within or below the bundle of His. In patients with a complete heart block and Stokes-Adams attacks, mortality is high. Pacemaker therapy greatly improves the survival prognosis, although it is somewhat worse as compared to the normal population due to the underlying cardiac disease.

The indication for pacing in the presence of AV blocks depends on the symptoms and prognosis. In this context it should be considered that the acquired forms of third degree AV block and advanced AV block are generally associated with symptoms and thus require pacing. Pacemaker implantation is also indicated in the rare form of a *symptomatic* Wenckebach block (Mobitz type I second degree AV block).

In contrast, the *congenital* complete AV block often remains asymptomatic for a long time. Exercise testing or atropin may result in disappearance of block, marker of a benign prognosis and, consequently, no need for permanent pacing. In a prospective study, however, the risk of Stokes-Adams attacks and sudden cardiac death was increased at every age and even in the absence of poor prognostic signs, so that prophylactic pacemaker implantation was recommended.[1] In the literature, a watch and wait approach is recommended and annual follow up examinations should be performed. Although reliable criteria for assessing the risks are lacking, a pacemaker should be implanted in the presence of associated anatomic heart disease, mean heart rates less than 50 $min^{-1}$, little or no change in the junctional rate with physical activity, asystoles at night, an escape rhythm with broad QRS complexes, frequent ventricular ectopies, a prolonged QT interval, cardiomegaly, limited left ventricular function, or enlarged atria.

Prognostic indications should also be observed in asymptomatic patients with an *acquired* AV block. In a third degree AV block, this includes broad QRS complexes, a slow escape rhythm, spontaneous asystoles, and frequent ventricular ectopies. Pacemaker implantation is indicated in the presence of a Mobitz II second degree AV block, a 2 : 1 block, and higher degree AV blocks when they are accompanied by QRS broadening. The prognostic indication is controversial in the case of an asymptomatic second degree AV block with narrow QRS complexes including a Wenckebach block with frequent blocks during the day. The recommendations of the BPEG regard this as a general indication, whereas the ACC/AHA recommendations define the asymptomatic second degree AV block as a relative indication and require evidence of a block within or below the bundle of His for the Mobitz I (Wenckebach) block.

Occasional AV conduction blocks, particularly at night or occurring simultaneously with an increase in the sinus cycle lengths, are primarily the result of increased vagal tone and usually do not require pacemaker therapy.

Class 1   The indication is unequivocal in third degree AV block, Mobitz II second degree AV block or „high degree" AV block, whether fixed or paroxysmal and symptomatic.

Class 2   Third degree and second degree AV blocks, 2 : 1 or higher grade blocks with narrow QRS complexes in asymptomatic patients. Pacing is advised, but needs scrutiny when AV block is asymptomatic, in distal Mobitz I second degree AV block, in symptomatic Mobitz I second degree AV block, or when a negatively dromotropic treatment needs to be prescribed, whether or not symptoms are present.

Class 3   Pacing is not indicated for *asymptomatic* first degree, or Mobitz I second degree AV block (Wenckebach type).

1 Michaëlsson M, Jonzon A, Riesenfeld T (1995) Isolated congenital complete atrioventricular block in adult life. A prospective study. Circulation 92: 442–449

## Bi- and Trifascicular Blocks

These are conduction disturbances affecting two or three branches or hemibranches of the His-Purkinje system. Bifascicular block combines

- Right bundle branch block and left posterior fascicular block
- Right bundle branch block and left anterior fascicular block
- Left bundle branch block with marked left axis deviation of the QRS complex

First degree AV block is present in nearly one quarter of such cases. Trifascicular block combines one of these findings with a prolonged HV interval, or alternating right and left bundle branch block, or right bundle branch block with alternating left posterior and left anterior fascicular block.

In bifascicular block, syncope is infrequent, rarely attributable to paroxysmal AV block, and often an isolated event in the patient's history. Second and third degree AV block is more likely in the context of syncope. Mortality is high, though often attributable to the underlying heart disease. Permanent pacing does not invariably control the symptoms, illustrating the difficulty in establishing their link with paroxysmal bradycardia. Therefore, in absence of typical Stokes-Adams attacks, intracardiac recordings are needed. An HV interval equal to or longer than 70 ms is considered to indicate a risk of progression of the conduction disorder toward Mobitz II second degree, or third degree AV block.

The test can be rendered more sensitive by atrial pacing maneuvers, or by drugs that are not contraindicated. Under such conditions, the appearance of Mobitz II second degree, or third degree AV block, or the prolongation of the HV interval beyond 100 ms are reliable indicators of a risk of spontaneous appearance of higher degrees of AV block.

Class 1   The indication for permanent pacing is unequivocal in cases of symptomatic alternating bundle branch block.

Class 2   The indication hinges on the type of symptoms and on the results of invasive electrophysiologic measurements in cases of asymptomatic alternating bundle branch block, of bifascicular block with or without first degree AV block, and with manifestations of transient cerebral ischemia.

Class 3   There is no indication for permanent pacing in asymptomatic bifascicular block with or without first degree AV block.

## Bradyarrhythmia in the Presence of Atrial Fibrillation

Patients with bradyarrhythmia in the presence of atrial fibrillation represent a very heterogeneous patient population. The arrhythmia is often associated with severe underlying damage to the myocardium. Also after pacemaker implantation, the survival prognosis remains significantly limited due to the underlying cardiac disease. Special consideration should be given to hemodynamic and drug – related factors when deciding on pacemaker therapy. Pauses up to 2.8 s during the day and 4 s during the night in the presence of chronic atrial fibrillation without clinical symptoms may be regarded as „normal findings" of a bra-dyarrhythmia. The diagnosis is based on the (Holter) ECG recording of a slow ventricular rate or long pauses. Atrial fibrillation can be a sign of a sick sinus syndrome, the latter being diagnosable only after cardioversion. In newly occur-ring atrial fibrillation a determination should be made whether cardioversion is possible and indicated. The indication for oral anticoagulant therapy in patients with atrial fibrillation must be observed.

Class 1    Atrial fibrillation with a slow ventricular rate or long pauses clearly associated with symptoms of reduced cerebral perfusion or heart fail-ure

Class 2    Atrial fibrillation with a slow ventricular rate (less than 40 min$^{-1}$) or long pauses (exceeding 3 – 4 s) and suspected correlation with clinical symptoms

Class 3    Asymptomatic bradyarrhythmia even when the rate drops below 40 min$^{-1}$ or individual RR intervals exceed 3 s

## Indications for Permanent Pacing in the Pediatric Patient

The indications to implant a permanent pacemaker in the pediatric patient have broadened as a result of technological progress in the form of smaller devices and better tolerated leads.

Class 1    Symptomatic congenital complete AV block and postoperative third degree AV block are absolute indications for permanent pacing.

Class 2    This class includes relative indications such as asymptomatic intra- or subhisian second or third degree AV block, asymptomatic congenital complete heart block with a slow ventricular escape rate, sinus node dysfunction that is symptomatic or associated with other rhythm dis-turbances requiring antiarrhythmic drugs, and the Kearns-Sayres syndrome with bifascicular block (autosomal, dominant transmis-sion).

Class 3    Permanent pacing is not indicated in asymptomatic congenital com-plete AV block with narrow QRS complex and a ventricular escape rate that is normal for age, asymptomatic Mobitz I second degree AV block, transient postoperative complete heart block, and asymptom-atic postoperative bifascicular block.

## Indications for Implantation of a Permanent Pacemaker for Sino-Atrial and Intraventricular Conduction Disturbances After Acute Myocardial Infarction

Complete heart block, a classic complication during the acute phase of myocar-dial infarction, mandates temporary, but rarely permanent pacing. The progno-sis of conduction disturbances is more favorable after an inferior than an ante-rior infarction.

In inferior infarction, AV block appears gradually, lasts at the most 2 to 3 weeks, and resolves completely. It carries no long-term risk in absence of intrahisian block, though a watchful follow up is in order. In anterior infarction, bundle branch block often precedes complete AV block, and bundle branch block, perhaps associated with fascicular block may persist on the long-term. Such conduction defects are indicative of the severity of the necrosis. In other cases, third degree block occurs abruptly, without prodrome.

Class 1    Permanent pacing is unequivocally indicated in fixed third degree AV block persisting at least 2 weeks after myocardial infarction.

Class 2    The indications are equivocal after an anterior infarction when bundle branch block persists after complete heart block, or in presence of left bundle branch block with first degree AV block or prolonged HV interval, particularly if negatively dromotropic drugs need to be administered.

Class 3    Permanent pacing is not indicated in transient complete heart block without residual bundle branch block, or for residual bundle branch block after anterior infarction without preceding transient complete heart block.


## Indications for Permanent Pacing in Cases of Syncope with Normal or Near Normal Electrocardiogram

This is a common medical problem. Besides arrhythmic causes, three cardio-circulatory mechanisms must be thoroughly investigated as possible causes of syncope.


### Intrahisian Block

Paroxysmal intrahisian block must be particularly suspected and looked for during periods of sinus acceleration, for example during exercise.


### Carotid Sinus Syndrome

The hypersensitive carotid sinus syndrome may present in two varieties that are reproducible during carotid sinus massage, though somewhat unpredictably:

- A cardioinhibitor response (90% of cases) with sino-atrial depression and cardiac standstill for at least 3 s. Some degree of atrioventricular block is also present in 50% of cases. In such patients, an associated vasodepressive component with a 10 to 60 mm Hg drop in blood pressure is often present (Morley and Sutton 1984).
- A pure vasodepressive response (5%–10% of cases) characterized by an abrupt fall in arterial pressure (greater than 30 mm Hg), without measurable slowing of the heart rate.

The history reveals the occurrence of syncopal or near syncopal episodes during daily activities such as head turning, shaving, wearing a tie, etc. Asystolic periods may be reproduced by head or neck motions during ECG monitoring. The relationship between symptoms and hypersensitive carotid sinus may be more difficult to establish in absence of precipitating maneuvers, and requires the performance of carotid sinus massage (for contraindications, see p. 169), keeping in mind the unpredictability of the response to the test. Only 5% – 10% of patients suffer from a true hypersensitive carotid sinus syndrome, and only in presence of symptoms is permanent pacing justifiable. This syndrome represents approximately 1% of all indications for pacing.

Class 1    Pacing is unequivocally indicated for recurrent syncope with positive response to carotid sinus massage due to pure, or strongly predominant, cardioinhibition.

Class 2    Pacing may be considered for recurrent syncope without obvious precipitating cause, but long pauses during carotid sinus massage, and in absence of treatment facilitating such pauses, or in mixed (cardioinhibition and vasodepression) carotid sinus syndrome.

Class 3    Permanent pacing is not indicated in asymptomatic carotid sinus hypersensitivity, in presence of pure vasodepressive responses, or in lightheaded or dizzy patients with cardioinhibition but no history of syncope.

### Vaso-Vagal Syndrome

The vaso-vagal syndrome is distinct from carotid sinus hypersensitivity. Its etiology remains unclear. One theory invokes an adrenergic surge causing ventricular mechanoreceptors (C fibers) overstimulation, triggering compensatory hypervagotonia. This syndrome is characterized by abrupt syncope occurring at rest in the upright position, with sudden drop in arterial pressure and excessive bradycardia, sometimes preceded by cholinergic symptoms. Syncope may be reproduced during upright tilt-table testing. Reproduction of symptoms during the test along with the development of bradycardia, or even prolonged asystole, is an indication for permanent dual chamber pacing for recurrent syncope refractory to medical management with beta adrenergic blockers, anticholinergic drugs, disopyramide, theophyllin or serotonin inhibitors. Successful temporary pacing during tilt table testing may confirm the indication. However some investigators showed recently that repetition of head-up tilt tests (a kind of readaptation) could cure this syndrome.

### Unexplained Syncope

Abstention from permanent pacing is usually in order when, after extensive investigations, no cause has been found to explain the symptoms. In rare cases, recurrent unpredictable episodes of syncope force the implantation of a pacemaker, particularly if the episodes result in injury (while keeping in mind the known benign prognosis of multiple episodes of unexplained syncope). In such cases, the implant of a device equipped with bradycardia monitoring and diagnostic functions should be chosen, such as the Theorema 90 (Sorin) or Chorus (ELA Medical) whose RAM include a surveillance program (see p. 305 ff., 393). Once a bradycardic episode has been documented, confirming the diagnosis, the pacemaker may be reprogrammed according to usual guidelines.

## Bradyarrhythmias Following Heart Surgery

Transient bradyarrhythmias following heart surgery occur frequently enough to appear to justify routine implantation of temporary epimyocardial pacemaker electrodes during the surgical procedure. The indication for pacing becomes manifest generally only after the 14th postoperative day. After this period, higher grade AV blocks will no longer recede, particularly when there is a high probability that they are the result of the surgical procedure (this applies particularly to replacement of aortic valves or correction of congenital defects such as atrial or ventricular septum defects). Due to findings in individual patients who again developed a total AV block in the late postoperative phase, prophylactic implantation of a pacemaker is recommended in the presence of AV blocks which had persisted for some time. Sinus node dysfunction, generally observed after coronary artery surgery, should normalize by postoperative day 14. In determining whether permanent pacemaker therapy is indicated after cardiac surgery, the physician should follow the guidelines detailed in the individual chapters relating to the specific arrhythmia.

Class 1    Second or third degree AV block resulting from surgery
Class 2    Sinus node dysfunction with resulting hemodynamic instability that precludes mobilization and rehabilitation of the patient
Class 3    As a rule, all bradyarrhythmias during the first two weeks postoperatively
           All bradyarrhythmias associated with multiple organ failure

### Bradyarrhythmias Following Heart Transplants

AV blocks following heart transplants are rare; the low number of cases does not permit a recommendation.

The decision to implant a permanent pacemaker due to sinus node dysfunction following heart transplant is often made too early and thus too frequently. The decision should be made two weeks after the heart transplant at the earliest, yet is best made one month postoperatively. The chronotropic insufficiency present in all patients who have received heart transplants and the intact ventriculo-atrial conduction, which can almost always be demonstrated, appear to favor implantation of a rate adaptive pacemaker system involving the atrium.

Class 1    Symptomatic sinus node dysfunction persisting after the first postoperative month

Class 2    Symptomatic sinus node dysfunction after the first two weeks postoperatively but before the end of the first month, with resulting hemodynamic instability that precludes mobilization and rehabilitation of the patient and which cannot be controlled with medication

Class 3    All bradyarrhythmias within the first two weeks postoperatively

## New Indications

There are five remaining, unclassified, less frequent indications. The first three are accepted by most authors.

### Complete Heart Block Induced by His Bundle Ablation

Following ablation of the His bundle, usually performed to control excessively rapid ventricular rates due to atrial tachyarrhythmias refractory to antiarrhythmic medications, a choice must be made with respect to the type of pacemaker to implant, i.e. VVIR versus dual chamber with automatic mode switch. The former does not ever offer AV synchrony; the second does offer AV synchrony if there is any hope to maintain sinus rhythm.

### Obstructive Hypertrophic Cardiomyopathy

The goal of permanent pacing is to decrease the intraventricular gradient by reversing the sequence of ventricular activation, to improve ventricular filling, and to decrease mitral regurgitation. Several preliminary studies have reported good long-term results as long as the AV delay has been programmed long enough to preserve the A wave of active ventricular filling, and short enough to allow exclusive ventricular pacing.

This double objective may sometimes be reached only at the cost of a prolongation of the spontaneous PR interval, either by the introduction, or increase, of treatment with beta adrenergic blockers, or by biatrial pacing associated with ventricular pacing to abolish the interatrial delay, or by His bundle ablation. With variable combinations of these three methods, a hemodynamic benefit becomes quite obvious, with persistence, or even growth of a long-term improvement. Rare failures are usually observed in elderly patients suffering from marked left ventricular diastolic dysfunction

The two remaining indications are in the realm of clinical research.

### Prevention of Atypical Atrial Flutter

Atypical atrial flutter with major interatrial conduction defects may be prevented by dual atrial pacing according to Daubert's method (see p. 195 f.)

## Non-Obstructive, Dilated Cardiomyopathy

The long-term results of permanent pacing remain scanty and contradictory. The indication is strictly hemodynamic and the goal is to enhance patient comfort. The goal seems to be more attainable in presence of ventricular mechanical asynchrony with AV valvular regurgitation. One other avenue of research consists of multisite pacing to resynchronize the contraction of the ventricles. Such indications are the product of recent technical advances and could not have been conceived without the progress made in leads development, as well as in the devices' software.

## 4.4
## Choice of Pacemaker Model

Several factors must be considered, particularly the patient's life style and the symptoms history. A close cooperation between the primary physician and the implanting center is therefore critical.

The choice of a pacemaker model is a logical process (Table 4.2). The kind of conduction disturbance, its frequency of occurrence, the adaptation of the sinus rate with exercise, the presence of atrial electrical or mechanical abnormalities, age, exercise capacity and overall health status, and the underlying heart disease are all elements to be considered when choosing a device. Consideration of all these variables implies a thorough understanding of the patient's physiologic status, and of the advantages and shortcomings of the various modes of pacing.

## Physiology of the Paced Patient

Nowadays, the growing complexity of pacemakers allows to restore an almost entirely normal hemodynamic profile, whatever physiologic situations the patient may encounter during daily life (Fig. 4.2). Several factors intervene in the hemodynamic improvement offered by the implanted pacemaker: maintenance,

---

▷

[a] For example AMS AAI/DDD, or AVD scanning
[b] For example fall-back, AMS: DDD(R) → DDIR or VDIR (= VVIR). Even in absence of overt arrhythmias, empirical observations have shown that the incidence of atrial arrhythmias in sinus node dysfunction is high. AMS is therefore recommended
[c] The difficulties in diagnosing isolated AV conduction abnormalities, the absence of atrial pacing, drug-induced sinus bradycardia, and the problems inherent to the single VDD lead will be discussed with particular attention
[d] The VVI mode (with rate < 45 BPM) is acceptable if AV block is very rare and in absence of retrograde conduction
[e] For example AMS AAI/DDD with hysteresis (with or without rate acceleration, or a reaction to a drop in heart rate)

**Table 4.2.** Recommendations in the choice of a pacemaker

| Diagnosis | Optimal mode | Acceptable mode | Unacceptable mode |
|---|---|---|---|
| **Sinus node dysfunction** | | | |
| Without atrial arrhythmia | AAI(R)<br>DDD(R) with special algorithms[a,b]<br>DDI(R) | | VVI(R)<br>VDD(R) |
| Bradycardia-tachy-cardia syndrome; paroxysmal atrial arrhythmias | DDD(R) with special algorithms[b]<br>DDI(R) | AAI(R) | VVI(R)<br>VDD(R)<br>DDD(R) *without* special algorithms[b] |
| **AV block** | | | |
| Fixed | DDD | VDD[c] | AAI(R)<br>VVI(R)<br>DDI(R) |
| Intermittent | DDD with special algorithms[a] | DDD<br>VDD[c] | AAI(R)<br>VVI(R)[d]<br>DDI(R) |
| **Binodal disease** | | | |
| Without atrial arrhythmia | DDD(R)<br>DDD(R) with special algorithms[b] | DDD | VVI(R)<br>AAI(R)<br>VDD(R) |
| With paroxysmal atrial arrhythmias, after AV node/His ablation + paroxysmal atrial arrhythmias | DDD(R) with special algorithms[b] | | VVI(R)<br>AAI(R)<br>VDD(R)<br>DDI(R)<br>DDD(R) *without* special algorithms[b] |
| **Chronic atrial arrhythmias** with AV conduction disorder | VVI(R) | | AAI(R)<br>DDD(R)<br>VDD(R) |
| **Carotid sinus and vaso-vagal syndromes** | DDD with special algorithms[e] | DDI + hysteresis<br>DDD + hysteresis | AAI(R)<br>VDD(R)<br>VVI(R) |
| **Hypertrophic obstructive cardiomyopathy** | DDD(R) with optimal AVD<br>VVI(R) if atrial arrhythmias are present | | AAI(R)<br>VVI(R) if rhythm is sinus<br>DDI(R)<br>VDD(R)[c] |

Programming of rate responsiveness is indicated only in cases of chronotropic incompetence or for rate smoothing or for automatic mode switch (AMS) in atrial arrhythmias

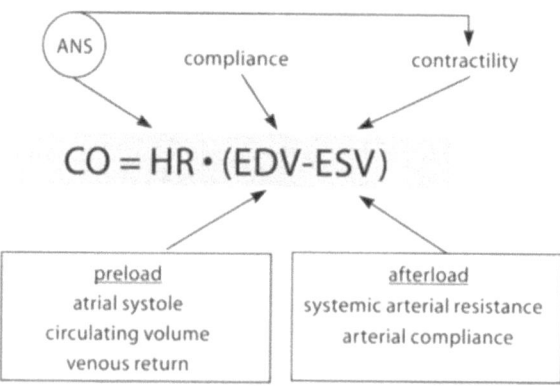

**Fig. 4.2.** The various parameters regulating cardiac output *ANS* autonomic nervous system; *CO* cardiac output; *HR* heart rate; *EDV* enddiastolic volume; *ESV* endsystolic volume

restoration and optimization of atrioventricular synchrony, observance of ventricular contraction synchrony, and rate acceleration with exercise.

Rate acceleration is the main determinant of the exercise-induced increase in cardiac output, and synchronous ventricular contraction is preferable to that associated with right ventricular pacing. Atrial systole contributes 10% to 15% of the resting cardiac output; its role, important in the beginning of exercise, later becomes less than that of heart rate in increasing cardiac output, though remaining essential in the regulation of the filling pressures.

### Heart Rate Increase with Exercise

With exercise, the increase in heart rate, which depends on the sinus rate, and the increase in myocardial contractility, are both mediated by circulating catecholamines. This process contributes approximately 75% of the increase in cardiac output. The remaining 25% results from an increase in filling facilitated by an increase in left ventricular compliance, an increase in venous return, and by an augmented atrial systole. In absence of an increase in heart rate, an increase in filling volumes, hence in ejection fraction, partially compensates to increase the cardiac output. One observes, nevertheless, a considerable reduction in exercise capacity, on the order of 25% – 30%, assuming that neither systolic nor diastolic ventricular functions are impaired, in which case exercise capacity is compromised even further. Therefore, in patients suffering from sinus node dysfunction and chronotropic incompetence, the implant of an AAI/DDD pacemaker may not be sufficient to restore normal physiology, which requires the addition of rate responsiveness. Consequently, in cases of sinus node dysfunction, rate responsiveness is advised a priori, recognizing that chronotropic incompetence may develop only gradually in the future.

### Atrioventricular Synchrony

The role of atrial systole is major. It contributes to endsystolic ventricular filling, and optimizes the filling pressures. It guarantees the closure of the atrioventricu-

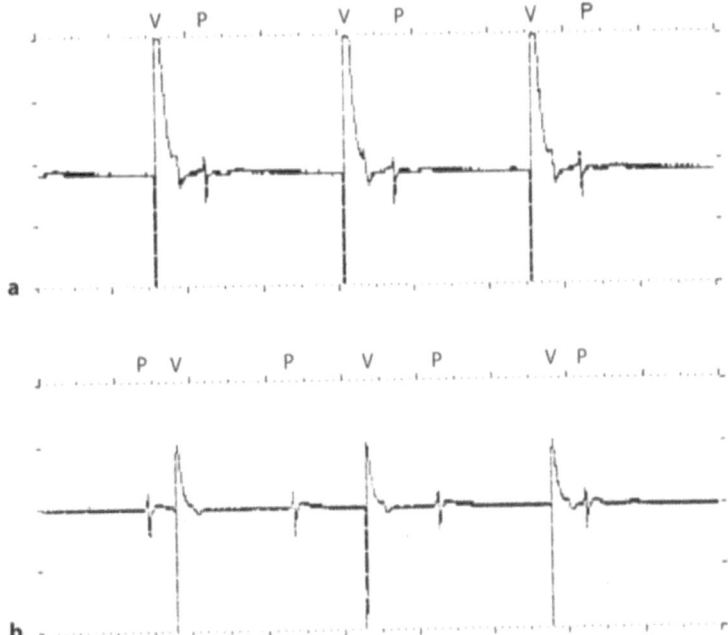

**Fig. 4.3.** Atrial intracardiac electrograms in VVI mode
**a** Ventricular pacing is regularly followed by a retrograde P wave
**b** Absence of retrograde conduction. The P waves do not follow ventricular pacing at predictable intervals
*P* P wave; *V* ventricular pacing

lar valves and participates in neuro-humoral reflexes and to the production of natriuretic peptides. Therefore, it contributes to pre- and afterload regulation, to inotropy (by the Frank-Starling mechanism), to ventricular filling and relaxation, and to myocardial oxygen consumption.

Loss of AV synchrony has important consequences, in the form of a decrease in cardiac output and an increase in ventricular filling pressures. The main expression of atrioventricular dissociation is 1 : 1 retrograde conduction from ventricular pacing (Fig. 4.3). A considerable drop in cardiac output and arterial pressure takes place, with inadaptation of systemic vascular resistances. Atrial systole takes place while the atrioventricular valves are closed, causing a marked increase in intraatrial pressure (canon A waves), atrioventricular regurgitation is promoted, and neuro-humoral reflexes are activated (Fig. 4.4).

These disturbances are the basis for the VVI pacemaker syndrome, present in 5%–10% of cases, most commonly in presence of preserved retrograde conduction, as well as for mitral and/or tricuspid insufficiency which perpetuate atrial dilatation, for the development or aggravation of congestive failure, and for exertional dyspnea from the absence of rate increase during effort. Moreover, in sinus node dysfunction, chronic atrial dilatation and AV dissociation caused by VVI pacing may lead to changes facilitating atrial tachyarrhythmias and second-

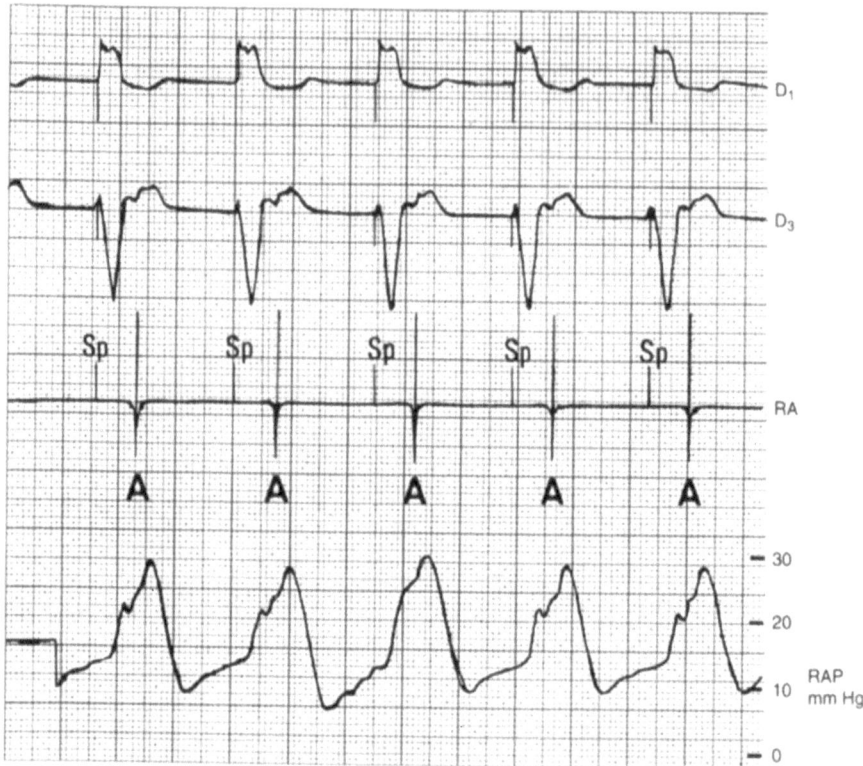

**Fig. 4.4.** Hemodynamic consequences of 1 : 1 atrioventricular conduction during VVI pacing. A canon A wave of approximately 20 mm Hg is measured on the atrial pressure channel, due to atrial systole occurring on a tricuspid valve closed by the prior ventricular contraction

ary thromboembolic complications. At 4 years, the incidence of established atrial fibrillation is 47% in VVI pacing, versus 6.7% in AAI and DDD modes, while the incidence of heart failure is 37% versus 15%, respectively. At 2 years, the incidence of thromboembolic events is 13% in VVI pacing, versus 4.5% with the other modes, while the differences at 4 years are no longer significant. These effects explain the favorable impact of AAI/DDD pacing, as opposed to VVI pacing, on the survival of patients with sinus node dysfunction. In contrast, in atrioventricular block, no conclusive large scale study is available, though a benefit has been shown with DDD pacing in a small series of patients suffering from cardiac decompensation at the time of pacemaker implantation.

Observance of AV synchrony may be critical in individual cases, particularly in the elderly (because of age-related changes in left ventricular compliance), and in presence of other alterations in ventricular filling and compliance (ischemia, hypertrophy), or of severe left ventricular dysfunction, all situations in which atrial systole contributes in a major way to filling of the ventricles.

The role of atrial systole becomes more important as a function of the extent of left ventricular dysfunction, particularly when atrial function is preserved. Conversely, if atrial function is reduced, and the atria are dilated, the contribution of atrial systole becomes minimal. However, a recent Austrian study has found a significant regression of NYHA functional class III and IV heart failure with dual chamber pacing and short AVD. These observations may be related to an optimization of the mechanical delay between left atrial and ventricular systoles.

Two factors enhance the effect of atrial systole as part of dual chamber pacing:

- Optimization of atrioventricular synchrony
- Preservation of ventricular contraction synchrony

### Optimization of Atrioventricular Synchrony

Physiologically, the PR interval shortens during exercise under the influence of circulating catecholamines. We have shown that the mean shortening is 4 ± ms for a 10 BPM increase in heart rate, a linear relationship with wide interindividual variations. Other authors have confirmed this shortening including in patients treated with beta adrenergic blockers, though of a lesser magnitude. The goal of modern pacemakers is to reproduce this natural model. This hemodynamic concept rests on two distinct phenomena.

As discussed earlier, an algorithm that shortens the AVD in DDD mode would allow a shortening of TARP, thus raising the 2 : 1 pacemaker AV block rate and making it possible to program a high maximal rate (see p. 84 f.). Chances of switching to the Wenckebach or even 2 : 1 mode when the sinus rate during exercise crosses the programmed maximal rate are minimized. Indeed, these detrimental AV associations are particularly noxious with respect to exercise capacity by causing a fall in cardiac output and arterial blood pressure, and by increasing filling pressures which cause dyspnea (Fig. 4.5).

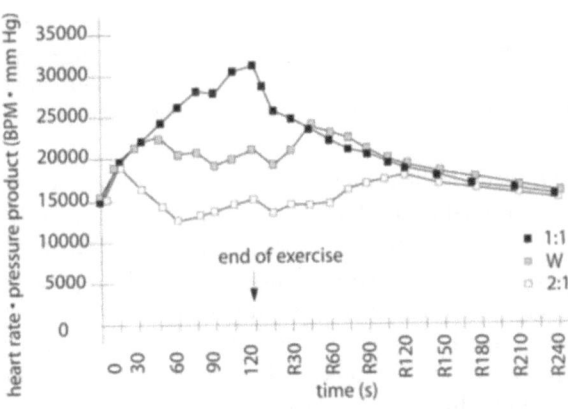

**Fig. 4.5.** Effects of various types of AV associations on the rate – pressure product. 1 : 1 association has a normal profile, in contrast to a marked alteration noted with a 2 : 1 ratio and, to a lesser extent, with Wenckebach periodicity
*R* Recovery

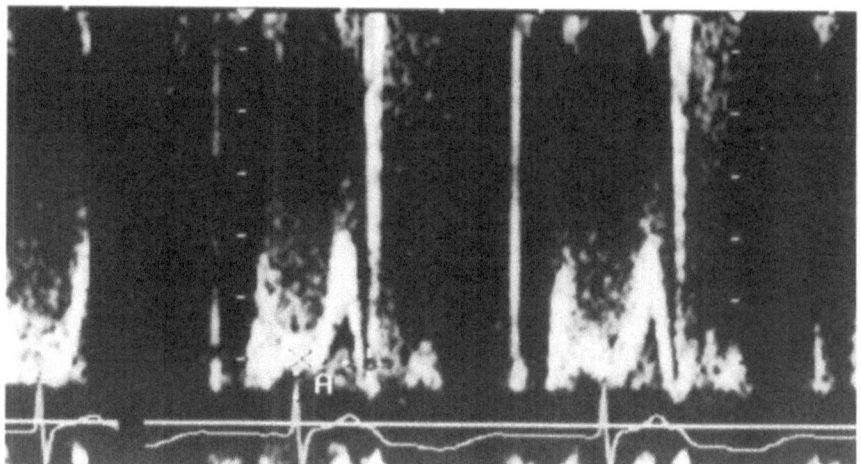

**Fig. 4.6.** Dual chamber pacing in a patient with complete heart block. At a programmed AVD of 110 ms, ventricular filling, as expressed by the Doppler transmitral flow pattern appears satisfactory, with a long diastolic period, and a complete A wave uninterrupted by ventricular systole

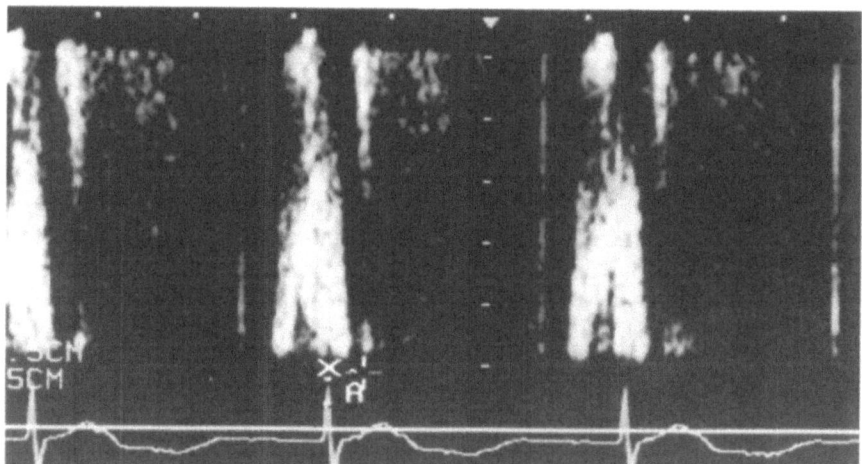

**Fig. 4.7.** Same patient as in Fig. 4.6. The AVD has been reprogrammed to 190 ms. A and E waves are superimposed; the diastolic period is shorten because of premature closure of the mitral valve. This filling pattern corresponds to a decrease in transaortic flow

The second phenomenon consists of optimizing the hemodynamic status on a beat-to-beat basis. It has been clearly demonstrated that a given sinus rate corresponds to an AVD associated with a better cardiac output. At rest, the optimal AVD ranges between 80 and 150 ms, while at peak exercise, its value is less distinct because of a lack of reliable methods of measurement. However, in experienced hands, doppler echocardiography or exercise spirometry are useful non-invasive tools. The metabolic benefit of a shortening of the AVD according to heart rate has now been validated with exercise spirometry.

Recent experimental work has also shown that a belated atrial systole (AVD < 50 ms) is prematurely interrupted by ventricular systole. If there is a quite optimal AV-delay (Fig. 4.6), the diastolic filling period is long. Conversely, if occurring too early (AVD is programmed too long), it is superimposed on the passive filling phase and shortens the period of diastolic filling (Fig. 4.7).

Therefore, at a given sinus rate, the optimal value will depend on the diastolic time available (itself a function of the ejection time), on the duration of atrial systole, on the interatrial and interventricular delay, and on the duration of the atrial and ventricular electromechanical intervals. In general, an AVD between 50 and 100 ms seems acceptable at peak exercise. In theory, the optimal AVD at a given heart rate in a patient with AV block should correspond to the longest filling time associated with complete atrial systole, uninterrupted by ventricular systole.

A simple, validated formula has been proposed to set an optimal resting AVD in patients with high degree AV block (e.g. it is measured with two different programmed AVD, paced in atrium and ventricle):

optimal resting AVD = [long AVD (170 ms) – short AVD (50 ms)] – [V spike – mitral closure interval with short AVD) – (V spike – mitral closure interval with long AVD)] + short AVD (50 ms).
(see also p. 359, Chap. 8)

The remaining factor in AVD optimization is the adjustment of the difference between an AVD after paced versus sensed P wave, allowing the maintenance of a constant left atrioventricular mechanical interval (Fig. 4.8). Its average value is between 70 and 75 ms.

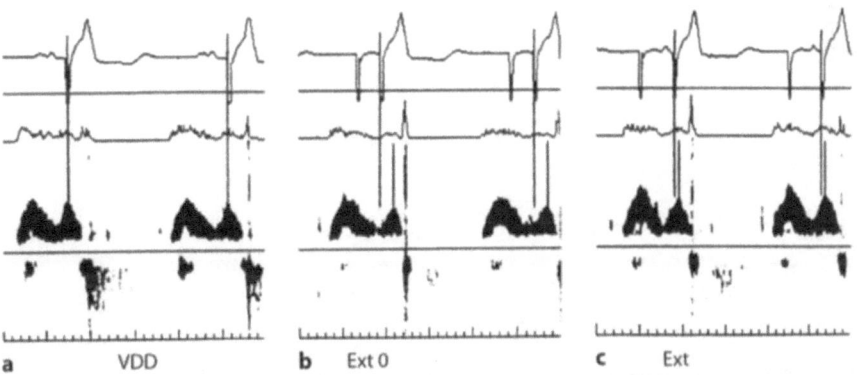

**Fig. 4.8a–c.** In a patient with AV block, the difference in AVD after paced versus sensed P wave intends to maintain a stable left atrioventricular mechanical sequence, whether the P wave has been paced or sensed

**a** In VDD mode, at the programmed AVD, the ventricular spike and the peak of the A wave are superimposed

**b** During AV sequential pacing with the same AVD, a delay between the spike and the peak of the A wave has become apparent (Ext 0)

**c** By programming this interval, nearly the same sequence as in VDD is observed during AV sequential pacing (Ext)

## Ventricular Contraction Synchrony

Since the ventricular lead is typically placed at the right ventricular apex, the sequence of ventricular activation is considerably altered, with the creation of a pseudo left bundle branch block. This has adverse hemodynamic consequences because of desynchronization of left ventricular contraction (the normal delay between right and left ventricular contraction is 40 to 60 ms, increasing to 150 ms with transseptal activation), and inversion of the sequence of activation, from the right ventricular apex, through the septum, to the left ventricular apex, and towards the ventricular free walls and proximal septum.

The higher the right ventricular pacing site towards the hisian junction, the least hemodynamically adverse is the effect of pacing. Recent studies have advocated the performance of pacing from the right ventricular outflow tract instead of the apex. The hemodynamic status of a heart paced from the apex is close to that of a patient with left bundle branch block. This results in an alteration of left

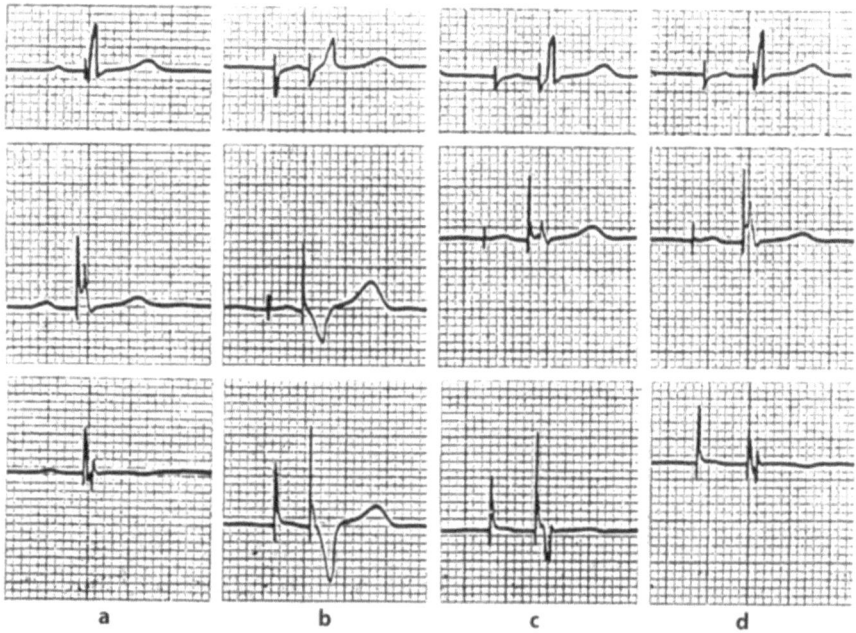

a                b                c                d

**Fig. 4.9.** In a patient with preserved spontaneous AV conduction, the difference between the 2 AVDs aims at maintaining the same sequence of ventricular contraction, whether the atrium is paced or sensed

**a** The AVD is programmed such that the ventricular spike appears in the beginning of the QRS without fusion in the VDD mode

**b** The atrium is paced with the same AVD and the QRS complex is nearly completely paced

**c** The programmed difference between the 2 AVDs is too short, resulting in ventricular fusion

**d** The AVD after paced P waves has been programmed correctly, resulting in the same QRS morphology as during VDD pacing

ventricular systolic function and relaxation with its impact on left ventricular filling and output, and an increase in myocardial oxygen consumption.

These abnormalities result in large part from a considerable decrease in septal segmental contraction. It is, therefore, important to preserve the normal ventricular activation process originating from the nodo-hisian junction. Several recent studies have shown a benefit from preserving normal AV conduction using different assessment methods, including hemodynamic measurements, angioscintigaphy, echocardiography, and exercise spirometry. These observations have increased the importance of various technical solutions, ranging from old features such as VVI mode with rate hysteresis, slow lower rate, DDI or DDD mode with long AVD, or AAI with a risk of long-term AV block development, or more recent ones, such as the automatic AVD hysteresis offered in the Ruby, Diamond (Vitatron) and Trilogy (Pacesetter) models, or automatic mode switch (see p. 397 and p. 398) found in the Chorus II, Chorum, and Talent (ELA Medical). These findings also explain the growing importance of a differential programming of AVD after paced versus sensed P wave (Fig. 4.9).

On the other hand, ventricular pacing appears hemodynamically beneficial in obstructive cardiomyopathy since the asynchrony of contraction minimizes the left intraventricular gradient by decreasing the dynamic obstruction via a mechanism that is still being debated. This model is of interest in that it seems to indicate that ventricular contraction originating from the right ventricular apex is the cause of a significant decrease in the pressure gradient (Fig. 4.10). This implies the programming of a very short AVD which allows complete capture of the ventricle, at the cost of a truncated left atrial systole. This raises the issue of artificially lengthening the atrioventricular conduction time, either by the usu-

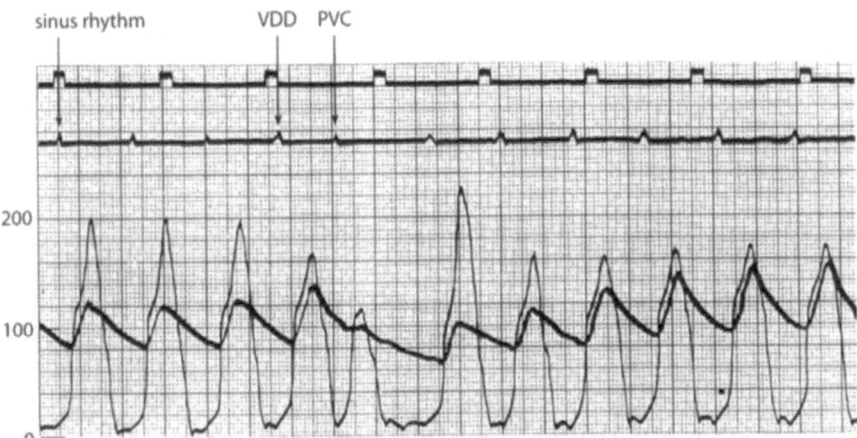

**Fig. 4.10.** Beneficial effect of DDD pacing with complete ventricular capture in obstructive cardiomyopathy. The left intraventricular gradient was 80 mm Hg at baseline. After postextrasystolic potentiation by a paced cycle unpreceded by a P wave (PVC) (in VDD mode, the pacemaker escapes as in VVI mode at the end of a pause), at which point the gradient is transiently increased, dual chamber pacing with 1 : 1 synchrony and complete ventricular capture results in the near elimination of the pressure gradient

sinus rhythm                              VDD pacing

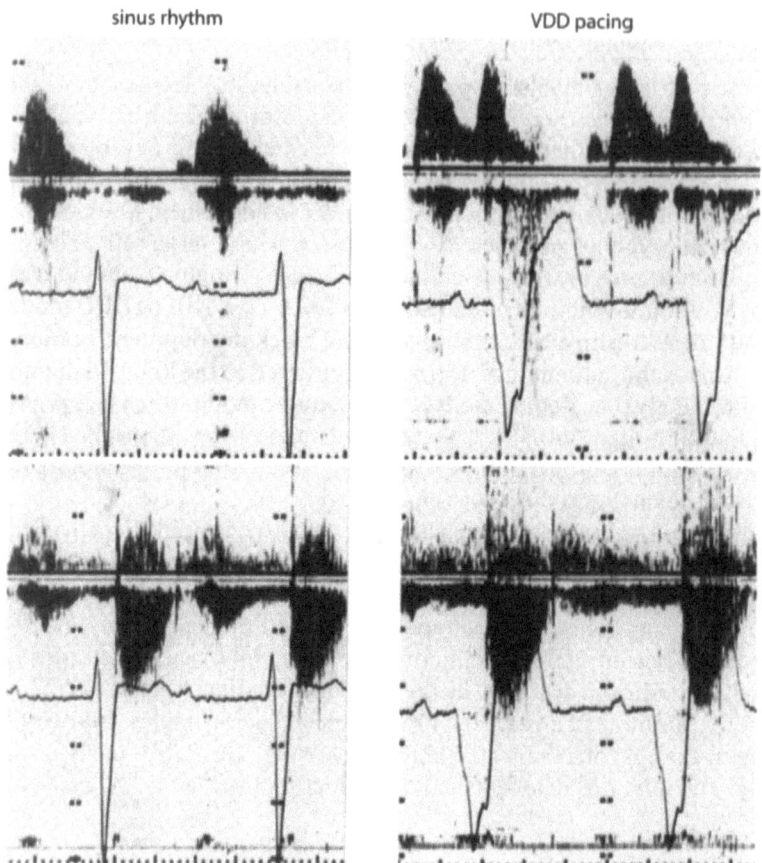

**Fig. 4.11.** *Left*: sinus rhythm with spontaneous AV conduction and very long PR interval, resulting in a single transmitral filling wave and short diastolic period (*top panel*) and modest aortic flow (lower panel). *Right*: VDD pacing restores a normal transmitral pattern with distinct E and A waves, and a longer diastolic period (*top panel*), resulting in a significant increase in aortic flow (*bottom panel*)

ally prescribed medications (beta adrenergic blockers, calcium antagonists), or biatrial pacing (which eliminates the interatrial conduction delay during the PR interval), or by irreversible ablation of the nodo-hisian junction.

First degree AV block with an inordinately long PR interval is another situation where ventricular pacing is preferable to spontaneous ventricular activation. In such cases, atrial systole takes place during the preceding ventricular systole, a phenomenon particularly noxious when the PR interval fails to shorten with exercise, mimicking the pacemaker syndrome in absence of pacemaker. Restitution of AV synchrony can successfully remedy this adverse process (Fig. 4.11).

The remaining concept, that of restoration of ventricular contraction synchrony with biventricular pacing, is still in the realm of clinical research. It is performed with a standard right endocardial pacing lead coupled with a left epicardial or transvenous left ventricular lead, both connected to the pacemaker's ventricular channel. The goal is to obtain synchronous pacing of both ventricles, to decrease the adverse impact of bundle branch blocks, particularly in presence of poor ventricular function, and to lessen the amount of valvular regurgitation. A few reports have been published which describe spectacular improvements in patients with endstage congestive heart failure. However, several technical problems remain to be solved.

### Atrial Resynchronization

This method has been advocated by Daubert for the prevention of certain atrial tachyarrhythmias, though it may also serve a hemodynamic purpose. In all cases of prolongation of the interatrial conduction time, optimal AV synchrony mandates the programming of a long AVD, which interferes with the programming of the 2:1 pacemaker AV block rate, hence with exercise hemodynamics, because of the obligatory reduction of the programmed maximal rate (Fig. 4.12). To achieve both goals (optimal AVD and high 2:1 pacemaker AV block rate) the atria can be resynchronized by implanting one lead in the standard right atrial position and another to pace the left atrium from the coronary sinus, both being connected to an AAT pacemaker, or to the atrial channel of a DDD pacemaker equipped with RAM software offering AAT pacing for all atrial sensed event (Fig. 5.27a). This results in a better ventricular filling and an increase in cardiac output (Fig. 4.13).

This technique is mostly indicated in patients with prolonged interatrial conduction times in presence of impaired ventricular function, whether from dilated or hypertrophic cardiomyopathy.

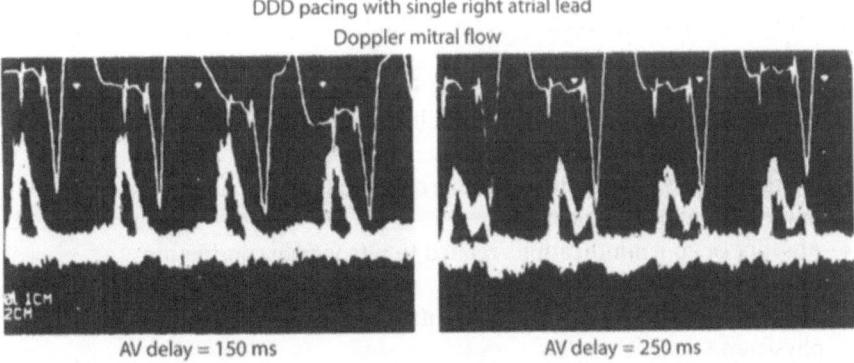

DDD pacing with single right atrial lead
Doppler mitral flow

AV delay = 150 ms          AV delay = 250 ms

pacing rate = 70 bpm

**Fig. 4.12.** Transmitral flow during DDD pacing for complete heart block with AVD set at 150 ms (*left*) and 250 ms (*right*). With the shorter AVD, the A wave is inapparent since it occurs during ventricular systole and closed AV valve. This causes a delay in left atrial systole with respect to atrial pacing, related to an inordinately long interatrial conduction time. Even with the longest AVD available, atrial systole is prematurely interrupted by ventricular systole. This constitutes an indication for atrial resynchronization

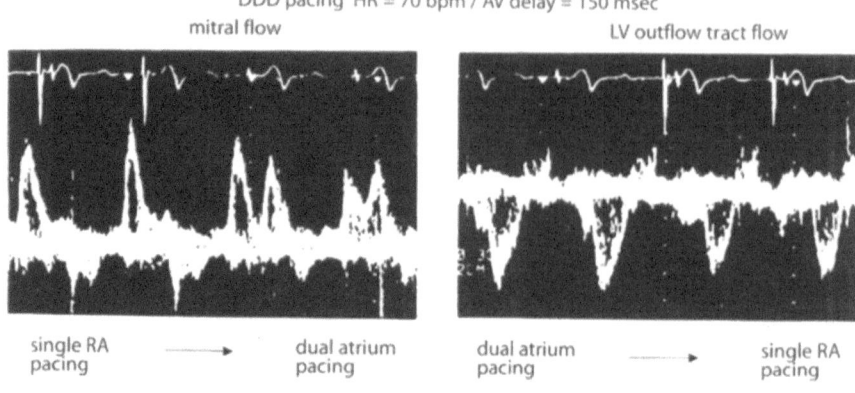

**Fig. 4.13.** Hemodynamic effects of biatrial resynchronization. *Left*: The transmitral flow, single during standard right atrial pacing, normalizes with biatrial pacing. *Right*: Transition from biatrial pacing to standard right atrial pacing results in a fall in transaortic flow

## Advantages and Disadvantages of Various Pacing Modes

A better understanding of the indications for permanent pacing and of the physiology of the paced patient allows a better appreciation of the advantages and shortcomings of the various pacing modes.

### Pure Atrial Modes

The advantages of pure, single chamber atrial pacing are the following:

- Physiologic pacing which preserves AV synchrony and the pattern of mechanical ventricular activation
- As a consequence, a hemodynamic improvement with higher ejection volume, optimization of ventricular filling, decrease in intracardiac pressures, and a reduction in myocardial oxygen consumption
- A preventive effect against atrial arrhythmias whose incidence is distinctly lower than with VVI pacing
- Absence of contraindications related to retrograde conduction
- Cost containment and ease of follow up since these devices allow only a limited number of individual adjustments, and can be followed by a „non-expert" physician.

The disadvantages of pure, single chamber atrial pacing are the following:

- Ventricular activity (R wave) may be sensed, causing ventriculo-atrial crosstalk.
- The use of this mode mandates the verification of the integrity of atrioventricular conduction. Its long-term future remains uncertain even after a baseline

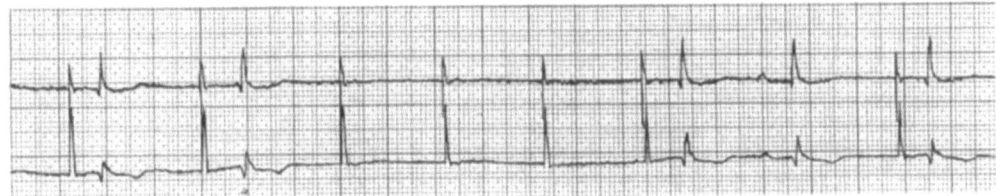

**Fig. 4.14.** Hazard of AAI pacing. During carotid sinus massage, several consecutive P waves are blocked with risk of syncope. Dual chamber pacing would be much more desirable

electrophysiologic study. A 24 h Holter monitor recording and the measure of the Wenckebach point (see p. 159) are only instantaneous indices of atrioventricular conduction. In absence of abnormalities at the time of implant, the risk of subsequent changes is estimated to be 1% annually (Fig. 4.14).

- In case of subsequent development of atrial fibrillation, an AAI pacemaker becomes useless since it cannot offer back up pacing for slow ventricular rates. This would also apply in case of frequent blocked atrial extrasystoles which might result in a slow ventricular rate (see Fig. 8.20).

CASE STUDY

*Example.* An AAI pacemaker has been implanted 5 years earlier for sino-atrial dysfunction in a 65 year old patient. In the interim, several poorly tolerated episodes of profound lightheadedness have developed. Their cause was found to be periods of atrial fibrillation and flutter with slow ventricular rate. These episodes needed to be suppressed with antiarrhythmic drugs which increased the risk of ventricular bradycardia during bouts of atrial tachyarrhythmias. A change in the pacing system was necessary, consisting of the addition of a ventricular lead and the substitution of a dual chamber device, resulting in disappearance of the symptoms. In the event of recurrent atrial arrhythmias, rate responsive ventricular pacing is offered by the pacemaker which automatically switches pacing from dual chamber to VVIR pacing, while during sinus rhythm AV synchrony is maintained most of the time.

In the AAIR mode, mention should be made of a complication representing a veritable AAIR pacemaker syndrome due to the paradoxical lengthening of the atrial spike to R wave interval as the rate responsive function accelerates the pacing rate (Fig. 4.15). This phenomenon may cause symptoms that are identical to those described with the VVI pacemaker syndrome. Its only remedy is the exchange of the pacing mode to DDDR.

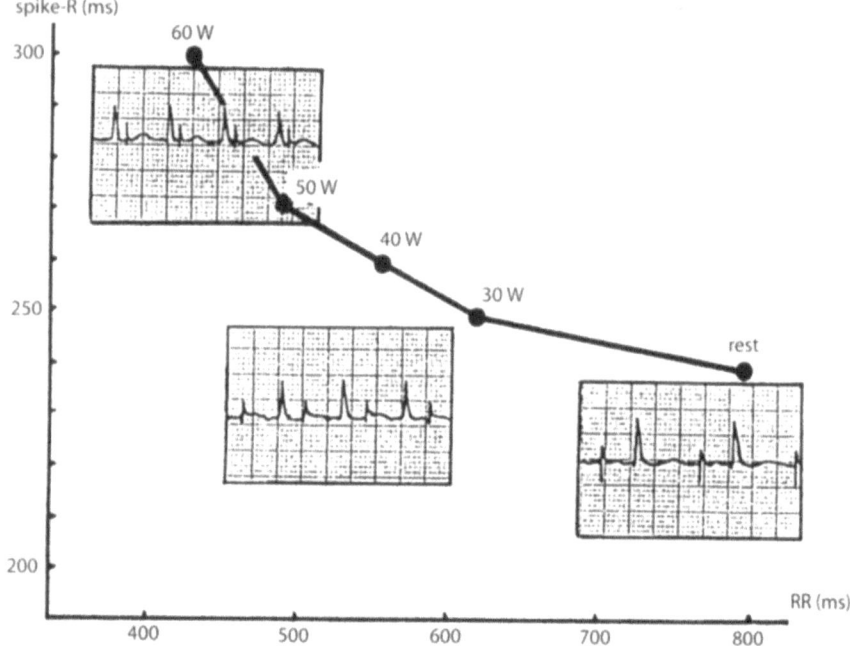

**Fig. 4.15.** Paradoxical lengthening of the atrial spike to R wave interval during exercise in patient who had received an AAIR pacing system

### Pure Ventricular Modes

Some of the advantages of single chamber ventricular pacing are obvious:

- Much information gathered in the past has shown a survival benefit from VVI pacing in cases of advanced atrioventricular block compared to nonpaced patients.
- This type of pacemaker is inexpensive and easy to implant.
- It is easy to program and to follow.

The disadvantages of single chamber VVI pacing are mostly those of the pacemaker syndrome already described earlier, particularly in presence of retrograde conduction, with symptoms ranging from bothersome pounding in the neck to precipitous drop in arterial pressure with loss of consciousness, such that the patient may be in worse health after than before the pacemaker implant (Fig. 4.4). VVI pacing also carries a higher risk of later development of chronic atrial fibrillation and secondary complications, such as thromboembolism and decreased exercise capacity, and, in patients with sinus node dysfunction, a higher mortality than dual chamber pacing.

VVIR pacing represents a clear improvement from a hemodynamic standpoint. However, the risk of pacemaker syndrome may be increased, particularly during exercise, because of retrograde conduction, expected to develop in nearly 40% of patients under such conditions.

## The Dual Chamber Modes

The advantages of dual chamber pacing stem from the flexibility and accurate programming of the system when appropriately chosen. The long-term hemodynamic benefits are attributable to the following:

- An increase in ventricular rate occurs with exercise. In presence of normal sino-atrial function, dual chamber pacing offers the most physiologic adaptation of the ventricular rate.
- A clear increase in the ejection volume and fraction has been measured.
- This results in an increase in cardiac output, while myocardial oxygen consumption is minimized.
- Better enddiastolic filling is obtained from active atrial systole, which usually persists on the long-term.
- Prevention of atrial arrhythmias is comparable to that noted with atrial pacing.

Its disadvantages are:

- Dual chamber pacemaker are more expensive despite their gradually lower cost due to increasing market competition.
- The devices are more difficult to program and require a greater knowledge of the various programming possibilities offered by the various models available.
- The implantation procedure is lengthened by the need to position two leads.
- Power consumption is greater than in single chamber devices.
- Complications are more likely, including AV crosstalk, ELT and other forms of pacemaker mediated tachycardia due to atrial tachyarrhythmias, etc..
- The use of these devices' full capabilities is time consuming.

The VDD mode offers the same advantages as the DDD mode. It eliminates the drawback of a second lead. This mode is contraindicated in cases of sino-atrial block since its function becomes VVI-like (see p. 118 f.), and in cases of sinus bradycardia because of the risk of retrograde conduction as the sinus rate falls below the lower rate. Moreover, the floating electrode may be associated with poor atrial sensing which converts the system to VVI mode. Such atrial sensing failures may be compensated for by rate smoothing, or by rate responsive sensors which can cushion the resulting drop in ventricular rate.

The DDI mode offers both AV synchrony during exercise and synchrony of ventricular contraction. ELT and other forms of pacemaker mediated tachycardias due to paroxysmal atrial arrhythmias are avoided. However, AV synchrony disappears with the development of complete heart block since the system switches to VVI pacing. This mode, indeed, offers AV synchrony only in absence of spontaneous atrial and ventricular activity (see p. 106 ff.).

To the above enumerated advantages and shortcomings, the rate responsive systems add those inherent to rate responsive sensors and their integration to the basic functions of dual chamber pacemakers (see p. 139 ff.).

## Pacing Mode Selection

### For Pure Sinus Node Dysfunction

The pacemaker needed for this indication should be technologically advanced and should offer:

- A lower rate in case of bradycardia as is found in AAI, DDI or DDD modes.
- Rate responsiveness for chronotropic incompetence as found in AAIR, DDIR and DDDR modes.
- Availability of inhibited mode (DDI(R)), or automatic mode switch (fallback), from DDD to VVI or DDI, or from DDD or DDDR to VVIR or DDIR, in the event of atrial tachyarrhythmias. The pacemaker should also be capable of antitachycardia burst pacing for the treatment of atrial tachycardias or flutter (see p. 157).

We consider the ideal pacemaker for this indication to be one of the following:

- An AAI system if AV conduction is intact (which mandates the performance of an electrophysiologic study).
- A DDD or DDI system since it may not be possible to verify the integrity of AV conduction. Measurement of the Wenckebach point is but one temporal assessment of AV conduction which does not accurately predict the possible subsequent development of AV block. Antiarrhythmic drug therapy may become necessary and cause AV conduction disturbances, or the underlying heart disease may progress. For these reasons, we prefer to implant dual chamber systems.
- A DDD pacemaker with automatic mode switch from AAI to DDD or with automatic AVD hysteresis, which combines the advantages of AAI mode with the safety of DDD in case of intercurrent AV conduction disorder.
- A pacemaker with antitachycardia pacing capabilities at the atrial level, an elegant method to interrupt noninvasively paroxysmal episodes of atrial tachycardia or flutter.
- A rate responsive system in case of chronotropic incompetence. The value of rate responsiveness becomes an issue when chronotropic incompetence is not apparent despite signs of sinus node dysfunction. Some consider that a nonresponsive system is adequate, though many would judge that the risk of subsequent development of chronotropic incompetence is high enough to justify the prophylactic implant of a rate responsive system. The same considerations apply to the choice between AAIR, DDIR or DDDR. In the case of AAIR, the atrial spike to R wave interval during exercise must be carefully assessed since it may lengthen abnormally and cause a variant of the pacemaker syndrome. In all cases, rate responsiveness should only be offered after it has been firmly established that it will improve exercise compared to the physiologic rate increase offered by spontaneous sinus activity.

The VVI mode is a priori contraindicated in sinus node dysfunction because of the abundance of literature showing its association with a higher incidence of atrial fibrillation and higher mortality. Moreover, it may cause symptoms that were not present before implantation of the pacemaker, in which case, the rate has to be programmed slow enough as to allow normal ventricular activation and avoid post pacing retrograde conduction. If retrograde conduction is known to be present, this mode is absolutely contraindicated, as is VVIR because of the likelihood of retrograde conduction during exercise, though inapparent at rest.

### For Isolated Atrioventricular Block

The pacemaker is mostly in charge of preventing bradycardia while preserving AV synchrony. The mode of choice is DDD. On the other hand, if the overall long-term prognosis is poor, or if the atrium cannot be used because of chronic arrhythmias, VVI mode is acceptable except if retrograde conduction causes significant hemodynamic difficulties. The VVIR mode is, in our opinion a poor choice since it does not offer AV synchrony and is associated with a high long-term risk of atrial arrhythmias.

In cases of paroxysmal AV block, the choices are wider: in exercise-related AV block, DDD mode seems natural, keeping in mind the risk of competition between paced and native QRS as long as AV conduction remains intact. If AV block is rare, some believe that VVI pacing is adequate, with a rate smoothing algorithm on stand by to improve patient comfort at the time of block, except in presence of retrograde conduction. However, our recommendation, in both cases, is the DDD mode with automatic mode switch. If the patient has first degree AV block, DDD mode is mandatory, particularly if the PR does not shorten with exercise. Single lead VDD pacing would be an acceptable alternative if sinus node function is preserved.

### For Binodal Disease (Sinus Node Dysfunction Plus at Least First Degree AV Block)

Unless limited by factors discussed earlier, dual chamber pacing is required: DDD in absence of chronotropic incompetence, keeping in mind that it often develops subsequently, in which case DDDR would be preferable (together with special algorithms).

### For Chronic Atrial Fibrillation with Ventricular Bradyarrhythmia

In presence of chronic atrial fibrillation, slow ventricular rate and preserved exercise capacity, VVIR restores a satisfactory performance profile. Otherwise VVI suffices.

### For Carotid Sinus Syndrome or Vaso-Vagal Syndrome

In cases of autonomic hyperactivity the conduction disorder occurs often at more than one level (paroxysmal binodal response). Pacing is required only sporadically, at the time of paroxysms since, outside of the episodes, conduction is usually intact. Single chamber atrial pacing is contraindicated because of the risk of AV nodal block at the time of vagal surge. VVI pacing is contraindicated because ventricular pacing induces already its own hypotensive effect in absence

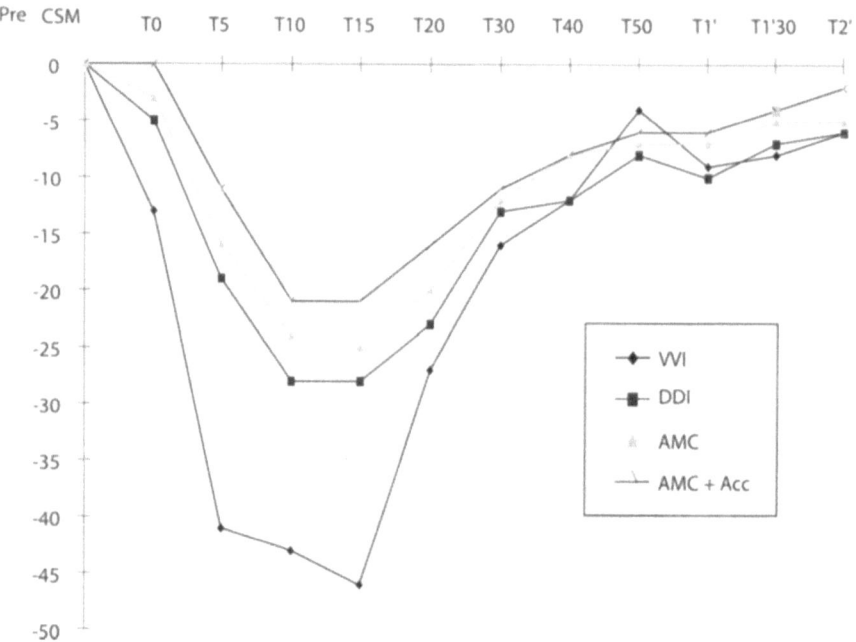

**Fig. 4.16.** Variations in systolic arterial pressure, expressed as a percentage of the baseline measurement, during carotid sinus massage (CSM) in 41 patients suffering from carotid sinus hypersensitivity. DDI pacing attenuates the fall in pressure which remains maximal in comparison with the automatic mode switch AAI/DDD (DDD/AMC) which delays the effect of CSM even further. With a superimposed acceleration of pacing rate (DDD/AMC + acceleration), CSM has a minimal repercussion. CSM was performed in random order according to a precisely rigorous technique (moderate pressure for no longer than 5 s)

of carotid sinus hypersensitivity, with a risk of exacerbation by retrograde conduction at the time of symptoms. Consequently, dual chamber pacing is indicated since it only is capable of preserving the hemodynamic status and of maintaining arterial pressure during the paroxysm. DDI pacing is the most natural since the pacemaker is only expected to intervene at the programmed lower rate, and to otherwise preserve spontaneous rhythm which, in-between episodes, is usually normal. Alternatively, DDD + special algorithms (AV-scanning) are provided in Diamond (Vitatron) or Trilogy (Pacesetter) devices. Programming of rate smoothing improves patient comfort in the event of an episode occurring in the midst of sinus tachycardia, thus avoiding abrupt variations of the atrioventricular paced rhythm. Ultimately, the best mode consists of DDD with automatic mode switch from AAI to DDD and rate acceleration (Fig. 4.16) as offered in the ELA Medical devices. A special algorithm is also available in the Thera, Kappa (Medtronic) pacemakers which monitor the fall in heart rate and respond by a sustained acceleration of the atrioventricular pacing rate.

# CHAPTER 5

# Implantation Techniques

Once a diagnosis has been made and a pacemaker model has been chosen, the patient needs to be advised and the system must be implanted.

## 5.1
## Preparation of the Patient

### Patient Information

The patient must, first of all, be informed of the various steps of the procedure, and of the usual postoperative course. A clear understanding of the sequence of events, even if it includes an explanation of risks and possible complications, should alleviate anxiety and reduce the amount of analgesics or tranquilizers needed to control it. Ideally, a descriptive booklet can be made available to the patient.

### Requirements of the Procedure

A trained operator is essential since the techniques of implantation, though not complex, include several potential hurdles which require much experience, particularly in system revision procedures, or when treating complications such as infections or erosions.

Ideally, pacemaker implants should be performed in centers equipped with operating rooms and intensive care unit to be ready for any complication. Cardiologists should be able to obtain help from surgeons in case of difficult venous access, and surgeons should be able to call on cardiologists for arrhythmias or unacceptable pacing thresholds. A single operator suffices with, perhaps, the assistance of a scrub nurse; however, safety is optimized by the presence of an anesthetist, or nurse-anesthetist, to monitor vital signs, watch the oscilloscope, and administer sedation or general anesthesia, if needed. A circulating nurse might be in charge of the fluoroscopy and of the surgical supplies.

## Implant Facilities

The implantable material is a foreign body which imposes the strictest aseptic precautions, of the same kind as those used in vascular surgery. The implant should be performed in an operating suite with resuscitation equipment, including a stand-by external defibrillator in flawless working conditions. Additional indispensable equipment includes fluoroscopy, intracardiac signals recorder, pacing system analyzer, and the usual monitoring devices such as surface electrocardiograph, blood pressure monitor and oxymeter.

## The Implantation Site

The most commonly used site of implantation is the prepectoral area. The side of implant is relatively unimportant and may be chosen by the patient. Some recommend that the operative site be contralateral to the dominant side, i.e. on the left for right-handed and vice-versa, which would reduce the risk of myosignal inhibition. Hunters should have the device implanted on the side opposite to that used to aim the gun.

Patients are often treated with intravenous infusions before the procedure. Care should be taken to not implant the pacemaker on the side of an infected perfusion site, which would markedly increase the risk of postoperative infection. The right-sided access is sometimes limited by difficulties in passing the lead through the right jugulo-subclavian junction, while the left may be hampered by the innominate-superior vena cava junction.

Finally, the operating room outlay and operator's preferences may have an influence on the site of implant. A subpectoral implant may be preferred in emaciated patients whose subcutaneous tissues may be fragile, or in patients who have had prior radiation therapy or mastectomy. For cosmetic or other reasons, the site chosen may be axillary, retromammary, abdominal, iliac and, in pediatric patients, intrathoracic.

## Preoperative Preparation

A preoperative chest radiograph, available in the operating room, and routine blood screening tests are mandatory. Coagulation studies should be obtained to exclude a serious bleeding disorder. Antiplatelet therapy should be stopped several days ahead of time, if possible. Heparin should be temporarily discontinued. Partial thromboplastin time should be less than one and one half times the control, prothrombin time above 50%, and INR should be below 2.0.

In patients at risk of asystole, prophylactic temporary pacing is recommended, either by placing a temporary pacing lead, or by applying a transcutaneous pacing system, the proper function of which should be verified. The latter method, though innocuous, is quite uncomfortable, and should be used only briefly in absence of other choices.

The site of operation is prepared outside of the operating room by shaving and cleaning the skin which should be rid of the adhesive left from previous monitoring electrodes, and painted with an antiseptic solution. All make up should be removed, and the hair should be covered with a cap. An intravenous infusion should be running on the side opposite to the implant.

The patient should be comfortably fastened to the operating table, with some elevation of the upper body in case of dyspnea, the head turned away from the surgical field. The monitoring electrodes should also be away from the surgical field and from the precordial area. Continuous oxygen should be administered to sedated patients. An intravenous dose of antibiotics should be given one hour before, and another one hour after, the procedure.

The immediate preparation of the surgical field should comply with the usual rules of surgical sterility. The field is again painted with the same antiseptic solution as earlier, and a disposable, waterproof sterile drape is used to cover the patient entirely, with a free space kept to allow unimpeded breathing. An adhesive sterile field is then applied to the surgical field where the delto-pectoral groove and supraclavicular area should be apparent, the latter in case the external jugular vein were needed.

## Choice of Implant Instrumentation

This choice is the result of the preoperative evaluation which lead to the indication for permanent cardiac pacing. The choice of pacing mode, hence of the pacemaker model, dictates the choice of lead(s). The lead(s) connector(s) must be strictly compatible with the pacemaker header. The choice of unipolar versus bipolar lead should be made before the implantation procedure by the physician who posed the indication, a choice that would be influenced only rarely by technical difficulties in implantation. The ultimate choice of the lead model is made by the implanting physician on the basis of maneuverability, size, fixation system, etc.

The choice is often between passive (tined) and active (screw-in) lead fixation. In the atrium, the *advantages* of the screw-in leads versus tined leads are the following:

- They are easier to manipulate, although they may get hung up during introduction, in which case they must be advanced while unscrewing. Retractable screw systems have been developed to avoid this problem.
- They are more stable, an advantage for operators with limited experience.
- They can be attached to any location, including where tined leads cannot be implanted.
- They are easier to remove, if necessary.

There are, however, a few *disadvantages*:

- Pacing and sensing thresholds are reputed to be less favorable at the time of implant.

- The post-traumatic current of injury interferes with the measurement of sensing parameters particularly in the atrium.
- Early threshold rises are more common, probably for similar reasons.
- There is a greater risk of myocardial perforation.
- The risk of phrenic nerve stimulation is greater if the electrodes is fixed on the lateral wall of the atrium.

Despite these drawbacks, one must recognize that the use of tined electrodes is often impossible in the atrium, especially after cardiac surgery, since outside of the appendage and the high lateral wall, trabeculations are absent. In contrast, tined leads can be implanted in the ventricle in nearly all cases.

We prefer a bipolar configuration, although an atrial bipolar, ventricular unipolar configuration is an acceptable alternative. We use active or passive fixation in the atrium, and tined leads in the ventricle, although we also implant screw-in leads in the ventricle to facilitate their extraction in case of late complication.

## Anesthesia

In a first implant of a pacemaker, a local anesthesia with lidocaine without adrenaline is sufficient to perform the incision and create the pacemaker pocket. General anesthesia is rarely necessary and usually reserved for psychologically unstable patients. In addition, the measurement of thresholds may be altered by anesthesia. Finally, general anesthesia may aggravate the circulatory embarrassment caused by bradycardia or by even brief pauses that are necessary during the analysis of the pacing system. Consequently, we occasionally prescribe some premedication, but use mostly conscious sedation when the patient is agitated, if the dissection is painful despite local anesthetic (device replacement with partial effectiveness of the infiltration in the scar tissue, or infection of the pacemaker pocket), if the procedure is lengthy, or if the patient is elderly. Though conscious sedation increases procedural comfort, one should keep in mind that patient cooperation is often needed, in deep breathing or coughing maneuvers, for instance.

## 5.2
## System Implantation

### Venous Access

Following local anesthesia inside the delto-pectoral groove and medial to the groove with a thin gauged needle, the incision is carried out at one of the following sites:

- In the delto-pectoral groove if one intends to access the cephalic vein in the first place, with the proximal incision beginning approximately 2 cm from the clavicle

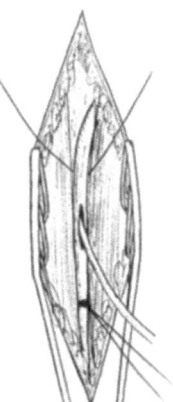

**Fig. 5.1.** Approach into the cephalic vein at the delto-pectoral groove and introduction of the pacing lead after upstream venous ligation, downstream subtending of the vein, and short venotomy

- Beginning at the delto-pectoral groove laterally, and extending medially and upward toward the mid portion of the clavicle, allowing puncture of either the cephalic or the subclavian vein
- 1–2 cm below the clavicle, and parallel to it, if the intention is to access the suclavian vein in the first place

The length of incision depends on the size of the pulse generator and should allow ample access to the vein. Careful hemostasis should be accomplished with the cauterizing scalpel.

If one chooses the cephalic vein access, the superior portion of the delto-pectoral groove is gradually entered in maintaining meticulous hemostasis plane by plane, with the assistance of a self-retractor. The vein is soon uncovered in the fatty tissue between the deltoid, laterally, and pectoralis major, medially, red muscle mass. The vein is progressively dissected, ligated upstream, and subtended downstream with an no resorbable suture (Fig. 5.1). If the vein is inaccessible because of being inexistent or too thin, one may, by dissecting the groove in the upward direction, find a sub-pectoral vein after partial resection of the clavicular insertion of the external head of the pectoralis major muscle. In that region, only few arterioles are encountered that may need hemostatic control.

Access and control of the vein that has been chosen regularly follow the same principles: ample approach, careful dissection, upstream ligation of all potential affluents, meticulous hemostasis. Once the vein has been exposed, all brisk movements must be avoided while a punctiform incision is performed which is widened in the axis of the vessel with either scissors or scalpel. The tiny introducer included with the kit facilitates the introduction of the lead with its stylet. In case of brisk bleeding, the vein may be clamped temporarily downstream at least 1 cm away from the venipuncture.

Once the lead has been introduced, the introducer is withdrawn and the vein unclampled. The stylet is slightly withdrawn to soften the extremity of the lead and facilitate its passage through the venous meanders and bifurcations, and minimize the risk of vascular trauma. An essential rule consists of carefully washing the operator's gloves with sterile saline solution, since the penetration of blood products inside the lead lumen and on the stylet may render all further manipulations difficult, or even impossible. If the lead is not advancing, the vein should be stretched with the upstream ligature, and to-an-fro movements performed in the axis of the vein while rotating the lead. If the lead continues to resist, the patient's shoulder may be lifted or pulled downward, or the stylet may be curved at its extremity and advanced fully to exert further pressure. In case of continued resistance, the vein must be dissected further downstream, and the same maneuvers repeated. If this fails, one may try to introduce a soft guide wire up to the subclavian vein, followed by a guiding sheath over the wire. In rare cases, the introduction of the lead requires the dissection of the vein up to its confluence with the axillary or subclavian vein.

When two separate leads must be introduced, of which one is of an active fixation variety, it is advisable to start with the screw-in lead, more difficult to advance than the tined lead. Once the screw-in lead has been advanced, the tined lead should pass more easily. If the screw-in lead cannot be advanced, the order is reversed, since the tined lead often opens the way for the second lead. This is, of course, possible only if the vein is wide enough. If it is wide enough, but the second lead cannot be advanced, an attempt can be made through a separate venotomy downstream from the original one. This technical difficulty has been largely minimized by the design of retractable screw electrodes.

Whichever technique is used, one must hold the first lead with its stiffening stylet in place in one hand, while the other lead is manipulated with the other hand with its stylet advanced at least up to the entrance point into the vein to exert enough pressure. In no case should force be exerted, especially with the stylet which may perforate both lead and vein. Usually, when the screw-in lead has been successfully advanced, it is immediately placed in the atrium. Its dislodgment during the manipulation of the ventricular lead, indicates that it was not properly fixed. If none of these maneuvers is successful, another approach needs to be attempted.

If a *subclavian puncture* is intended in the first place, the technique is that of Seldinger: it consists of introducing a soft „J„ wire through a needle mounted on a syringe, followed by an introducer sheath mounted on a dilator, introduced over the wire inside the vein. We prefer the use of a 10.5 Fr introducer kit which includes a stiff dilator and a sturdy, though pliable sheath which curves through the venous meanders without buckling. Two thin unipolar, or any thick bipolar, lead passes easily through this sheath. A bigger size introducer may be needed for VDD leads.

The puncture of the subclavian vein under local anesthesia requires a rigorous technique if one wants to avoid serious complications, including the inadvertent puncture of the artery, of the pleural dome, or of a nerve. The patient should be relaxed, the shoulder directed downwards, with the arm along the side and the head turned to the opposite direction. The needle is introduced two finger breadth below the clavicle, at the junction of its lateral and middle thirds. The needle is advanced slowly through the skin incision after removal of the retractor, with gentle suction on the syringe, under the clavicle, aiming towards the

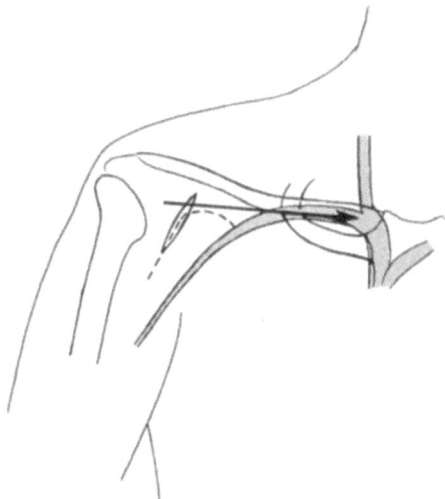

**Fig. 5.2.** Technique and landmarks for subclavian puncture

manubrium which can be felt through the sterile drape (Fig. 5.2). As soon as the needle is under the clavicle, it must remain horizontal and aim in the same direction.

Despite adequate landmarks, the vein may not be reached. With the assistance of fluoroscopy, and according to the same principles, the needle is advanced towards the head of the clavicle, along its inferior margin, towards the manubrium, staying horizontal with respect to the operating table. We have encountered no complication from puncturing the subclavian vein tangentially to the posterior aspect of the clavicle. Another technique, however, has been described which consists of puncturing the subclavian vein in its extrathoracic segment, at the junction between medial 1/4 and lateral 3/4, at a 40° angle relative and after identification of the first rib. This approach is reported to put less mechanical strain on the leads and to minimize the risks related to the venipunture.

In case of persistent difficulties, the subclavian vein can be visualized by injecting contrast material in the cephalic vein.

Once venous return is observed, the syringe is removed and venous back flow must be visualized, fluctuating with respiration, though avoiding introduction of air. A soft, usually „J" shaped, guide wire can then be introduced and advanced toward the right atrium. On occasion, the wire curves up toward the internal jugular vein. One must, then, rotate the „J", or form a loop to drop the guide into the vena cava. A dilator is then advanced over the wire and the dilator is withdrawn, mounted on a sheath, and both sheath and dilator are readvanced over the wire (Fig. 5.3). The dilator is removed while leaving the wire in place, if possible. The pacing lead is introduced and advanced into the heart, and the sheath is removed while keeping the wire in position. If a second lead needs to be placed via the subclavian approach, the wire can be reused to place a second introducer and follow the same steps as those used for the first lead (Fig. 5.4).

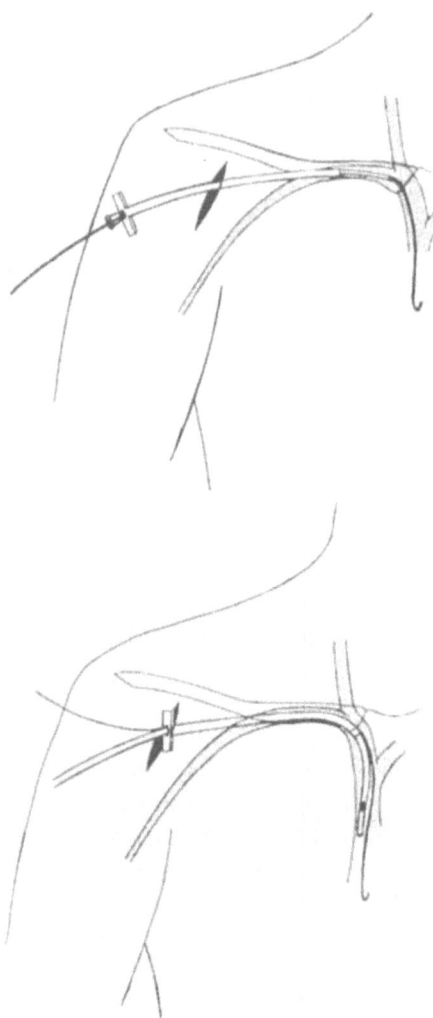

**Fig. 5.3.** Introduction of the introducer sheath mounted on the dilator over the guide wire introduced through the needle after subclavian vein puncture

**Fig. 5.4.** Introduction of the lead through the sheath after withdrawal of the dilator, leaving the guide wire in place. The guide left in place allows a second introduction of the sheath to pass the second pacing lead

However, some operators prefer a second, separate puncture of the vein to introduce the second lead.

One can also attempt the isolation of the external jugular vein which is easy to find and visible under the skin, most often above the medial third of the clavicle, in a triangle contained between the anterior and posterior heads of the sternocleiodomastoid muscle, and the clavicle below. We use this approach only when the cephalic and subclavian veins cannot be used, which is virtually never. This route carries a theoretical long-term risk of lead fracture at the preclavicular level. In addition, the area remains often painful. This approach is discouraged in violinists, wind instruments players and singers because of local mechanical strains. Under local anesthesia, a 3- to 4-cm incision is made one or two finger widths parallel to the superior edge of the clavicle. The vein can be found under the cutaneous neck muscle layer. The technique is then similar to that described for the cephalic vein. At the end of the procedure, the lead must be covered with the muscle layer before closing the skin.

One can often use *collateral veins* if the external jugular vein is too small, as long as they have an infraclavicular course. Very rarely, other venous approaches must be considered such as axillary or subclavian dissection, or internal jugular vein which must be performed by a trained surgeon.

If these routes are not accessible, because of subclavian or innominate thrombosis, the alternate side must be used. This is why we like to inject contrast material in an antecubital vein before implantation in case of suspicion of venous thrombosis, or when replacing or adding a lead.

On occasion, both sides are inaccessible because, for example, of infection on one side and thrombosis on the other. In such cases, the surgical implantation of an epicardial lead must be performed through the diaphragmatic sterno-costal triangle, after resection of the xyphoid process. A left lateral thoracotomy allows access to the left ventricle. Other indications for an epicardial approach include patients with prosthetic tricuspid valves, congenital anomalies, tricuspid atresia, or right-to-left shunts and risks of systemic thromboembolism. This approach does not allow dual chamber pacing.

Some authors have described the placement of endocavitary pacing leads via right atriotomy through a thoracotomy and, more recently, we have described the implant of dual chamber systems by video-surgery and pleuroscopy. Such procedure remains exceptional, as does the venous iliac approach with implant of the pulse generator in the iliac fossa.

## Lead Placement

Whether to position the ventricular or atrial lead first remains the choice of the operator. Once the lead is in the axillary or subclavian vein, few difficulties are usually encountered. If after entering the cephalic vein, the lead drifts upstream, the stylet should be withdrawn to soften its tip, then advanced to form a loop. The rigid segment of lead containing the stylet will carry the loop toward the subclavian vein (Fig. 5.5). If this fails, the lead must be withdrawn to the venous bifurcation, then bend the stylet to allow a torsion maneuver and redirect the lead in the proper direction pushing it without forceful motion.

If one starts with the *ventricular lead*, it is often necessary to withdraw the stylet by a few centimeters to soften it. The lead is advanced to enter the right ventricle, the stylet readvanced and the lead positioned at the apex with gentle, continuous forward pressure. More often, a loop must be formed in the right atrium, and then widely advanced into the right ventricle. This avoids trauma to the tricuspid valve, but may cause ventricular extrasystoles. One must then withdraw the lead while advancing the stylet and, in most cases, the lead tip falls into the ventricular cavity, straightens out, pointing toward the apex. One, then, simply

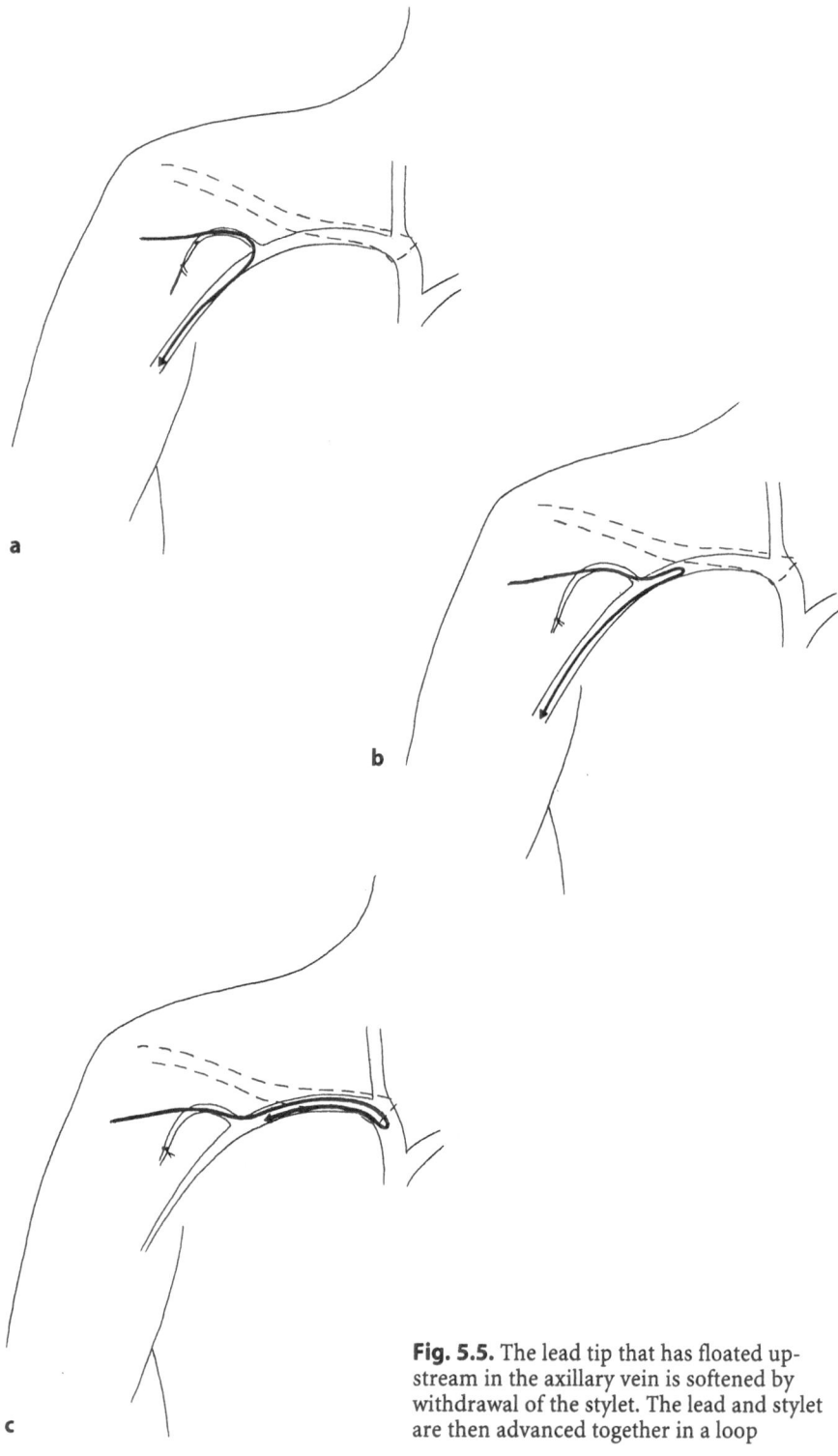

**Fig. 5.5.** The lead tip that has floated upstream in the axillary vein is softened by withdrawal of the stylet. The lead and stylet are then advanced together in a loop

needs to advance the lead which, which may migrate toward the outflow tract (Fig. 5.6). Withdrawing the lead will usually cause it to drop into the apex (Fig. 5.7). In some instances, the lead does not straighten out and hangs up at the tricuspid orifice, particularly if it is stiff, as some bipolar leads may be. In such cases, it is advised to preform the stylet in a regular curve over its distal 10 cm which facilitates the passage through the tricuspid valve. Once the lead is in the ventricle, the curved stylet is replaced by a straight one.

In some cases, poor thresholds mandate to look for a less typical lead position. One can use a stylet highly curved in its distal 2 cm, as a hook to guide the lead and use the torque that has been created. With this technique, one can position the lead in various locations such as the posterior wall of the ventricle, where thresholds are often excellent (in absence of previous infarction), under the septo-marginal trabeculation (arciform band), or against the septum, which bends the lead upward after removal of the stylet (Fig. 5.8).

In exceptional situations, a tined lead must be replaced by an active fixation lead. These include poor thresholds in the entire ventricle because of previous infarction or dilated cardiomyopathy, massive right ventricular dilatation and

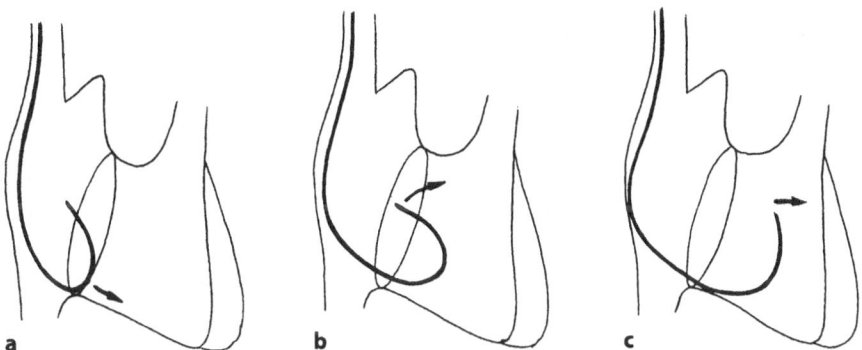

**Fig. 5.6.** Passage of the lead in a loop through the tricuspid valve, the lead being without stylet in its last 10 cm

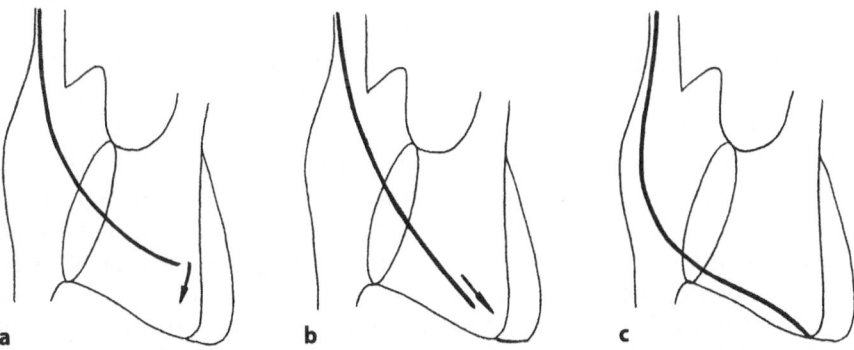

**Fig. 5.7.** The stylet is advanced while the lead is being withdrawn: the lead tip straightens out and drops toward the right ventricular apex

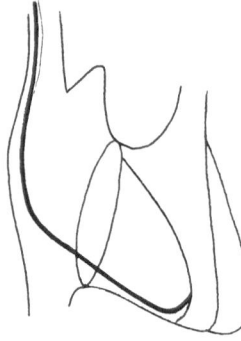

**Fig. 5.8.** Lead placement under the septo-marginal trabeculation

unattachement of the tines, or deliberate placement of the lead in an unusual site such as the outflow tract. The introduction maneuvers, however, are the same.

If one wishes to implant the lead in the outflow tract, it must be advanced into the pulmonary artery, then gently withdrawn back into the right ventricle. The tip is positioned at the anterior margin of the ventricle in the pulmonic infundibulum where it is fixed. To verify its stability, one can gently pull on the lead and perceive a subtle rhythmic tension with each cardiac contraction, confirming that it is properly attached. Both lead and stylet should, then, be readvanced to maintain this position.

To verify the placement of the electrode in the right ventricle (because the heart may be displaced by pleuro-pulmonary disease, be congenitally anomalous, have a vertical droop, or be pointing forward), the lead can be advanced into the pulmonary artery before being placed at the apex. This will exclude its position in the coronary sinus, a spontaneous course often followed from the right atrium. In addition, when pacing from the right ventricular apex, the QRS is positive in lead I, negative in leads II and III, and has a left bundle branch block morphology on the surface electrocardiogram. Rarely, the lead may cross a patent foramen ovale and finds its way to the apex of the left ventricle, in which case the QRS morphology will be that of right bundle branch block (Fig. 5.9). We discourage leaving the lead in such position because of the risk of thromboembolism.

Once the ventricular lead is in place, the *atrial lead* may be positioned. Any manipulation of this second lead may dislodge the first one. One must, therefore, manipulate one lead with one hand, while the other, with its stylet, is kept immobile. An active fixation lead is most commonly placed in the antero-lateral region of the right atrium or in the atrial appendage. Once the lead is in the atrium, the straight stylet is replaced by a „J"-shaped stylet preformed by the manufacturer. If this stylet is not adequate, one can preform a „J" shape from a straight stylet. The curve needed depends on the estimated size of the atrium and should be widely U shaped. This offers the necessary torque control after reintroduction of the stylet (Fig. 5.10). If the lead is located in the appendage, it will have a typical rhythmic motion with each cardiac cycle (Fig. 5.11).

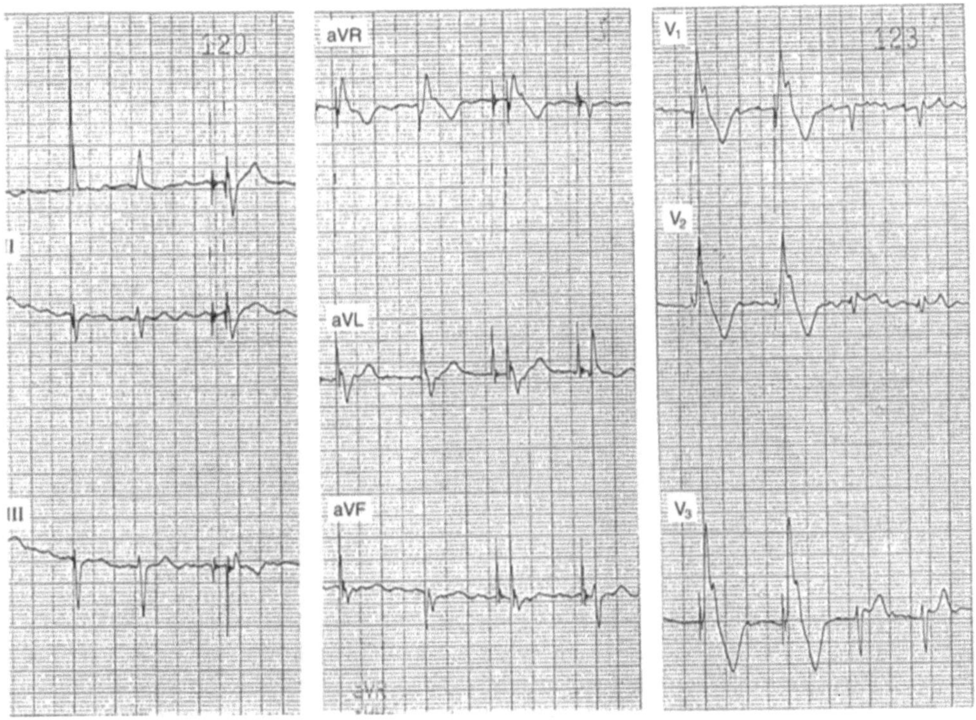

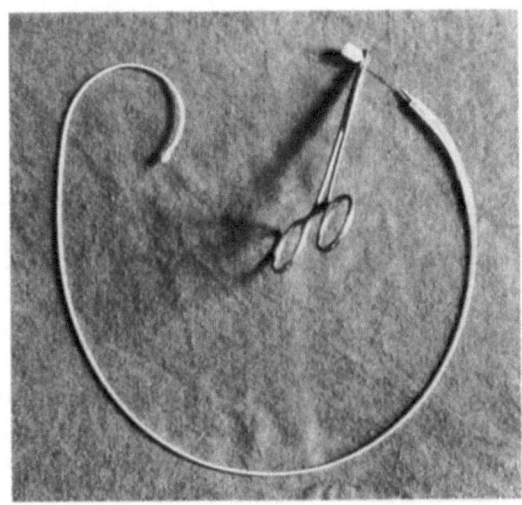

**Fig. 5.9.** Right bundle branch block morphology of the QRS from left ventricular placement of a lead through a patent foramen ovale

**Fig. 5.10.** The hemostat clipped to the proximal end of the stylet determines the orientation of the „J" shape. The lead can be oriented inside the heart chamber by rotation of the hemostat together with the stylet

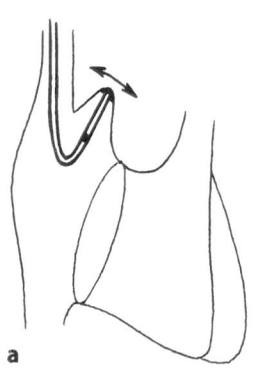 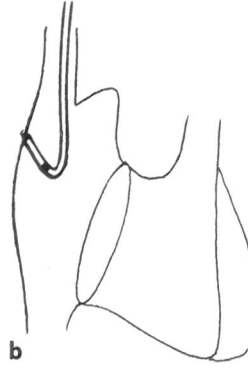

**Fig. 5.11. a** Typical motion of a lead implanted in the atrial appendage **b** Ideal position of an active fixation pacing lead

If not in the atrial appendage, the lead should be placed as close to the sino-atrial node as possible to obtain very short spike-to-P wave intervals during atrial pacing.

If one intends to place the right atrial lead in a high septal position in a patient who has an interatrial conduction defect (and one prefers not to implant 2 atrial leads), or if the implantation of a left atrial lead at the coronary sinus ostium was not successful (see below), the following maneuver is recommended, using an active fixation lead: The stylet is tightly U-shaped. The lead is introduced into the right ventricle, thus oriented towards the left. It is then gradually withdrawn while being redirected posteriorly. When crossing the tricuspid annulus, it passes near the His bundle. Then reaching the atrial side, the U-shaped stylet directs the lead upward, in the angle between the superior vena cava on the right, the roof of the atrium above, and the septum below and to the left. The lead can be affixed in that position, with pacing thresholds in that area being usually slightly higher than those measured at the appendage or on the atrial free wall. The advantage of this lead placement is to decrease the amount of interatrial conduction delay.

Whatever the lead position is, once perpendicularly positioned against the wall, the lead should be screwed in by rotating its body clockwise while keeping the stylet stationary. After a few turns (five to six), a resistance is noted. The lead should be freed and will spontaneously rotate counterclockwise over the stylet. The latter is withdrawn over a few centimeters and a gentle tug is applied to the lead to verify its proper fixation, and then, readvanced. If a loop has developed, it should be uncoiled by advancing the lead in an anticlockwise fashion. Then its attachment is confirmed.

When using a retractable screw, the lead body is usually kept stationary while turning one of its components with a special tool, or by using the stylet like a screwdriver. While these models are easier to introduce, they sometimes have the disadvantage of getting locked after several extrusions and withdrawals of the screw during multiple fixation attempts. This is the reason for the development, by CPI, of an olive-shaped, mannitol coated electrode („Sweet Tip") which facilitates its introduction, but requires to wait at least 5 min before attempting

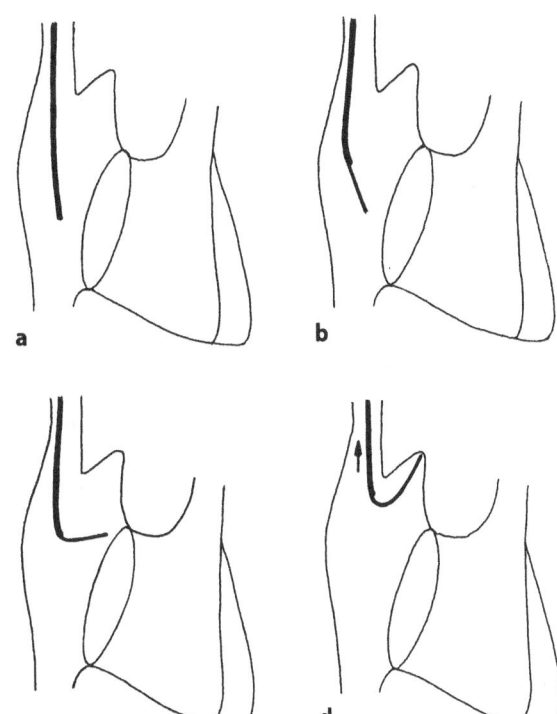

**Fig. 5.12a–d.** The preformed „J" shape of a lead may be more or less open as a function of the position of the stylet with respect to the „J"
**a** Stylet advanced to the end of the lead which is straight
**b** Partial withdrawal of the stylet resulting in slight curvature of the lead
**c** Further withdrawal with greater curvature
**d** Even more withdrawal resulting in hook-shaped lead

to screw it in. A similar system is offered by Intermedics, which requires a shorter waiting period.

When the lead is attached to the lateral atrial wall, a high output pacing test should be performed to confirm the absence of phrenic nerve stimulation, which would mandate repositioning of the electrode.

For the atrium, preshaped „J" leads are also available. After withdrawal of the stylet, the lead keeps its „J" shape to facilitate its placement and stability in the appendage. These leads, however, have drawbacks:

- They are stiffer than the active fixation leads.
- Their curve cannot be modified to accomodate the atrial size.
- They can only be positioned in the appendage.

The introduction technique is quite specific. The lead is advanced with a straight stylet into the body of the right atrium. The stylet is withdrawn over a few centimeters, which causes formation of the „J" shape, more or less according to how much of the stylet has been withdrawn (Fig. 5.12). This allows to control the aperture of the „J" angle. The appendage is then hooked in a forward motion, while gently withdrawing lead and stylet together. Penetration of the appendage is indicated by the typical rhythmic motion of the lead tip.

Whichever models are used, the stylets are removed from both leads. The patient is asked to breathe deeply, then cough, to confirm the stability of the system. The measurements to be performed next will guide the rest of the procedure, i.e. keeping the leads in position, or look for better pacing/sensing parameters.

## Intraoperative Measurements

These measurements are critical since they determine the long-term integrity of the pacemaker functions. The best possible values must be looked for (Table 5.1).

Intraoperative measurements require special instrumentation. The threshold testing device must offer a wide range of values, as do the pacing system analyzers 5311 by Medtronic and the ERA 300 by Biotronik. These testing devices allow dual chamber pacing, as well as the measurement of intracardiac slew-rate, recording of electrograms, and offer safety pacing in the ventricle while measurements are made in the atrium. The batteries of the instrument must be fully loaded.

The measurement procedure is as follows: The stylet is withdrawn by approximately 10 cm for a quick, preliminary check, but must be completely removed for final measurements. The electrical contact should simulate that of the actual pacemaker can; it is recommended to use a dummy device in close contact with the subcutaneous tissues. Contact dependent on a wound retractor may yield values up to 50% higher than actual. One must also avoid all contacts between lead connector or stylet and patient's skin, or between stylets, since they also may alter the measurements (Figs. 5.13, 5.14).

**Table 5.1.** Intraoperative measurements

| | | Thresholds Sensing amplitude (mV) | Sensing slew rate (mV/ms) | Pacing threshold (V) at 0.5 ms |
|---|---|---|---|---|
| **Atrium** | | | | |
| | Best | 3.0 | 1.0 | 0.5 |
| | Acceptable (after several repositionings) | 2 | 0.5 | 1.0 |
| **Ventricle** | | | | |
| | Best | 10 | 1.5 | 0.5 |
| | Acceptable (after several repositionings) | 6.0 | 1.0 | 1.0 |

Mandatory impedance measurements at 5 V/0.5 ms (350–1200 Ω, depending on the lead model). Mandatory pacing at 10 V (to look for diaphragmatic stimulation). Mandatory verification of measurements stability during deep breathing and coughing (variation < 20%).

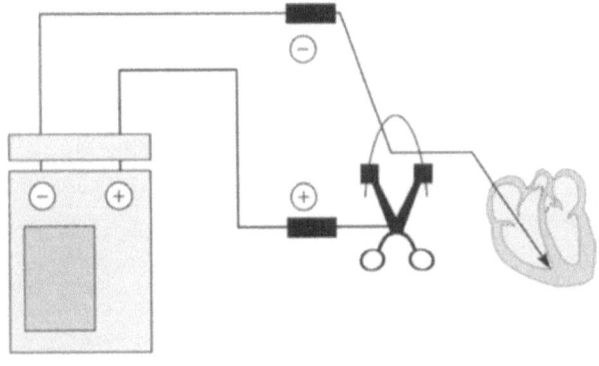

**Fig. 5.13.** Unipolar pacing measurements. The pulse is delivered between the distal electrode and the pacing can. In absence of a permanent can, it is essential to use a dummy device or the retractor serving as the reference electrode. The negative pole is connected to the distal electrode, and the positive pole to the retractor. The best reference electrode remains a dummy device with a volume equivalent to that of commonly used pacemakers

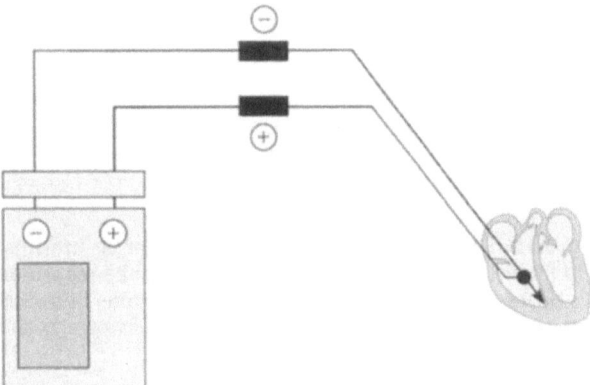

**Fig. 5.14.** Bipolar pacing measurements. The pulse is delivered between the lead's distal and proximal electrodes. No dummy device is needed. The distal electrode is connected to the negative pole, and the proximal to the positive pole

### Sensing

Once the leads have been properly positioned, slew-rates of P and R waves are measured. Pacing is inhibited to allow the appearance of spontaneous signals. In a pacemaker dependent patient, the pacing rate is slowed to a low value, and brief periods are allowed without pacing at all. A slow ventricular pacing rate is needed to perform the atrial measurements. An electrogram amplitude of 2 mV and a less than 20% beat-to beat variation in slew rate indicate adequate lead stability, to be confirmed during deep breathing and coughing. For ventricular sensing, a signal at least 6 mV in amplitude should be measured.

Measurement of the slew-rate is critical since it determines the sensing properties of the pulse generator to be implanted. Its value should be above 0.5 mV/ms in the atrium, and 1 mV/ms in the ventricle. This measurement by the electronic device should be verified by a high speed recording of the intracardiac

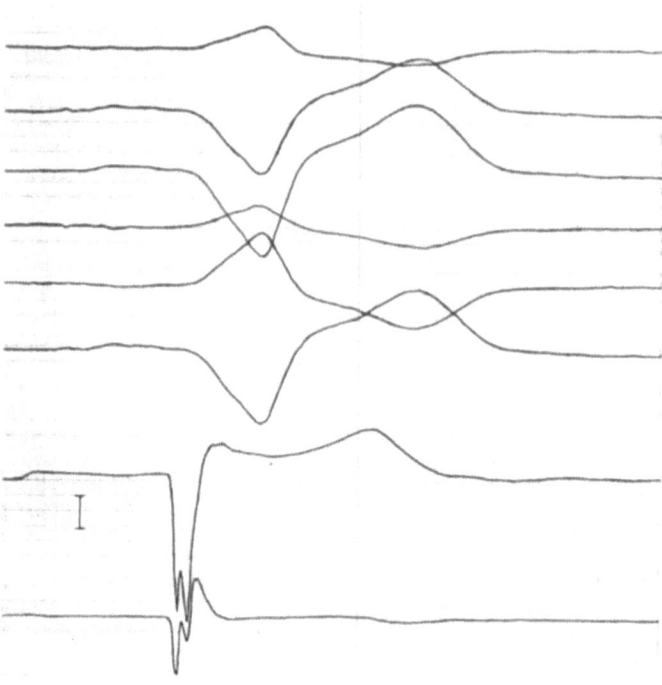

**Fig. 5.15.** The signal recorded by the ventricular electrode is of poor quality, low voltage and fragmented (filtered signal). The lead must be repositioned. The *six top tracings* are the surface ECG. The *seventh tracing* is the non-filtered (0.05 to 1 kHz) intracardiac signal. The *last tracing* is the same signal, filtered between 30 and 100 Hz. Recording speed: 500 mm/s. Amplitude scale: 1 cm = 2.5 mV

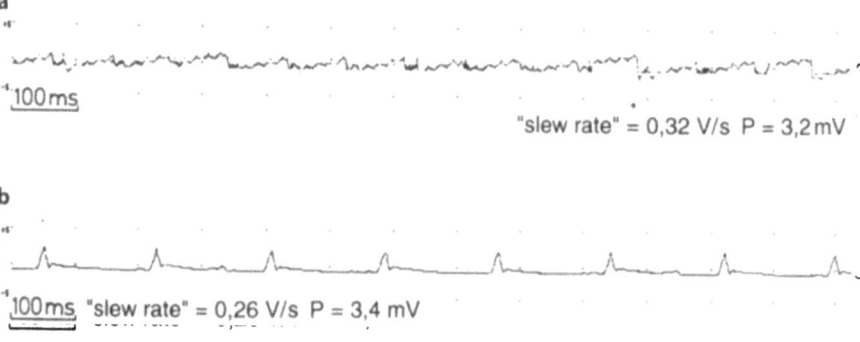

**Fig. 5.16. a** The connection to the pacing system analyzer is not correct. The signals have a slow slew-rate (0.32 mV/ms) though the amplitude is adequate (peak-to-peak = 3.2 mV), in fact due to artifacts
**b** After establishing a proper connection, similar slew-rate and amplitude values are recorded from atrial flutter waves. Proper connections are, therefore, essential to correctly interpret the results. It also confirms the importance of recording the intracardiac signal

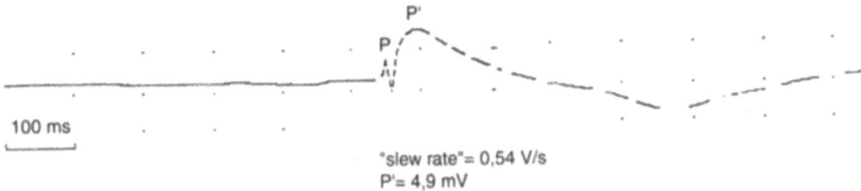

"slew rate"= 0,54 V/s
P'= 4,9 mV

**Fig. 5.17.** Endocavitary signal from a screw-in electrode with large current of injury recorded by a pacing system analyzer
*P* Patrial depolarization signal; *P'* injury signal

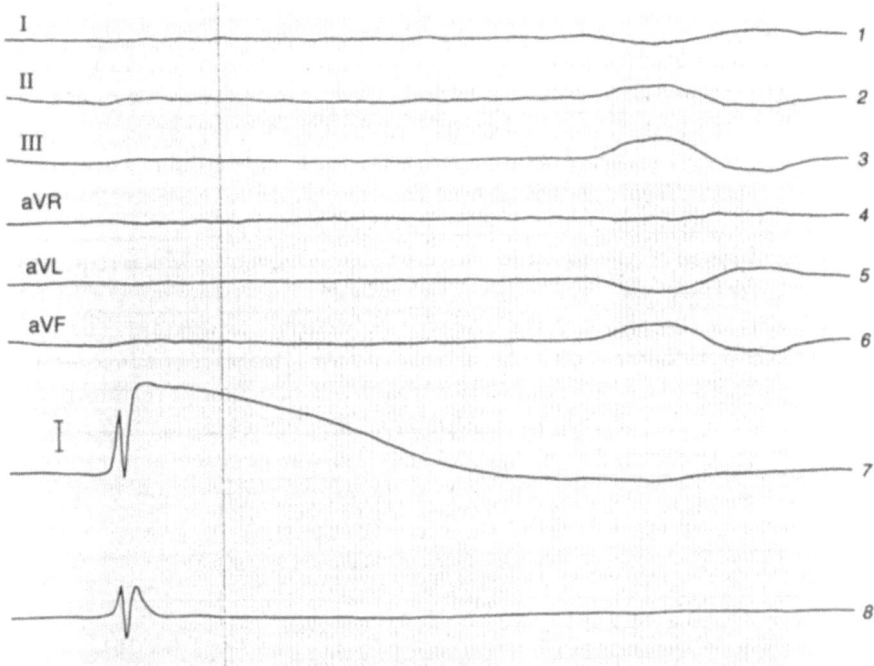

**Fig. 5.18.** This signal, recorded from the atrial lead, is of good quality, showing rapid slew-rate, high amplitude and ST segment elevation. The *top six tracings* are surface ECG leads. *Tracing 7* is unfiltered (between 0.05 and 1 kHz) atrial electrogram. The *last tracing* is the same signal filtered between 30 and 100 Hz. Recording speed = 500 mm/s. Amplitude scale: 1 cm = 2.5 mV

electrogram, if such system is available. If the slew-rate is too low, amplification of the signal may be insufficient for the sensing filter to enable proper sensing by the pacemaker (Fig. 5.15).

Intracardiac recordings also allow the elimination of possible artifacts (Fig. 5.16), which may mislead the threshold sensing device, for example the current of injury caused by the screw-in electrode (Fig. 5.17). Its amplitude may be sizable, with a steep ascent which completely obscures the atrial signal, and is only detectable on a high speed intracardiac recording (Fig. 5.18). After having scre-wed-in the active fixation lead, it is recommended to wait at least 5 min for the current of injury to subside before proceeding with measurements. This current of injury is likely to be observed regularly, even when using tined leads. It is an indication of a close contact of the electrode with the endocardium. Its absence has been correlated with a higher incidence of lead dislodgment, an additional reason to record the intracardiac electrogram intraoperatively and verify the quality of the spontaneous signal.

### Pacing

The pacing rate should be programmed above the spontaneous heart rate. At a pulse duration of 0.5 ms, the pacing threshold should be below 1 V. The imped-ance of each lead is measured at a pacing rate of 100 BPM, and an output of 5 V. Usual atrial values range from 350 to 800 $\Omega$, while in the ventricle impedance normally varies between 500 and 1200 $\Omega$. An inordinately high impedance usu-ally indicates a poor contact of the electrode with the endocardium. The stability of these measurements should also be confirmed during deep breathing and coughing.

Recognition of *retrograde conduction* is a classic maneuver which requires to pace the ventricle while recording atrial activity. The retrograde conduction time separates the pacing spike from the right atrial electrogram. The atrial potential should follow ventricular pacing, and the retrograde conduction time remains usually fixed. One looks for retrograde conduction at various pacing rates. In actual practice, we have abandoned this maneuver for two reasons. First, it has been shown that retrograde conduction can be absent at rest and only develop during exercise. Second, state-of-the-art pacemakers now offer func-tions which automatically terminate ELT, making this information less critical than in the past.

### Verification of Absence of Diaphragmatic Pacing and Lead Stability

High output pacing (10 V/1 ms) should be performed in each paced chamber, in unipolar, and bipolar configuration if a bipolar lead is used, to confirm the absence of diaphragmatic pacing. If it is present, the lead must be repositioned. This complication may occur later on at lower pacing outputs, and its develop-ment necessitates a reintervention. These various precautions are the best guar-antee of successful long-term pacing. The importance of verifying the leads sta-bility during deep breathing and coughing at the end of the procedure is particu-larly emphasized.

## Attachment and Connections of the Leads

Once the electrical and anatomic characteristics of lead placement have been found satisfactory, one must verify that enough endovascular length is available to allow sometimes considerable stretching by changes in posture or deep breathing (Fig. 5.19). The leads are tied to the vein if the approach was from a peripheral vessel, or the pectoralis major muscle fascia if the subclavian approach was used. A last radiographic check is performed after the leads have been fastened. The ligatures should never be tied with excessive force, which may disrupt the insulation or fracture the lead (Fig. 5.20). The protection sleeve does not eliminate the importance of avoiding crushing the lead when securing it with a ligature which should be strong, though atraumatic. Conversely, a week ligature may facilitate the „twiddler syndrome", or the progressive coiling of the lead upon itself or around the pulse generator, resulting in the dislodgment of the lead, even without manipulation of the device by the patient.

The pacemaker pocket is, then, prepared. This can also be done before venous insertion, giving an opportunity to verify hemostasis through the procedure. Using finger or a sponge, the fascia of the pectoralis major muscle is separated from the muscle itself in a medial prepectoral and suclavicular direction. In an emaciated patient, the pocket should preferably be subpectoral. Hemostasis is accomplished with electrocautery, paying attention to all walls of the pocket. If hemostasis is complete, no drain is necessary. Otherwise, a drain should be inserted at this point.

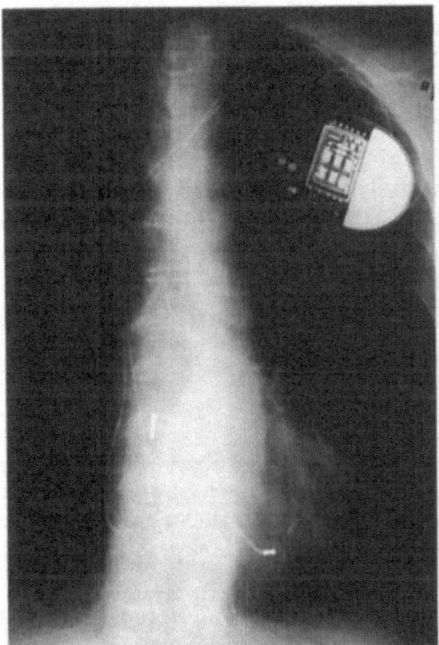 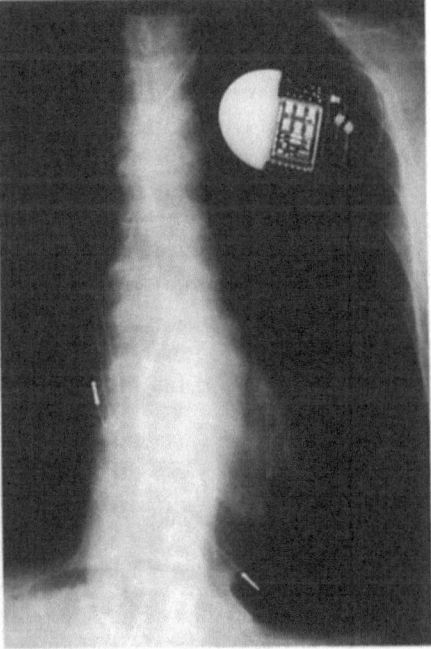

a                                                            b

**Fig. 5.19a,b.** Leads position in supine (**a**) versus upright (**b**) position in the same patient. In the upright position, considerable stretching of the lead system has occurred

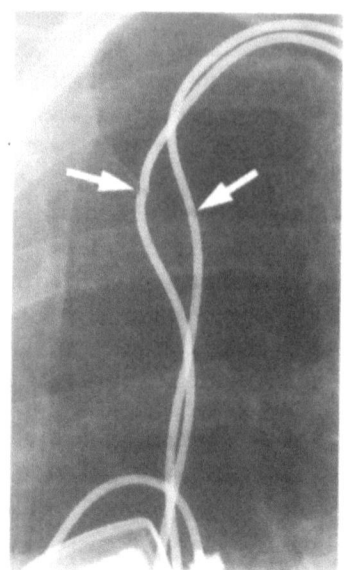

**Fig. 5.20.** Leads crush by ligatures at site of fixation

For cosmetic reasons, the pacemaker pocket can be created in the submammary space, and the lead system is tunneled from the subclavian area to the pacemaker. The latter should be inserted in a pouch and tied at several points to the pectoralis fascia. For similar cosmetic reasons, we prefer a subpectoral implant since the contact of foreign material with glandular tissue may cause severe inflammatory reactions.

At the time of connecting the lead to the device header, errors responsible for long-term complications must be thoroughly avoided. The lead connectors must be cleaned before carefully and fully inserting them into their corresponding receptacles. An illustration is usually provided on the pacemaker can to show the proper insertion of atrial and ventricular leads, respectively. After verification of the insertion of the pins past the points contact, the latter is established with the tools provided by the manufacturer, usually by a set screw or a clip. Screwing should be tight enough to establish electrical contact and secure the pin, but not so tight as to damage the Allen screw of the connector (Fig. 5.21).

> **!** To avoid a confusion between atrial and ventricular lead, one can verify the lead serial number usually inscribed within the insulation material. One can also pace the corresponding chamber before making the connection with the header (Fig. 5.22).

The connection may be hampered by the use of a lead of a different brand than the pacemaker, even when they are theoretically compatible. Other anomalies that may result in long-term pacing/sensing failure include:

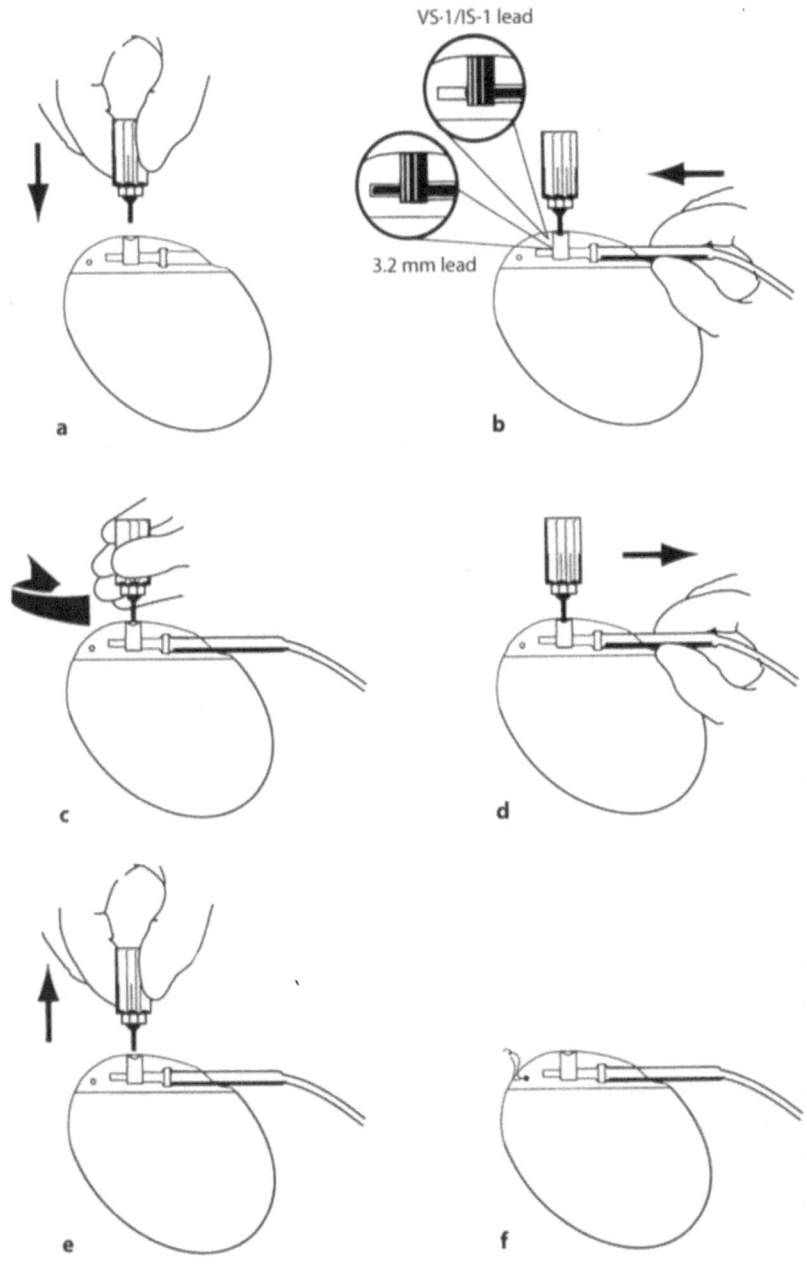

VS-1/IS-1 lead

3.2 mm lead

a    b    c    d    e    f

**Fig. 5.21.** Proper procedure to tighten the lead connections (drawings by Telectronics)

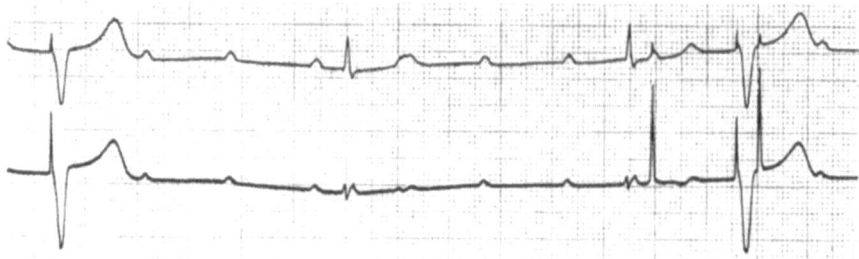

**Fig. 5.22.** Pacing leads reversal in a dual chamber pacemaker header. The pacemaker is inhibited by the P waves which are sensed in the ventricular channel

- Improperly screwed Allen screw.
- Defective housing of the screw giving the impression of having fully screwed in the Allen screw.
- Incomplete insertion of the pin. This is more likely to occur with the use of lubricant (piston effect) in a hermetically sealed connector.
- Mismatch between various 3.2 mm leads and pacemakers with side locks whose insulator compressibility is superior to that of the leads.
- Possible injury to 3.2 mm unipolar leads inserted into a 3.2 mm bipolar pacemaker when the set screw of the positive pole is tightened down on a lead without protection ring at that site.

These two last complications are, unfortunately, not the only problems one might encounter when using pacemaker and lead of different brands as long as no world wide standard has been adopted. One should add:

- Terminal pin too long to fit into the connector housing; it can be shortened with a metal cutting tool (Fig. 5.23).
- Improper seal when a lead without sealing rings is inserted into a housing without sealing rings. A spare sleeve is recommended rather than adhesive (Fig. 5.23).
- Most difficult insertion of a lead with sealing rings into a header (of a different brand) with poorly fitting sealing rings (Fig. 5.24).
- Delayed complications with some 3.2 mm lead models from fracture at the junction of the conductor coil (soft) and the connector pin (stiff). This is observed when this junction remains unprotected by an insufficiently deep housing of the connector pin, causing mechanical strain and fracture at this weak point (Fig. 5.25).

The excess length of the leads is, then, coiled and placed under the pacemaker can to minimize the risk of damage at the time of pulse generator replacement. The entire system is inserted into the pocket with the active side of the can facing upward in a prepectoral position, versus downward in a subpectoral position, if the system is unipolar. If pectoral muscle stimulation is noted, the connections must be inspected again, and possibly insulated with silicone rubber, including at the point of insertion of the connector pins. Some operators fasten the can to

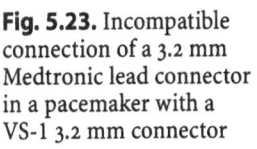
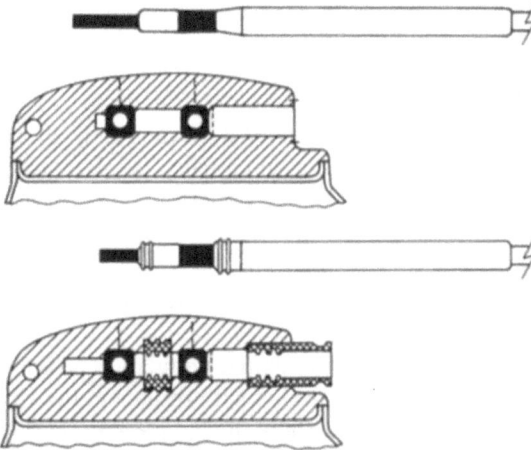

**Fig. 5.23.** Incompatible connection of a 3.2 mm Medtronic lead connector in a pacemaker with a VS-1 3.2 mm connector

**Fig. 5.24.** Difficult connection between a VS-1 3.2 mm lead and a CPI/Medtronic 3.2 mm pacemaker connector

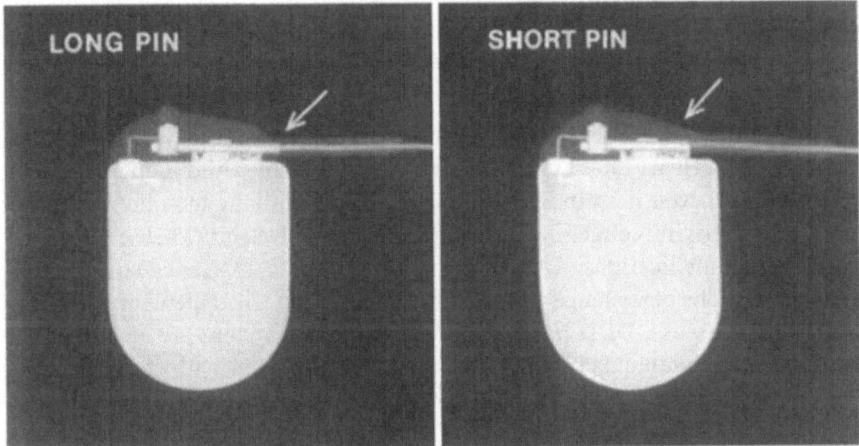

**Fig. 5.25.** Risk of conductor fracture in a lead whose stiff connecting segment protrudes (*left*) outside the pacemaker epoxy header (photograph from Vitatron)

the fascia to prevent its migration toward the axilla, which we perform systematically in subpectoral implants. After removal of the temporary pacing lead under fluoroscopic control, the wound is closed in layers. The skin should be neatly sutured for cosmetic reasons, contributing to better patient acceptance. A subcuticular stitch is preferred. The pacemaker is, then, programmed according to the measurements just made, and the clinical requirements of each individual case.

## The Post-Implant Period

After implantation, the patient should remain under monitored surveillance for at least several hours. A pacemaker dependent patient should remain under intensive surveillance for 24 h, not to miss a lead dislodgment or any other event causing pacing failure. A chest radiograph is obtained routinely after 24 h. If a drain has been left in place, it should be removed no later than 48 h later. Wound dressings are changed no more often than every 2 days. The patient is encouraged to ambulate and to not allow „freezing" of the shoulder, with the assistance of mild analgesics. The subcuticular stitch is removed within 8 to 10 days.

## 5.3
## Pacemaker Implant in the Pediatric Patient

Cardiac pacing in the pediatric population poses specific problems related to the size of the instrumentation with respect to the size of the patient, body growth, and long-term tolerance of the implanted materials.

The approaches to implantation are the same as in the adult. Economy of venous access is of utmost importance in an individual in need of lifetime pacing. Consequently, a decision must be made regarding the need for dual versus single chamber pacing since a risk exists of crowding the cardiac chambers with pacing leads over the years.

Instead of a fixed rate pacemaker, no less than a rate responsive system should be implanted. Heart rates are considerably higher in the child than in the adult. Furthermore, even if an indication does not exist initially for rate responsiveness, an underlying congenital heart disease may evolve, or the patient may need cardioactive medications. AAI pacing is satisfactory in presence of normal AV conduction. The persistence of normal AV conduction will depend on the underlying heart disease. DDD pacing is preferable, unless there are atrial tachyarrhythmias, the patient is small (which may pose problems with crowding of the venous circulation), or venous access is limited. Since DDD and VVIR pulse generators are currently of the same size, it is no longer an important determinant in the choice of pacing mode. If dual chamber pacing is necessary, a VDD system may be considered only if the patient has reached an adult size, even though, in a child, a non functional lead should be removed if at all possible. Finally, the pulse generator should be as small as possible, while offering a reasonable battery life expectancy.

More and more intracardiac leads are implanted, even in small children. Likewise, because of their advantages and current size, bipolar leads can be used without inordinate difficulties. Finally, steroid eluting leads are recommended.

We give preference to active fixation leads which allow a wider choice of pacing sites in hearts that often are congenitally anomalous, and which are easier to extract than tined leads. In all cases, one must take into consideration further growth of the patient, the number of leads already implanted, potential future extraction problems, and alterations of the tricuspid valve.

Conversely, intracardiac leads are contraindicated in presence of right-to-left shunt because of risks of systemic embolization, in cases of high pulmonary vascular resistance, since even a small pulmonary embolism may be catastrophic, and in presence of a prosthetic tricuspid valve.

## 5.4
## Pacemaker Implantation in the Cardiac Transplant Patient

The donor heart is deprived of the neural input which normally modulates the heart rate. Remnants of the recipient heart are present since the posterior part of the right atrium is left in place. A suture line prevents a priori all conduction between recipient and donor tissue. The rhythm of the recipient heart is faster and dissociated from that of the donor's atrium. The choice of pacemaker is influenced by the observation that most transplant patients develop systemic hypertension in the first year, causing changes in left ventricular compliance. Hence, it is preferable to implant a dual chamber system to guarantee an optimal AV synchrony.

Several options are available when a pacing system needs to be implanted. A lead is placed in the native atrium and another in the donor's atrium. An SST pacemaker

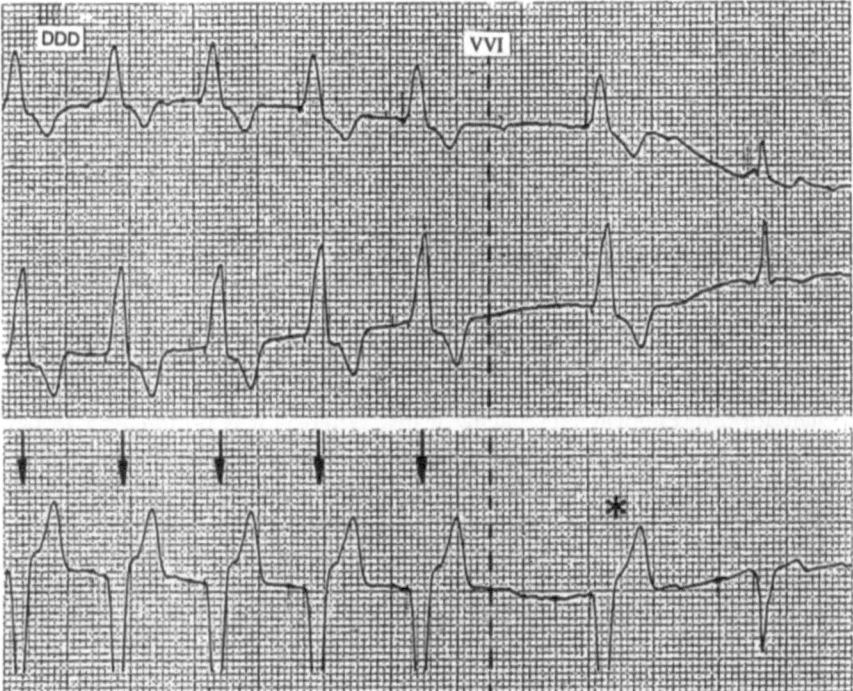

**Fig. 5.26.** Dual chamber pacing in a transplanted patient. The atrial lead is in the recipient's heart and the ventricular lead in the donor's heart ventricle. The donor's atrium has no implanted lead. In DDD mode, sensing of the recipient's atrium, whose rate is rapid, is tracked in the ventricle. This is associated with retrograde conduction in the donor's heart (*arrows*). The pacemaker cannot sense this retrograde conduction since its atrial lead is in the recipient's atrium. When switching from DDD to VVI mode, ventricular pacing occurs at the lower rate. No retrograde P wave is apparent on the surface ECG (*) since the atrium of the donor heart seems refractory at this point, when the retrograde conduction time is shorter at this slower heart rate. The last event is a ventricular fusion

is connected to the transplanted heart which tracks the recipient atrium's rhythm in absence of AV conduction defect. Another option consists of using a dual chamber system, with the lead implanted in the donor heart's atrium connected to the ventricular channel and the AVD set at o ms. The end results is the same, though the function of the pacemaker is more complex. In both cases, the stability of sinus rhythm in the recipient heart should be considered, as well as the likelihood of development of atrial fibrillation and its consequences, or the risk of subsequent development of AV block.

The second solution consists of implanting an atrial lead in the recipient atrium and a ventricular lead in the transplanted heart. The latter tracks the recipient atrium, at the risk of retrograde conduction occurring in the donor's heart (Fig. 5.26). The third solution, which we favor, is to implant an atrial or dual chamber rate responsive system solely in the donor's heart, with rate responsiveness programmed on the basis of the information provided by the pacemaker sensor. The last, least desirable, option is the implant of a single chamber, rate responsive, ventricular pacemaker. The ultimate choice depends mostly on the quality of the thresholds measured, which are often altered in the donor's as well as in the recipient's atria.

Whichever implant strategy has been chosen, the physician performing the biopsies must be mindful of the existing leads to avoid their dislodgment if they have been implanted recently, or their damage by mismanipulation of the bioptome.

## 5.5
## Pacemaker Implantation in Special Cases

### Presence of a Left Superior Vena Cava

Catheterization of a persistent left superior vena cava may complicate the implantation of endocavitary pacing leads. Whereas it is no longer a serious problem for the implant of a right atrial active fixation lead, implant in the ventricle may be more tedious. By preshaping the last 10 cm of the stylet, providing an approximately 130° angle, one can, by leaning on the lateral wall of the atrium, advance both the lead and its stylet through the tricuspid valve. An active fixation lead is recommended.

### Right Heart Chambers Dilatation

This requires the use of active fixation leads. No particular difficulty is expected in the atrium as long as the stylet is widely curved to reach the atrial wall. Much greater difficulties may be encountered in the ventricle from frequently associated tricuspid regurgitation which forcefully whips the unattached lead. The following maneuver may be helpful: the straight stylet is preshaped in a „J" as in preparation for an atrial fixation. By advancing the lead, the „J" tends to cross the tricuspid orifice and progresses toward the outflow tract. After exchanging the „J" for a widely curved stylet which is withdrawn over a few centimeters, the distal end of the lead will bend backwards, dropping it towards the apex. As soon as contact is established, the lead can be fixed. This may be helped by the exchange of the curved stylet for a straight one.

If one wishes to position the lead in the outflow tract, the procedure is simplified since the widely curved stylet facilitates the passage through the tricuspid valve, and the lead tends to hang up at the anterior rim of the pulmonic infundibulum.

Besides the difficulties in lead placement in dilated right heart chambers, the main challenge consists of obtaining acceptable pacing and sensing thresholds, which often involves testing at several locations.

## Tricuspid Annuloplasty or Prosthetic Tissue Valves

The challenge is even greater since the orifice size is markedly reduced with respect to the cardiac chambers, and the struts of a tissue valve may further restrict the progress of a pacing lead toward the ventricle. Such situations, however, do not represent contraindications to the implant of an endocavitary system.

## Planned Cardiac Surgery

In case of a planned cardiac operation, the surgeon would be well suited to implant the pacing system intraoperatively. However, surgery is often considered as a distant option as, for instance, in the case of evolving valvular disease. In such cases, it may be advisable to not implant a lead in the right atrial appendage which is often cannulated to establish artificial heart-lung circulation. Such situations, fortunately rare, require thoughtful strategic planning before implantation of the pacemaker.

## Biatrial Pacing

Biatrial pacing via the coronary sinus was introduced by Arthur Moss in 1968, in preliminary attempts to implant dual chamber pacing systems at a time when leads were not properly designed to be implanted in the right atrium. With the development of right atrial leads, this technique was temporarily abandoned, though later revitalized by a new pacing indication, i.e. biatrial pacing.

Biatrial pacing may be indicated:

- Preventively, in patients with interatrial conduction defects and atrial arrhythmias.
- For hemodynamic purpose, in patients with interatrial conduction defects associated with hypertrophic obstructive or dilated cardiomyopathy.
- In patients whose right atrium cannot be paced or sensed properly because of major changes in the atrial tissue. In such cases, left atrial pacing replaces right atrial pacing.

The technique relies on a specially designed lead (Medtronic 2188) which has a double 45° distal angulation. The aim is, on one hand, to obtain stability of the lead within the coronary sinus and, on the other hand, to maintain permanent contact of the distal electrode with the left atrial wall, despite the absence of terminal screw or tines on the lead. Catheterization of the coronary sinus is easy when it is wide and in the absence of right atrial dilatation. The electrode is pressed inside the triangle contained between the tricuspid annulus anteriorly, and the inferior vena cava inferiorly. After withdrawing the stylet by 1 cm, the lead is oriented posteriorly and advanced in a 45° oblique direction between the left lateral border of the spine and the horizontal surface of the left hemidiaphragm. After the lead has entered the coronary sinus, its position is confirmed in the LAO view where it is visible along the left postero-lateral border of the cardiac shadow. When the cannulation is difficult, help can be obtained from examination of the intracardiac electrograms. The lead is in the coronary sinus when the atrial electrogram appears at the end of the P wave of the surface ECG, accompanied by a high amplitude R wave of left ventricular origin.

The next step consists of finding a stable position with satisfactory pacing and sensing thresholds, along with a left ventricular R wave as small as possible. The best position is in the distal coronary sinus, though most leads are actually left in the middle segment. A more proximal position is unstable, unless the lead can be wedged, usually in a small vein draining from the posterior left atrium. This requires the lead to be bent upward and posteriorly toward the left atrium (Fig. 5.27a). The lead stability should be confirmed during deep breathing and coughing maneuvers. The techniques of implantation of the right-sided leads are as described earlier; they should be placed as high as possible.

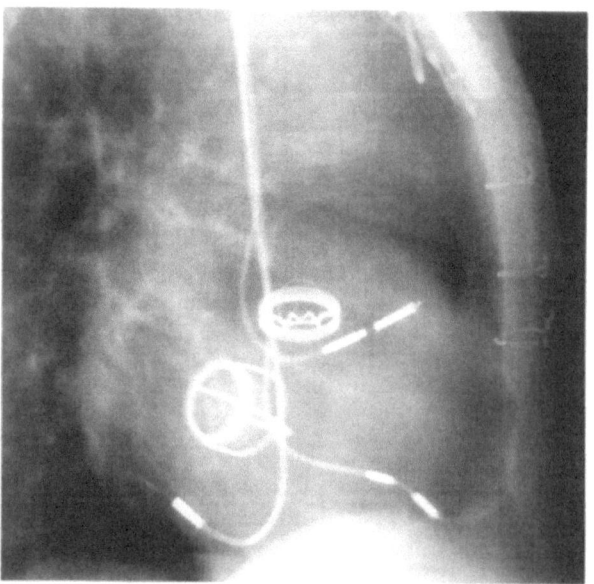

**Fig. 5.27. a** Lateral chest radiograph showing the leads implantation sites of a triple chamber system. One lead is implanted in the high, anterior right atrium (*top right*) another is in the coronary sinus (*bottom left*), and the third is located at the right ventricular apex (*bottom right*)

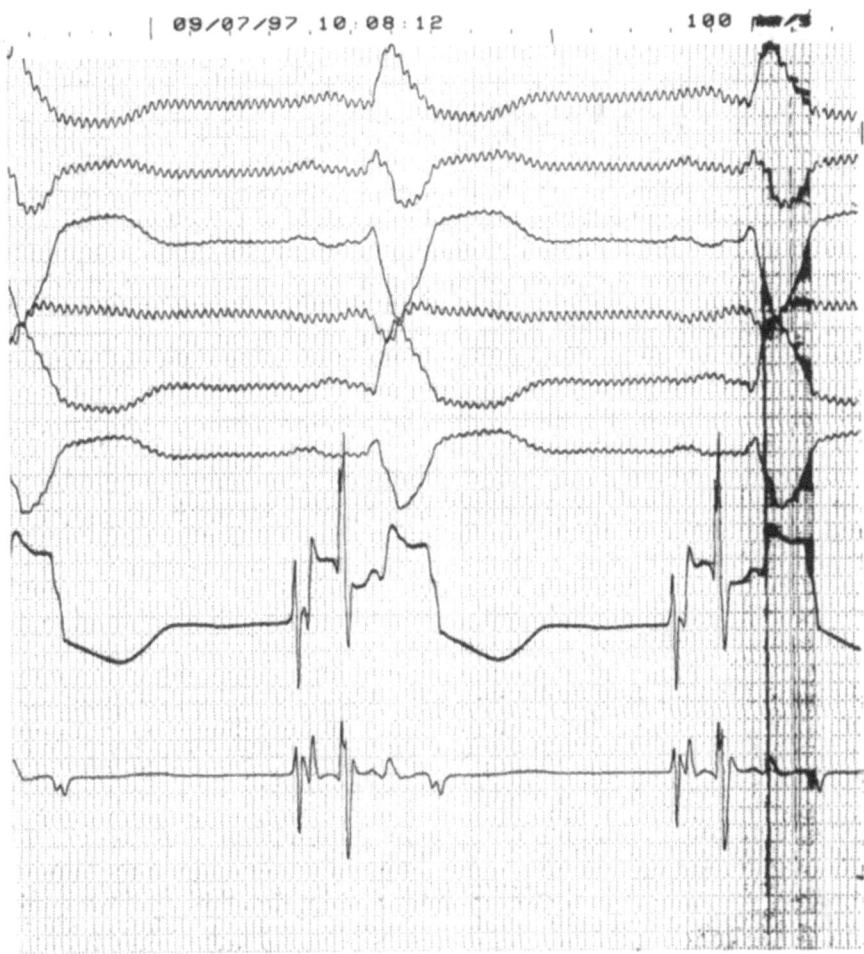

**Fig. 5.27. b** The intracardiac recording of the atrial electrograms (right atrium: cathode; left atrium: anode) reveals a 120 ms interatrial conduction delay, indicative of an interatrial conduction disorder

In the method described by Saksena, the atrial pacing system consists of two right atrial leads, one placed in the upper atrium and another in the ostium of the coronary sinus. Since it is a straight screw-in lead, it is the preshaped stylet (similar to that of the Medtronic 2188 lead) which helps in the cannulation of the coronary sinus. The distal angle must be tighter to achieve more pressure by the electrode on the myocardium at the time of fixation of the lead. Once in the coronary sinus, the electrode must be withdrawn back to the ostium and screwed into the roof of the first centimeter of coronary sinus. Although pacing and sensing thresholds are often high, the lead stability is guaranteed by the active fixation mechanism.

The next step consists of interfacing both atrial leads to the atrial channel of the pulse generator. A Y connector is currently indispensable (Fig. 5.27b). It should preferably be double bipolar, i.e. the distal electrodes should be connected to the pulse generator's cathode and the proximal electrodes to the anode. The disadvantage of these adapters is to cause an inordinately low lead impedance, the source of considerable waste of pacemaker power. One might, therefore, prefer to use an adapter which connects the pulse generator's cathode to the right atrial lead, and the anode to the left atrial lead. This, however, is usually associated with a significant rise in pacing threshold at the anode, which may be quite problematic since the maximal pacing output of the pacemaker may be insufficient to achieve capture at the anode.

What is currently much needed is a pacemaker with separate connections allowing the independent control of each lead.

Finally, the pacemaker must be able to synchronize both atria with a DDT-like atrial triggered mode responsive to all atrial sensed events, including atrial extrasystoles. This function should preferably be assumed by a RAM algorithm, which must also be capable of dealing with VA crosstalk since the left atrial lead also records a left ventricular electrogram.

## Left Ventricular Pacing

This pacing modality is in the investigational stage; its current application pertains to NYHA class IV (possibly III) heart failure due to dilated cardiomyopathy associated with ventricular contraction asynchrony. The implant of the left ventricular lead may be performed in two different ways:

- Either from an epicardial approach via video-assisted thoracoscopy, which mandates the use of specific pacing leads, and which is potentially dangerous in these patients who often suffer from multi-organ failure. The lead must be externalized through the rib cage and tunneled to the pulse generator.
- Or via the transvenous approach, with the major advantage of avoiding general anesthesia and left lung exclusion needed for the epicardial approach. Although the implant procedure may be lengthy, it does not involve more risk than that of a traditional implantation. The technique requires dexterity, patience and some good fortune.

The preferred leads currently in use are the long (65 cm) Medtronic 2188 and the 2187 models, the latter being still under evaluation.

The aim is to place the distal electrode over the mid postero-lateral left ventricular wall, wedged in a venous tributary of the coronary sinus. If multiple lateral venous accesses are available, the lead will be left at the site where the left ventricular electrogram is the latest with respect to the QRS complex on the surface ECG.

Retrograde angiography of the coronary sinus venous network is helpful for orientation. The coronary sinus must first be catheterized as described earlier. This initial procedural step is already delicate, as it may be hampered by regularly encountered right atrial dilatation, and attempts to exchange the stylet (to

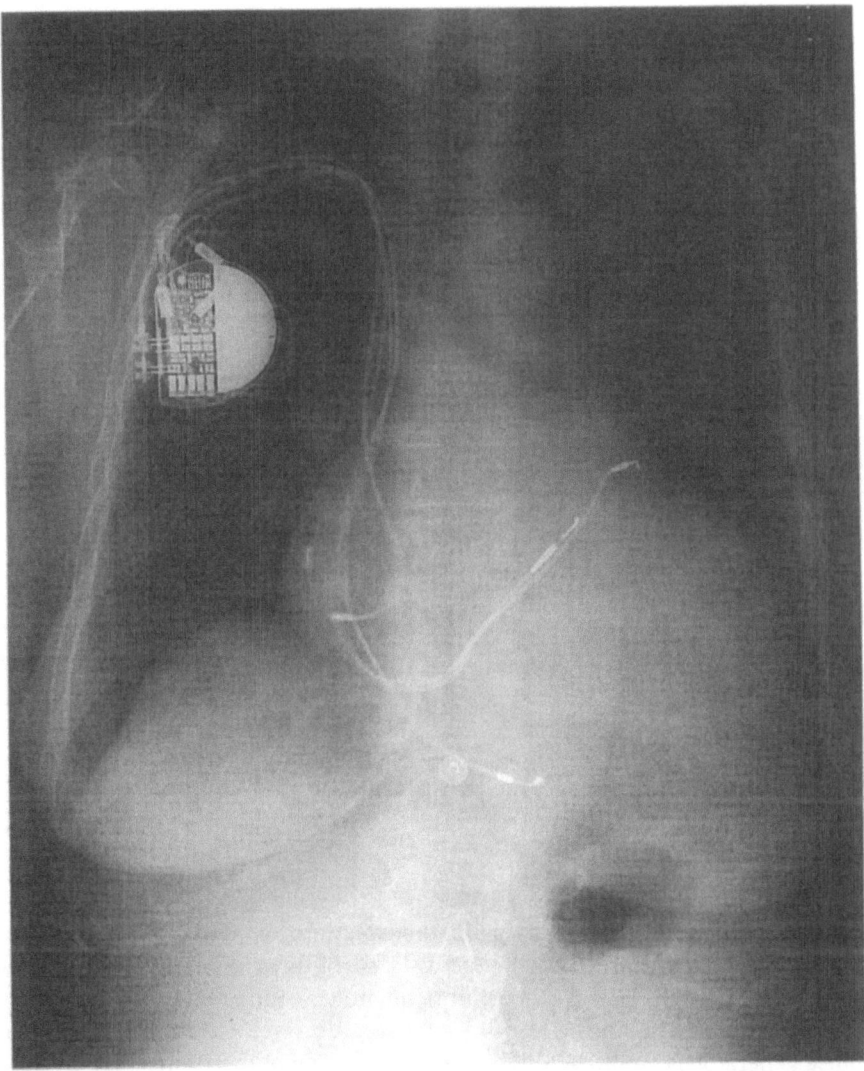

**Fig. 5.28. a** Antero-posterior chest radiograph showing the implantation sites of the various leads in a case of four-chamber pacing: the right atrial lead is in a conventional location; a lead was placed in the coronary sinus for pacing/sensing of the left atrium; the left ventricular lead was introduced via the coronary sinus and wedged near the ostium of a high antero-lateral vein; the right ventricular lead was placed in an infero-lateral position

modify its shape) invariably lead to dislodgment of the lead out of the coronary sinus. A double angulation should, therefore, be chosen from the onset. The lead is then advanced to a zone near the ostium of the lateral vein to be catheterized. To-and-fro and rotational motion of the lead usually succeeds in bringing it to that ostium, at which point it must be advanced after softening its tip (after withdraw-

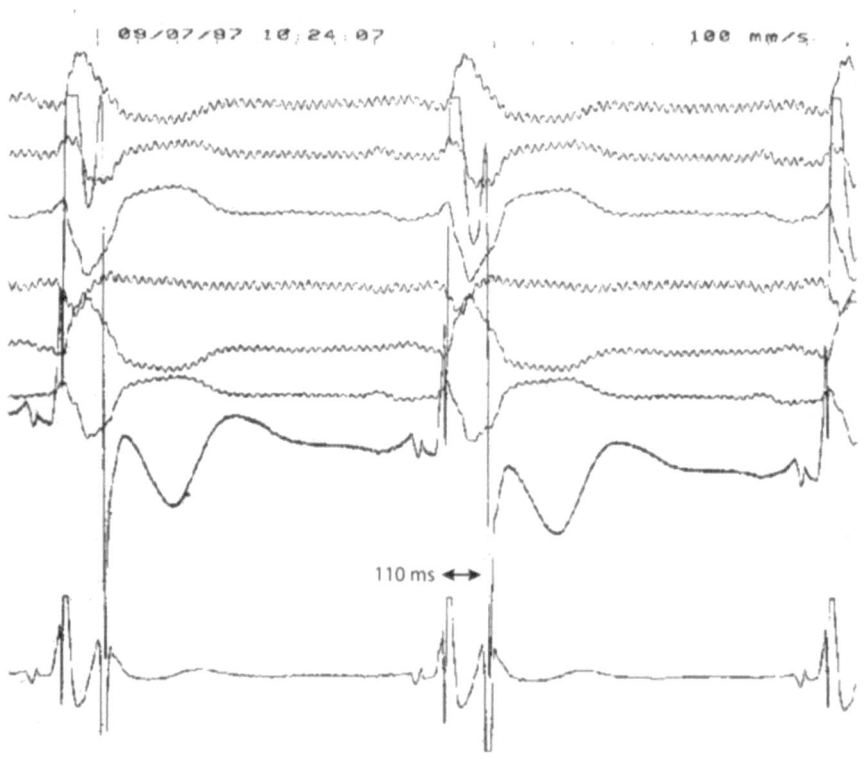

**Fig. 5.28. b** The intracardiac recording of the ventricular electrograms (right ventricle: cathode; left ventricle: anode) reveals an 110 ms interventricular delay, indicative of an interventricular conduction defect

ing the stylet by 1 cm) and applying further rotational motion. Once in the vein, the lead must be advanced until wedged. Measured thresholds are often excellent distally (far from the lateral vein ostium), but not as good proximally, sometimes forcing repositioning of the lead. Interfacing of the ventricular leads with the pulse generator is facilitated by the high amplitude of the ventricular electrograms. A double unipolar or double bipolar adapter usually allows the maintenance of an excellent long-term pacing impedance. This configuration is applicable for triple or quadruple chamber pacing: RA (+ LA), RV + LV (Fig. 5.28).

In case of chronic atrial fibrillation, pacing is limited to the ventricles with a traditional dual chamber device. One ventricular lead is connected to the pacemaker's atrial channel, the other to the ventricular channel. The shortest AVD must be programmed. Refractory periods and upper rates are set to avoid a Wenckebach-like „AV" (or rather RV – LV) association, by programming as high as possible an upper rate, identical refractory periods in both ventricles (equal to the period corresponding to the 2 : 1 AV block rate), and the rate responsive function must be activated. Indeed, biventricular pacing must be uninterrupted. In case of atrial fibrillation, it is often necessary to ablate the His bundle in order to achieve this goal.

# CHAPTER 6

# Complications

This chapter will begin by briefly reviewing the complications that have been largely eliminated with the introduction of transvenous pacing systems. The first approach consisted of a left thoracotomy through the fourth intercostal space. Access to the left heart was found through pleural and pericardial cavities. Inherent risks consisted of postoperative pneumo- or hemothorax, systematically prevented by the use of chest tubes. The epigastric approach appeared next in two variations: the first was a midline, supra-umbilical technique requiring removal of the xyphoid process which may be quite hemorrhagic; the second was a left abdominal approach along the lateral margin of the abdominus rectus muscle. In each, the pericardium was reached transdiaphragmatically, which carries risks similar to that of a thoracotomy.

Other problems were related to the pacemaker pocket. The original implantation sites were retromammary with the leads crossing the rib cage subjected to the stress of respiratory movements, and the development of marked tissue sclerosis from the presence of glandular tissue near the pacemaker.

When placed in the abdominal region, between peritoneum and posterior layer of the abdominus rectus muscle, the device is well protected, but may migrate into the abdominal cavity through a peritoneal tear. If placed over the muscle, transcutaneous erosion may occur. The least complicated implant site seems to be between the rectus muscle and its posterior fascia.

Complications occurring in more recent times will be divided into early and late occurrences.

## 6.1
### Intra- and Postoperative Complications

These complications will be best avoided or diagnosed by a close early surveillance, including wound inspection and identification of possible drainage, heart and lung auscultation, daily electrocardiogram, chest radiograph, and early testing of the pacemaker.

## Complications at the Implant Site

### Hematoma

Hematomas occur within hours or days of typically lengthy and tedious implants with suboptimal hemostasis. They are, of course, facilitated by anticoagulants or antiplatelet agents taken at the time of procedure, or resumed too early thereafter. If the implant can be postponed, antiplatelet agents should be withheld for several days. Warfarin type anticoagulants should regularly be replaced by heparin, whose administration should be suspended, or significantly decreased in the hours preceding the operation.

Progressive swelling of the pocket, sometimes associated with inflammatory signs, should raise the suspicion of hematoma. A compressive dressing may, on occasion, halt its progression. In absence of spontaneous resolution, or in case of expansion with painful cutaneous distension, its evacuation by needle aspiration under strictly sterile conditions may be attempted, though not always successful because of location of the pocket. If an open reintervention is necessary, it must be performed as a sterile surgical procedure during which, after evacuation of the hematoma, the source of bleeding may or may not be identified. In a patient in need of anticoagulation, oral treatment should best be postponed for 48 hours. Despite these precautions, a secondary hematoma may form infrequently.

*Recommendation.* Prevention is essential. Use electrocautery (only before insertion of pacemaker system) to control bleeding sites. Placement of a drain is unnecessary. Use compressive bandages in patients at risk.

### Pectoral Stimulation

Pectoral stimulation is caused by a current leak within the pacemaker pocket; it is often facilitated by the presence of fluid in the pocket, by a subpectoral position, or by an improper orientation of the pacemaker can, with its active surface apposed to the muscle. This phenomenon tends to subside with disappearance of the fluid. On occasion the current leak originates from a lead insulation failure, from a connector or from an adaptor. Corrective measures include a decrease in pacing output, reprogramming to a bipolar pacing, if feasible, or, in few cases, reintervention to seal all connections with silicone rubber.

*Recommendation.* Always gently manipulate the implantable instrumentation. Never expose a polyurethane lead to electrocautery. Carefully seal all screw housings and adaptors.

## Infection

Often heralded by local or regional (scapula) discomfort, infection may take two main forms:

- Local signs are predominant (redness, increased local heat, skin distension, fluctuance, etc.). Such findings should prompt a needle aspiration for microbiologic examination.
- Systemic signs and symptoms are on the forefront, whereas local findings are subtle, or even absent. In the worst case, the clinical picture is that of septicemia which suggests lead-induced endocarditis with or without tricuspid valve involvement. A complete echocardiographic evaluation, including transesophageal imaging is in order. In presence of infection, explantation of the entire implanted material is the rule, in conjunction with the administration of systemic antibiotics, targeting staphylococcus species, while waiting for the bacteriologic results of local aspiration specimens, or of blood cultures. The infected lead should be extracted by direct traction, and its tip cultured.

*Recommendation.* Keep in mind that the management of infections is primarily preventive. During implantation, rigorous precautions, comparable to those applied to the surgical implant of prostheses, must be taken. They impose to work in an environment prohibited to infected patients.

- Favor early morning cases, when the room is the cleanest.
- The patient must be afebrile, rid of all infectious sources.
- Carefully prepare the surgical field before entrance into the operating room: ban make up and jewelry, cleanse, shave and disinfect the skin, and avoid the placement of an intravenous perfusion on the anticipated side of the implant.
- Limit the number of operating room workers and insist on the observance of the same rigorous sterile precautions.
- Completely cover hair, beard, footwear.
- Verify the expiration date of all sterile materials.
- Strictly observe surgical hand washing techniques.
- Wear two layers of gloves; change gloves in lengthy procedures.
- Use prophylactic antibiotics.
- Change surgical scrub suit in-between cases.
- Have operating room floor scrubbed between cases.

## Complications Related to Vascular Access

### Lead Implantation in a Left-Sided Chamber

This complication may result from the introduction of the pacing lead through the subclavian artery during an attempt to puncture the vein. Though the color of the blood and the blood pressure are quite different, these differences are not always apparent. The course of the lead is midline; the most obvious finding is that of right bundle branch block QRS complex morphology on the electrocardiogram during pacing (see Fig. 5.9, p. 215). The main potential risk consists of local thrombus formation and secondary peripheral or cerebral embolization. We have not encountered this complication.

> *Recommendation.* It is important to understand clearly the landmarks of a subclavian puncture in a patient, supine on the table, with the ipsilateral arm along the body, shoulder downward, and the head turned to the opposite direction.

### Pneumothorax, Hemothorax and Hemomediastinum

Pneumothorax and hemothorax result mainly from an inadvertent puncture during an attempt to enter the subclavian vein. They are more likely to occur when the penetration of the vein is difficult (Fig. 6.1), and develop either immediately or within days of the implant. They are usually small and infrequently require suction or drainage. Localized subcutaneous emphysema may be present. A chest radiograph should be systematically obtained after each procedure which include an attempt to enter the subclavian vein.

Hemomediastinum is rare, occurs under similar circumstances, and is usually associated with the two previously described complications.

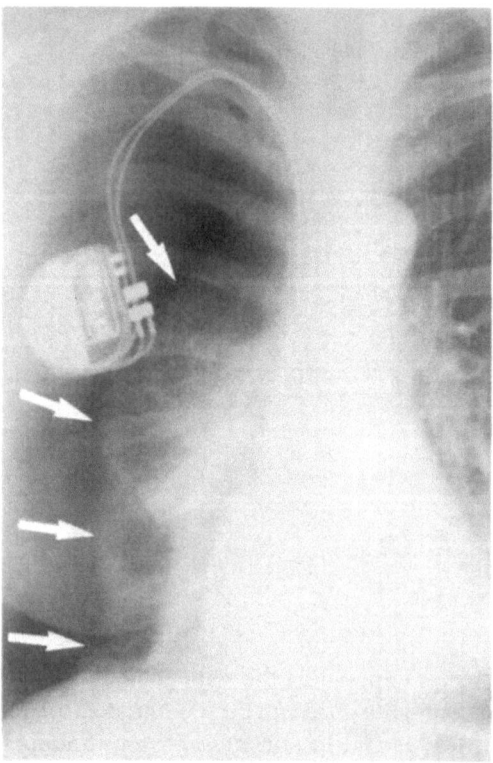

**Fig. 6.1.** Pneumothorax, hemothorax and hemomediastinum are uncommon, but justify obtaining a postoperative chest radiograph after attempts to puncture the subclavian vein

## Air Embolism

This may occur during lead implantation, at the time of venotomy and lead introduction, particularly when using the subclavian approach. This risk may be minimized by lowering the head of the table, by occluding the introducer sheath before introducing the lead, and by asking the patient to withhold breathing at this very moment. Introducer sheaths with valves eliminate this complication.

## Venous Thrombosis

Thrombosis develop primarily in the veins used to introduce the lead(s), usually the subclavian or cephalic veins. The risk increases with the number of leads in the vein. It is often undetected and only diagnosed much later from the development of venous collateral circulation at the shoulder or on the neck. It rarely causes signs of acute upper extremity phlebitis in the form of a swollen, inflamed, cyanotic and painful upper extremity, ipsilateral to the site of implant, accompanied by fever and sinus tachycardia. This thrombosis is rarely complicated by pulmonary embolism. Acute occlusion of the superior vena cava does not occur in absence of preexistent anomaly, and should prompt treatment with antithrombotic agents, heparin, or even a surgical intervention.

Deep vein, femoral thrombosis is possible when a temporary pacing lead was used, particularly if it was left in place for several days.

*Recommendation.* To limit this risk, some operators use small perioperative doses of heparin. Because of its insidious development, it is recommended to look for it systematically in instances where a lead needs to be added or exchanged.

## Cardiac Complications

### Rhythm Disturbances

Arrhythmias can be expected mostly at the time of lead implantation. Elderly patients with chronic ischemic heart disease, often with electrolytes abnormalities or treated with cardioactive medications, are prone to ventricular arrhythmias, themselves facilitated by bradycardia. They tend to occur upon crossing the tricuspid valve, or during placement of the lead in the right ventricle. In other cases, bigeminal extrasystoles appear systematically after each paced ventricular beat, probably from mechanical stimulation by the lead on the tricuspid valve; they mandate lead repositioning.

Atrial arrhythmias also may occur at the time of atrial or ventricular lead implantation, as well as several days later. During the procedure, if the patient is in atrial fibrillation while the intent is to implant an atrial or a dual chamber system, it may be necessary to proceed with cardioversion in order to examine the quality of atrial thresholds during sinus rhythm. This carries a risk of systemic embolization which may sometimes be delayed. Another option is to implant the lead in the atrium during atrial fibrillation, to start anticoagulation, and to proceed with medical or electrical cardioversion 3 weeks later. (Caution: electrical cardioversion may irreversibly damage pacemakers and may cause inflammatory and chronic fibrotic changes at the electrode-tissue interface resulting in a rise in pacing and sensing thresholds, see p. 260). This may be complicated by poor atrial thresholds when finally measured, requiring lead repositioning, a situation which we have never encountered.

> *Recommendation.* Because of the ever present risk of ventricular tachyarrhythmias, an external defibrillator ready to be used should always be available in the implantation room.
>
> In case of atrial fibrillation at the time of atrial or dual chamber pacemaker implant, we suggest implanting the atrial lead, followed by anticoagulation and delayed cardioversion.

## Asystole

Since the indication for cardiac pacing is usually a conduction disturbance, one must be prepared for the development of asystole at any time during the procedure. Asystole is particularly likely in patients with complete heart block and slow ventricular escape rate, and tends to occur at the time of tricuspid valve crossing or after the onset of pacing. This risk, of course, is even more likely at the time of pulse generator replacement in a pacemaker dependent patient.

> *Recommendation.* To face this potential complication, one should always be ready to pace by having prepared, in the first place, the material needed for external pacing, an infusion of isoproterenol, or by having placed the transthoracic external pacing system or a temporary transvenous pacing electrode.

## Myocardial Perforation and Tamponnade

Myocardial perforation is a more common complication than generally appreciated, particularly with thin or screw-in leads; it may or may not have one or more consequences: rise in pacing and/or sensing threshold(s), and a small or moderate pericardial effusion which should be looked for systematically with echocardiography at the slightest suspicion of perioperative perforation. In the worst case, fortunately rarely, tamponnade develops with tachycardia, dyspnea, pleuritic chest pain, and Kussmaul sign, requiring urgent drainage. This complication should be feared if, during the procedure, one notices the lead to be located to the left of the cardiac silhouette, or to be inching up along the left heart border. In other cases, perforation is caused by an active fixation lead. When performing intraoperative measurements, one may discover very high thresholds, a large difference in the quality of pacing versus sensing, a wide difference in measured unipolar versus bipolar thresholds, diaphragmatic pacing at low pulse strength, or pericardial type chest pain reported by the patient. In all cases, the lead must be repositioned.

*Recommendation.* Gently manipulate the leads during implant; do not overscrew active fixation leads.

## Complications Related to the Pacing System

In the immediate postoperative period, these complications are mostly related to the leads.

### Diaphragmatic Pacing

This trivial complication must be resolved rapidly because of the discomfort it causes the patient. It is due either to direct stimulation of the phrenic nerve by an active fixation lead at the lateral right atrial wall, or by diaphragmatic muscle stimulation from the proximity of the ventricular electrode at the ventricular apex. It can sometimes be resolved by reprogramming a lower pacing output while leaving a safe margin; in other cases a reintervention is necessary to reposition the pacing lead.

*Recommendation.* The importance of high energy pacing during lead implant is reemphasized. Diaphragmatic pacing observed during the procedure should prompt repositioning of the lead.

### Lead Dislodgment

An early dislodgment of the atrial lead is always possible, especially if the lead is tined, if the implant conditions are atypical (as in the case of massively dilated right heart chambers), if the lead is taut and moves with forced inspirations, or if it has not been properly screwed in. A dislodgment of the ventricular lead has become quite rare. At fluoroscopy the electrode can be seen floating inside the heart chamber, the pacing/sensing thresholds are unstable, or impedance rises markedly. A microdislodgment should be suspected in cases of sudden rise in sensing and/or pacing thresholds without apparent radiologic change (Fig. 6.2).

*Recommendation.* Verify the attachment of the lead by applying gentle tug after implantation, and return some extra length. Tie the lead to the entrance vein or affix to the muscle fascia.

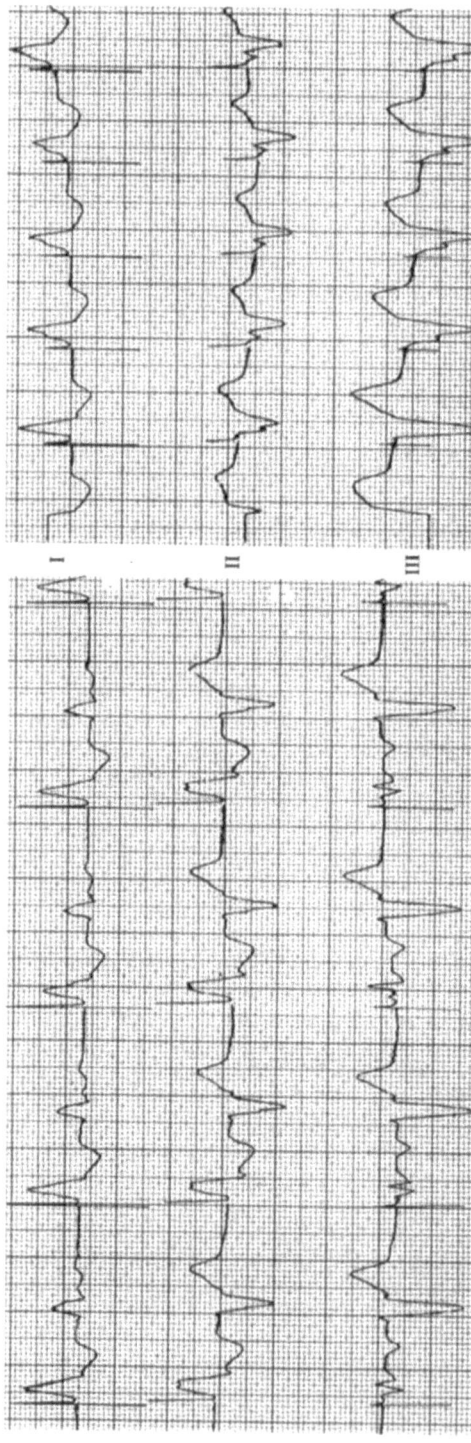

**Fig. 6.2.** DDD mode, 70 BPM, AVD=150 ms. Migration of the atrial lead into the right ventricular outflow tract. *Left:* the atrial stimulus causes high right ventricular pacing. No ventricular pacing. *Right:* Magnet application over this pacemaker model induced V00 mode associated with right ventricular apical pacing. Note the different axis of the paced events on the left and right side

## Pacing and Sensing Threshold Rise

The postoperative inflammatory process explains most of the time the nearly systematic increase in pacing and sensing thresholds. In the worst case, one may observe exit or entrance (see p. 428 and 21 ff., 27 ff.) block. The increase in pacing threshold, a common phenomenon, may begin within a few days in the atrium and resolve within 6–8 weeks. In the ventricle, the threshold rise is delayed and subsides over 3–6 months. As a consequence, it is advised to set relatively high pacing output (5 V) and sensitivity during the first several months, and reprogram at 6 months. Threshold rise is usually attenuated by the more biocompatible carbon electrodes and by the steroid-eluting leads. Short of steroid-eluting leads, systemic corticosteroid administration, in the form of prednisone, 1 mg/ kg per day may be given. If, after a few days, the thresholds have not changed, steroid treatment should be discontinued. Consideration should, then, be given to reintervene to reposition the electrode, or replace it by a steroid-eluting electrode. If, conversely, systemic steroid therapy is successful, it should be continued in the same dosages for 2 weeks, then slowly tapered to avoid a rebound phenomenon.

Interruption of electrical continuity is a much less common complication, as in the case of lead crush from excessively forceful tying of a ligature, or inadvertent, partial section of the lead insulation. A rare cause which appears hours or days after implantation consists of the insufficient tightening of the Allen screw(s) that are responsible for the electrical contact between the lead and the pulse generator. This intraoperative mistake necessitates a reintervention. An air space between the device and the subcutaneous tissues should be thoroughly avoided, particularly since most pacemakers are provided in a unipolar configuration (included the polarity programmable bipolar devices), and since most devices are coated with insulation material with a conductive window that needs to be facing upward (toward the skin).

CASE STUDY

*Example.* A pacemaker dependent patient undergoes upgrade of his system with implant of an atrial lead. The preexistent ventricular lead is judged to be operating flawlessly. A post implant ECG confirms proper function of the system. A few hours later, the patient suffers from severe fainting spells due to complete pacing cessation. The pacemaker appears inactive. The impedance of both leads is greater than 3 KW. However, by simple pressure on the skin overlying the pulse generator, all functions return to normal, including the impedance of both leads. Release of the pressure immediately results in the pacing failure observed earlier. The problem was resolved by needle aspiration of the air left in the pocket at the end of implant.

*Recommendation.* The inflammatory reaction is difficult to prevent, other than by the use of carbon or steroid-eluting leads. Do not crush the leads with the fixation sutures. Tighten firmly, though not excessively, the connectors' set screws. Evacuate all air from the pocket.

## Postoperative Autonomic Dysregulation

Disturbances in systemic pressure regulation may appear after the implant of a pacemaker, particularly if profound bradycardia was present before. If a dual chamber system has been implanted, it may be advisable to program a slow VVI or DDI mode for 2 to 3 days before returning to the program that has been planned for the long-term. In general, in the hypertensive patient, the systemic blood pressure needs close surveillance, and the hypertensive treatment may have to be revised.

CASE STUDY

*Example.* A DDD pacemaker was implanted in an 80 year old patient suffering from severe light-headed spells caused by AV block and a ventricular escape rhythm at 30 BPM. Before implantation systemic hypertension related to bradycardia at 200/90 mm Hg was present. After implantation of a DDD pacemaker, the pacing rate was that of the atria, at 90 BPM. In the immediate postoperative period the blood pressure regulation was markedly disturbed. The pacemaker was reprogrammed to DDI at a rate of 60 BPM and, 24 h later, reprogrammed further to a rate of 70 BPM. Two days later, the DDD mode was reinstituted, the blood pressure stabilized at 140/80 mm Hg, and the circulatory instability did not return.

These complications, taken as a whole, militate against the implantation of pacemakers on an outpatient basis, as has been proposed by some. This practice may be acceptable in patients whose conduction disorders are paroxysmal, provided their pacing system can be tested early after implant. It would seem dangerous in a pacemaker dependent patient.

## 6.2
## Late Complications

Late complications may be local or regional, and may be due to leads, pulse generator, or device programming

## Local or Regional Complications Related to the Site of Implantation

### Infection

Pacing system infection may develop for months or years after implantation. Even if delayed, it may have been caused by contamination during the procedure. The infection propagates along the insulating sleeve, or through the lead's lumen if the insulation has broken down, or via the lymphatic or venous network. Or it may have been introduced via an other route. It is rarely the cause of septicemia or other systemic presentation, and is usually due to staphylococcus epidermidis or, rarely, to a fungus or enterococcus. The background clinical presentation often includes low grade fever and sweats. Local manifestations are either absent, or consistent with impending erosion, i.e. discomfort, increase in pocket size, skin discoloration. Occasionally the infection presents as an insidious form of endocarditis, or recurrent bronchitis without other precipitating factors. Transesophageal echocardiography is of major importance to identify the presence of vegetations along the lead system, or signs of right-sided endocarditis. The diagnosis may also become apparent after needle aspiration of the pocket content, or at the time of device replacement prompted by impending erosion or suspicion of purulent collection. The operative strategy will vary widely according to the sites that may already have been used earlier, of the availability of venous access which must be fully assessed preoperatively, and, above all, on the dependency of the patient on pacing. The various options available are described on p. 375 ff.

> *Recommendation.* Always think of pacing system infection in the face of inflammatory or septic manifestations. Prevent secondary infections by recommending the same precautions as for patients with artificial heart valves.

One has to keep in mind that, if an infected system is not explanted, the complication will be fatal in two thirds of cases.

### Migration of the Pacemaker Can

Migration of the pulse generator is uncommon. Some operators use a non resorbable suture to fasten it to the underlying muscular fascia.

> *Recommendation.* The construction of a new pocket should be considered before erosion of the surrounding cutaneous tissues. If the pacemaker is in a subpectoral location, it must be attached to the overlying muscle layer.

### Pacemaker Pocket Erosion

Extrusion of the pacing system has become much less common since the pulse generators have become smaller and rounded. It is often facilitated by a considerable weight loss. Erosion usually occurs during the first year after implantation and begins by mere skin redness. On palpation, which often causes discomfort, thinning of the cutaneous layers and abnormal adhesion of the can is noted. Such findings may also be present at the level of the lead connections, or even along the subcutaneous course of the leads. They should systematically prompt a reintervention before frank extrusion (Fig. 6.3), to bury the material as deep as possible, at times in a subpectoral location, particularly in recurrent cases which may be due to an intolerance of the can alloy.

> *Recommendation.* Advise patients to avoid friction by garments (suspenders, brassieres etc.) and to avoid prolonged sun exposure. Protection with a towel can prevent cutaneous erosion, the starting point of complete extrusion of the system. At the abdominal level,[1] belts are the main culprits. In impeding erosions, the use of ointments is futile; reintervention is mandatory.

---

1 This site of implantation is more of historical interest

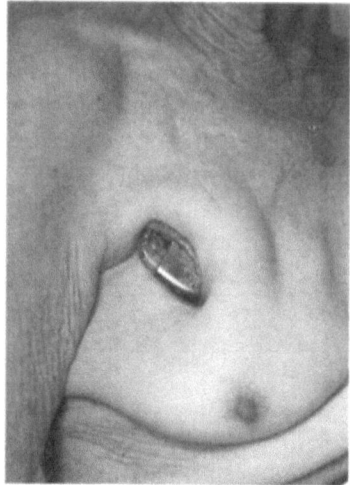

**Fig. 6.3.** Pacemaker pocket erosion with partial exposure of the pulse generator

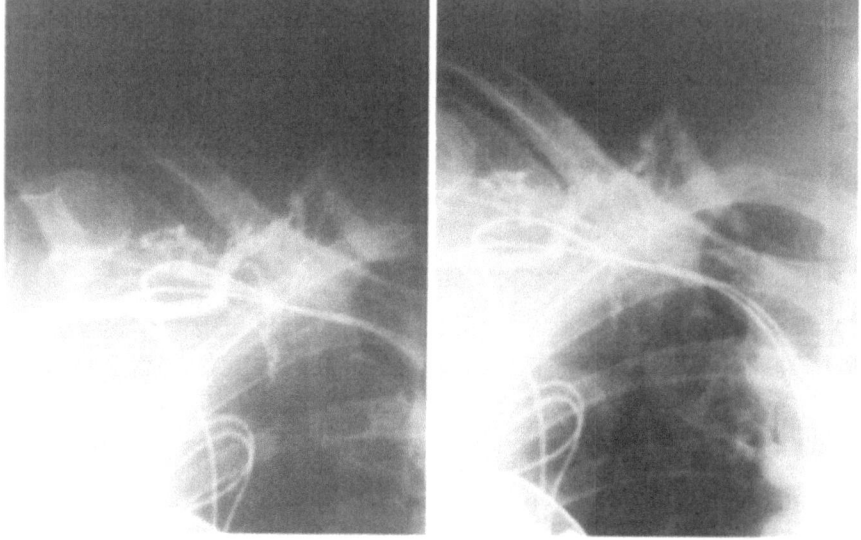

**Fig. 6.4.** Subclavian vein thrombosis around pacing leads

## Venous Thrombosis

Often asymptomatic, venous thrombosis is suspected on the basis of collateral circulation which has developed on the shoulder ipsilateral to the site of implant. Prospective studies have found thrombosis to be present in up to 10% of cases, more often when two or more leads have been introduced in the same vein. The innominate and subclavian veins, rarely the superior vena cava, are the main vessels involved. Chronic occlusions need no particular treatment, but represent a loss of venous access and may pose technical difficulties if a new lead needs to be implanted, or one needs to be extracted. Venography is helpful in identifying the veins that are available in such situations (Fig. 6.4). Venoplasty has been proposed to allow the introduction of new leads without changing the site of implant.

## Lead-Related Complications

### Secondary Dislodgment

Now quite rare, secondary dislodgment causes loss of pacing and sensing, along with a rise in pacing impedance. A particular form is known as the „twiddler syndrome," caused by the patient's manipulating the pulse generator, or by a loose fixation of the lead at its entrance point into the vein, both related to a pocket that is too large for the can. In either case the lead is pulled away from its site of endocardial attachment. At reintervention, the segment of lead contained in the pacemaker pocket must be examined thoroughly. The lead should not be reused if either the conductor or the insulation have been damaged, or if it was found to be tightly coiled, since it may be associated with mechanical weakening resulting in complications months or years later.

*Recommendation.* In psychiatric patients, besides meticulously securing the lead at its entrance point, consideration should be given to performing a subpectoral implant.

### Changes in Pacing and Sensing Threshold

Outside of physiologic fluctuations in pacing threshold due to, for instance, meals (increase) or physical activity (decrease), anomalies in pacing and/or sensing threshold may force the surgical revision of the system, sometimes several years after establishment of a chronic threshold (3 – 6 months post implant). If the rise in threshold(s) is due to a fibrotic process following the initial inflammatory reaction, administration of corticosteroids generally offers only short-term ameliorations. Conversely, some rises in threshold may be due to metabolic disorders such as diabetes or electrolyte imbalance (see p. 25) whose resolution restores the baseline conditions. Exceptional situations may also cause acute, transient elevations of the pacing threshold (Fig. 6.5).

*Recommendation.* Handle leads with care at implant. Always look for inflammatory or infectious sources, endocrine or metabolic disorders, or introduction of new drug therapy.

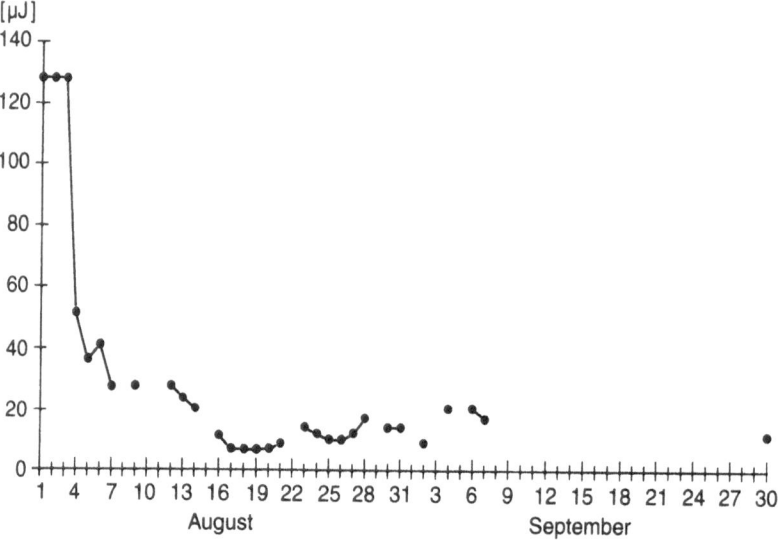

**Fig. 6.5.** Evolution of ventricular capture threshold (in µJ) in a 42 year old patient who had undergone dual chamber pacemaker implantation 18 months earlier with pacing thresholds measurements consistently below 1 V during follow up. On 1 August, she presents with loss of ventricular capture due to a marked increase in pacing threshold in the context of a corynebacterium diphteriae infection. Sixteen weeks after the onset of antibacterial treatment the pacing threshold has nearly returned to its baseline. Six months later the patient has remained clinically stable and without recurrence of infection

## Insulation Failure (Fig. 6.6 and 6.7)

This complication may have various manifestations. Striated muscle, typically pectoral, stimulation is common from the current leak through the insulation defect along the course of the lead. The differential diagnosis is an infiltration of body fluids into a leaky connector. This rather minor complication may, nevertheless, require a reintervention to restore hermeticity. This can be avoided by observing absolute compatibility of the 3.2 mm connectors between pacemaker header and lead. Whichever the cause may be, pectoral stimulation should be an alert in a patient who has a bipolar lead and whose pacemaker is programmed in a bipolar pacing configuration, or a patient who has a unipolar lead but no pectoral stimulation up to that point.

Another diagnostic finding of insulation failures electrocardiographic:

- Increase in the pacing spike in bipolar pacing. In bipolar pacing, if the insulation defect is around the anodal conductor, a marked increase in the pacing spike will give the appearance of unipolarity.
- Decrease in the pacing spike in bipolar pacing. If the insulation defect is internal, between anodal and cathodal conductors, the short-circuit will prevent the delivery of an important proportion of electrical charge at the electrodes, considerably decreasing the pacing spike amplitude on the surface ECG.

- Decrease in the pacing spike in unipolar pacing. In unipolar pacing, the insulation failure will cause considerable decrease in the pacing spike amplitude.

This also implies a fall in pacing impedance (e.g. < 300 $\Omega$), considered significant if greater than 20% compared to steady-state measurements. This causes an increase in power consumption by the pulse generator. Photoanalysis of the spike is key in detecting early insulation failure. Measurement of the spike amplitude in three orthogonal leads allows the determination of the pacing vector. Insulation failures deviate the axis and change the amplitude of the spike by a growing amount as the defect is situated further away from the distal electrode. As a result of the current leak caused by the defect, and in presence of stable output requirements to achieve successful pacing, the pacing threshold rises.

> *Recommendation.* A decrease in pacing impedance should raise the suspicion of insulation failure.

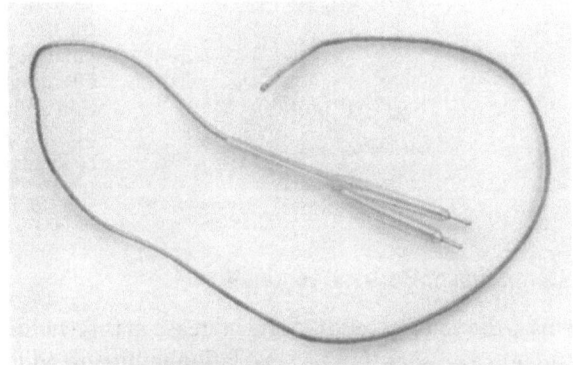

**Fig. 6.6.** Considerable alterations of the lead, with multiple bends of the conductor and insulation failures

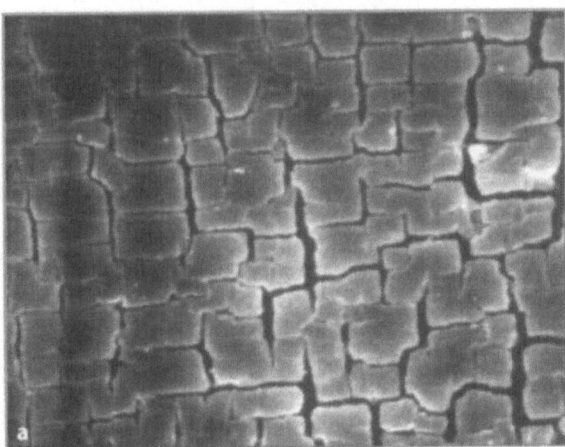

**Fig. 6.7. a** Scanning microscopy showing the surface of a 80 A polyurethane lead. The whole surface cracking weakens the insulation properties of the material

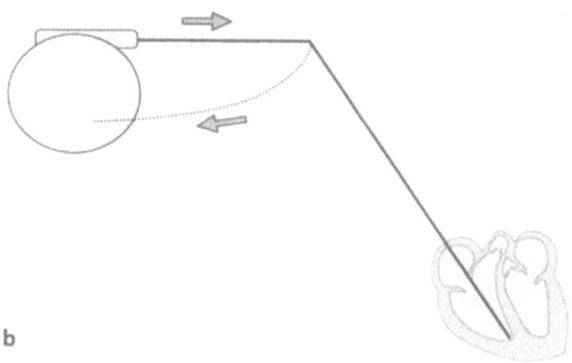

b

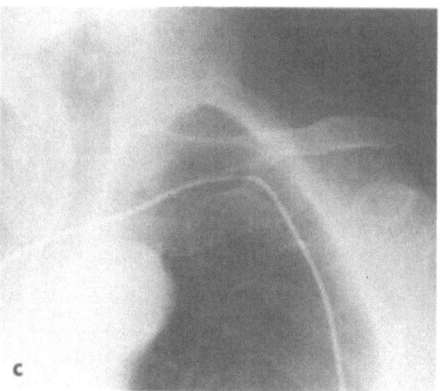

c

**Fig. 6.7. b** Insulation failure causing a decrease in the total impedance of the circuit. The absence of insulation at any point along the lead causes a short-circuit resulting in failure to pace and, in some cases, pectoral stimulation if the current leak occurs at an extravascular point of the lead
**c** Radiographic appearance of insulation and external conductor fracture on a bipolar pacing lead at the costoclavicular space

### Interruption of Electrical Continuity

This is the leading cause of late increase in thresholds. Causes of the interruption are the same of as those of insulation failure, to which should be added fracture of the conductor at the pulse generator header when the stiff portion of the lead connector protrudes outside of its receptacle. This causes stress at the junction of the lead connector, which is stiff, with the lead body, which is soft. Similar risks exist at connectors of lead extensions or at points where the lead may have been repaired.

Fracture of the conductor has become rare since the introduction of multifilar leads. It is diagnosed as a loss of pacing and sensing functions on the surface electrocardiogram, perhaps associated with a return of symptoms experienced by the patient before implantation of the pacing system. Pacing spikes may be completely absent on the ECG. Telemetry of modern devices can assist in the diagnosis by displaying event markers confirming the delivery of pulses by the pacemaker without apparent spike on the ECG. The lead impedance is markedly elevated or even infinite (Fig. 6.8).

If the fracture is limited to the anodal conductor of a bipolar lead, unipolar pacing may be preserved. However, this persistence of cathodal electrical

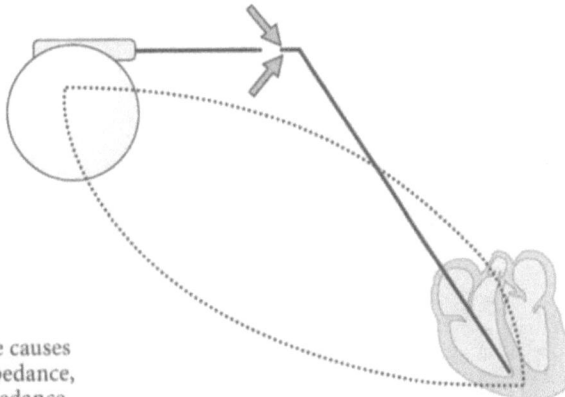

**Fig. 6.8.** A conductor fracture causes a marked increase in lead impedance, hence, of the total circuit impedance

conduction does not allow the preservation of the lead which should be replaced. The conductor fracture may be visible on a radiograph at any point along the course of the lead (see Fig. 6.7c). It is much more difficult to see on a bipolar lead. Finally, the interruption of electrical continuity may be intermittent.

CASE STUDY

*Example.* A patient wearing a pacemaker is hospitalized for recurrent syncope. Upon testing of the device, the surface ECG is normal, including normal pacing and sensing parameters, until a distinct motion of the shoulder causes intermittent pacing exit block. Several radiographs fail to show a lead fracture which became apparent macroscopically only after it had been extracted and stretched (Fig. 6.9).

This clinical case illustrates the importance of various helpful maneuvers to establish the diagnosis. If a fracture is suspected, the patient should be instructed to perform arm and shoulder motions, and to breathe deeply under fluoroscopy or during electrocardiographic recording. The lead impedance increases markedly.

If the fracture is extravascular and has occurred in a unipolar silicone lead, it can be repaired with dedicated kits, provided the rest of the lead appears intact on close scrutiny. In all other cases, it must be replaced. The abandoned lead must be capped to insulate it before burying it.

Epicardial leads are less reliable than endovascular leads and must, therefore, be closely watched, or perhaps systematically replaced after 10 years (Fig. 6.10).

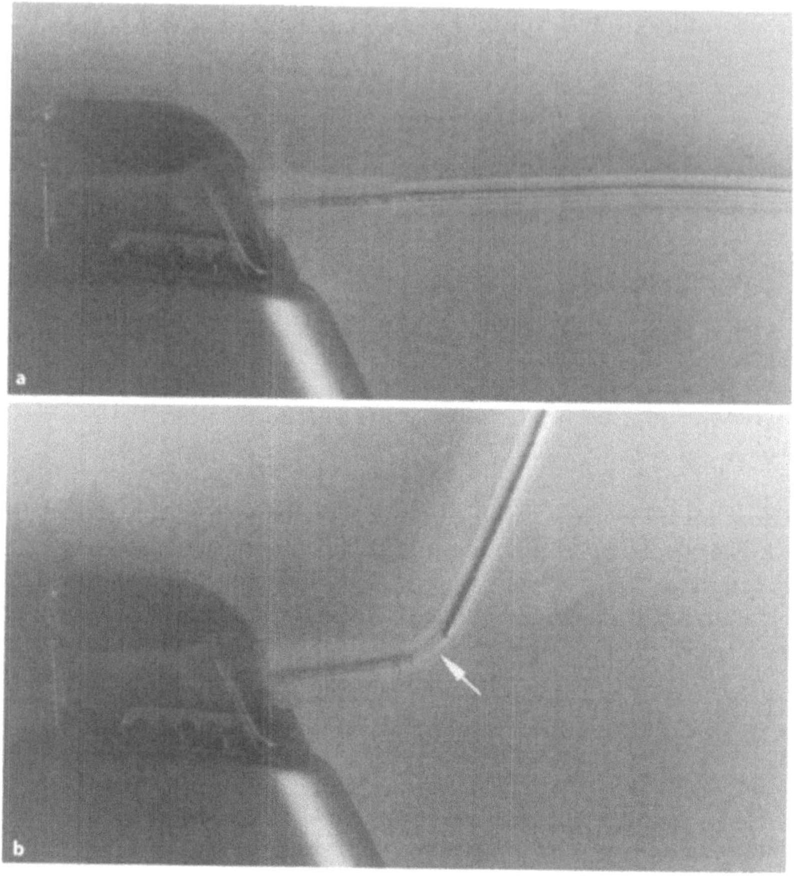

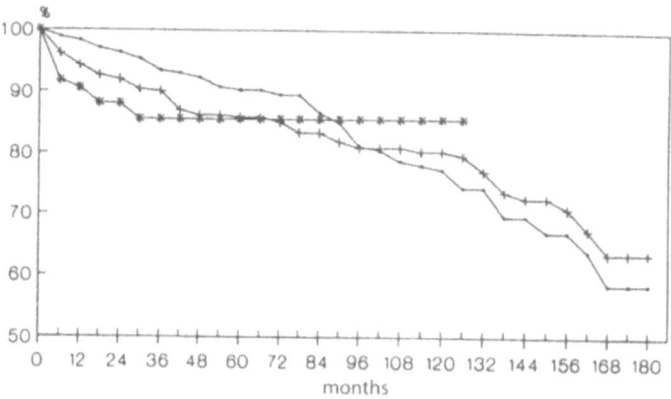

**Fig. 6.9.** A lead fracture may not be apparent without stretching
**a** Without stretching
**b** With stretching

**Fig. 6.10.** Cumulative survival of various epicardial leads. After 10 years of implantation, leads must be closely monitored

## Mechanical Complication Related to the Lead

This recent complication pertains to the Telectronics Accufix lead which contains a retention wire contained in the outer insulation, separate from the conductor, and gives the lead its „J" shape. The difference in stiffness between the insulator and the sharp wire may lead to protrusion of the latter and perforation of the heart muscle with risk of tamponnade.

## Recommendations Relative to the Accufix and Encor Leads

Patients who have received an Accufix lead should receive special attention in order to prevent complications due to the protrusion of the retention wire. Regular, high resolution fluoroscopic examinations are necessary, preferably with cine or video recordings. One should look for:

- An obvious protrusion of the wire (Fig. 6.11).
- A crack in the insulation indicating a fracture of the wire inside the insulation.
- A bulge in the insulation above the wire fracture. An appearance of „green stick" fracture has been described.
- Excessive amplitude of the „J" motion.

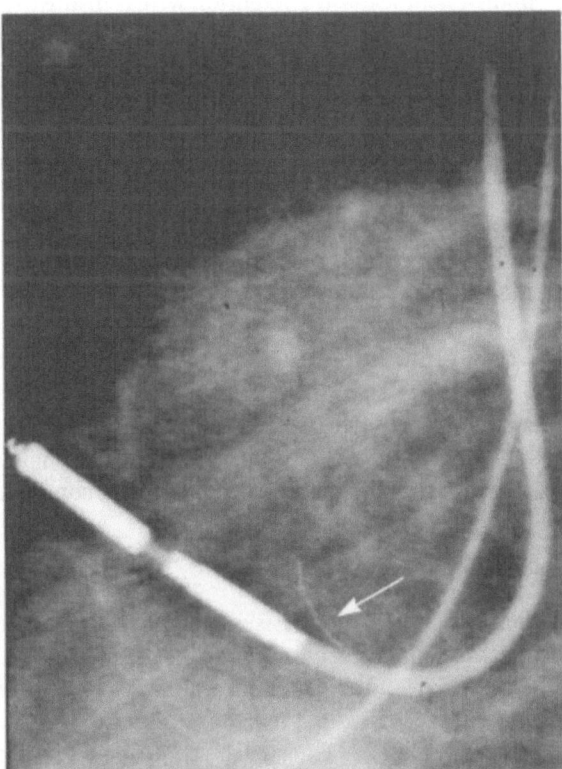

**Fig. 6.11.** Protrusion of the retention wire of a J-shaped Accufix lead. It can dangerously injure the atrial myocardium

Multiple views should be examined, including antero -posterior, lateral and 45° angles. Several situations may present: Extraction must be performed in all patients younger than 40 years, women of child-bearing age, or if open heart surgery has been scheduled. Extraction should be considered it the generator needs to be replaced or the system revised because of sensing or pacing failure. It must, of course, be extracted if the system is infected. Extraction is advised in patients between 40 and 60 years of age.

Past 60 years of age, five situations are possible:

- No suspicion of fracture; the patients must be reexamined every 6 months.
- A fracture is suspected without protrusion: the risks must be balanced with those of extracting the lead. Shorter intervals between examinations may be scheduled by the physician.
- Fracture is suspected with protrusion: extraction of the lead is advised.
- A fracture with migration is present: these patients should be the object of a joint consultation between cardiologist and cardiothoracic surgeon. Decisions should be made on a case-by-case basis.
- The „J" is open or subject to excessive stress: extraction is recommended.

The decision to extract the lead should take in consideration the risks of the procedure, the patient's preference and life expectancy, and the cumulative radiation exposure.

In the Encor leads, the retention wire is inside the conductor, and the risks are less, though instances of protrusion have been observed. All patients with this lead model should have a fluoroscopic examination to assess its status. If a protrusion is observed, the lead should be extracted. If the lead is bent between the two electrodes, or if the „J" is fractured, additional fluoroscopic surveillance should be scheduled at regular 6-month intervals.

## 6.3
## Complications Related to the Pulse Generator or the Programmed Mode

### Sources of Interference

Electrical interference consists of currents of non-cardiac origin which interfere with the sensing and pacing circuits of the pacemaker. They may be endogenous, i.e. coming from the patient, or exogenous, coming from the outside.

### Endogenous Interference

Endogenous interference arises from physiologic signals (generally myosignals), or electrical signals originating from the pacemaker or other electrically active prosthesis, for example a defibrillator. Whatever their origin, the pacemaker is incapable of recognizing their source if these signals have not been rejected by its filters and amplifiers. They will be confused with cardiac physiologic signals and cause various behaviors depending on the programmed mode of the pacemaker.

In the single chamber back up mode, and in the DDI mode, the pacemaker will be inhibited, and its escape interval will be reset by each sensed interfering signal. In DDD mode, sensing of the signals limited to the ventricle causes inhibition of ventricular pacing; if sensing is limited to the atrium, inappropriate acceleration of ventricular pacing will occur from tracking of each interfering signal that has been sensed; if sensing occurs at both levels, the pacemaker will be seemingly shut down (see p. 270 and p. 337).

*Recommendation.* To minimize these inappropriate inhibitions, use bipolar sensing.

### Exogenous Interference

### Physical Characteristics of Exogenous Interference

Exogenous interference may cause three types of disturbances:

- *Induced disturbances* which transmit the interference to the lead, or directly to the pulse generator, without direct contact. The lead acts as an antenna, and the disturbance occurs by magnetic induction or capacitive coupling;
- *Conducted disturbances* which require cutaneous contact. Signals generating currents on the order of 20 µA or voltages near 0.2 V can inhibit the pulse generator, particularly if their frequency is within the bandpass of the filters of the pacemaker's sensing circuit.
- *Ionizing radiations*, associated with emissions of photons or electrons, can modify the atomic structure of semi-conductors, and of components used in pacemaker circuitry.

Currents that may interfere with pacemaker circuits originate from four sources: galvanic, magnetic, electromagnetic, and magnetostatic.

- *Currents of galvanic origin* are observed when two poles of a current source and the body form a closed circuit. One of the most common examples consists of electrocautery.
- *Magnetic currents* originate from the physical properties expressed in the law of Faraday: any magnetic field varying over time is accompanied by a current whose voltage is proportional to the surface of influence and to the frequency and intensity of the field (a unipolar pacemaker and its lead encompass a surface of $500 - 600$ cm$^2$). Such interference is observed in the vicinity of electrical conductors such as antitheft or airport security systems, arc welding sites, etc. Interference caused by lithotripsy may be of the same type.
- *Electromagnetic interference* are of high frequency waveforms emitted from a distinct source. Their penetration into the body is inversely proportional to their frequency, and their effects vary as a function of their power, frequency of emission, and distance between source and pulse generator. In this type of interference, the lead generally behaves as an antenna. Police radar and remote control devices (radio, TV and VCR) are harmless such electromagnetic current sources. On the other hand, medical diathermy, military high

power radar, some CB radios, and industrial microwave ovens may interfere with pacemakers.

- *Currents of magnetostatic origin* are emitted by nuclear magnetic resonance imagers (MRI), and electrical drills. Other sources such as digital scanners, loud-speakers, and non-cellular telephone receivers, are innocuous.

### Situations of Exposure

*Home and Day-To-Day Environment*

Home appliances, most of which are now innocuous, are the most common source of concern and inquiries by pacemaker patients. At a distance of 0.1 meters from the transformer at the back, a domestic microwave oven is harmless, even with its door open and safety turned off. In contrast, induction ovens and stove plates emit powerful interference against which no effective protection currently exists, and it is advised to stay at least 2 m away from such appliances. Additional potential harmful sources include motors included in some toys (train sets), starter circuits of internal combustion engines, and home water purifiers.

Patients wearing pacemakers should identify themselves at airports before crossing the security gates, though very little risk is incurred with the systems currently in use in Western countries. One should keep in mind that no safety or warning is included in the antitheft systems used by department stores. To achieve maximal security, these gates may, at times, emit powerful signals which may interfere with pacemakers. Therefore, it is strongly advised to cross these systems rapidly, and avoid multiple crossings or standing in their vicinity. Television transmitters are harmless outside of the posted safety zone. Powerful radio transmitters may be a problem depending on the wavelength that is emitted. A few recent studies have shown possible interference from cellular telephones; it is advised to not use the phone on the side of the pacemaker, and not store the instrument (if it is on active or standby mode) in a pocket near the pulse generator. Navigation radars should be avoided and safety limits around commercial and military radars should be respected.

Ultimately few situations of daily life represent a hazard, if mere prudence is wisely applied.

*The Workplace*

Since significant interference may occur in some special work environments (internal combustion engine, arc welding, powerful radars, etc.), job reassignments may be indicated in occasional cases, although, in general, safety guidelines applicable to the overall working force are sufficient to protect the majority of pacemaker patients. In case of persistent uncertainty, a 24 h ambulatory ECG may provide the answers needed.

*The Medical Environment*

Most risks of external interference to pacemaker function are incurred in the medical environment. Since they are foreseeable, and given the health implications for the patients and medical-legal implications for the physician, these risks should be fully understood and all measures should be taken to prevent them.

*Electrocautery*

Electrocautery represents the main cause of electrical interference. A significant number of patients wearing permanent pacemakers become surgical candidates. All complications described earlier may be encountered. More rarely, exit block may develop from microcoagulation burns due to currents transmitted by the pacemaker lead (cardiac surgery). In practice, the pacemaker and the electric scalpel should be kept as far apart as possible and, if possible, both should be used in a bipolar configuration, with the operating table properly grounded. The electrical knife should be preferably set on the coagulation rather than cutting mode. The power should be set as low as possible, and the knife used in brief pulses rather than continuously. Other precautions include monitoring of the ECG, programming the pacemaker to an asynchronous or triggered mode at maximal output, having a programmer available in the operating room, and verifying, immediately after the procedure, that the device has not been reprogrammed, and again several days later since delayed changes in pacing and sensing thresholds have been reported.

*Magnetic Resonance Imaging*

MRI has several potential adverse effects: Exposure to a continuous magnetic field may cause the device to switch to an asynchronous mode by closing the reed switch. This may depend on the spatial orientation of the pulse generator, and on its separation from the magnetic source. No effect may be apparent on the pacemaker in a supine patient.

The magnetic gradient and high frequency field may have various effects:

- No effect on the pacemaker which has switched to an asynchronous mode induced by the magnetic field, a mode which is self-protected
- Complete inhibition by the high frequency field
- Partial inhibition with slowing of the pacing rate, observed with unipolar systems
- Acceleration of the pacing rate to a frequency equal to that of the high frequency signal

In few cases, the pacemaker may have an unpredictable behavior, with no apparent effect of the MRI initially, followed, after a few minutes by asynchronous pacing or partial inhibition. This is due to the development, at the electrodes, of current perfectly synchronous with the high frequency of the MRI system, which causes different effects on different pacemakers.

Because of these many unpredictable adverse effects, MRI is absolutely contraindicated in pacemaker patients.

*Lithotripsy*
Despite all its theoretical effects, lithotripsy is not particularly risky. The shock wave is produced by an electrical arc synchronized with the ECG to avoid the induction of ventricular fibrillation. The shocks are triggered by the ventricular stimulus in VVI mode, and by the atrial stimulus in DDD mode, in which case there is a risk of inhibition of the ventricular channel. The pacemaker should therefore be programmed in VVI or V00 mode. Lithotripsy is feasible if the pacemaker is not in an abdominal position. Rate responsiveness pacemakers based on activity are at risk of destruction of the quartz, or of an acceleration to the maximal rate responsive rate; therefore, the rate responsive function should be off during the procedure.

*Direct Current Shocks*
DC shocks from cardioversion, defibrillation or fulguration may irreversibly damage pacemakers, despite their programmation in a bipolar configuration. This may be due to damage to various components, including those controlling sensitivity, rate, refractory periods, and programming memory, or to the quartz of activity sensors. In other cases, the shocks may cause inflammatory and chronic fibrotic changes at the electrode-tissue interface resulting in a rise in pacing and sensing thresholds.

In all cases, the shocking electrodes must be placed away from the pulse generator, the electrical field should be antero-posterior, as to be perpendicular to the axis lead -pacemaker, and the shock strength should be kept to a minimum, with consideration of the patient's body habitus. Programming the pacemaker to an asynchronous mode is recommended, though this will not protect its circuits. Complete testing of the pacemaker should be performed at the end of the procedure.

*Transcutaneous Nerve Stimulation*
This treatment exposes to little risk of reprogramming or inhibition, though its safety should preferably be verified by the recording of a 24 h ambulatory ECG.

*Radiation Therapy*
Progress in pacing technology over the last two decades, instead of protecting pacemakers against ionizing radiation has rendered them more vulnerable. This is due to the development of sophisticated electronic circuitry and new semiconductors. Radiation directly affect the transistors. Since the energies absorbed are well below those known to be damaging, the use of radiation therapy is not contraindicated. However, the effects are cumulative, and caution must be observed with respect to possible heating of the materials.

The following precautions are critical:

- Avoid the direct exposure of the pulse generator under the field of irradiation. In some cases, the pulse generator will need to be relocated to an other site.
- Alternatively, one may protect it with a lead shield, which can reduce 10-fold the dose delivered.

- In case of unavoidable exposure, the maximal calculated dose should not exceed 5 Gray for a state-of-the art pacemaker, although cases have been reported of exposures reaching 10 Gray without apparent damage to the device.
- Never expose the patient to a betatron because of risk of electromagnetic interference.
- Avoid excessive heating of the can, which may be damaging as much for the circuitry as for the tissues surrounding the device.

**Protection Against Sources of Interference**

Several methods may protect against interference. From a general preventive point of view, the public should not be exposed to magnetic fields stronger than 1 millitesla (mT). Power stations or electrical heaters emit fields on the order of 30 µT at a distance of 30 cm. Household appliances emit a field of approximately 1 µT at 3 cm. A transformer of 100 KVA creates a field of 20 µT at 1 m. It has been shown that a field of 20 µT could induce a 1 mV potential at a unipolar lead. However, in general a field of a few microtesla switches the pacing system to the noise reversion mode.

In addition, the public should not be exposed to electrical fields above 5 kV/m. These recommendations are applicable to pacemaker patients. Stronger fields are likely to switch the pacing system to the noise reversion mode for the duration of exposure. In daily life high power lines have no effect on cardiac pacemakers.

Protections against sources of interference are mostly technological:

- Better shields of the pacemaker can.
- Interposition of diodes (Zener) which, by being connected to the input into the pulse generator, limit surges in sensing voltages (in which case the current is diverted to the lead).
- Improvements in filters which pass signals strictly of cardiac origin.
- Incorporation of a reed switch which protects against intense magnetic fields. Its efficacy depends on its spatial position relative to the field. It triggers a connection with safety circuits.
- Bipolar configuration, which diminishes the influence of endogenous (myo-signals) and exogenous galvanic and magnetic forms of interference. In bipolar configuration, the risk of interference is tenfold less than in unipolar, though the protection against exogenous signal is far from complete.
- Incorporation of safety modes, which are surveillance programs written in the pacemaker ROM. They are better protected and activated in case of alteration of the ongoing program.
- Presence of algorithms against noise which force asynchronous pacing when signals above a threshold determined by the manufacturer are sensed. In order to recognize noise, the pacemaker must be inhibited for one cycle before reversion to the asynchronous mode.
- Observance of the CENELEC norm, a norm that must be respected by all manufacturers. It takes in consideration all the construction characteristics of

pulse generators. With respect to interference, two parameters are included: amplitude and frequency of the signal. The norm distinguishes two protection thresholds: the first defines those kinds of interference that may disturb proper device function; the second defines those that may damage or reprogram the device.

These protective measures do not replace the information provided to the patient. In practice, patients should be advised not to use equipment that contains electrical coils. Household appliances are mostly protected, except induction plates that should be strictly avoided. It is the medical environment that represents the highest risk for pacemaker patients. Electrocautery may be quite dangerous, particularly for pulse generators near end of life, even when used at a distance from the can.

## Changes in Pacing Rate

We have seen that certain kinds of interference may change the pacing rate. Pacemaker run-away, much feared in the past, has become extremely rare, since modern devices successfully limit the upper rate, minimizing the effects of this noxious complication.

## Shut Down

This signifies complete cessation of device function due to a breakdown of the electronic circuits. This is, of course, quite dangerous in a pacemaker dependent patient.

## Battery Depletion

Rapid depletion of the battery has become rare as well. This dysfunction must be distinguished from normal depletion. Therefore, regular surveillance is necessary, at shorter intervals when the surveillance indicators (see Chap. 7) begin to drift. One should remember that a nearly depleted device may not be reprogrammable, and that programming with telemetry may halt the pacemaker because of the temporary increase in power consumption that it causes.

In conclusion, the prevention of complications imposes a systematic observance of the proper rules of implantation. The quality of the surgical procedure, which is seemingly simple, hinges on a number of „tricks", astute maneuvers and skillful gestures with which the operator should be familiar.

Likewise, interference of all kinds invade the pacemaker patient's living space. Without causing undue fear of exposure to these potentially harmful forms of interference, the best prevention remains information to the patients and to the medical and paramedical community.

# CHAPTER 7

# Patient Follow-Up

This chapter repeats elements already presented in previous sections, this time in the perspective of the usual practical and clinical considerations that apply to the long-term surveillance of pacemaker patients.

The goals of follow-up in cardiac pacing are the following:

- Optimal adjustment of the programming to the particular hemodynamic and electrophysiologic needs of each individual patient
- Preservation of device life expectancy by setting the pacing output according to the thresholds measured and the required margin of safety
- Identification and treatment of complications

## 7.1
## General Principles

The surveillance of pacemaker patients requires a close cooperation between the referring physician and the implanting center. The primary care physician provides as much information as possible relative to the patient's medical condition and history, while the implanting center assumes a technical role and steers the long-term pacing strategies as a function of advances in technology. Dedicated programmers are necessary to verify the optimal workings of all functions and to reduce the risk of complications. While the follow-up of previous generations single chamber pacemaker was simple, that of state-of-the-art dual chamber, particularly rate responsive, devices has become much more complex.

Surveillance of the pacemaker, which is both clinical and electrocardiographic, aims to verify the patient's tolerance with respect to the device and its activity, to detect possible complications, and to identify the presence of battery end of life indicators. Complementary tests, including Holter monitoring, exercise testing and echocardiography may be needed.

The organization of a pacemaker outpatient clinic presumes a thorough familiarity with the various models, particularly the rate responsive ones, the indications for their replacement, and their response to interferences.

The *frequency of visits* depends on the implanted model. Dual chamber and rate responsive devices should be followed more closely to offer the patient the greatest benefits of an optimal programming. As others, we perform the first test

and programming of the pacemaker, along with a chest radiograph, on the day
after the procedure. With rate responsive systems, adjustment of the rate
response is postponed until the patient has become able to exercise, usually 2 – 3
days later, depending on the underlying heart disease and the pacemaker model
implanted. However, it is often worthwhile to wait 1 – 3 months, until the healing
process is well completed, to adjust the final settings. We also perform a check
before the patient's discharge from the hospital. Some cardiologists militate in
favor of the implantation of pacemakers on an outpatient basis, arguing that
complications are rare and that it can be safely performed in non pacemaker
dependent patients. We do not share this opinion, because the in-hospital period
is a time particularly favorable to better understand the patient's health status,
and examine the impact of pacing on hemodynamics. At the end of hospitalization, the programming requirements are better defined. It is also an ideal time to
educate the patient and alleviate persistent anxiety over the newly implanted
„foreign body" over which no immediate control can be exerted. During this
period, hemodynamic status, wound healing and body temperature are monitored. The cutaneous stitch(es) is removed on the tenth day. An identification
card is provided to the patient with the instruction to carry it at all times. It provides precious information in case of accident or serious intercurrent illness.

The next visit is scheduled after complete wound healing 1 – 3 months later, at
which time the system is reprogrammed to optimize sensing threshold and rate
responsiveness. Such adjustments should include exercise testing, particularly
in the case of rate responsive pacing. Reprogramming of the pacing output is
postponed until the end of the first 6 months, at which time the pacing threshold
should have stabilized, with, as a main goal, conservation of battery power while
respecting the usual 100% margin of safety. Subsequent appointments should be
scheduled at 6 months intervals, with interim electrocardiograms recorded by
the primary physician. When the pulse generator battery approaches end of life,
visits should be increased to three or four times a year. The same recommendation applies when a manufacturer recommends close surveillance of a specific
device.

A computerized data base is quite helpful by allowing a global surveillance of
the pacemaker patients at a given center, and by pointing to an inordinately high
complication rate caused by a lead or a pulse generator. It also tracks, before the
advent of complications, patients who, otherwise, might have been lost to follow-
up, or those who need to be quickly notified of a manufacturer's recall of a defective product. A recall is a recommendation, by the manufacturer, to systematically replace an item because of the observation of an unacceptably high incidence of failure or dysfunction. However, if a repetitive and statistically significant anomaly of a lead or pacemaker model is noted in a given center, the
implanting physician(s) may decide independently to proceed with the systematic replacement of the item. Such decision must be supported by objective data
unrelated to poor device programming, or inaccurate interpretation of electrocardiographic or telemetric data. If a decision to replace has been made, the
highest risk patients, for instance those who are pacemaker dependents, should
be scheduled early. On the other hand, the manufacturer's recommendation may

be limited to closer surveillance of a particular product's series because an anomaly has been detected in, for instance, a particular batch of electronic components. As a reminder, in the United States, the observation of a device or lead dysfunction, or failure, should be reported to the device section of the Food and Drug Administration and in Europe to the governmental administration in charge of controlling medical devices.

The follow up may be simple enough as to be assumed by the referring physician, or complete, requiring the expertise and equipment of the implanting center.

## 7.2
## Simple Follow-Up

The equipment necessary for a simple follow-up visit consists of a sphygmomanometer, an electrocardiographic recorder, a magnet, and a universal testing device known as „miniclinic" which measures the heart rate, the pacing pulse duration, and the AVD of dual chamber pacemakers, but cannot be used for programming. Interrogation should focus on the following:

## History

Historical inquiries should probe into the patient's general health, specific cardiac (dyspnea, palpitation, angina pectoris, exercise tolerance) and cerebral (lightheadedness, syncope) manifestations, and signs of diaphragmatic or pectoral muscle stimulation. Development of any of these symptoms during follow-up will require particular attention.

### Syncope and Near Syncope

Continuation or recurrence of these symptoms may signal an inaccurate original diagnosis (syncope due to several mechanisms) or a poor choice of pacing system or programming (e.g. VVI mode in a mixed form of carotid sinus syndrome). If such explanations have been excluded, one must look for pacing dysfunction in a pacemaker dependent patient. The circumstances in which the symptoms appear should be carefully defined. If they are movement-related, an attempt should be made to reproduce them:

- By mobilizing the can or leads through the skin, looking for intermittent contact due to poor connection, electrode fracture, etc.
- By deep breathing.
- By isometric exercise of the upper extremity on the ipsilateral side of the pulse generator to examine the presence of myosignal inhibition. This is particularly applicable to systems in a unipolar configuration.

Other situations may suggest exogenous interferences from environmental electrical sources, for instance the exposure to an electronic antitheft system. If the diagnosis remains unclear after the exploration of these various mechanisms, the investigations should be completed by the recording of a 24 h ambulatory ECG while the patient goes about the activities usually associated with symptoms.

### Dyspnea

The development of dyspnea in a paced patient may be due to cardiac insufficiency from spontaneous evolution of the underlying disease, or to the inappropriate choice of pacing system or programming. The most severe form of the latter is a component of the pacemaker syndrome which occurs in 5% – 10% of patients paced in VVI mode, and in which dyspnea at rest or during exercise or orthopnea are usually associated with other manifestations such as asthenia, atypical angina, near syncope or syncope, vasomotor dysregulation, bothersome neck pulsations, etc. This disorder may appear at various intervals after pacemaker implantation, early or late. If one examines the patient during a symptomatic period, hypotension, aggravated by orthostatic maneuvers is often present. The ECG typically shows ventricular pacing with 1 : 1 retrograde conduction. The treatment of this syndrome consists of either reprogramming the pacemaker to a slower rate with hysteresis to allow escape of normal sinus rhythm, or to the implantation of an atrial lead to convert the system to dual chamber pacing.

One other form of the pacemaker syndrome pertains to the AAIR mode. Up to one third of patients paced in this mode are unable to adapt their spike-R interval during exercise, such that, as the RR interval shortens, the P wave shifts closer toward the preceding R wave, causing the atria to contract against closed atrioventricular valves. The diagnosis can be made readily during exercise testing. The treatment consists of decreasing or withdrawing medications which depress AV conduction, to reprogram the upper pacing rate to a lower value, or, as a last resort, to upgrade the pacing system to DDDR.

The last form of pacemaker syndrome is encountered with DDD and DDDR pacemakers. When the AVD is programmed too long, the effects are the same as those just described in AAIR mode; when programmed too short, the atrial systole is suddenly interrupted by ventricular contraction, causing AV regurgitation, and the ventricles are completely paced, causing asynchrony of ventricular contraction which can be avoided by programming a longer AVD.

The development or aggravation of dyspnea in a paced patient may also prompt the examination of other possible mechanisms:

- Chronotropic incompetence, common with sino-atrial dysfunction. It may develop gradually over the months or years following pacing system implantation (see p. 186). Dyspnea and fatigue are limited to conditions of exercise. An exercise test, preferably with exercise spirometry, will confirm the diagnosis.
- Chronotropic incompetence caused by inappropriate programming in the so-called „physiologic" modes. This may be due to the setting of too low an upper

rate in DDD mode, resulting in Wenckebach behavior or even 2 : 1 pacing at low levels of exercise (see p. 89 ff.). Similarly, during rate responsive pacing, excessive limitation of the sensor maximal rate, or the programming of too shallow a slope of rate responsiveness may lead to the equivalent of chronotropic incompetence with all its associated symptoms.

- A pacing system dysfunction, whether paroxysmal or fixed, involving sensing, pacing, or both, may cause bradycardic symptoms to reappear, as, for instance, in the case of atrial sensing failure in the DDD mode with return of AV dissociation. The diagnosis is simple when the dysfunction is fixed, but may be more difficult when intermittent, particularly when exercise-related. In patients paced in DDD mode, monitoring of the atrial electrogram by telemetry often reveals a decrease in signal amplitude in the standing position, during deep breathing, or with exercise. Once recognized, this dysfunction can often be corrected by reprogramming a higher atrial sensitivity.

### Palpitation

Palpitation may develop from rhythm disturbances unrelated to the pacing system. Occasionally, in paced patients, especially those with VVI pacemakers, the onset of pacing is perceived as an uncomfortable feeling, particularly in the weeks that follow the implant. In such cases, reprogramming of the back up pacing rate to a lower value, or the use of hysteresis to lessen the chances of competition between spontaneous and paced rhythm, will usually suffice to alleviate the symptoms.

On occasion, in cases of 2 : 1 atrioventricular block, alternans of narrow and completely paced QRS complexes may occur and be poorly tolerated. The AVD should be shortened to obtained fixed ventricular pacing and stable ventricular contraction patterns from cycle to cycle.

On the other hand, other arrhythmic symptoms may be attributable to the pacing system:

- Run-away pacing caused by electromagnetic interferences (see p. 331), by pacemaker failure (rare nowadays with reliable rate-limiting features), and tachyarrhythmias caused by poor setting of the rate responsive function or poor function of the sensor are such examples.
- Ventricular pacing tracking atrial arrhythmias: in triggered dual-chamber modes (VDD, DDD, DDDR), in absence of spontaneous AV conduction, the pacemaker synchronizes ventricular pacing with each sensed atrial event (atrial extrasystoles, flutter, fibrillation, etc.). The electrocardiogram reveals either a regular tachycardia at a rate below or equal to the programmed upper rate and n : 1 association, or Wenckebach behavior, or ventricular paced complexes irregularly associated with the unpredictable sensing of atrial events (atrial fibrillation). This risk is now minimized by mode switch algorithms which dissociate ventricular pacing from atrial activity as soon as an atrial rhythm above a certain rate appears, for as long as that rate persists (see p. 402 ff.).

- ELT represents an other form of tachycardia induced and perpetuated by the pacemaker in modes synchronized to the atrium; this has been discussed in detail in Chap. 3 (see p. 95 ff.). Once ongoing, ELT requires electronic treatment. The mere application of a magnet, temporarily converting the pacing mode to D00 may suffice; occasionally reprogramming of the device is necessary. However, some state-of-the-art pacemakers are now capable of diagnosing and automatically terminating the tachycardia without the intervention of medical personnel. In some cases, the Holter memory of the device will provide the only confirmation of such events.

## Chest Pain

Chest pain are often reported by paced patients, particularly the elderly. Besides the disorders already mentioned (pacemaker syndrome, hypertrophic cardiomyopathy, etc.), the presence of angina pectoris due to excessively rapid ventricular pacing rates aggravating underlying coronary insufficiency, must always be kept in mind. This complication is specific to rate responsive pacemakers. Such systems, or at least the programming of a rapid sensor maximal rate, are a priori contraindicated in patients suffering from coronary artery disease.

In dual chamber pacing, the risk is linked to ventricular synchrony with sensing of rapid atrial rhythms, whether sinus or ectopic. This may be prevented by limiting the upper rate; however, it has the disadvantage of inducing early Wenckebach behavior, or even 2 : 1 mode, which may be poorly tolerated. A better solution, if left ventricular function allows it, is to prescribe a medication with chronotropically negative effects, a beta adrenergic blocking drug for instance, to limit the acceleration of the sinus rate.

## Pectoral Stimulation

This is a common complication in the post implant period when the pacing configuration is unipolar. It usually disappears promptly, though it sometimes forces a reduction in the pacing output. In presence of a normal pacing lead impedance, the phenomenon is due either to a reversal of the can position inside the pocket with its electrically active surface against the muscle (in which case an attempt can be made to turn the can over transcutaneously, a maneuver which may be painful) or to a small current leak at the pulse generator header which rarely requires a reintervention to seal the connector. It may also be due to an insulation failure, associated with a decrease in impedance, which mandates a reintervention to replace or repair the lead. Pectoral stimulation in presence of a bipolar system is highly suggestive of an insulation failure and requires a revision of the system.

## Diaphragmatic Stimulation

This complication is unusual if, during the implant, care was taken to verify its absence during high output pacing. If it is observed, the lead position must be changed. With active fixation atrial leads, the electrode has been placed near the phrenic nerve on the lateral right atrial wall. If the culprit electrode is ventricular, it has usually been placed at the very apex of the right ventricle. A reduction in pacing output does not always solve the problem. In addition, the delayed development of diaphragmatic pacing may be indicative of myocardial perforation, usually accompanied by an increase in thresholds, a pericardial type chest pain, or even pericardial effusion. The lead must be repositioned.

## Physical Examination

A physical examination in search of signs of cardiac insufficiency, inspection of the lower extremities, palpation of the peripheral pulse, and measurement of the arterial pressure is mandatory. Such examination allows to clarify the symptoms listed earlier, and to better evaluate the clinical repercussions of a possibly inappropriate programming of the pacing system. The examination must be systematic and meticulous. The skin in the area of the pocket must be inspected, looking for dystrophic signs or abnormal adhesion of the can, suggesting an impending erosion, of cutaneous necrosis, forerunner of the extrusion of the implanted material, or of local signs of infection (tenderness, redness, heat, swelling), perhaps accompanied by signs of systemic infection. In presence of any of such symptoms, the prescription of ointments, antibiotics, or antiinflammatory agents is futile; instead, the patient should be immediately referred to the implanting center for a pocket revision (in absence of infection) or, in the worst case, explantation of an infected system.

## Resting Electrocardiogram

Long recordings may be needed to evaluate the behavior of the pacing system with respect to the patient's spontaneous rhythm, as well as the integrity of sensing and pacing. The influence of breathing and patient motion should also be examined. Isometric exercises of the upper extremities are performed in search of either myosignal inhibition or, conversely, of an acceleration of ventricular pacing by a dual chamber pacemaker if sensing of the myosignals is limited to the atrial channel (Fig. 7.1). Spontaneous rhythm is often associated with repolarization abnormalities which cannot be accurately interpreted since they may be secondary to recent ventricular pacing (Fig. 7.2).

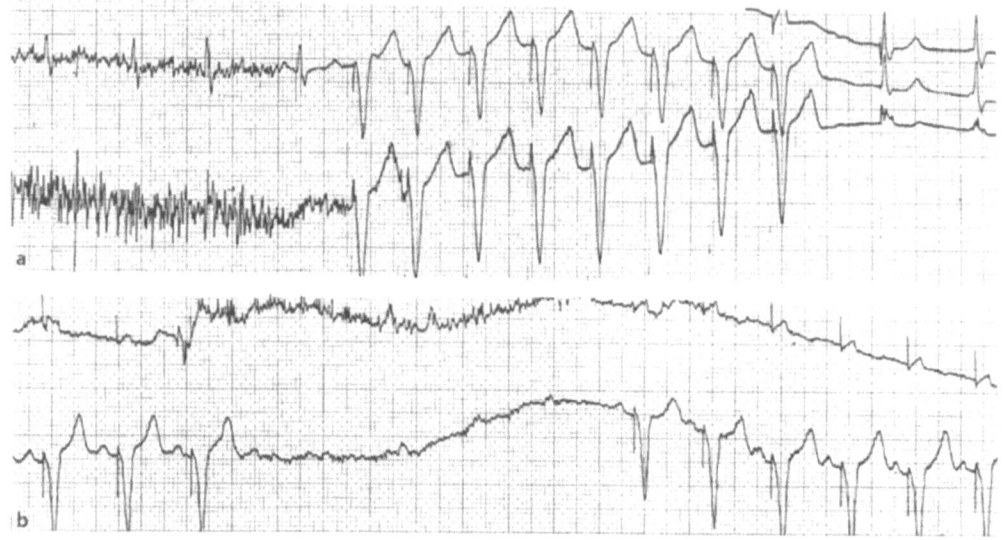

**Fig. 7.1.** Myosignal inhibition of the pacemaker must be systematically looked for
**a** Sensing of myosignals by the atrial channel causing rapid ventricular pacing because of
the interpretation of the myosignals as being of atrial origin
**b** Myosignal sensing by the ventricular channel resulting in complete inhibition of pacing

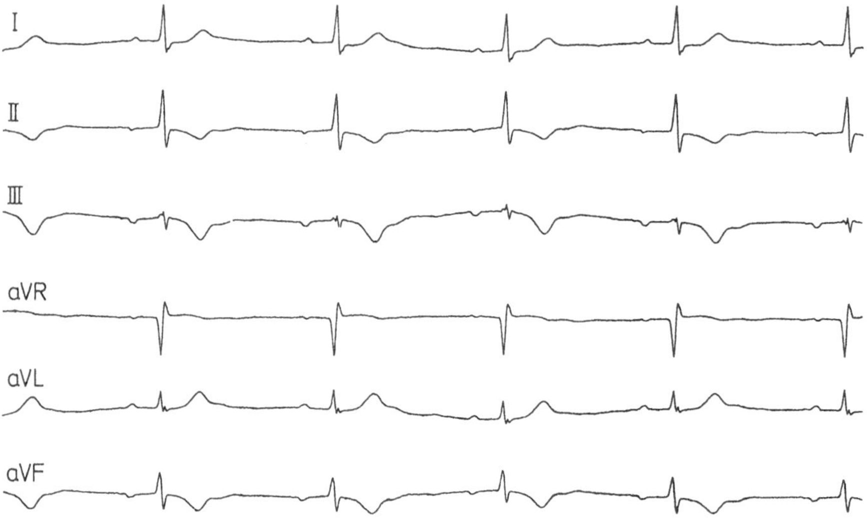

I

II

III

aVR

aVL

aVF

**Fig. 7.2.** Repolarization changes in the form of inverted T waves after spontaneous depolarization should not be, a priori, be considered pathologic in a paced patient

## Verification of Proper Pacing Function

Proper pacing can only be confirmed if the pacing rate is above the spontaneous rate and/or if, in dual chamber pacing, the AVD is shorter than the natural atrioventricular conduction time (when ventricular pacing is to be tested). If spontaneous rhythm prevails, carotid sinus massage may allow the pacemaker to escape after slowing of the sinus rate or, in dual chamber pacing, after lengthening of the PR interval (Fig. 7.3a). A magnet can also be applied over the pulse generator (Fig. 7.3b), which may revert to fixed, asynchronous pacing in various ways according to the model that has been implanted (see p. 381). The pacemaker may escape at the programmed lower rate or at a different rate, or in a mixed fashion, with a few cycles at a rapid magnet rate, followed by pacing at the lower rate. AVD is often shortened during magnet test to verify proper ventricular pacing, and the pacing output may or may not remain the same as that which is programmed. Finally with some pacemaker models, asynchronous pacing will be delivered for a precise number of cycles after removal of the magnet. If the pacing spike falls in the natural refractory period of the myocardium, no capture will be observed, which does not mean that the system is ineffective.

> **!** During magnet test, since the mode is switched to S00 or D00, a pulse may fall in the vulnerable period and trigger serious arrhythmias.

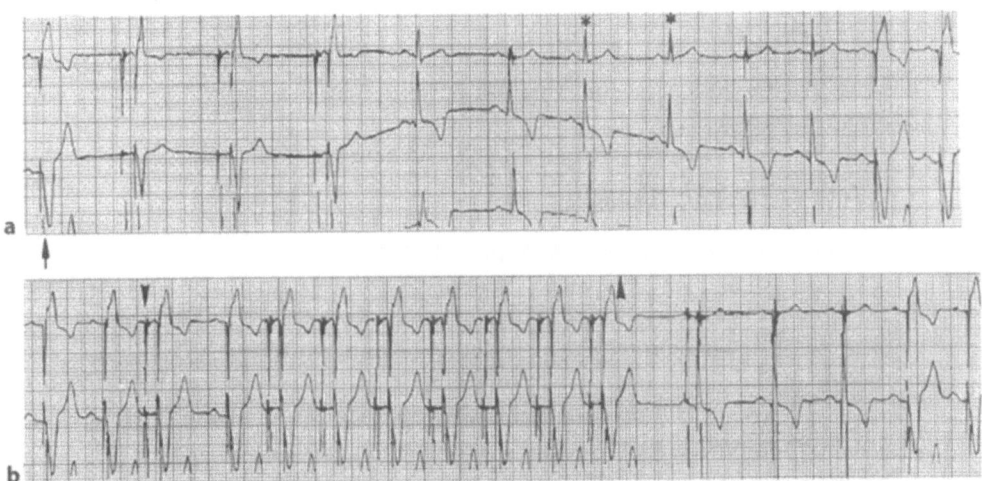

**Fig. 7.3.** During a simple follow-up visit, carotid sinus massage (begun at the *arrow*) resulting in slowing of the spontaneous rhythm, and application of a magnet, both reveal effective ventricular and atrial, pacing
**a** Carotid massage
**b** Magnet application

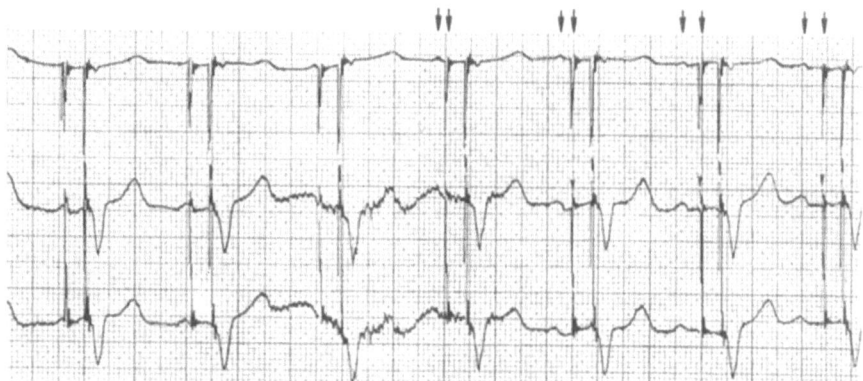

**Fig. 7.4.** Usefulness of moderate exercise to verify proper sensing. In this example, the test discloses failure to sense (*arrows*): an atrial spike is delivered after each P wave in the last 4 cycles of the tracing

### Verification of Proper Sensing

Sensing may only be tested if the spontaneous cardiac rhythm is faster than the pacing rate and/or, in dual chamber pacing, if the AVD is longer than the AV conduction time (for ventricular sensing). Moreover, no magnet should be placed over the pulse generator during this test. If pacing prevails, moderate exercise (sit ups on the examination table) often causes enough heart rate acceleration to inhibit the pacing system (Fig. 7.4).

In spite of all these maneuvers, no information is gathered relative to the sensing or pacing safety margins. One can only confirm that the system senses and paces properly.

### Elective Replacement Determination

A „miniclinic" of the Paceview type placed on the patient's thorax allows to measure the pacing rate or the pacing interval, and the stimulus duration(s) (along with the AVD with dual chamber pacing), particularly when a magnet is applied over the pulse generator. Values of magnet rate and/or stimulus duration(s) are specific of the device tested and are indicated on their respective specification cards. A decrease in the pacing rate and/or an increase in pulse duration are the usual signals of elective replacement and correspond to an increase in the internal impedance of the battery, indicating end of life.

When the pulse generator has been implanted for a long time, it is recommended to leave the magnet in place for over one minute, as one may observe a drift in the values measured as a consequence of higher power consumption, since magnet testing often increases the pacing rate (Fig. 7.5; see also Appendix).

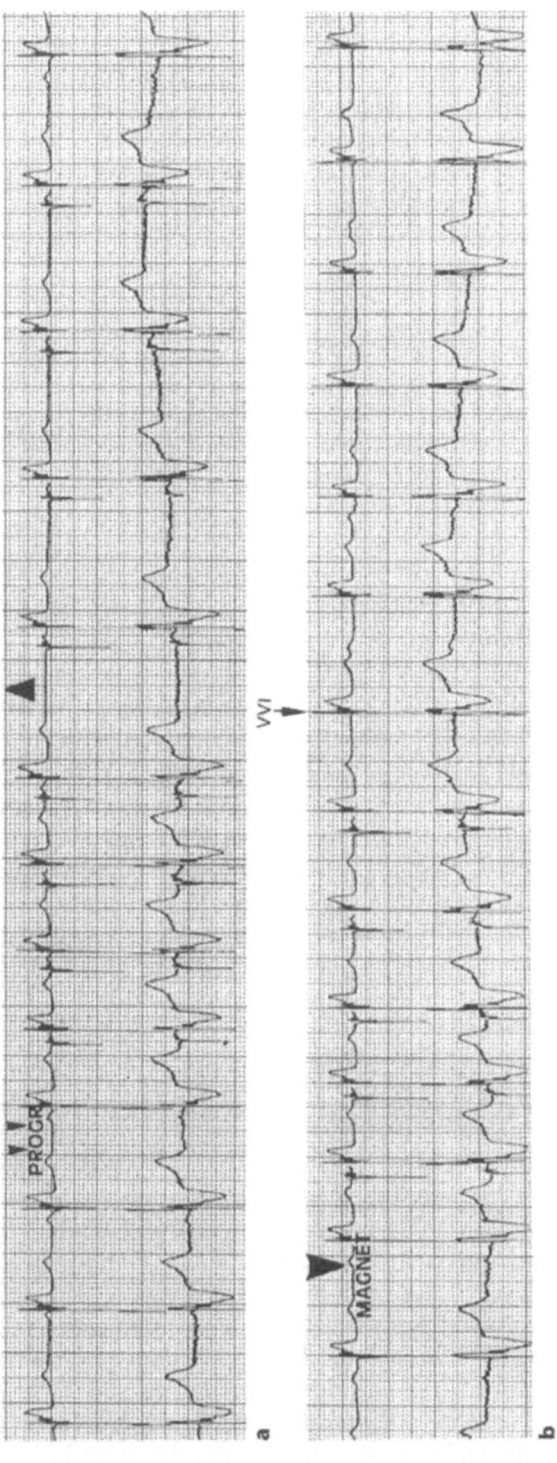

**Fig. 7.5.** Magnet test to determine the battery depletion. It is important to leave the magnet in place for over 1 min, particularly when the battery is approaching end of life

**a** The pacing system is DDD, but the patient presents in VVI mode. After reprogramming (*PROG*), normal DDD function is restored

**b** Upon magnet application (*MAGNET*), the pacemaker switches again to VVI or V00 mode (*VVI*). The power consumed during reprogramming, followed by acceleration of the pacing rate from application of the magnet, has caused reversal to safety pacing at the battery end of life

## Transtelephonic Interrogation

Interrogation of the pacemaker over the telephone is of great help when the patient resides away from the pacemaker clinic. It allows to gather succinct and reliable information, equivalent to a simple magnet test. However, in case of transmission failure, or at the approach of end of life, a complete test must be performed at the specialized center. To our knowledge, a complete transtelephonic test of the pacemaker is not currently feasible. However, the ability to modify certain pacemakers softwares has been reported. One can reinitialize a pacemaker as in the following example.

CASE STUDY

*Example.* A 72 year old patient has received a Vitatron Quintech DDD 931 pacemaker for complete heart block. A few years later, she underwent an aortic valve replacement operation during which her pacemaker was deinitialized. In the postoperative period, the device was reinitialized transtelephonically from the Netherlands without difficulty, allowing its subsequent reprogramming.

## 7.3
## Comprehensive Follow-Up

Comprehensive follow-up visits must be scheduled at a specialized center. A multichannel electrocardiographic recorder, interfaced with an oscilloscope, is preferred to provide continuous visualization of the ECG tracing. Clear understanding of the event markers and electrograms is necessary for the interpretation of the pacemaker function. Some devices have a „magnet off" function which facilitates certain steps of the procedure. An external defibrillator must be available in the examination room, since torsade de pointe may occur when the pacing rate is programmed down during testing of the sensing functions, or after a ventricular pause during testing of the pacing function. Serious arrhythmias may also be triggered upon application of the magnet which switches the device to an asynchronous mode.

A comprehensive test involves temporary reprogramming to measure sensing and pacing thresholds, and to optimize the rate response, the AVD of dual chamber systems, the refractory periods, etc. It also involves the interrogation of all the pacemaker memories. These tests should be scheduled twice yearly, and may need to be performed more frequently in case of intercurrent adverse events such as exposure to exogenous interferences, myocardial infarction, metabolic or electrolyte disturbances, the introduction of drug therapy which may modify thresholds, etc.

A comprehensive test begins with simple measurements, as described earlier. A programmer dedicated to the device under examination is used throughout the procedure. The device memories should be interrogated before programming since, with certain models, any programming may erase the information that had been memorized. In other models, all counters and statistics must be cleared at the very end of the test. In all cases, the examination is completed with the printing and verification of all the programmed parameters.

## Telemetry

Telemetry is essential since it provides diverse information pertaining to events that have occurred since the last interrogation.

### Is the Device Programming Identical to What It Was at the Last Visit? (Fig. 7.6)

If such is not the case, four possibilities should be considered:

- The pacemaker was reprogrammed by another physician.
- The pacemaker reprogrammed itself automatically according to the specific instructions of its algorithms, an event which is displayed at the time of interrogation.
- The pacemaker was deprogrammed by exposure to interferences; though rare, its exact cause must be identified. The pacemaker is usually found operating in a safety mode.
- The pacemaker is operating in a mode corresponding to the end of life of the battery which needs to be replaced; in such cases, the end of life (EOL) indicators are listed.

```
292-09 SN 176640                    17 JUL 97 10:34
          SUMMARY OF INITIAL / CURRENT VALUES
                                 INITIAL     CURRENT
          MODE:                  VVI-R       VVI-R


          SLEEP RATE:                 50          50 MIN-1
            BEDTIME:             11:30 PM   11:30 PM
            WAKETIME:             7:30 AM    7:30 AM
          PACING RATE:                55          55 MIN-1


          SLOW WALK RATE:             85          85 MIN-1
          MAXIMUM PACING RATE:       135         135 MIN-1


          VENT. PULSE AMPLITUDE:     2.5         2.5 V
          VENT. PULSE WIDTH:        0.30        0.30 MS
          VENT. POLARITY:         UNI/BI      UNI/BI

          VENT. SENSITIVITY:         7.0         7.0 MV
          VENT. AUTOSENSING:          ON          ON


          VENTRICULAR REFRACTORY:                320         320 MS

        * EXERCISE RATE RESPONSE:                  9           5
```

**Fig. 7.6 a–e.** Programming parameters **a** Printout of the programmed parameters of the Intermedics Marathon pacemaker

```
Vitatron                Release 4.07.00
------------------------------------------

Date     : 1997-07-04   Time : 09:52

Physician:.............................

Hospital :.............................

------------------------------------------

Type                    Diamond II DDDR
Connector                   IS-1 bipolar
Serial number              15 02 431
Patient code
Implantation date          1997-04-21
Battery                          GOOD
Battery impedance                <2 kΩ
Impedance when depleted         9.3 kΩ

------------------------------------------
                PARAMETERS
Mode                               DDDR
Lower rate                  55 min-1
Night rate drop              5 min-1
Start night                  22:30
End night                    06:30
Maximum tracking rate       140 min-1
Maximum sensor rate         120 min-1
Flywheel                          OFF
Mode switching                   AUTO
Maximum AV delay             180 ms
Adaptive AV delay              MEDIAN
AV hysteresis                     OFF

                    Atrium : Ventricle
                    ----------+----------
Pulse amplitude      2.5  V :   2.5  V
Pulse duration       0.3 ms :   0.3 ms
Pace polarity        UNI     :   UNI
Sensitivity          1.0 mV :   4.0 mV
Sense polarity       BI      :   BI
Lead impedance       450  Ω :   500  Ω

Refractory period                260 ms
Atrial blanking                  250 ms
ASP interval                     300 ms
Ventricular blanking              30 ms
Ventricular safety pacing          ON
PVC->Astim                        OFF

------------------------------------------
              RATE RESPONSE
Sensors                        QT=ACT
T sensitivity                  1.0 mV
Activity threshold             MEDIUM
Slope                           AUTO
```

**Fig. 7.6. b** Printout of the programmed parameters of the Vitatron Diamond pacemaker. The instantaneously measured battery impedance and that when depleted are listed

**ELA Medical**
CSO 2.50A V3 PROGRAMMER

7/10/1997 10:37
Ref/R4/B1.8A/2.10+

**PACEMAKER:**
    Model                    =    CHORUM 7234
    Serial number            =    640RA010
    Implant date             =    5/5/1997
        Battery resistance   <    100 ohms
        Magnet rate          =    96.0 min-1
        At BOL : 96 min-1 - At ERI :        78.4 min-1
        AV DELAY modified by Algorithm.

**PATIENT:**
        Patient's name       =
        Birth Date           =    12/24/1941
        Symptoms             = DIZZY SPELLS
        Indications for implant=
                             SICK SINUS SYNDROME - BRADY-TACHY
                             CHRONOTROPIC INCOMPETENCE
        Etiology             =    ISCHEMIC

**Ventricular lead**
    Model                    =    4024   - MEDTRONIC
    Implant date             =    5/5/1997
    Threshold(Ampl/Width)    =    0.5 V / 0.50 ms

**Atrial lead**
    Model                    =    4024   - MEDTRONIC
    Implant date             =    5/5/1997
    Threshold(Ampl/Width)    =    0.4 V / 0.50 ms

**PARAMETERS:**

| MODE: | DDD/AMC | |
|---|---|---|
| **RATE & TIMING PARAMETERS** | | |
| BASIC RATE | 60 | min-1 |
| REST RATE | 60 | min-1 |
| MAXIMUM RATE | 132 | min-1 |
| HYSTERESIS | 0 | % |
| **ATRIOVENTRICULAR DELAY** | | |
| REST AVD | 125 | ms |
| EXERCISE AVD | 78 | ms |
| AV DELAY EXT | 31 | ms |
| **REFRACTORY PERIODS** | | |
| ABS.REF.PERIOD | 203 | ms |
| BLANKING | 47 | ms |
| **ALGORITHMS** | | |
| FALLBACK | YES | |
| ELT PROTECTION | REPROG | |
| SMOOTHING | OFF | |
| ACCELERATION | OFF | % |

**Fig. 7.6. c** Printout of the programmed parameters of the ELA Medical Chorum pacemaker. The measured magnet rate and that at elective replacement time are listed

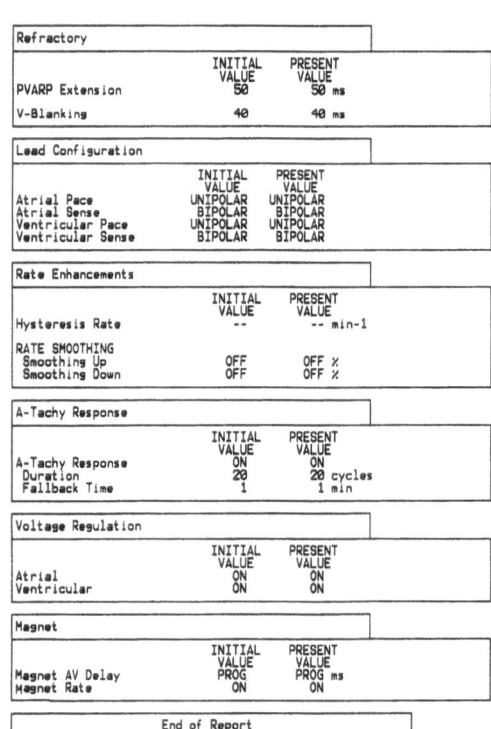

```
Cardiac Pacemakers, Inc.                                    VIGOR

                          15-JUL-97      09:27
Institution:     KRANKENHAUS PEISSENBERG
                                        Programmer:    000360
1230 Generator:   Serial   404680    2880 Software:       3.0
```

```
Session Net Change Report

                          INITIAL     PRESENT
                           VALUE       VALUE
Mode                       DDDR        DDDR
Lower Rate Limit             50          50 min-1
Upper Rate Limit            135         135 min-1
AV Delay (paced)             --          -- ms

ATRIAL
 Pulse Width               0.30        0.30 ms
 Amplitude                  2.5         2.5 V
 Sensitivity               0.50        0.50 mV
 Refractory-PVARP          250         250 ms

VENTRICULAR
 Pulse Width               0.30        0.30 ms
 Amplitude                  2.5         2.5 V
 Sensitivity                4.0         4.0 mV
 Refractory                250         250 ms
```

```
AV Delay

                          INITIAL     PRESENT
                           VALUE       VALUE
Dynamic AV Delay            ON          ON
 Maximum Delay             180         180 ms
 Minimum Delay             100         100 ms

Sensed AV Offset           -60         -60 ms
```

```
Sensor

                          INITIAL     PRESENT
                           VALUE       VALUE
Max Sensor Rate            120         120 min-1

Activity Threshold        MEDIUM      MEDIUM
Reaction Time               30          30 sec
Response Factor              8           8
Recovery Time                5           5 min
```

```
Refractory

                          INITIAL     PRESENT
                           VALUE       VALUE
PVARP Extension             50          50 ms

V-Blanking                  40          40 ms
```

```
Lead Configuration

                          INITIAL     PRESENT
                           VALUE       VALUE
Atrial Pace              UNIPOLAR    UNIPOLAR
Atrial Sense             BIPOLAR     BIPOLAR
Ventricular Pace         UNIPOLAR    UNIPOLAR
Ventricular Sense        BIPOLAR     BIPOLAR
```

```
Rate Enhancements

                          INITIAL     PRESENT
                           VALUE       VALUE
Hysteresis Rate             --          -- min-1

RATE SMOOTHING
 Smoothing Up              OFF         OFF %
 Smoothing Down            OFF         OFF %
```

```
A-Tachy Response

                          INITIAL     PRESENT
                           VALUE       VALUE
A-Tachy Response            ON          ON
Duration                    20          20 cycles
Fallback Time                1           1 min
```

```
Voltage Regulation

                          INITIAL     PRESENT
                           VALUE       VALUE
Atrial                      ON          ON
Ventricular                 ON          ON
```

```
Magnet

                          INITIAL     PRESENT
                           VALUE       VALUE
Magnet AV Delay            PROG        PROG ms
Magnet Rate                 ON          ON
```

```
              End of Report
```

**Fig. 7.6. d** Printout of the programmed parameters of the CPI Vigor DR

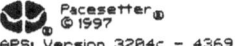

Pacesetter ®
© 1997
APS: Version 3204c - 4369

Microny®SR+

15 Jul 1997 08:47
Last programmed on: 15 Jul 1997
MODEL: 2425T    SERIAL: 6225 47800

PATIENT: _____

PHYSICIAN: _____

Patient I.D.:                    Implant Date: 6 May 1997
Lead Type: Bipolar               Lead Chamber: Ventricle

**Fig. 7.6. e** Printout of
the programmed
parameters of the
Pacesetter Microny.
The parameters listed
under „INITIAL" are
those obtained at first
interrogation of the
device, at the begin-
ning of the visit;
those listed under
„PRESENT" are those
currently in effect
(d,e). Programming
modifications are
indicated by *arrows*

( PROGRAMMED PARAMETERS )

|  | INITIAL | PRESENT |  |
|---|---|---|---|
| Mode | VVIR | VVIR | |
| Autocapture Function | OFF → | ON | |
| Sensor | ON | ON | |
| Basic Rate | 55 | 55 | min⁻¹ |
| Hysteresis Rate | OFF → | 10 | bpm |
| Refractory | 300 | 300 | msec |
| Pulse Width | .31 | .31 | msec |
| Pulse Amplitude | 2.4 → | AUTO | Volts |
| P/R Sensitivity | 7.5 | 7.5 | mVolts |
| ER Sensitivity | 1.6 → | 2.5 | mVolts |
| Vario | OFF | OFF | |
| Maximum Sensor Rate | 130 | 130 | min⁻¹ |
| Slope | 11 | 11 | |
| Reaction Time | FAST | FAST | |
| Fast Response | ON | ON | |
| Recovery Time | MEDIUM | MEDIUM | |

→ INITIAL value differs from PRESENT value

```
292-09 SN 176640            17 JUL 97 08:59
VVI-R           TELEMETRY DATA
  PACING RATE                       55 MIN-1
  PACING INTERVAL                 1091 MS
  CELL VOLTAGE                     2.79 V
  CELL IMPEDANCE                  ‹2.5 KOHMS
  CELL CURRENT                    11.9 UA
                               VENT. UNI/BI
  SENSITIVITY                      7.0 MV
  LEAD IMPEDANCE                   567 OHMS
  PULSE AMPLITUDE                 2.46 V
  PULSE WIDTH                     0.30 MS
  OUTPUT CURRENT                   4.2 MA
  ENERGY DELIVERED                 2.9 UJ
  CHARGE DELIVERED                1.28 UC


292-09 SN 176640            17 JUL 97 09:20
          AUTOSENSING DATA


                              VENTRICLE
  MAXIMUM SENSITIVITY
          REACHED:                7.0  MV

  MINIMUM SENSITIVITY
          REACHED:                7.0  MV


292-09 SN 176640            17 JUL 97 09:19
   CARDIAC JOURNAL DATA SUMMARY    VVI-R


  PERCENT OF TIME VENTRICLE WAS PACED:      48 %


  PERCENT OF TIME THAT SENSOR CONTROLLED
  RATE......................................48 %
```

**Fig. 7.7. a** Additional information from telemetry. Information obtained from telemetry by an Intermedics Marathon pacemaker. Autosensing data is also provided: maximal and minimal amplitudes are shown

**Battery Status and End of Life Indicators** (Fig. 7.7; see also Appendix)

The battery replacement indicators vary from one pulse generator to the other. Besides the decrease in magnet rate, or even the increase in pacing stimulus duration, the approach of end of life of a lithium battery is manifest by an output voltage of 2.3 V or below, and a battery internal impedance reaching 10 K$\Omega$, whereas a new battery puts out 2.8 V and has an internal impedance below 1 K$\Omega$.

Two consecutive periods are distinguished. First, a recommended, or elective replacement time, defined by the onset of drift of the parameters described earlier. At this point a period of a few weeks or months remains before total exhaustion of the battery leading to shut down of the pulse generator. The length of this time interval is difficult to estimate and depends on the degree of dependency of the patient on the pacemaker, of the power consumed to pace, and on the size of the battery. A small battery will deplete much more rapidly than a larger one at the approach of end of life. Accordingly, when a drift of the indicators is noted with a small battery, we recommend a much closer surveillance, at the least every

```
╭─────────────  MEASURED DATA  ─────────────╮

    Measured Rate ──────────────────────── 116.3  min⁻¹
    Test Rate ──────────────────────────── 99.7  min⁻¹
    Sensor Indicated Rate ──────────────── 55  min⁻¹
    Pulse Amplitude ────────────────────── 2.42  Volts
    Pulse Current ──────────────────────── 3.6  mAmperes
    Pulse Energy ───────────────────────── 2.4  μJoules
    Pulse Charge ───────────────────────── 1.8  μCoulombs
    Lead Impedance ─────────────────────── 673  Ohms
    Battery Voltage ────────────────────── 2.78  Volts
    Battery Current ────────────────────── 5.6  μAmperes
    Battery Impedance ──────────────────── < 1.0  KOhms
```

```
╭──────────────  TEST RESULTS  ──────────────╮

    VARIO Capture Thresholds (V):
        0.30  0.30
        Max. Capture Thresholds (V):   0.30
        Min. Capture Thresholds (V):   0.30
        Test Pulse Width: .31 msec

    AUTOCAPTURE Threshold Test:
        Capture Threshold: =0.60 Volts
        Test Pulse Width: .31 msec

    P/R Sensitivity:
        Proposed P/R Sensitivity: 7.5 mVolts
        Sense Margin: 182.5%
        P/R Signal: 21.19 mVolts
        ─────────────────────────────────
        Original P/R Sensitivity: 7.5 mVolts
        Sense Margin: 182.5%

    ER Test:
        ER Signal: 4.31 mVolts
        ─────────────────────────────────
        Proposed ER Sensitivity: 1.6 mVolts
        Sense Margin: 169.7%
        Original ER Sensitivity: 1.6 mVolts
        Sense Margin: 169.7%
        ─────────────────────────────────
        Polarization Signal: 9.12 mVolts
        % Of Proposed ER: 570%
```

**Fig. 7.7. b** Information obtained from telemetry by a Pacesetter Microny pacemaker. Note that the results of the sensing and pacing threshold tests appear with their respective calculated safety margins, additional auto-capture and evoked response measurements.
*ER* evoked response; see also p. 66

3 months, or the rapid replacement of the generator. In our opinion, when the battery is small, the most reliable criterion is the evolution of its internal impedance, and we proceed with replacement of the pulse generator as soon as it reaches $4-5$ K$\Omega$, trading the saving of, at the most, a few months for the elimination of a risk that remains difficult to estimate.

Elective replacement indicators may also become temporarily manifest when the battery is subject to high power consumption, for example rapid, rate responsive, dual chamber pacing; this may even lead to the temporary switch of pacing to a safety mode, VVI or asynchronous. In such cases, close surveillance is also advised. This behavior, however, must be distinguished from the switch to safety pacing caused by external interference. The pacemaker can usually be reprogrammed by reinitialization; if not, particularly if the device can be neither programmed nor interrogated, it should be rapidly replaced, after having verified that both the programmer and its wand are functioning properly.

```
                    MEASURED DATA
Output status:
    +-------------+----------+-----------+
    :Status type  : Atrium   : Ventricle :
    :Pace polarity: Unipolar : Unipolar  :
    +-------------+----------+-----------+
    :Impedance [Ω]:    450   :    500    :
    :Amplitude [V]:    2.5   :    2.5    :
    :Current  [mA]:    5.5   :    5.0    :
    :Energy   [µJ]:     4    :     4     :
    +-------------+----------+-----------+
```

```
Pulse Duration threshold:
    +-----------+------------+-----------+
    : Output [V]: Atrium [ms]: Ventr [ms]:
    : Polarity  : Unipolar   : Unipolar  :
    +-----------+------------+-----------+
    :   2.5     :   <0.10    :   <0.10   :
    +-----------+------------+-----------+
```

```
Amplitude threshold:
    +-----------+------------+-----------+
    : Pulse [ms]: Atrium [V] : Ventr [V] :
    : Polarity  : Unipolar   : Unipolar  :
    +-----------+------------+-----------+
    :   0.3     :   0.45     :   0.65    :
    +-----------+------------+-----------+
```

```
              ELECTROGRAM AMPLITUDES
P wave:
    Atrial sense polarity            BI
    P wave amplitude             4.0 mV

R wave:
    Ventricular sense polarity       BI
    R wave amplitude          >12.0 mV

T wave:
    +-----------+------------+
    : Paced rate : T amplitude :
    :  [min-1]   :    [mV]    :
    +-----------+------------+
    :   100     :    2.4     :
    +-----------+------------+
```

```
                  INTERVALS
QT analysis:
    +-----------+------------+
    : Paced rate : QT interval :
    :  [min-1]   :    [ms]    :
    +-----------+------------+
    :   100     :    332     :
    +-----------+------------+
```

**Fig. 7.7. c** Information obtained from telemetry by a Vitatron Diamond pacemaker. The measured T wave amplitude is listed

```
Histogram                        V Rate
Holter                           24 HOUR
Atrium paced                       61 %
Ventricle paced                    99 %
T waves sensed                     85 %
AV synchrony                       99 %
PVC's                              551
PVC's                            4/day

                                DD:HH:MM
Time since last follow up        122
Atrial rate > 140 min-1 Path     0:00:00
Atrial rate > 140 min-1 Phys     0:00:00
Atrial rate < 140 min-1 Path     0:00:26
```

a

b

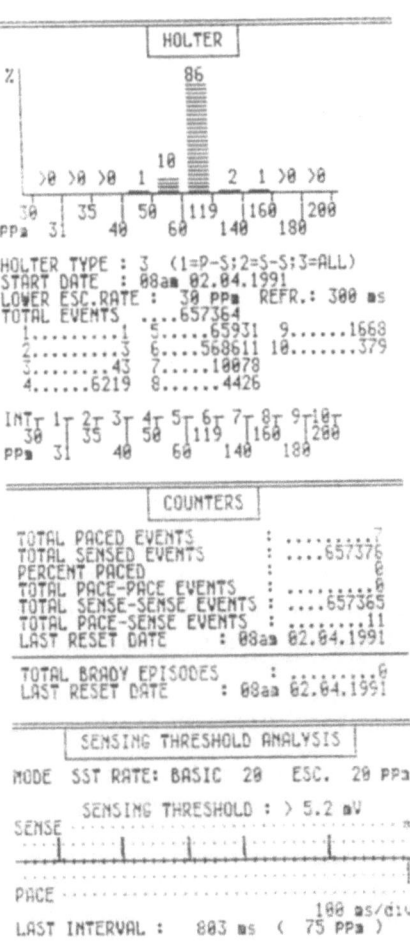

**Fig. 7.8.** Statistical information
**a** Statistics offered by the Vitatron
Diamond pacemaker. The main information consists of a count of ventricular extrasystoles and of abnormal atrial rhythms
**b** Statistics offered by the Sorin Theorema 90 pacemaker

```
STATISTICS:
  MODE                              DDD
  RATE RESPONSE                    RRauto
  Last reset date    : 6/27/1997

  Programmings                      0

PACED BEATS
  A. Paced Beats          294993   42 %
  V. Paced Beats          196952   28 %
  Cardiac Cycles          695848
  AV   no sensor    :        357
       with sensor  :     131489   19 %
  AR   no sensor    :      34447    5 %
       with sensor  :     128700   18 %
  PR                      303358   44 %
  PV                         478
  CP                         720
  PVC                       1829
  PAC                        265
  R                        30562    4 %
  V    no sensor    :      10288    1 %
       with sensor  :      54341    8 %

  FALLBACK
  Fallback Mode Switch        2
  Total time in fallback  0d22h26m16s

  ELT PROTECTION
  Detected PMTs               6

ATRIAL MEASUREMENTS:
  Voltage         =   3.38     V
  Current         =   6.44    mA
  Impedance       =    524    ohms
  Energy          = 13.26  uJoules

VENTRICULAR MEASUREMENTS:
  Voltage         =   2.25     V
  Current         =   4.29    mA
  Impedance       =    523    ohms
  Energy          =  2.35  uJoules
```

**Fig. 7.8. c** Statistics offered by an ELA Medical pacemaker. The display includes the number of activation of certain algorithms such as fall-back, and number of ELT episodes („PMT") detected

Some pacemaker models have occasionally an aberrant behavior at the approach of end of life, despite the absence of criteria for elective replacement. One might, for instance, observe intermittent sensing failure despite the finding of satisfactory intracardiac signals at the time of generator replacement, after which normal function of the system returns.

**Information Stored in the Pacemaker's Memory**

Modern pulse generators are capable of storing large amounts of information in their memory which may include all or some of the following:

- Statistical data (Fig. 7.8) which help programming the pacemaker by analyzing the percentage of paced versus sensed events. This may lead to reprogramming of the pacing rate and AVD (in dual chamber) to offer both physiologic and safe pacing, and spare the battery by minimizing the number of paced events. This information allows also a better understanding of the underlying

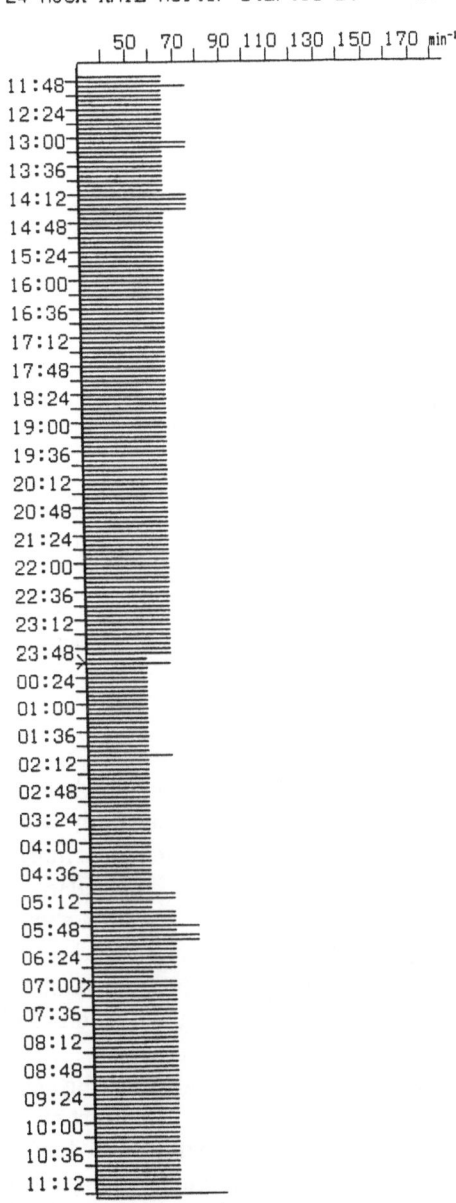

```
Vitatron                    Release 4.07.00
-------------------------------------------

Date : 1997-07-28           Time : 11:34

Type                        Diamond II DDDR
Serial number                  15 14 028
Holter information read at         11:44
Start night                        00:00
End night                          07:00

24 HOUR RATE Holter started at:    11:42
```

**Fig. 7.9.** 24 h display of heart rate
**a** Holter type information provided
by a Vitatron Diamond pacemaker

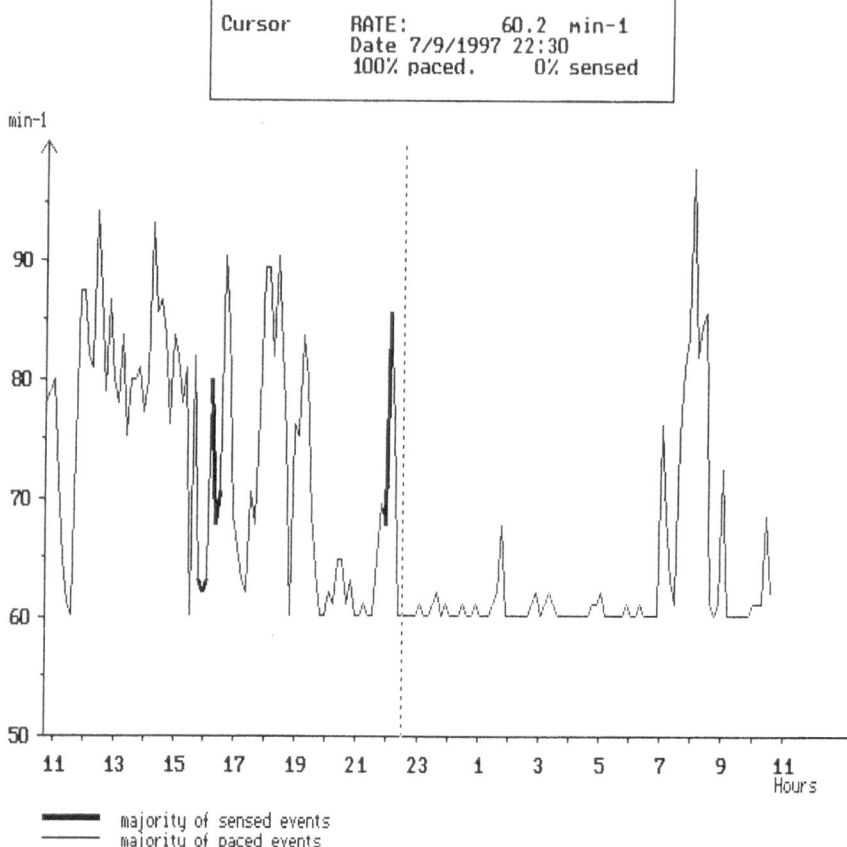

**Fig. 7.9. b** 24 h heart rate curve retrieved by telemetry of an ELA Medical Chorum pacemaker. It is apparent that the patient woke up at 7:00 a.m. The ratio of sensed events/paced events is inferior to 1%

atrioventricular conduction and chronotropic function. This type of data is offered by the majority of currently available pacemakers. Some models provide additional information that is more specific: the number of occurrences of distinct events such as ventricular, or sometimes atrial extrasystoles, the number of episodes of tachycardia above rates and duration that can be programmed (with, sometimes a marker channel or diagrams, or electrograms for corresponding episodes), the number of activation of safety features (pacing in the safety window, activation of protection algorithm against ELT or atrial tachyarrhythmias, etc.).

- A 24 h display of the heart rate (Fig. 7.9), with possible distinction between paced and sensed events, or a heart rate curve calculated by the rate responsive function, are frequently offered by state-of-the art pacemakers.
- Long-term event histograms display the distribution, since the last interrogation, of sensed versus paced events. The display may be purely cumulative, or

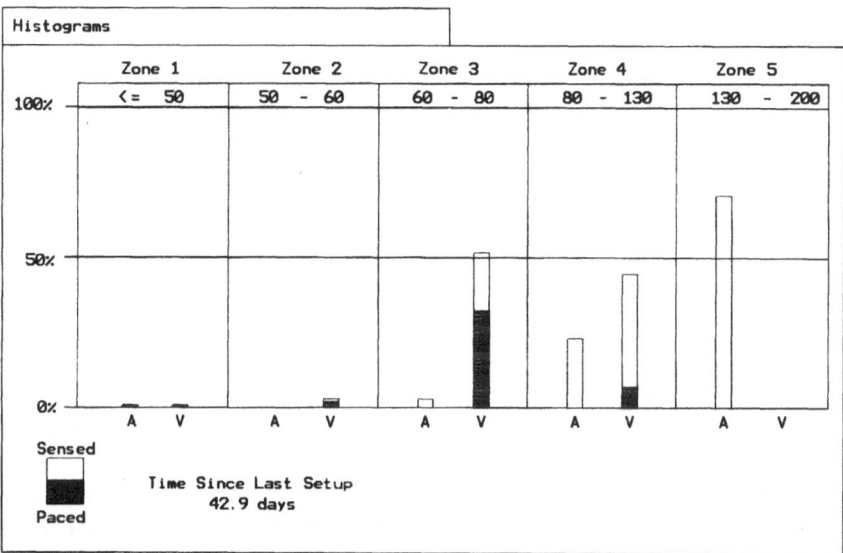

**Fig. 7.10 a–h.** Long-term event histograms
**a** Information obtained by telemetry of a CPI Vigor DR pacemaker. A histogram-like print-out is provided, along with the percentage of sensed versus paced events in each cardiac chamber

divided in programmable time intervals, or limited to the last 24 h. Other combined histograms may be programmed to gather chronological information on selected items such as interatrial, interventricular or atrioventricular intervals, ventricular extrasystoles, etc. (Fig. 7.10a–e).

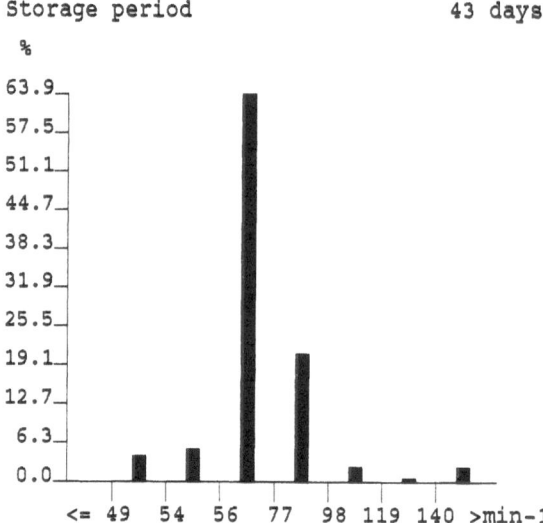

Storage period                         43 days

| Atrial rate [min-1] | Number of events | Percent [%] |
|---------------------|------------------|-------------|
| <=    49            | 685              | 0.0         |
| 49  -  54           | 176204           | 4.2         |
| 54  -  56           | 225953           | 5.4         |
| 56  -  77           | 2649040          | 63.9        |
| 77  -  98           | 871297           | 21.0        |
| 98  - 119           | 97968            | 2.4         |
| 119 - 140           | 26912            | 0.6         |
|     > 140           | 98741            | 2.4         |

**Fig. 7.10. b** Atrial rate histogram recorded by a Vitatron Diamond pacemaker

- Long-term histograms of rate response provide information on the sensor by displaying the heart rate variations that would have been induced by the sensor (Fig. 7.10f–h).
- A Holter function activated during an exercise test may assist in programming a given parameter such as the rate response (Fig. 7.11a).
- A simulation function based on the data memorized by the device (Fig. 7.11b,c) helps programming the rate response when the patient has performed a single exercise test.
- An autocalibration curve may show the evolution of the rate response parameter over time (Fig. 7.11d).
- Marker channels of programmable sequences of events (Fig. 7.12) may be automatically memorized according to programmed instructions (see also Fig. 7.21).

Besides the memorized information, the pacemaker may display event markers and intracardiac electrograms, which facilitate distinguishing anomalous functions from normal behavior, and helps examining the next question.

INT V: Ventricular events
Period = 1 week

| Bound (ms) | < 234 | >= 234 < 297 | >= 297 < 359 | >= 359 < 422 | >= 422 < 609 | >= 609 < 797 | >= 797 < 1000 | >=1000 |
|---|---|---|---|---|---|---|---|---|
| min$^{-1}$ | > 256 | <= 256 > 202 | <= 202 > 167 | <= 167 > 142 | <= 142 > 98 | <= 98 > 75 | <= 75 > 60 | <= 60 |
| 1 | 0 | 1 | 2 | 33 | 104489 | 318948 | 297818 | 62237 |
| 2 | 0 | 0 | 8 | 118 | 66833 | 267213 | 269283 | 139657 |
| 3 | 0 | 0 | 0 | 1 | 18113 | 294140 | 305647 | 115179 |
| 4 | 0 | 1 | 0 | 15 | 31951 | 297804 | 235193 | 167156 |
| 5 | 0 | 1 | 9 | 679 | 182220 | 284556 | 263335 | 77712 |
| 6 | 0 | 0 | 12 | 105 | 129731 | 384263 | 231653 | 62652 |
| 7 | 0 | 0 | 7 | 16 | 91315 | 357369 | 301375 | 37598 |
| 8 | 0 | 0 | 0 | 3 | 69514 | 359299 | 309980 | 40124 |
| 9 | 0 | 0 | 0 | 7 | 70371 | 330350 | 310949 | 58987 |
| 10 | 0 | 0 | 2 | 13 | 85861 | 337999 | 272841 | 80908 |
| 11 | 0 | 1 | 33 | 233 | 62437 | 372458 | 296601 | 51141 |
| 12 | 0 | 0 | 8 | 40 | 83162 | 348040 | 293024 | 55246 |
| 13 | 0 | 0 | 1 | 0 | 51386 | 341953 | 294365 | 73191 |
| 14 | 0 | 0 | 76 | 300 | 88251 | 358523 | 297613 | 43181 |

INT A: Atrial events
Period = 1 week

| Bound (ms) | < 250 | >= 250 < 297 | >= 297 < 359 | >= 359 < 422 | >= 422 < 609 | >= 609 < 797 | >= 797 < 1000 | >=1000 |
|---|---|---|---|---|---|---|---|---|
| min$^{-1}$ | > 240 | <= 240 > 202 | <= 202 > 167 | <= 167 > 142 | <= 142 > 98 | <= 98 > 75 | <= 75 > 60 | <= 60 |
| 1 | 122226 | 19283 | 10225 | 3031 | 103573 | 304775 | 279815 | 61378 |
| 2 | 108 | 9 | 35 | 99 | 66825 | 267497 | 270297 | 138350 |
| 3 | 8 | 3 | 13 | 31 | 17480 | 294941 | 306862 | 113750 |
| 4 | 30 | 7 | 26 | 72 | 31887 | 298229 | 235737 | 166196 |
| 5 | 157616 | 21447 | 17742 | 4916 | 181095 | 270642 | 235602 | 76325 |
| 6 | 23375 | 3832 | 2485 | 678 | 129523 | 381852 | 228868 | 61455 |
| 7 | 40 | 5 | 40 | 125 | 91251 | 359316 | 302103 | 35493 |
| 8 | 2 | 15 | 29 | 98 | 70708 | 359159 | 310493 | 38924 |
| 9 | 9 | 16 | 44 | 117 | 70708 | 331682 | 311038 | 57620 |
| 10 | 5 | 5 | 32 | 120 | 85830 | 338335 | 273545 | 79899 |
| 11 | 100175 | 14008 | 8112 | 1897 | 62833 | 370674 | 274753 | 49868 |
| 12 | 43 | 24 | 64 | 75 | 84042 | 347046 | 295138 | 53580 |
| 13 | 5 | 53 | 37 | 84 | 51506 | 342401 | 295380 | 71849 |
| 14 | 144647 | 20676 | 11328 | 2915 | 88531 | 350552 | 270614 | 41609 |

**Fig. 7.10.c** Holter type information provided by an ELA Medical Chorus II pacemaker. Programmable event histograms (A and V intervals), are displayed in weekly intervals (*rows*) and ranges of cycle lengths (*columns*). In the analysis of the atrial intervals (INT A), it is apparent that in weeks 1, 5, 6, 11 and 14 a large number of short atrial intervals is listed, due to atrial arrhythmias without corresponding ventricular acceleration, confirming the proper function of the fall-back algorithm

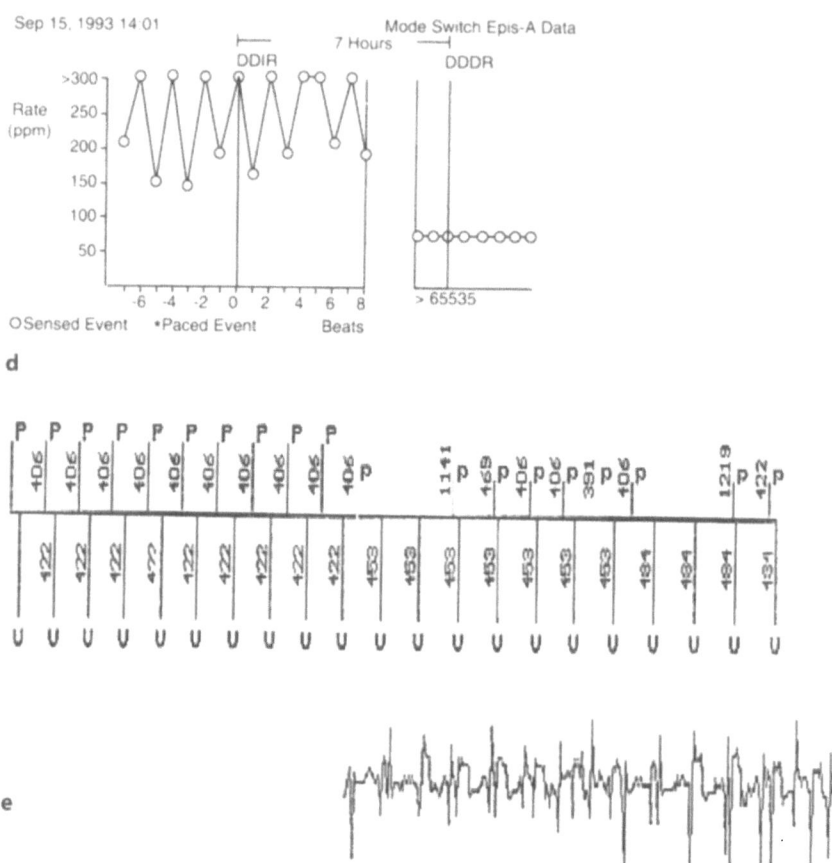

**Fig. 7.10. d** A display of successively sensed atrial beats from Thera DR in a patient with an atrial tachycardia. The „W" pattern occurs in the diagnostic printout from the programmer. Alternate atrial beats which fall into blanking provide beat-to-beat intervals which are approximately twice the actual tachycardia cycle length (Medtronic document) **e** Recording of an events markers chain with the corresponding atrial electrogram, which reveals an atrial tachycardia triggering the mode switch function. One can see during the first half of the recording that there is a detection of a fast atrial rate (PP intervals: 406 ms) leading to a Wenckebach AV association (the ventricular pacing interval is limited to 422 ms) . During the second half, pathological P waves become refractory ones (*p*) which means the triggering of a mode switch. The ventricular pacing rate progressively slowers. Some of the P waves are missing because they fall into the post-ventricular atrial absolute refractory period. The atrial endocardial electrogram confirms the presence of an atrial tachyarrhythmia

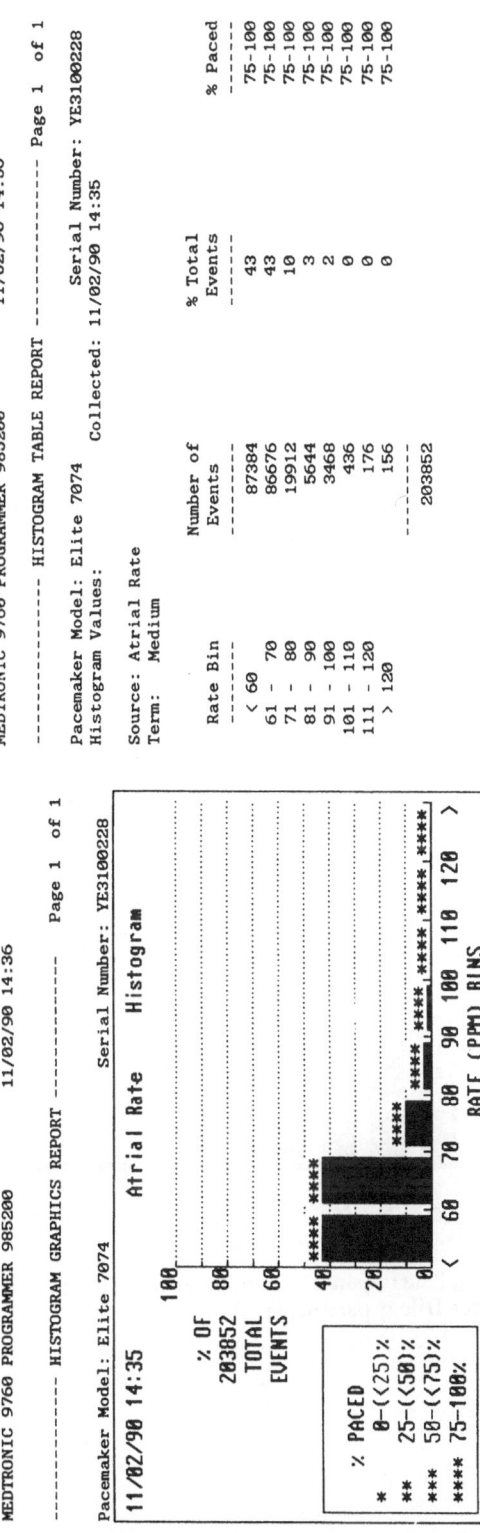

**Fig. 7.10. f** Information retrieved by telemetry on the rate response function of a Medtronic Elite 7074 pacemaker. The rate response curve was judged satisfactory

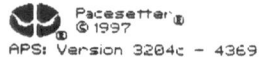

## TRILOGY™ DR+

Pacesetter®
© 1997
APS: Version 3204c – 4369

11 Jul 1997 07:49
Last Programmed on: 14 May 1997
MODEL: 2364      SERIAL: 199843

PATIENT: _____

PHYSICIAN: _____

Atrial Lead Type: BIPOLAR
Ventricular Lead Type: BIPOLAR

2:1 Block Rate at 201 ppm

### SENSOR INDICATED RATE HISTOGRAM

Total Time Sampled: 62d 20h 33m 44s
Sampling Rate: 1.6 seconds

Sensor _____ ON
Rate _____ 50 ppm
Maximum Sensor Rate _____ 110 ppm
Slope _____ 8 (Normal)
Threshold _____ 1.5
Reaction Time _____ FAST
Recovery Time _____ MEDIUM
    Measured Average Sensor _____ 2.5

Note: The above values were obtained
when the histogram was interrogated.

| Bin Number | Range (ppm) | Time | | | | Sample Counts |
|---|---|---|---|---|---|---|
| 1 | 45 – 52 | 17d | 20h | 59m | 0s | 950,363 |
| 2 | 52 – 59 | 27d | 5h | 20m | 12s | 1,447,392 |
| 3 | 59 – 67 | 7d | 6h | 43m | 4s | 387,067 |
| 4 | 67 – 74 | 6d | 22h | 16m | 45s | 368,372 |
| 5 | 74 – 81 | 2d | 18h | 40m | 4s | 147,695 |
| 6 | 81 – 88 | 0d | 15h | 27m | 1s | 34,228 |
| 7 | 88 – 96 | 0d | 2h | 29m | 28s | 5,519 |
| 8 | 96 – 103 | 0d | 0h | 35m | 56s | 1,327 |
| 9 | 103 – 110 | 0d | 0h | 2m | 15s | 83 |
| | | | | | Total: | 3,342,046 |

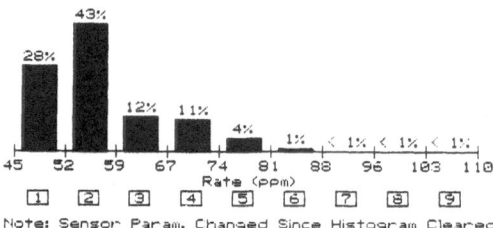

Percent of Total Time

Note: Sensor Param. Changed Since Histogram Cleared

**Fig. 7.10. g** Rate response histogram retrieved by telemetry since the last interrogation of a Pacesetter Trilogy pacemaker

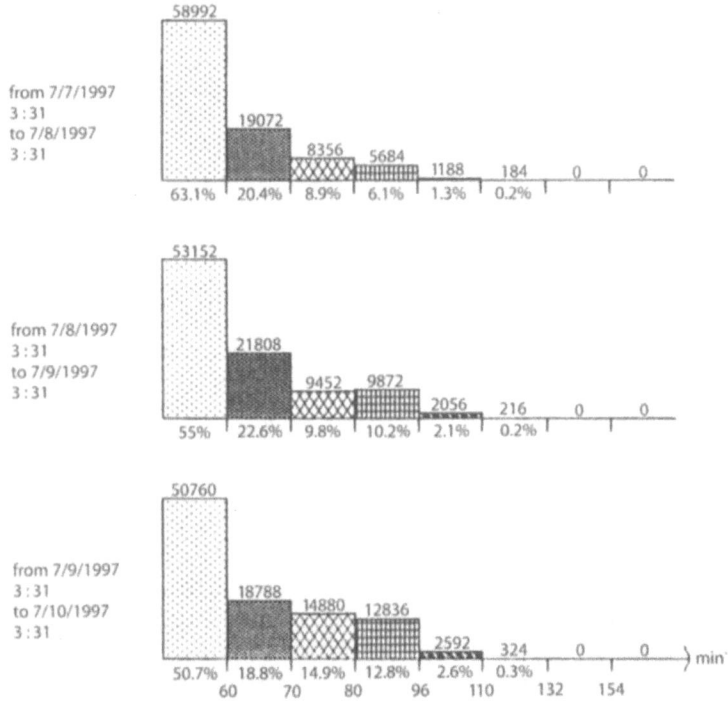

**Fig. 7.10. h** Rate response histogram over 3 days preceding the interrogation of an ELA Medical Chorum pacemaker

## Exercise Test Report

Pacemaker Model: Medtronic.Kappa KDR401/403   Serial Number: PER201937                                                   Date of Visit: 08/04/97

| Patient Name: | ID: | Chart Number: |
|---|---|---|

**Exercise Test   Collected: 08/04/97 11:44:54 AM**

|  | During Exercise | CurrentValues * |
|---|---|---|
| Mode | DDDR | DDDR |
| Lower Rate | 60 ppm | 60 ppm |
| ADL Rate | 95 ppm | 95 ppm |
| Upper Sensor Rate | 110 ppm | 110 ppm |
| Upper Tracking Rate | 130 ppm | 130 ppm |
| Optimization | On | On |
| RR Sensor | Integrated | Integrated |
| ADL Rate Setpoint | 12 | 12 |
| Upper Sensor Rate Setpoint | 32 | 32 |

* Note: Current values depicted by Exercise Test Graph

**Additional Data**

| Maximum Achieved Rate | 110 bpm |
|---|---|
| Maximum MV Counts | 49 |
| Maximum Activity Counts | 5 |

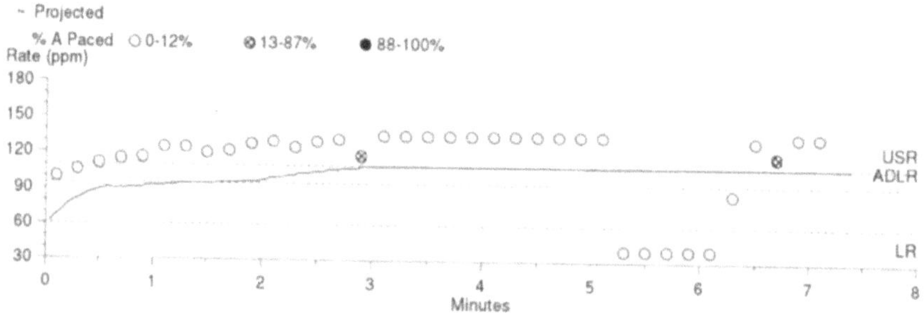

**Fig. 7.11a – d.** Short-term Holter type function and simulation tests
**a** Heart rate curve retrieved by telemetry of a Medtronic Kappa pacemaker which displays only the rates computed by the rate response algorithm

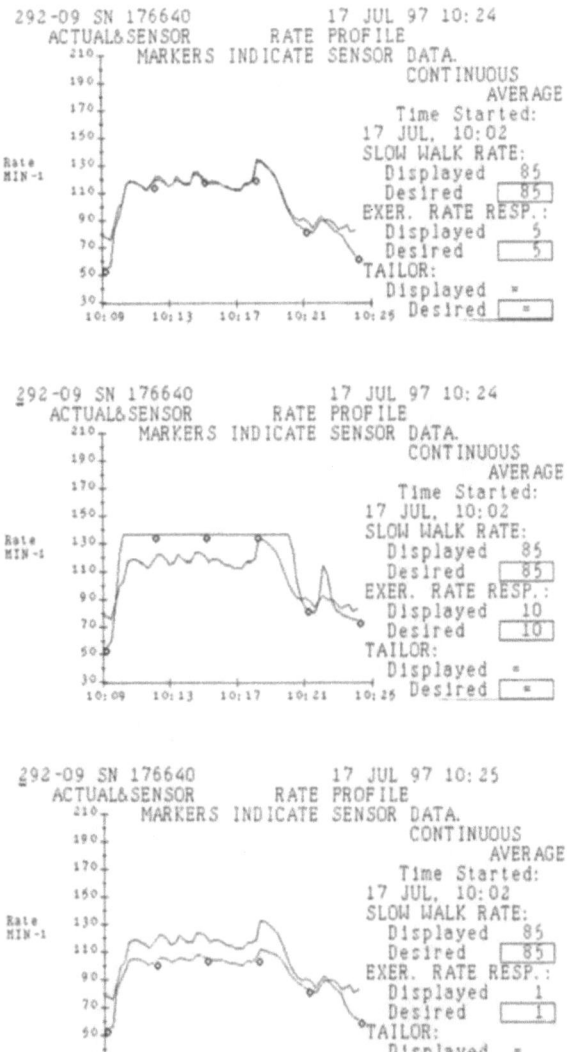

**Fig. 7.11. b** Information on rate responsive function retrieved by telemetry of an Intermedics Marathon pacemaker, using the simulation function. The pacemaker memorizes the computed heart rate response (*markers* indicate sensor data) and displays it on the programmer screen. The programmer also shows the actual heart rate for comparison with the computed heart rate response. After modifying the rate response parameters of the device, the programmer recalculates the heart rate which would have been dictated by the pacemaker given the new sensor settings. One can then choose the slope of rate responsiveness and other parameters that best fit the patient: *Top tracing*: rate response during exercise test with slope set at 5. *Middle tracing*: rate response during exercise test with slope set at 10. *Bottom tracing*: rate response during exercise test with slope set at 1

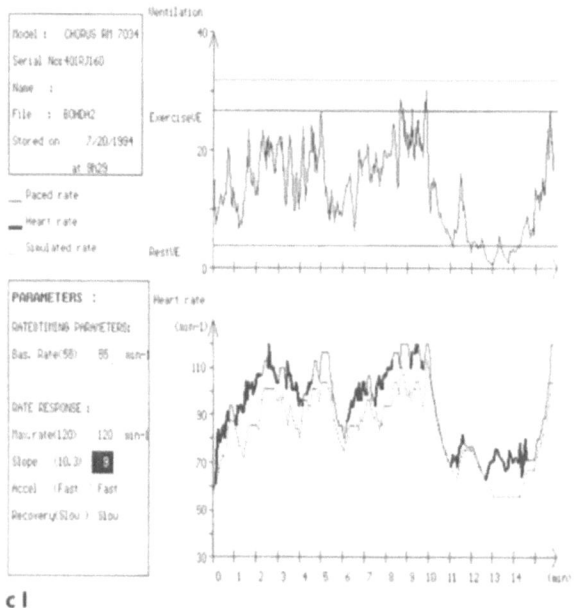

c I

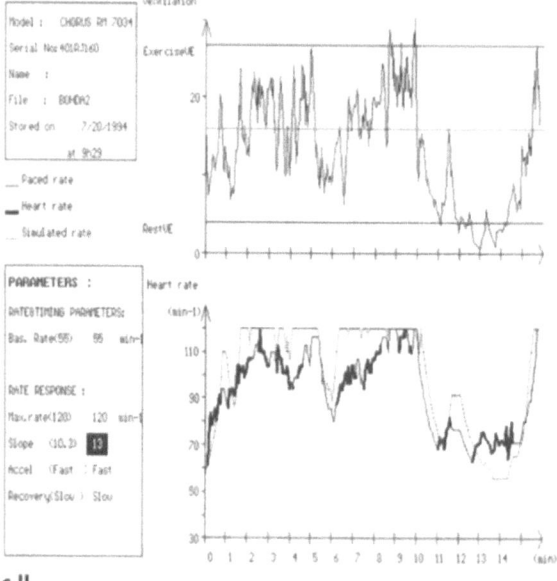

c II

**Fig. 7.11. c** Information on rate responsive function retrieved by telemetry of an ELA Medical Chorus RM pacemaker. The principle is the same as that of the Marathon. In each panel, the *upper tracing* displays the thoracic impedance curve correlated with minute ventilation, and the *lower tracing* displays the sinus (*fat solid line*) and paced (*thin solid line*) rate, along with the simulated curve, calculated according to the programmed rate response parameters (shown in the *left lower box* of each panel). Changes in the programmed parameters generate new calculated curves displayed on the programmer screen:
c I: rate response measured during exercise with a slope set at 9
c II: rate response measured during exercise with a slope set at 13: at this setting, the rate responsive function would be completely in charge of driving the heart rate

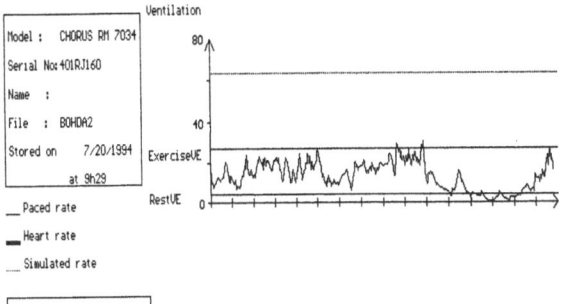

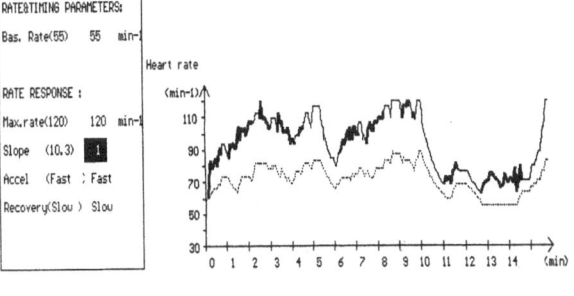

**Fig. 7.11. c III** Rate response measured during exercise with a slope set at 1: this form of programming could be used as a rate smoothing function
Note: scales vary among various graphs

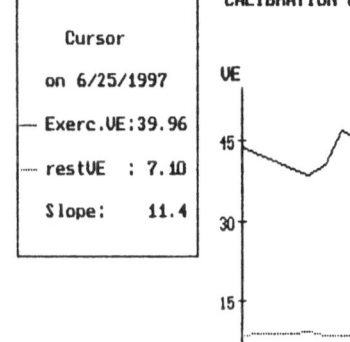

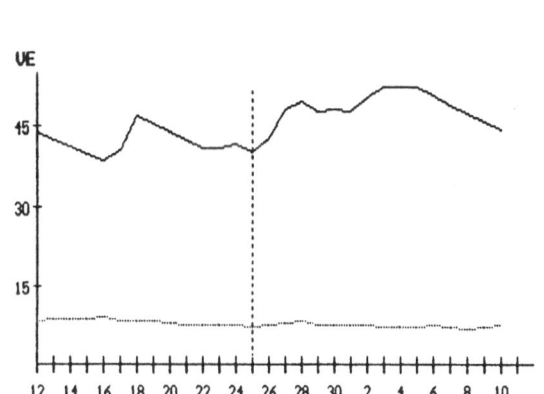

**Fig. 7.11. d** Graph showing variations in the programming of the slope of rate responsiveness (*bottom graph*) relative to changes in the highest and lowest measured minute ventilation values (*top graph*). The system (ELA Medical Chorum) is able to adapt to the day-to-day changes in the patient's functional status

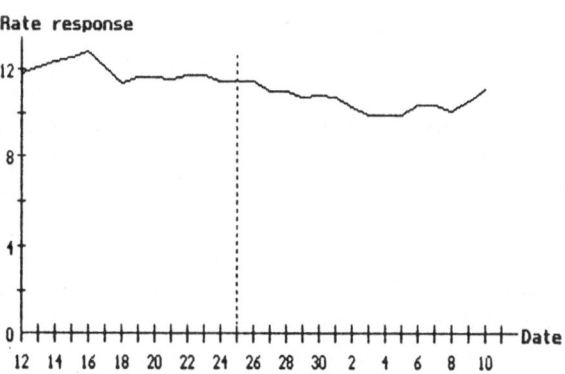

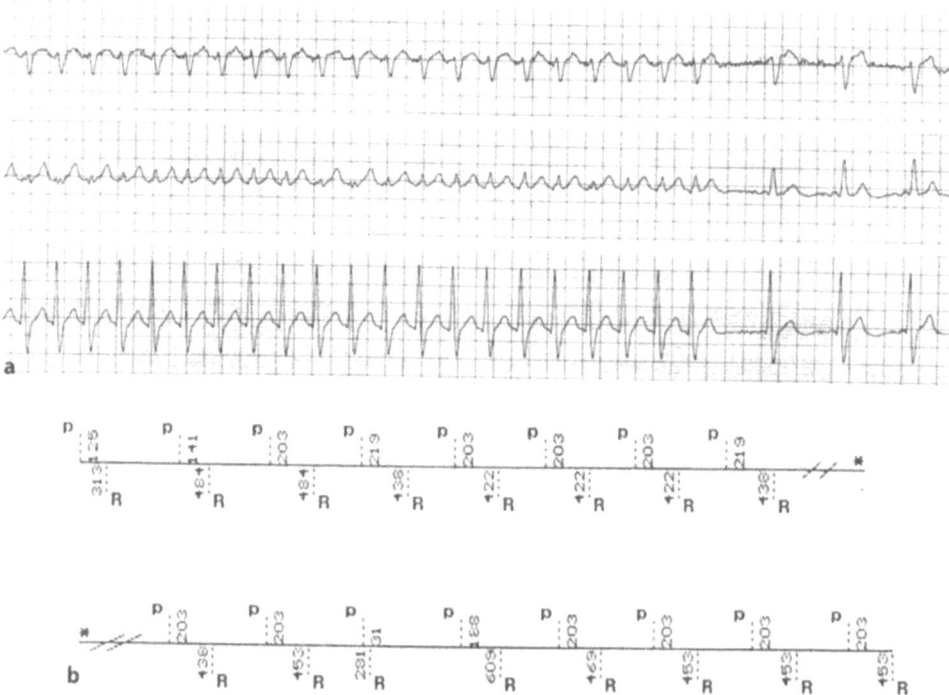

**Fig. 7.12.** Event markers stored in the pacemaker's memory
**a** Supraventricular tachycardia recorded at the onset of treadmill exercise
**b** Event markers corresponding to the tachycardia recorded, stored in memory and displayed on the programmer screen (Chorus II, ELA Medical)
*p* P wave in refractory period; *R* spontaneous R wave

## Electrical Integrity of the Lead System

### Conductor Fracture

When, in a unipolar pacing mode, a marked permanent or intermittent loss of amplitude of the stimulation spikes is observed in several simultaneous electrocardiographic leads, a fracture of the conductor or a connection defect should be suspected. This observation is generally accompanied by pacing failure and rise in lead impedance. If the pacemaker is inhibited by non cardiac events in absence of exogenous or myosignal interference, the most likely explanations consist of intermittent discontinuity of the conductor, causing so-called fracture potentials from intermittent short-circuit of the conductor wires, a failure of the internal insulation of a bipolar lead, or intermittent loss of electrical contact at a loose connector. In such cases, photoanalysis of the spike waveform may reveal abnormalities, irregularities of the plateau phase, for example (Fig. 7.13). Impedance rises, and the intracardiac electrogram recordings show abnormal potentials that are detected on the marker channel and reset the pacemaker. Normal lead

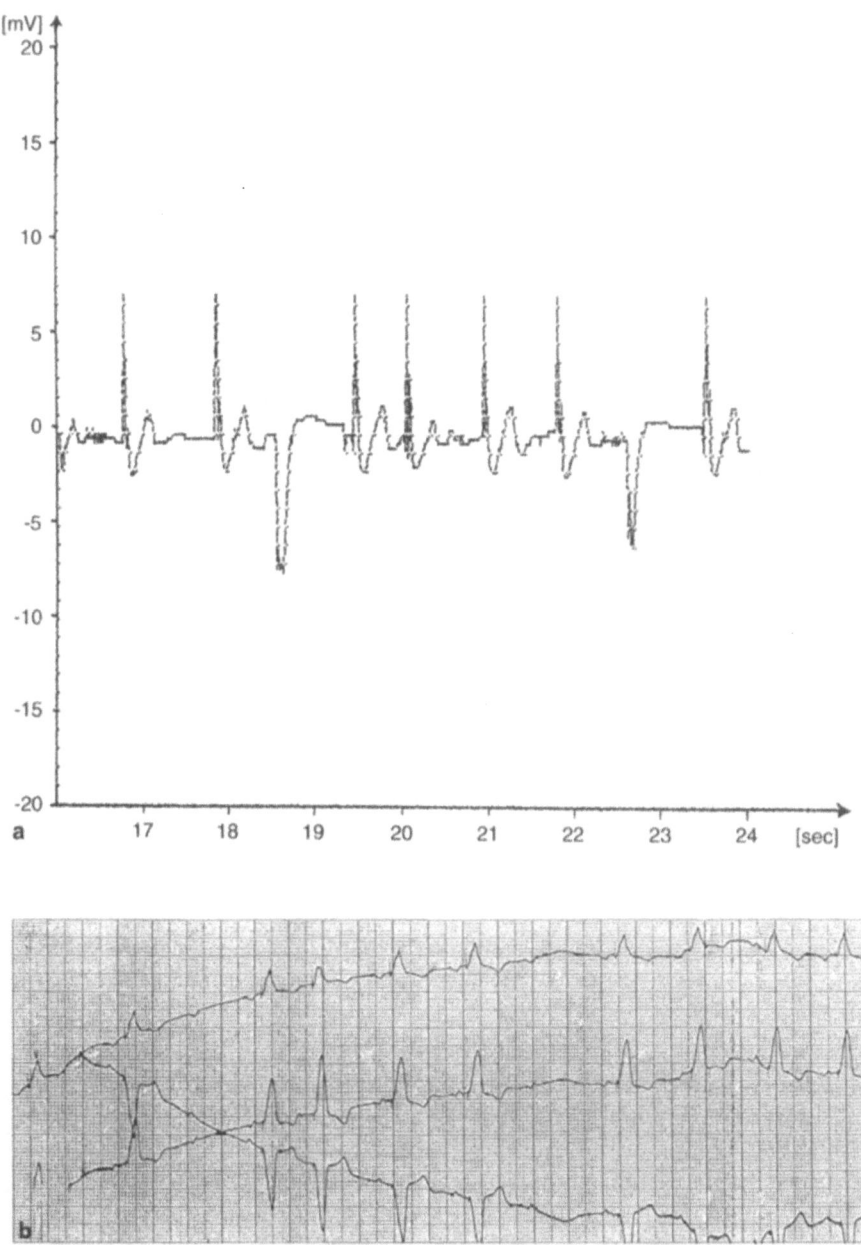

**Fig. 7.13a,b.** Electrical noise generated by a conductor fracture cause potentials interpreted as spontaneous cardiac events by the pacemaker, causing inappropriate inhibition
**a** In this case, the ventricular lead is the culprit, and the pulse generator (Chorus II, ELA
Medical) senses artifacts shown on the intracardiac ECG
**b** without corresponding signal on the surface ECG

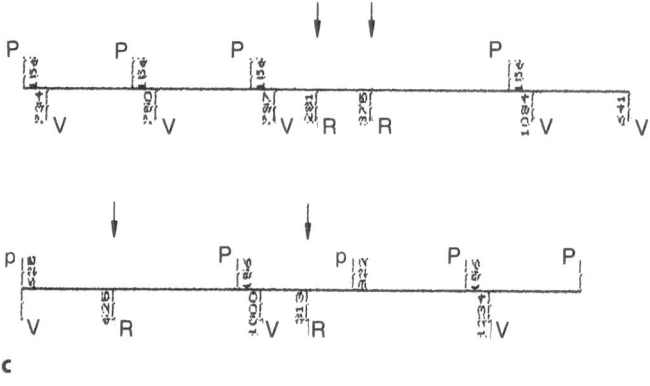

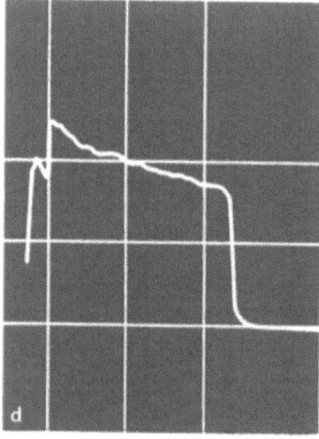

**Fig. 7.13. c** Same phenomenon detected by the marker channels stored in memory
*P* P wave outside refractory periods; *p* P wave in refractory period; *R* spontaneous R wave; *V* ventricular pacing spike
The „R" markers correspond to artifacts due to the conductor fracture (*arrows*) and sensed by the pacemaker
**d** Current generated by conductor fracture identified during high speed oscilloscopic examination of the pacing spike; note the irregularity of the plateau phase

impedance values range from 300 to 1000 Ω. Beyond 1500 Ω, or when impedance rises markedly between two follow-up visits, a conductor fracture should be suspected. On the other hand, in case of intercurrent myocardial infarction involving the site of electrode implantation, impedance values above 1000 Ω may be measured.

Chest radiographs obtained at various angles perpendicular to the axis of the lead may disclose a conductor fracture as a loss of continuity. This is usually found at the site of subcutaneous ligation of the lead, or between clavicle and first rib from prolonged mechanical stress, particularly when a relatively thick lead has been introduced via the subclavian approach.

### Insulation Failure

If the insulation is damaged in its extravascular segment, the patient will often present with pectoral muscle stimulation. If pacing is bipolar, the amplitude of the pacing spikes increases to a size near that of unipolar spikes. The axis of the pacing spike is deviated from its usual position, and photoanalysis shows a rapid

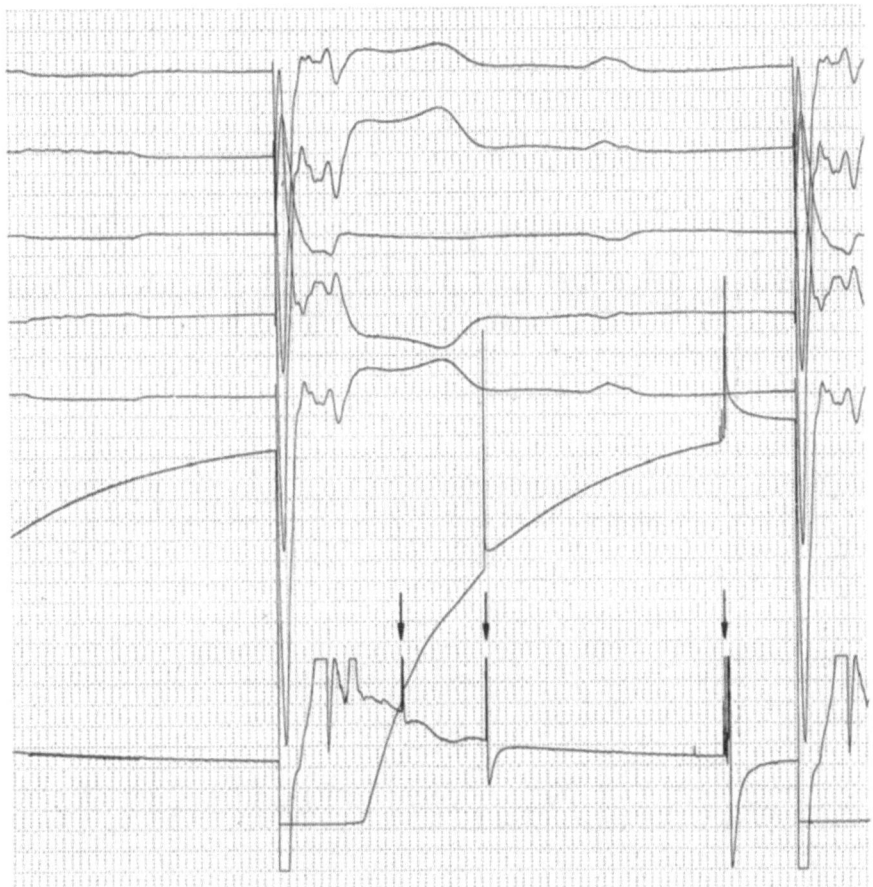

**Fig. 7.13. e** Electrical noise generated by conductor fracture identified on endocavitary ECG recording (*arrows*) during pacing via the same lead. Recording speed = 100 mm/s

decay of the plateau phase. Lead impedance is low (< 300 Ω), causing an increase in power consumption. In the case of a bipolar lead, impedance must be measured in bipolar configuration to examine the integrity of both conductors.

The most common causes of insulation failure are those already described in the previous chapters, as well as the incessant rubbing of two leads implanted next to each other. Various maneuvers, including transcutaneous massage of the can, coughing, deep breathing, and changes in body or arm position may disclose the abnormality during recording of the electrocardiogram, event markers, or photoanalysis.

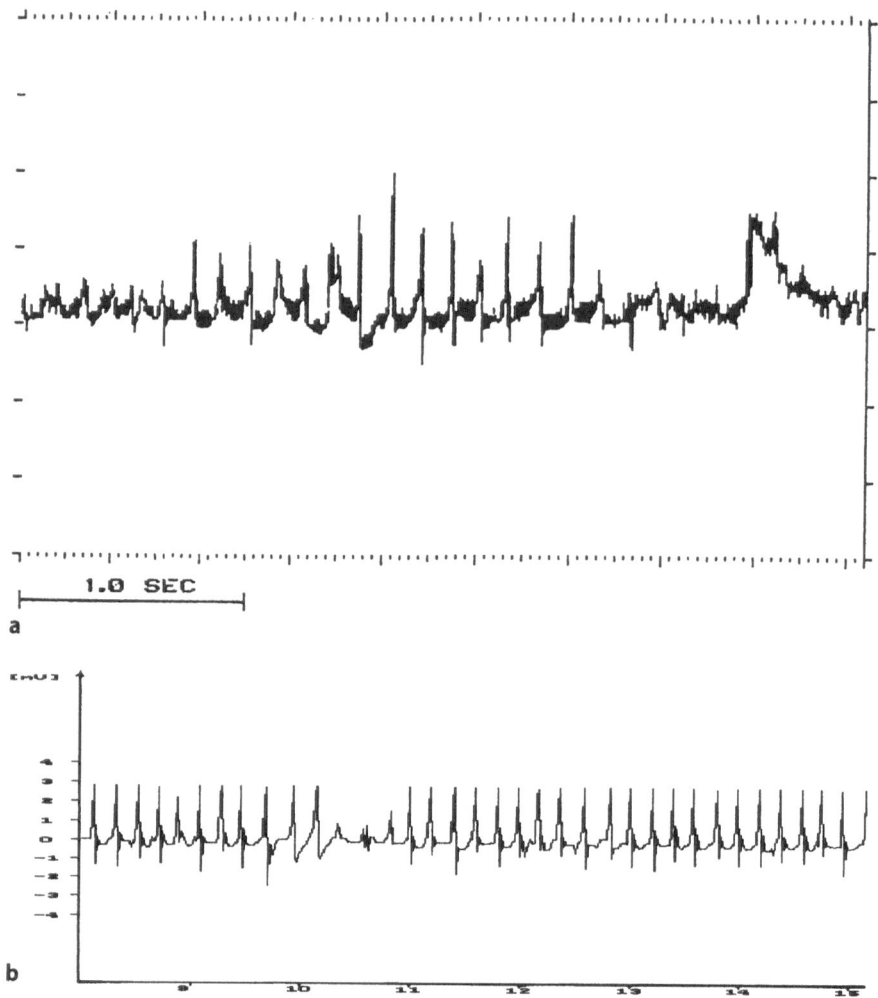

**Fig. 7.14a,b.** Intracardiac electrograms
**a** Intracardiac atrial electrogram during atrial fibrillation. Note the marked variability in signal amplitude
**b** Intracardiac atrial electrogram during atrial flutter. Note a more stable atrial electrogram amplitude

## Intracardiac Events Displayed by the Pacemaker

Intracardiac events may be analyzed with the assistance of intracardiac electrograms and event markers (Figs. 7.14–7.16). These analytical tools facilitate the interpretation of surface electrocardiographic tracings which, nowadays, is often complicated by the specific functions of each pacemaker model.

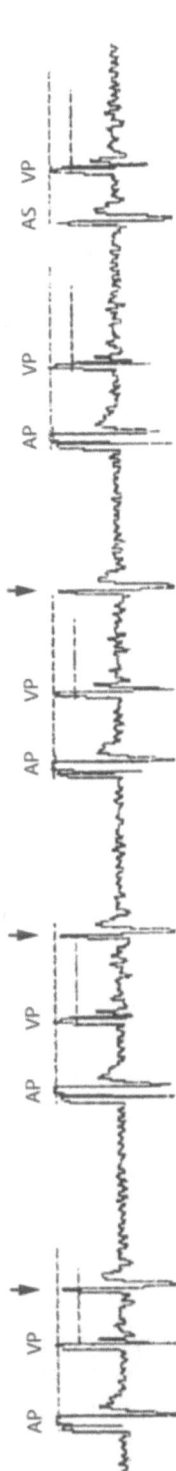

**Fig. 7.15.** Intracardiac atrial electrograms retrieved from an Intermedics Relay pacemaker showing failure of atrial pacing. Following two apparently normal AV sequences, a sinus P wave signal (not sensed) appears with a gradually longer VP interval (*arrows*). This signal is initially not sensed because it falls in PVARP. When it is finally detected (*AS*), it induces a paced ventricular event at the end of the AVD
*AP* atrial pacing; *AS* atrial sensing; *VP* ventricular pacing

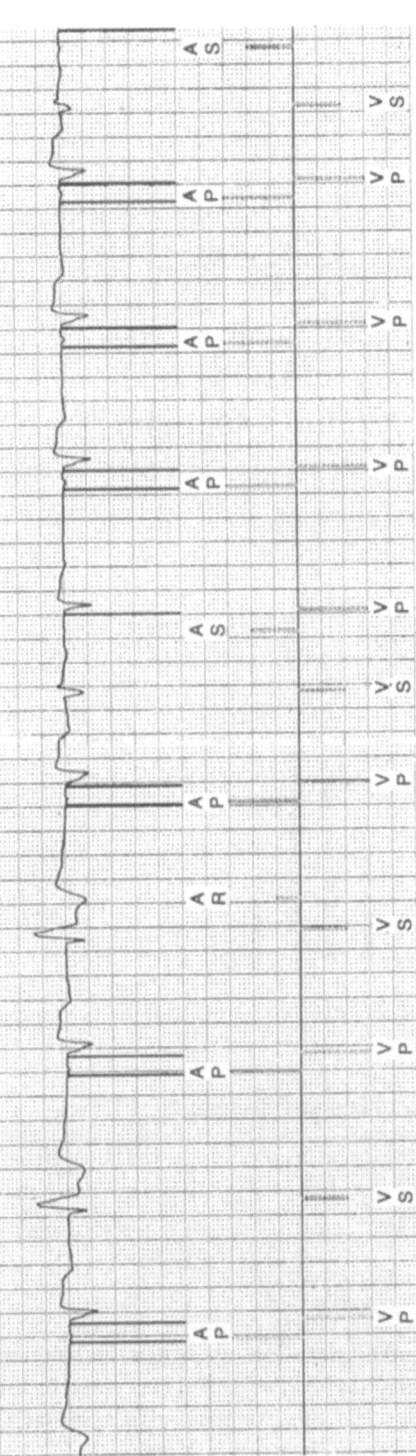

**Fig. 7.16.** Event markers recorded from a Medtronic Elite 7074 pacemaker confirming proper device function
*AP* atrial pacing; *VP* ventricular pacing; *VS* ventricular sensing; *AR* atrial sensing during refractory period

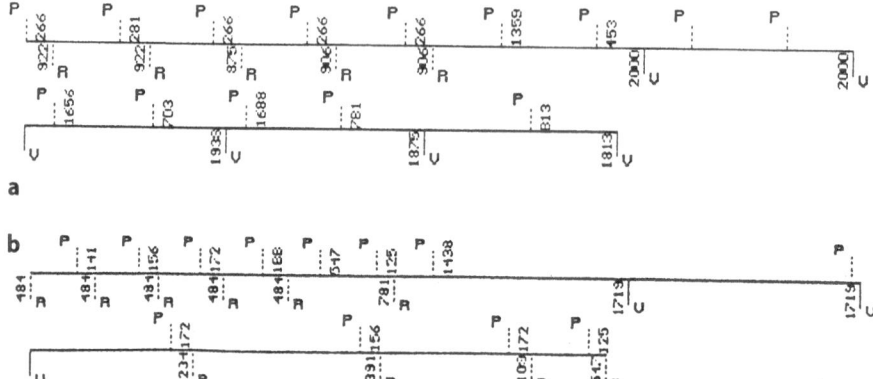

**Fig. 7.17. a** Episode of complete heart block disclosed by a special diagnostic program loaded in the RAM of an ELA Medical 6234 pacemaker
**b** Episode of sino-atrial block retrieved via the same function. PR and RR intervals are shown
*P* spontaneous P wave; *R* spontaneous R wave; *V* ventricular pacing spike

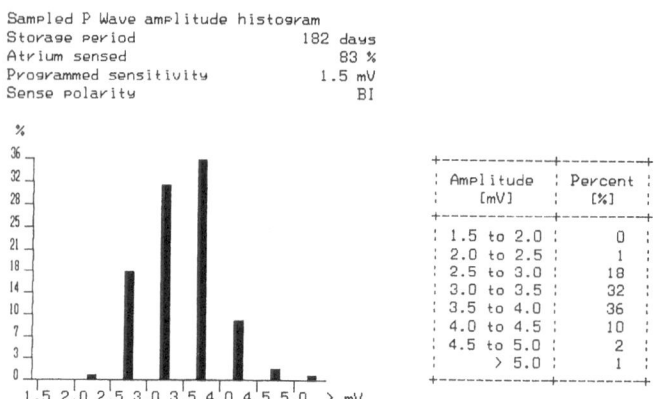

Sampled P Wave amplitude histogram
Storage period                    182 days
Atrium sensed                        83 %
Programmed sensitivity            1.5 mV
Sense polarity                         BI

| Amplitude [mV] | Percent [%] |
|---|---|
| 1.5 to 2.0 | 0 |
| 2.0 to 2.5 | 1 |
| 2.5 to 3.0 | 18 |
| 3.0 to 3.5 | 32 |
| 3.5 to 4.0 | 36 |
| 4.0 to 4.5 | 10 |
| 4.5 to 5.0 | 2 |
| > 5.0 | 1 |

**Fig. 7.18.** Spontaneous P wave amplitude histogram retrieved from a Vitatron Diamond pacemaker

### Economy of Energy Consumption

Telemetry measurements allow the optimal programming of the pacemaker. They allow a closer estimate of the safety margin that needs to be programmed (Fig. 7.7).

### Final Interrogation

At the end of the follow-up visit, a final interrogation allows to verify that all programming has been effectively accepted by the device, as instructed by the physician. This last interrogation also summarizes the results of all the tests performed during the examination.

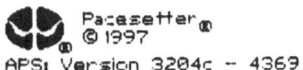

Pacesetter®
© 1997
APS: Version 3204c – 4369

Microny®SR+

8 Jul 1997 08:10
Last programmed on: 16 May 1997
MODEL: 2425T    SERIAL: 6225 47800

PATIENT: _____

PHYSICIAN: _____

Patient I.D.:
Lead Type: Bipolar

Implant Date: 6 May 1997
Lead Chamber: Ventricle

```
(              Stimulation Threshold              )
```

Total Time Sampled: 10d 16h 0m 0s
Samp. Rate: 1 hr
Samp. Mode: FREEZE
Samp. Source: THRESHOLD
Threshold Searches: 2756
Diagnostic Data Cleared: 16 May 1997 09:53

```
                    30 Hr              Sample Counts
                    ——                     256
                   Scale

Volt
  4.8
  3.9
  3.0
  2.1
  1.2
  0.3 |
      5:16:09    5:18:21    5:21:09    5:23:21    5:26:03    5:28:21    5:31:09
         5:17:15    5:20:03    5:22:15    5:25:03    5:27:15    5:30:03
                                                              mnt:day:hr
```

**Fig. 7.19.** Pacing threshold measured over 10 days by the Pacesetter Microny pacemaker

### Results of Long-Term Diagnostic Data

This discussion cannot be comprehensive, particularly since additional diagnostic functions will emerge in the near future. Pacemakers now have a function of surveillance in addition to their therapeutic role (Fig. 7.17). Some models, such as the Sorin Theorema 90, offer special diagnostic functions, providing rate histograms which show the escape of the pacemaker at very slow rates, perhaps indicative of long cardiac pauses, confirming the appropriateness of the implant, particularly in a patient presenting with sudden syncope and a negative diagnostic evaluation. With that in mind, the loading in RAM of a special „bradycardia"

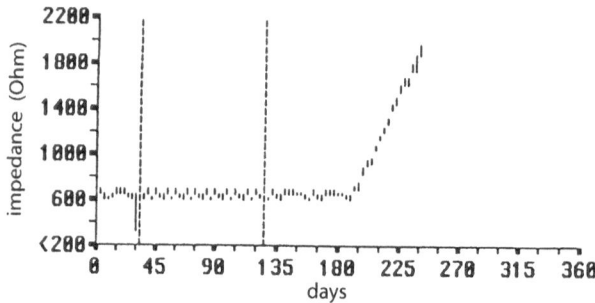

**Fig. 7.20.** Pacing impedance histogram retrieved from a Medtronic Thera pacemaker during long-term follow-up

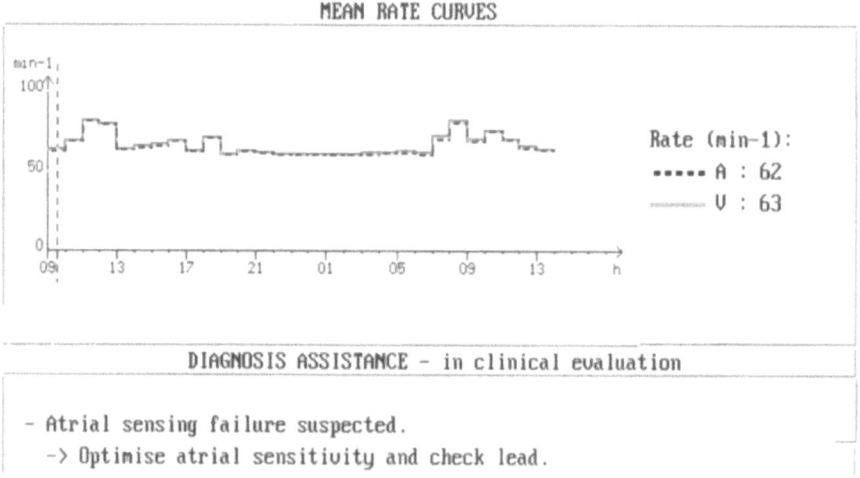

**Fig. 7.21. a** The pacemaker diagnostic function warns the physician against a possible defect in atrial sensing. The curves of atrial and ventricular mean rates show no abnormalities in the last 24 h.

program has been developed by ELA Medical, including dual chamber analysis and storage in memory of the marker channel when a bradycardic episode is sensed by the pacemaker. This manufacturer offers a separate algorithm which memorizes a marker channel and an electrogram for tachycardias specified in the program.

Finally, some data are specific for certain implanted models, such as the P wave histograms of the Vitatron pacemakers which allow the reliable reprogramming of an optimal atrial sensitivity (Fig. 7.18), or the gathering of long-term measurements of threshold and loss of capture, in a chronologic and in an amplitude histogram format by the Pacesetter Microny (Fig. 7.19), or the evolution of the lead(s) impedance by the Medtronic Thera and Kappa (Fig. 7.20). The sum of the telemetry data provided by a given pacemaker should be used to its fullest

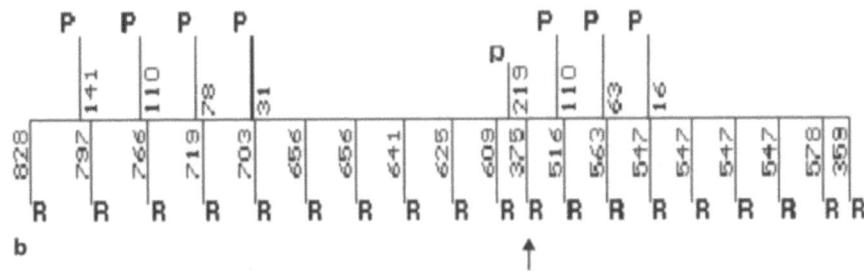

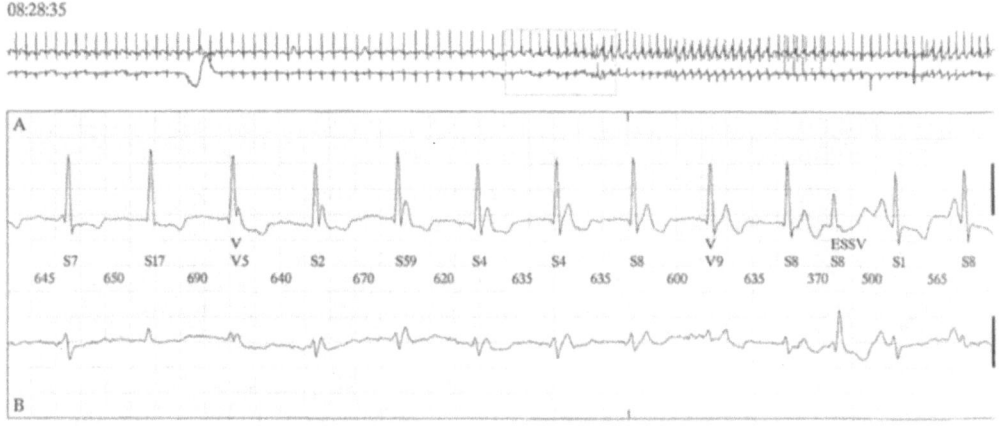

**Fig. 7.21. b** However, the pacemaker has memorized one atrioventricular events markers chain. The atrial events are shown above the horizontal line with the PR intervals and the ventricular events below with the RR intervals

*P* P waves outside refractory periods; *p* P wave in refractory periods; *R* spontaneous R waves. Some of the P waves are not visible. This sequence appears during the acceleration of the ventricular rate with a progressive shortening of the PR intervals

**c** Holter ECG trace recorded at the same time as the events markers chain of Fig. 7.21b. This figure shows a fast junctional rhythm with AV dissociation. The ventricular rate is faster than the atrial one, therefore, the P waves slowly fade behind the QRS complexes, then reappear after the QRSs (*p*) until the AV node comes out of its refractory period leading to a ventricular capture. This event explains why one of the R waves comes early at 375 ms with a 219 ms PR interval (see *arrow*)

since, together with the clinical information, they may lead to a more precise diagnosis, or even directly to a therapeutic intervention.

An attempt at automatic interpretation of the data stored in the pacemaker memory (AIDA system) has been developed by ELA Medical. Abnormal events (related to the patient, such as arrhythmias, or related to sensing or pacing failure of the system) cause distinct profiles of the memorized information. The analysis is, therefore, expected to recognize these specific profiles, and puts on an alert for the physician, along with recommendations regarding appropriate corrective measures (Fig. 7.21). This represents a practical tool which may also be

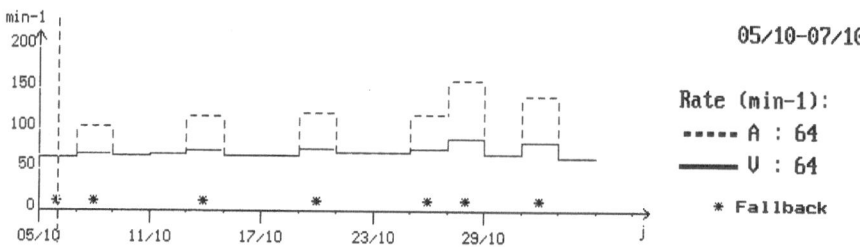

MEAN RATE CURVES

05/10-07/10

Rate (min-1):
····· A : 64
——— V : 64

* Fallback

DIAGNOSIS ASSISTANCE - in clinical evaluation

The spontaneous ventricular rate may be high following fallback mode switching.
- Total time in fallback mode :  3 d 22
- Number of episodes of fallback mode switching : 9
- Tachy episodes available in F3 (time) : 7
d   - Mean duration of fallback : 12 h 06 (min:28 sec, max:1 d 01)

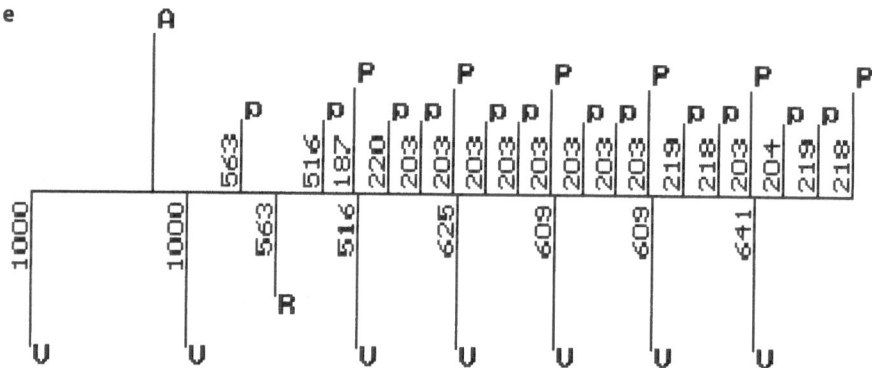

**Fig. 7.21. d** In this example, the „diagnosis assistant" reveals possible atrial tachyarrhythmias. Nine episodes were stored, only seven of them are available in the memory for events markers chain analysis. The total time in mode switch is given as well as the mean, minimal and maximal lengths of the nine episodes
**e** In order to confirm a presumed diagnosis of atrial tachyarrhythmias (Fig. 7.21d), the events markers chains must be analyzed. The PP intervals are shown and their stability and values mean the onset of an atrial flutter
*A* atrial pacing; *P* P wave outside refractory periods; *p* P wave in refractory periods; *V* ventricular pacing; *R* spontaneous R wave

used as a learning device for physicians unfamiliar with this type of pacemaker. A complete examination of the pacemaker should be included in the patient's medical record, and the information should be passed on to the referring physician to guarantee a comprehensive follow-up. A check list tailored to the specifications of each pacemaker should be prepared in order not to forget the smallest detail.

# CHAPTER 8

# Practical Guide to Programming

The examination of the main functions of a pacemaker will be presented with the assistance of examples, and a practical and clinical goal in mind. The complex functions already presented in Chap. 3 and its appendix will not be reviewed here. The gathering of information necessary for a reliable device examination and optimal programming implies a thorough knowledge of the implanted model and its programmer (Figs. 8.1, 8.2). Before proceeding with testing, it is most important to print the current values of the various parameters in order to easily retrieve them in case one wishes to restore them at the end of the test, as well as the power consumption of the device with respect to the programmed parameters. Consequently, all data retrieved from telemetry must be printed since they may be erased during the reprogramming needed to test the sensing and pacing functions.

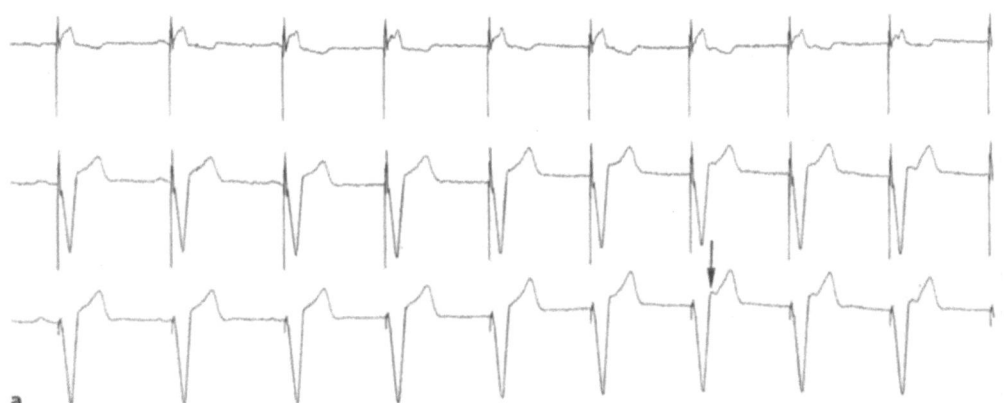

a

**Fig. 8.1a,b.** VDD mode
**a** When P waves are present, the pacemaker delivers a synchronous ventricular spike. When P waves are absent by the end of the escape interval (from slowing of the atrial rate below the programmed lower rate), the pacemaker delivers a stimulus in the ventricle only, associated with retrograde atrial activation (*arrow*). The VDD mode breeds a VVI behavior in presence of sinus bradycardia. Given the type of programming, this represents normal function

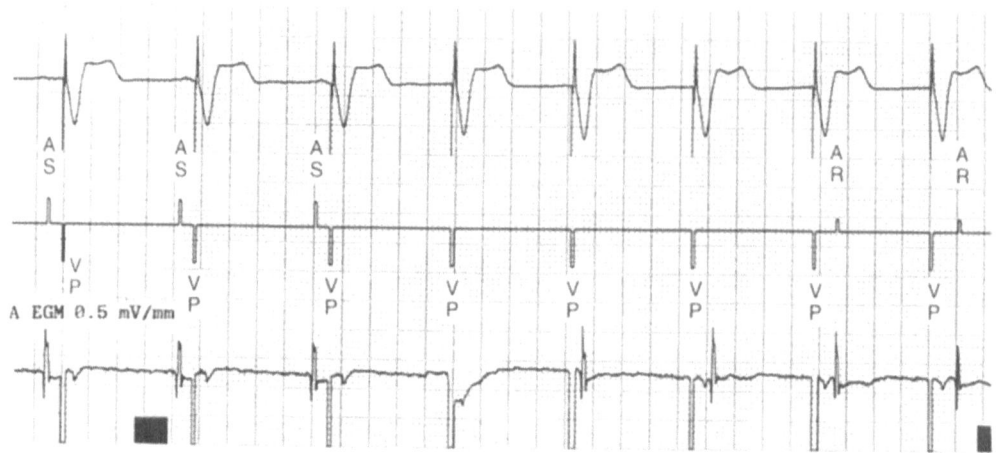

**Fig. 8.1.b** Simultaneous recording, via the programmer, of surface ECG, event markers and atrial intracardiac electrogram corresponding to the ECG tracing shown in (a)
*AR* atrial sensing during refractory period; *AS* atrial sensing; *VP* ventricular pacing

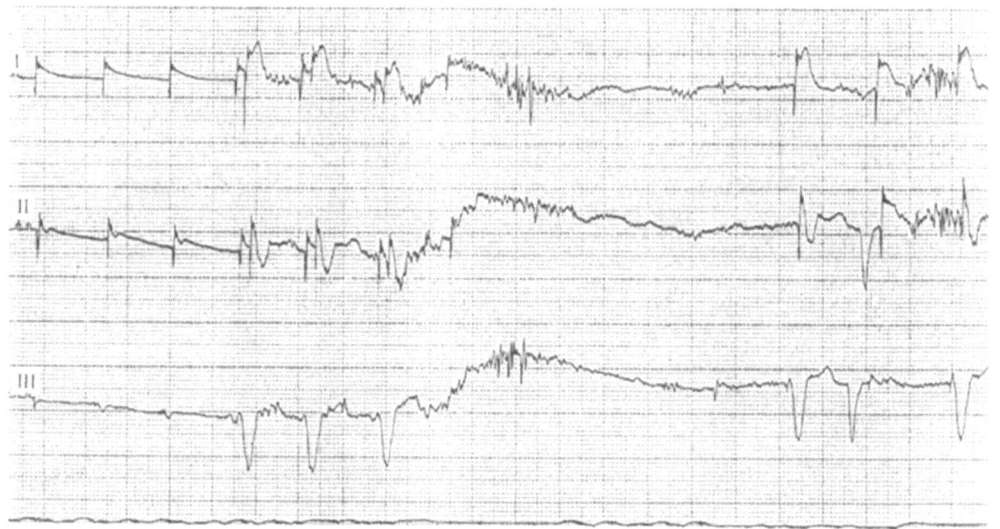

**Fig. 8.2.** The programmer head is not properly placed over the pulse generator, causing ventricular inhibition

# 8.1
# Programming of a Single Chamber Pacemaker

## Sensing

We prefer to manually control sensing by successive programming of the various sensitivity levels available rather than use automatic programs. At threshold, sensing must be 100% effective, included during deep breathing.
The sequence is as follows:

Program a slow back up pacing rate (30 BPM). If the spontaneous heart rate is below 30, the patient may be considered pacemaker dependent and sensing threshold cannot be measured. With some models the slowest lower rate is 40, 50 or more beats per minute. This makes measurements of the sensing threshold quite difficult, or impossible.

Decrease, step by step, the sensitivity (i.e. increase the programmed value) until failure to sense is observed in the form of intermittent or fixed asynchronous pacing. The sensing threshold is the value, expressed in millivolts, at which the pacemaker is capable of reliable sensing, just below that associated with asynchronous behavior (Fig. 8.3). Unfortunately, measurement of sensing threshold may be quite imprecise since some pacemakers do not allow the programming of very low sensitivity (> 4 mV in the atrium and > 10 mV in the ventricle, for example; Fig. 8.4).

The reliable sensing of extrasystoles, when present, must be verified at the threshold level, after verifying that they fall outside the programmed refractory periods (Fig. 8.5). The Biotronik system offers a highly reliable measure of real time and a cycle-by-cycle display of sensed events of the programmer screen (Fig. 8.5d).

One must be aware of the appearance of fusions, pseudofusions, and pseudo-pseudofusions (Fig. 8.6). A fusion is caused by a stimulus occurring before the pacemaker had a chance of sensing a spontaneous event. This results in the superimposition of the spontaneous complex and the pacing spike. In pseudofusion, the pacing spike is positioned at the very beginning of the complex and does not contribute to myocardial depolarization, because pacing is ineffective. To differentiate these various patterns, the pacing rate must be increased. In the case of pseudo-pseudofusion in dual chamber pacing, an atrial spike is delivered coincident with a spontaneous QRS complex, as in the case of ventricular extrasystoles occurring at the end of the AV interval, in a junctional rhythm, or in failure to sense the atrium with a dual chamber pacemaker, etc. (Fig. 8.7).

Test unipolar and bipolar configuration (to avoid exogenous forms of interference, the bipolar configuration is preferred). Programming must be at twice the measured threshold to allow a safe margin. In the atrium, an even higher sensitivity may be necessary to guarantee proper sensing during effort, and an exercise test should be performed for confirmation. Caution must be exercised before programming polarity because very few systems verify the polarity of either lead or pulse generator before programming. If the lead is unipolar and the system is bipolar, sensing and/or pacing may be ineffective (Fig. 8.8). The

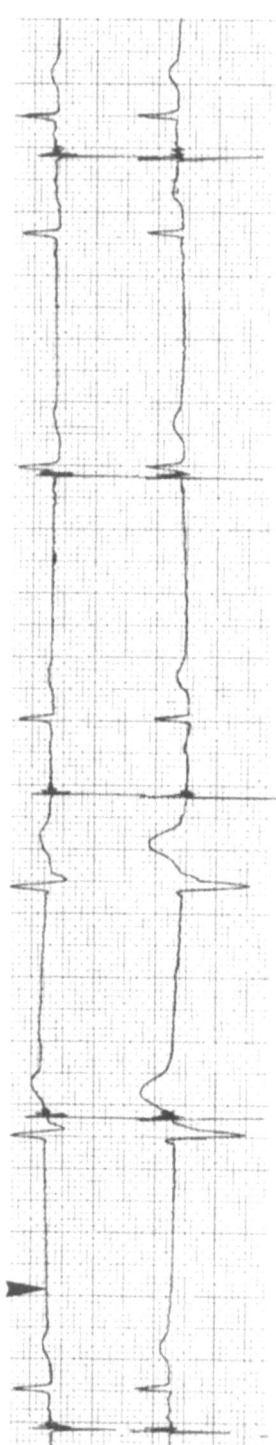

**Fig. 8.3.** AAT mode, atrial sensitivity = 0.8 mV, lower rate reprogrammed from 70 to 30 BPM (*arrow*), pulse duration reduced from 0.3 to 0.2 ms. Atrial sensing failure, because spontaneous P waves should be detected and atrial spikes should be delivered simultaneously; additionally intermittent atrial pacing failure

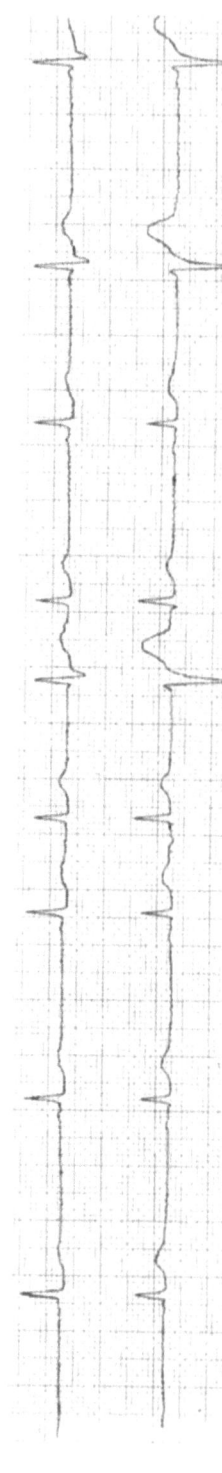

**Fig. 8.4.** VVI mode, 30 BPM, ventricular sensitivity = 7 mV. The absence of pacing spike indicates proper ventricular sensing. The actual sensitivity is unknown since it could not be programmed to a higher value

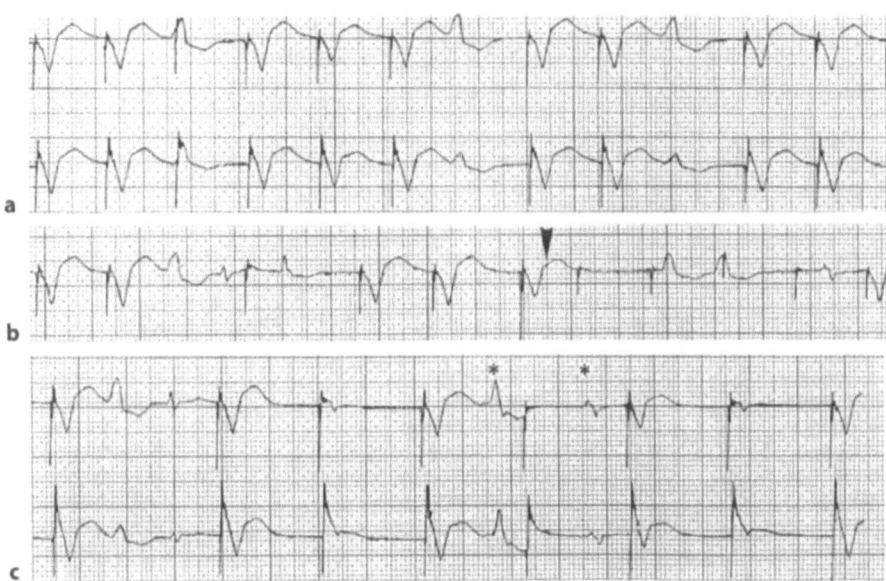

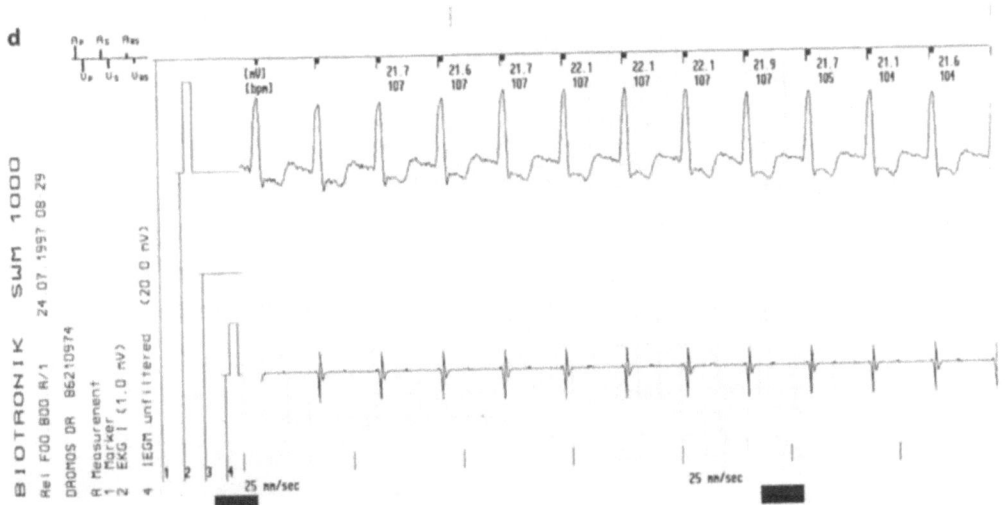

**Fig. 8.5. a** Programmed in VVI mode at 100 BPM and a pulse strength of 5 V/0.25 ms, there is stable ventricular pacing and proper sensing of ventricular extrasystoles
**b** Reduction of the pacing output to 2.5 V results in loss of pacing capture
**c** At a sensitivity of 2.5 mV, intermittent loss of sensing occurs when the R wave morphology changes (*)
**d** The Biotronik system offers a highly reliable measure of real time and a cycle-by-cycle display of sensed events of the programmer screen

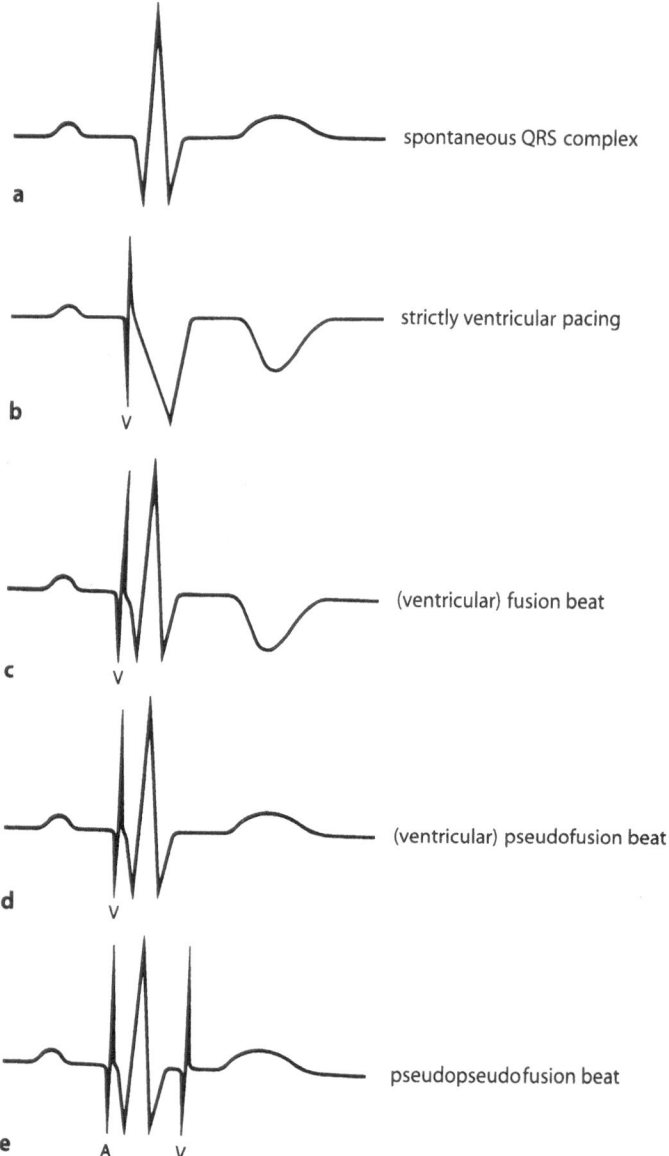

spontaneous QRS complex

**a**

strictly ventricular pacing

**b**

V

(ventricular) fusion beat

**c**

V

(ventricular) pseudofusion beat

**d**

V

pseudopseudofusion beat

**e**    A    V

**Fig. 8.6. a** Spontaneous QRS complex
**b** Exclusive ventricular pacing: the QRS complex and the T wave are unlike the spontaneous event
**c** Fusion complex: the ventricular myocardium is depolarized by both the pacing stimulus and by the spontaneous wavefront. The QRS and the T wave have a configuration intermediate between a spontaneous and a paced complex
**d** Pseudofusion: the pacing spike has no effect on ventricular depolarization which is entirely spontaneous. Neither the QRS nor the T wave are modified
**e** Pseudo-pseudofusion: the atrial stimulus coincides incidentally with the spontaneous QRS complex
*A* atrial stimulus; *V* ventricular stimulus

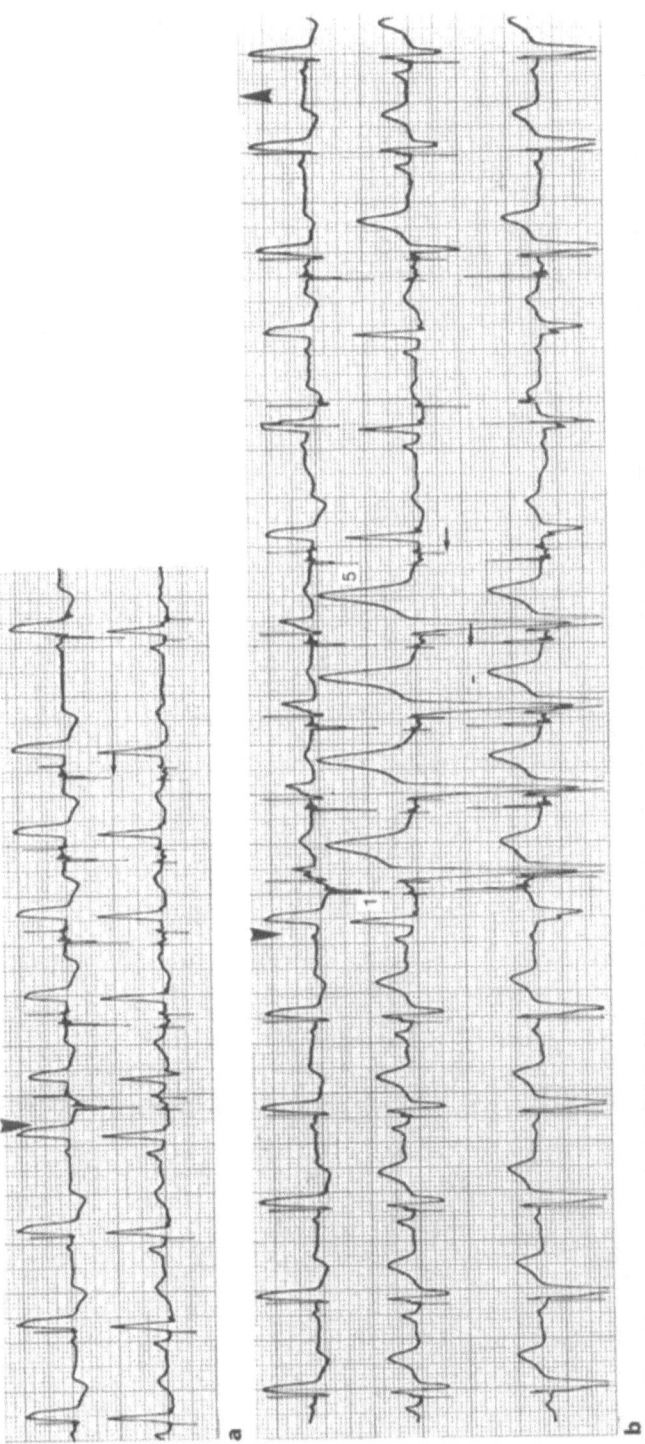

**Fig. 8.7.** DDD mode, 60 BPM, AVD = 170 ms, with magnet application 100 ms, atrial sensitivity = 2.8 mV, ventricular pacing output = 2.7 V

**a** Pulse duration: 0.1 ms. Before magnet application, the ventricular spikes fall in the beginning of the QRS. Atrial sensing is preserved, but ventricular capture cannot be ascertained. With magnet application (*arrow*: acceleration of the rate for five cycles; D00, AVD shortened), the spikes become separate from the spontaneous QRS complex, unmasking loss of ventricular capture. Atrial pacing is preserved and followed by spontaneous AV conduction

**b** Pulse duration: 0.2 ms. By increasing slightly the pacing output, ventricular capture is regained except for the fifth complex under magnet (5) since the pulse duration of the fifth complex is automatically reduced by 50% with this pacemaker model (Intermedics Cosmos). The ventricular pacing spike of the fifth complex is therefore, once again, subthreshold

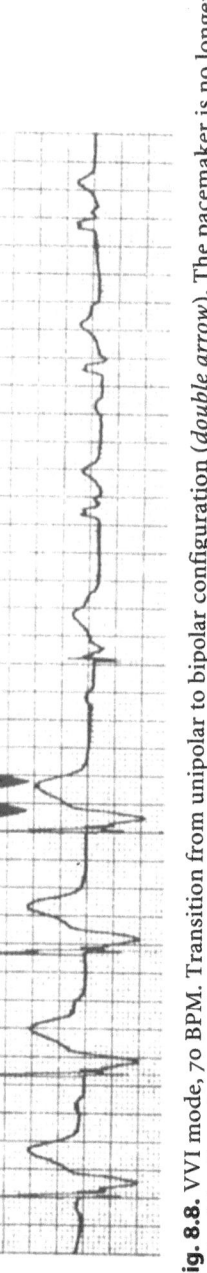

**Fig. 8.8.** VVI mode, 70 BPM. Transition from unipolar to bipolar configuration (*double arrow*). The pacemaker is no longer functioning since the lead is of a unipolar variety. Caution must be exercised when reprogramming the polarity

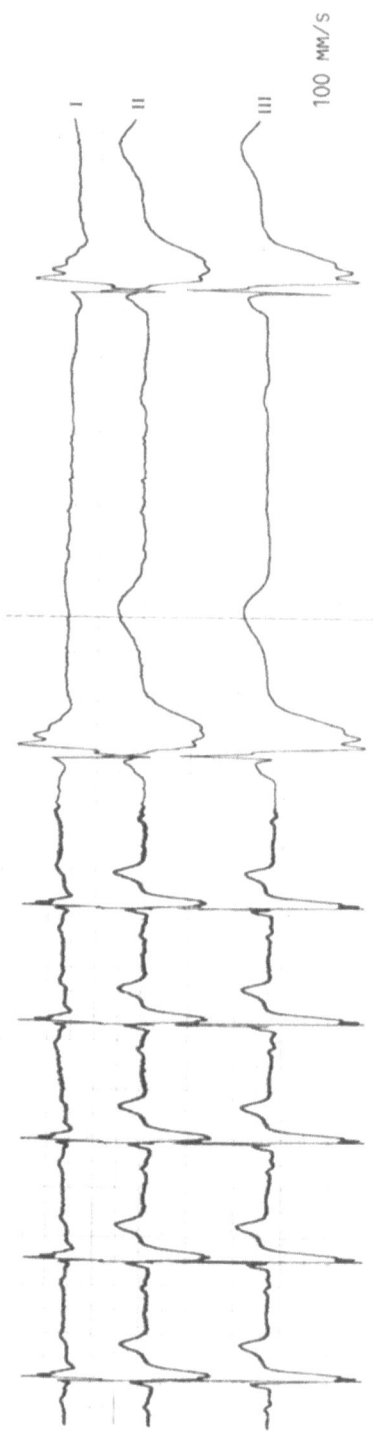

**Fig. 8.9.** Delayed sensing of the R wave, well visible in the VVT mode (*second half of the tracing* is at 100 mm/s paper speed)

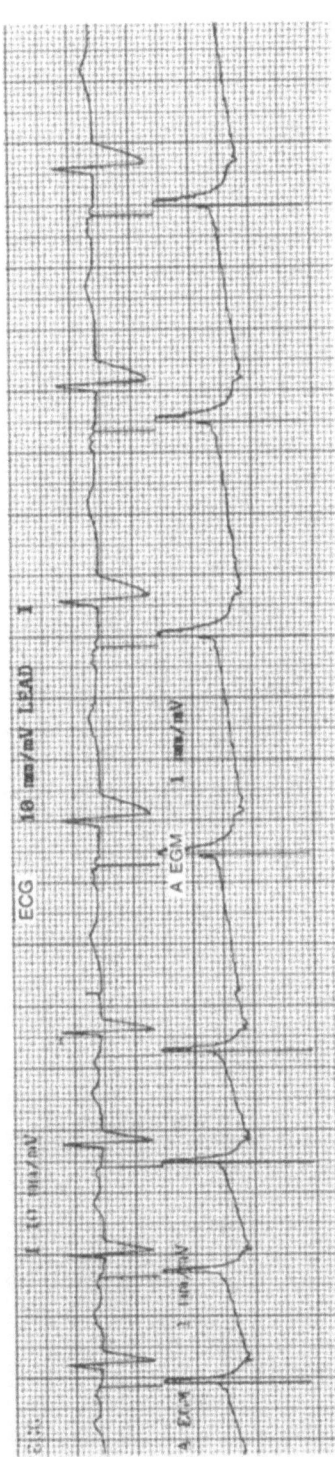

**Fig. 8.10.** The AAT mode discloses delayed sensing of the P wave. The electrode has been implanted in the left atrium, away from the sinus node (corrected transposition of the great vessels). Paper speed initially at 25 mm/s, then 50 mm/s

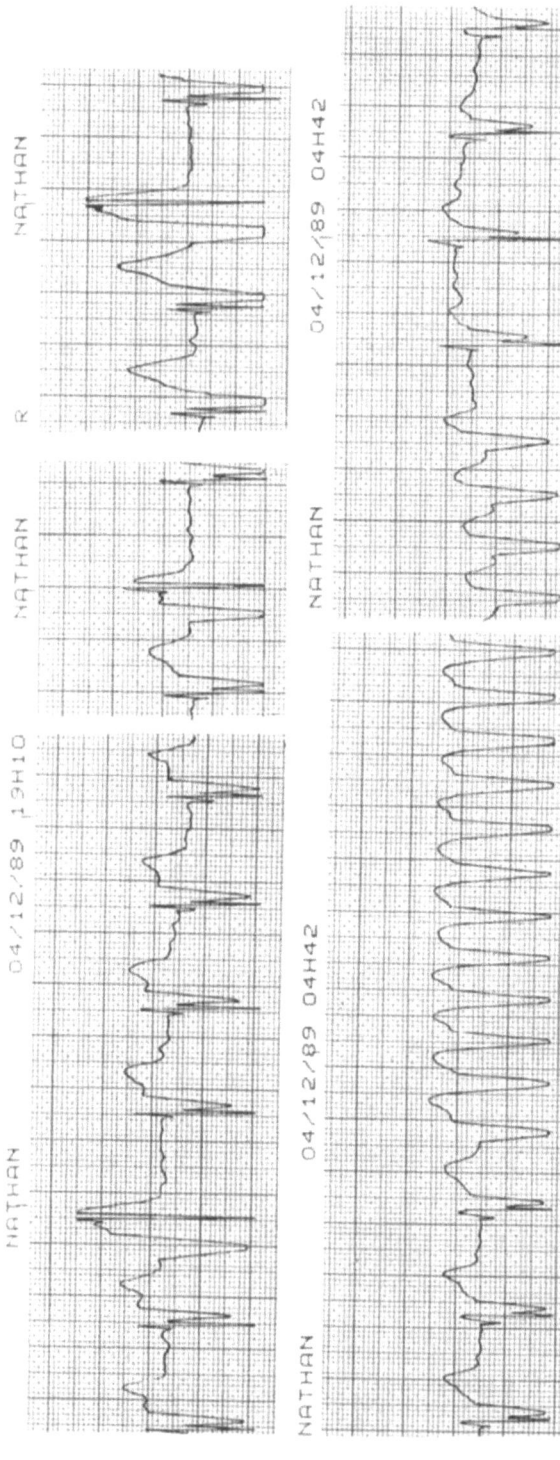

**Fig. 8.11.** Ventricular sensing failure with ventricular spikes falling in the T wave of extrasystoles, a dangerous occurrence in a patient suffering from spontaneous episodes of ventricular tachycardia

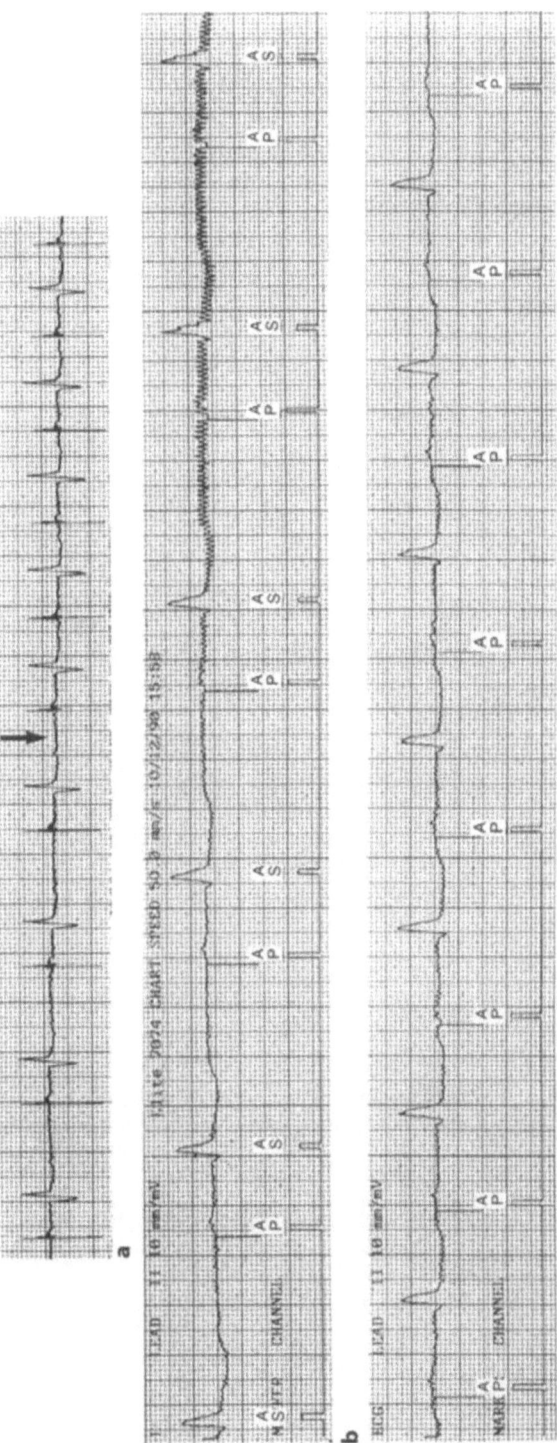

**Fig. 8.12a–c.** AAI mode, 80 BPM

**a** The atrial pacing rate is below the programmed rate as a result of resetting by the R wave (far field sensing = sensing of R wave in the atrium). By reprogramming from an initial unipolar configuration to bipolar (*arrow*), pacing at 80 BPM is restored

**b** Event markers in bipolar configuration confirming sensing of the R wave

**c** Event markers in bipolar configuration. There is no more R wave sensing

*AP* atrial pacing; *AS* atrial sensing

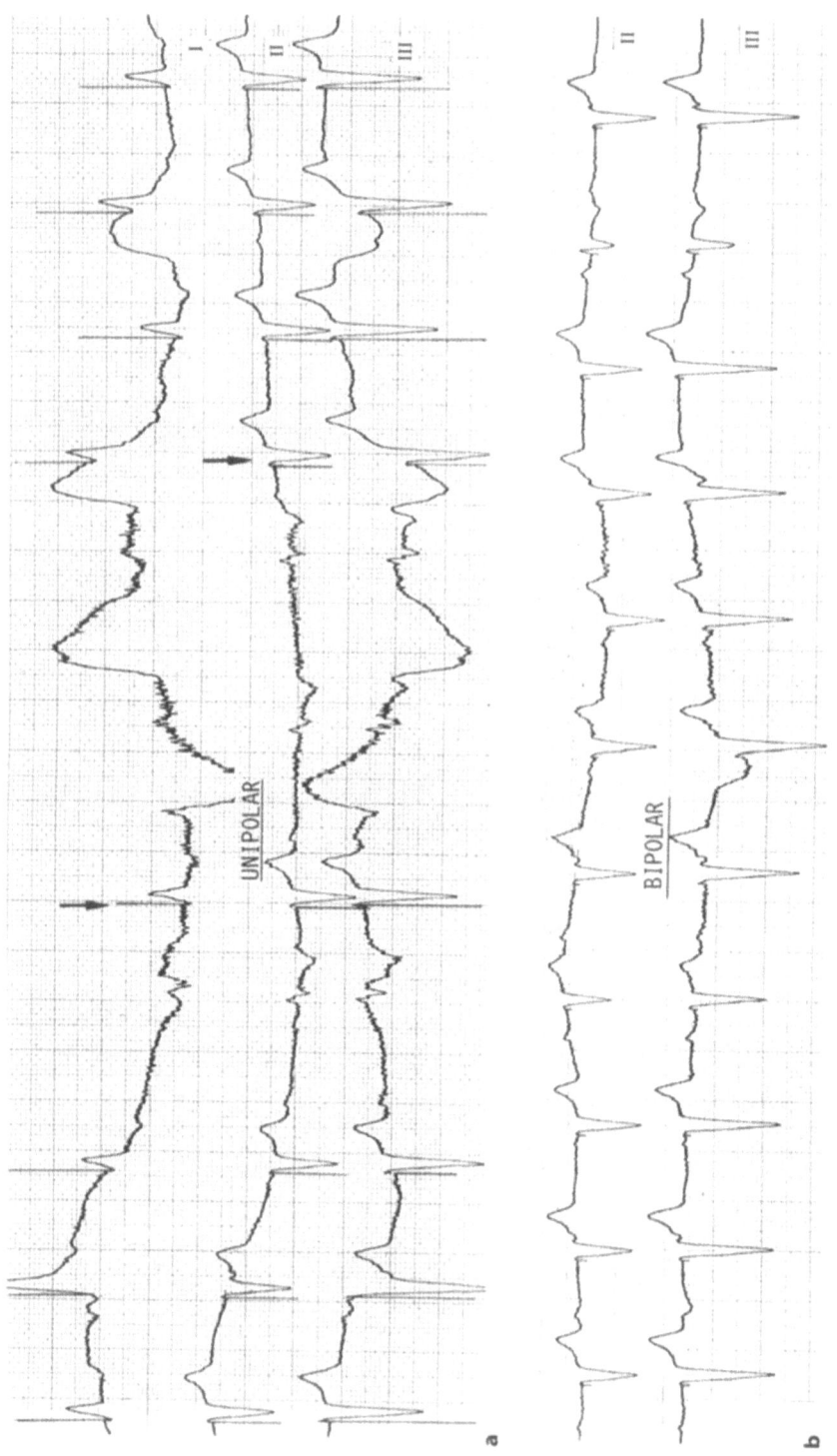

**Fig. 8.13. a** Myosignal inhibition of a VVI unipolar pacemaker
**b** No further inhibition after reprogramming of the system to a bipolar configuration

Kappa pacing system is capable of automatically programming the pacing/sensing polarities according to the type of leads that is connected to the pulse generator. However, any hermeticity defect due to incompatible connectors may cause the inappropriate programming of a polarity that does not correspond to that of the lead (e.g. bipolar for a unipolar lead).

Sensing may also be evaluated by using the SST mode which triggers the delivery of a stimulus with each sensed event. Pacing is, thus, used as a marker of sensing, which allows to demonstrate delayed sensing and avoid inaccurate interpretations (Figs. 8.9, 8.10).

Ventricular sensing failure (normal QRS sensed, PVC not sensed) with ventricular spikes falling in the T wave of extrasystoles may be a dangerous situation (Fig. 8.11) and may cause ventricular tachyarrhythmias.

Resetting by T wave in VVI mode (see also Fig. 8.29), and by R and T in AAI mode must be excluded next (Fig. 8.12). Adjustment of sensitivity allows to discriminate events that need to be sensed from those who do not, while maintaining a satisfactory safety margin. Otherwise, the refractory period must be lengthened, or the system converted to bipolar configuration, which does not always correct the problem.

VA crosstalk is a major problem in modern dual chamber pacing since inappropriate mode switch may be triggered by double counting in the atrium. The only reliable protection against it consists of lengthening the absolute PVARP, which is not possible with all models.

Once sensitivity has been programmed, absence of myosignal sensing must be confirmed by isometric exercises, particularly if the system is unipolar. If resetting by myosignals is noted, sensitivity must be reprogrammed to eliminate it while making all efforts to observe the appropriate safety margin, or preferably, sensing should be switched to bipolar (Fig. 8.13). If the problem cannot be resolved, the pacemaker can be programmed as a single chamber device in SST or DDT mode which triggers delivery of pulses upon sensing of myosignals. This solution is recommended in pacemaker dependent patients, even though it is potentially arrhythmogenic by triggering pacing at unpredictable coupling intervals. If the SST mode is chosen, long refractory periods or, depending on the model, a limitation of the upper rate need to be programmed to avoid excessively rapid heart rates upon sensing of interferences.

Electrograms and event markers, when available, are most useful to clarify the causes of pacemaker resetting.

## Pacing

Automatic programs to set the pacing parameters are quite useful. The automatic program to determine the pacing threshold can be interrupted either by removing the programmer head, or by pressing a programmer's key. The lower rate must be above the spontaneous rate in the chamber being tested (Fig. 8.14). If an automatic or temporarily manual function is not available, the pacing output must be programmed manually (as permanent function), very cautiously in

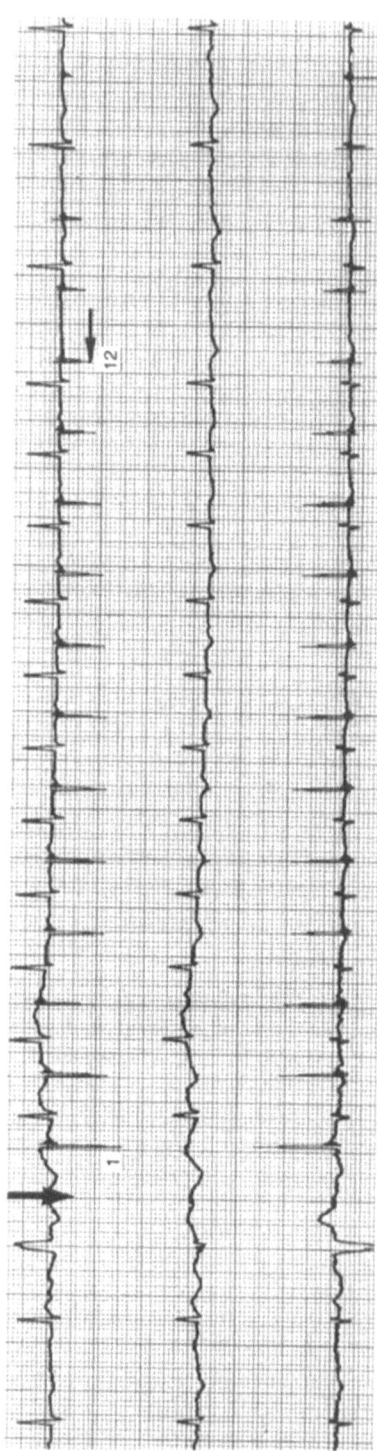

**Fig. 8.14. a** Automatic threshold measurement, driven by the programmer, while the pulse generator is programmed in AAI mode. The 12th spike is ineffective. The decrements were steps of 0.25 V, between 4.75 V and 0 V

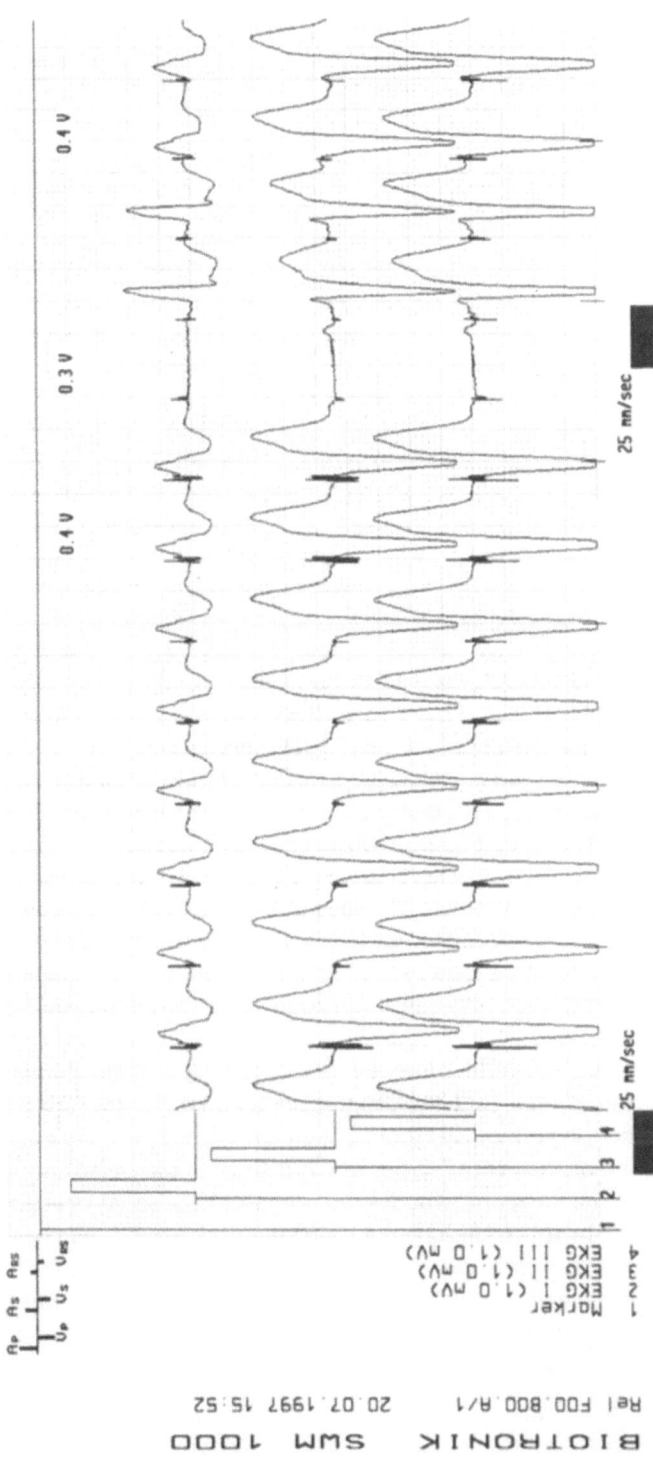

**Fig. 8.14. b** Threshold determination by temporary programming. The pacing output may be manually controlled by reducing or increasing it with the programmer (Biotronik). In this example (threshold test with temporarily VVI mode), the pulse duration was decreased from 0.4 V to 0.3 V and back to 0.4 V. Pacing remains effective at 0.4 V, but not at 0.3 V. When the pulse strength is increased back to 0.4 V, ventricular capture is restored. The tracing is a complete, real time recording obtained via the programmer. Note the similar morphology of the paced and the spontaneous QRS complex in this patient with left bundle branch block

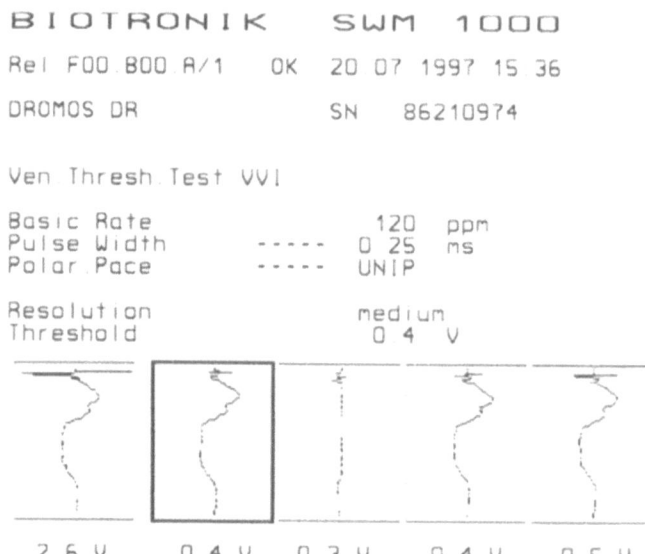

BIOTRONIK    SWM 1000

Rel F00.800.A/1    OK  20.07 1997 15.36

DROMOS DR              SN    86210974


Ven Thresh.Test VVI

Basic Rate                  120  ppm
Pulse Width      - - - - -  0.25 ms
Polar Pace       - - - - -  UNIP

Resolution                  medium
Threshold                   0.4  V

2.6 V      0.4 V      0.3 V      0.4 V      0.5 V

**Fig. 8.14. c** Test summary

the pacemaker dependent patient, keeping in mind that an emergency safety function is always available (Fig. 8.15). However, the onset of this function may be quite slow with some pacemaker models and programmers.

We advise to test threshold by varying voltage instead of pulse duration since doubling voltage offers a 100% safety margin, which is not the case when doubling the pulse duration (see p. 23, Fig. 2.6). Moreover, it is theoretically preferable to establish a rheobase-chronaxie curve, by determining the pacing threshold in volts at various pulse durations, to identify the pulse duration at which power consumption at twice threshold is the lowest (Fig. 8.16). In actuality, with modern leads, chronaxie is typically found between 0.2 and 0.5 ms. Consequently, threshold is usually determined at a pulse duration in the neighborhood of 0.3–0.5 ms.

If a safety margin twice threshold cannot be obtained at 0.3–0.5 ms, a longer pulse duration is programmed (but usually not longer than 1.0 ms) until a safety margin at twice the voltage threshold has been reached. During automatic threshold testing of the „vario" type, which decreases the pulse amplitude from one cycle to the next, one should keep in mind the Wedensky effect: the threshold measured by this technique is a little bit lower than if it had been tested step-by-step, over several cycles, or starting from a subthreshold value. Consequently, in a pacemaker dependent patient, our routine consists of programming the pulse amplitude above twice the value measured during automatic threshold testing.

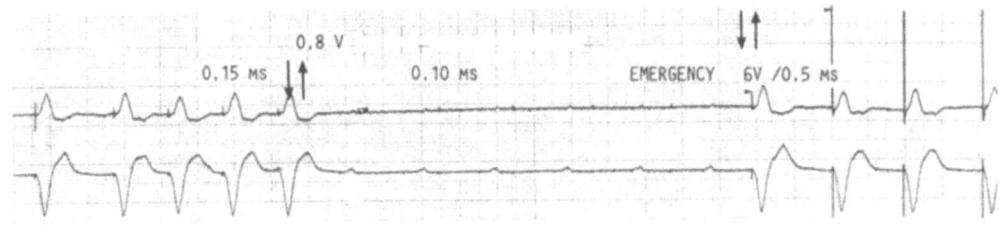

**Fig. 8.15.** Capture threshold test by permanent programming: Caution must be exercised when proceeding with manual determination of the capture threshold in a pacemaker dependent patient. *EMERGENCY* indicates that the emergency function key had to be pressed

**Fig. 8.16.** The Thera models (Medtronic) allow the determination of chronaxie-rheobase curves from two measurements of the pacing threshold and propose the programming of the optimal pacing value with respect to the lowest power consumption (at least twice the amplitude at the chronaxie: here 1.5 V/ 0.3 ms) as well as observance of the safety margin

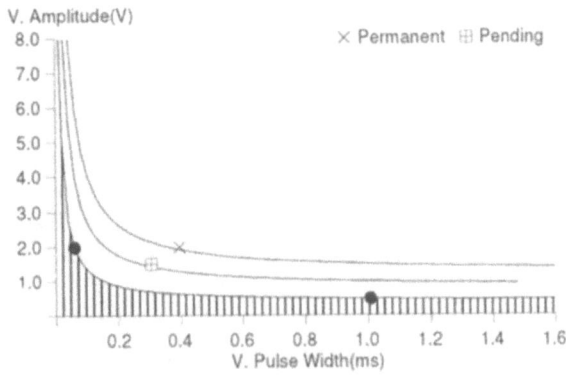

> **!** As a rough rule for 100% safety margin the pulse duration should be programmed near to the chronaxie, the pulse amplitude at least at twice the voltage threshold.

Once all pacing parameters have been finally programmed, the telemetry data are analyzed. After the basic pacing and sensing functions have been tested, eventually also on exercise, as especially sensing failure may become evident (see Fig. 8.51), the setting of escape interval and refractory periods come next.

## Escape and Pacing Interval Setting

Several reasons may explain a pacing rate different from the programmed lower rate:

- If the escape rate is below the programmed lower rate:
  - Resetting of the pacemaker by cardiac events such as T wave in VVI mode, or R wave or T wave in AAI mode (Figs. 8.17 – 8.20). As discussed earlier, the correction of such problems involves reprogramming of the sensitivity, refractory period or sensing polarity. In AAI mode, however, blocked atrial

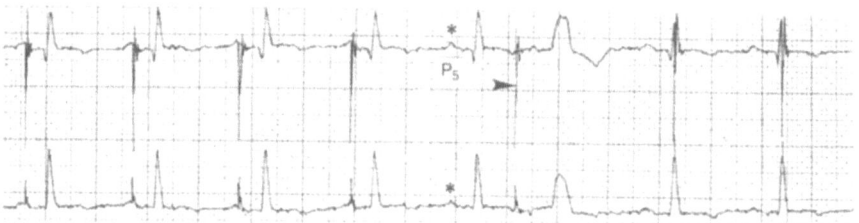

**Fig. 8.17.** AAT mode, 30 BPM. At a sensitivity of 0.5 mV, sensing of the P wave is delayed. The R wave is not sensed and falls in the refractory period. By reprogramming the sensitivity to 0.75 mV, the pacemaker no longer senses the P waves (starting with *P5*), delivers an effective stimulus (*horizontal arrow*) which is conducted to the ventricles with left bundle branch block, and then senses the R wave, because the R wave is now outside of the atrial refractory period. The R wave amplitude in the atrium here is much higher than that of the P wave

extrasystoles, occurring outside the refractory period cause an apparent slowing of the atrial pacing rate, which should be recognized as normal function. Electrograms or event markers may help resolve this problem.

- Programming of rate hysteresis, interval added to the escape interval after each sensed event in the same chamber to facilitate the emergence of a spontaneous rhythm (Figs. 8.21, 8.22).
- Application of an automatic program of the „search hysteresis" type, as offered by Intermedics (Fig. 8.23) and recently also by Pacesetter.
- Programming of a bradycardia diagnostic function.
- Programming of a sleep rate.
• If the escape rate is above the programmed lower rate:
  - Programming of a rate smoothing function (or of Flywheel, Vitatron) after an increase in the lower rate by a spontaneous rhythm at a rate above the lower rate.
  - Programming of a rate responsive function, with the sensor dictating an increase in the pacing rate.

In both instances, the lower rate should return to its programmed value within a few minutes if the patient is resting. The principles behind the programming of the lower rate were described on p. 74.

## Refractory Period

The refractory period should be programmed as short as possible to guarantee proper sensing of rapid rhythms in the implanted chamber. On the other hand, its programming should be long in case of crosstalk, or when using the SST mode to avoid too rapid an acceleration of the pacing rate by myosignals.

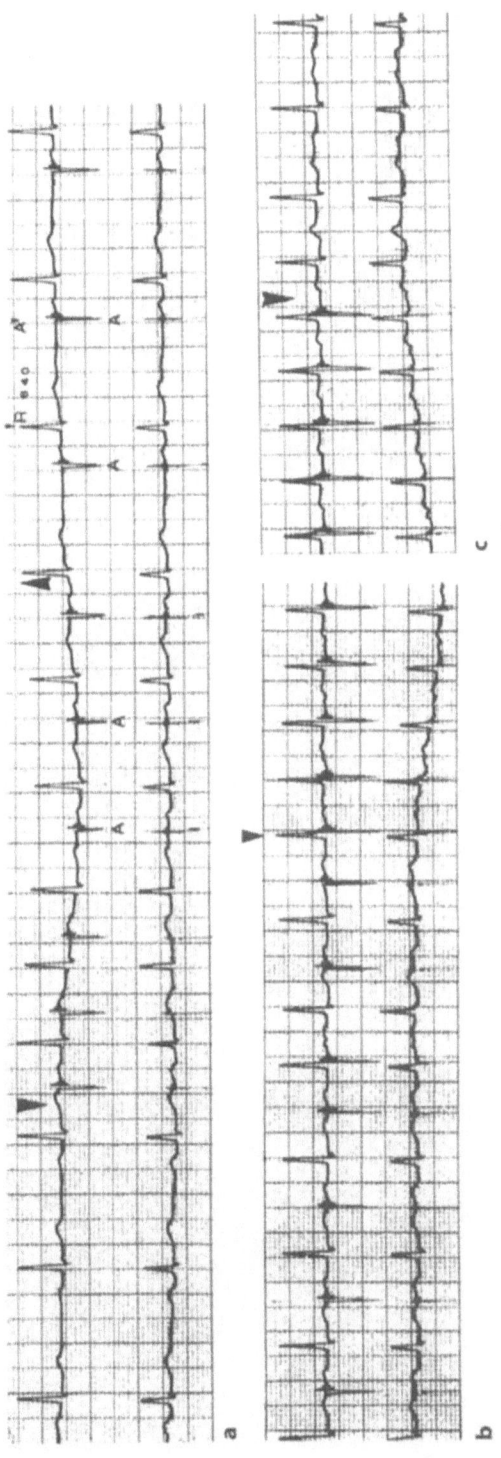

**Fig. 8.18. a** AAI mode, 70 BPM, 5 V/0.5 ms, sensitivity = 1.25 mV, refractory period = 325 ms, unipolar configuration, spontaneous rate < 70 BPM. Resetting by R wave. During magnet application, (*downward arrow*), the rate is 70 BPM. Upon removal of the magnet (upward arrow), the rate decreases due to sensing of the R wave. The RA (R wave – atrial spike) interval is 840 ms (=70 BPM). As the AR (Atrial Spike – R wave) interval must be added to the pacing interval, the result is a slowing of the pacing rate
**b** Same settings as in (**a**), AAT mode. Sensing of the R wave (downward arrow) causes a sustained atrial tachycardia
**c** Programming of a bipolar configuration (downward arrow) eliminates the phenomenon. Sensing of the R wave has ceased despite the simultaneous programming of a refractory period at 220 ms

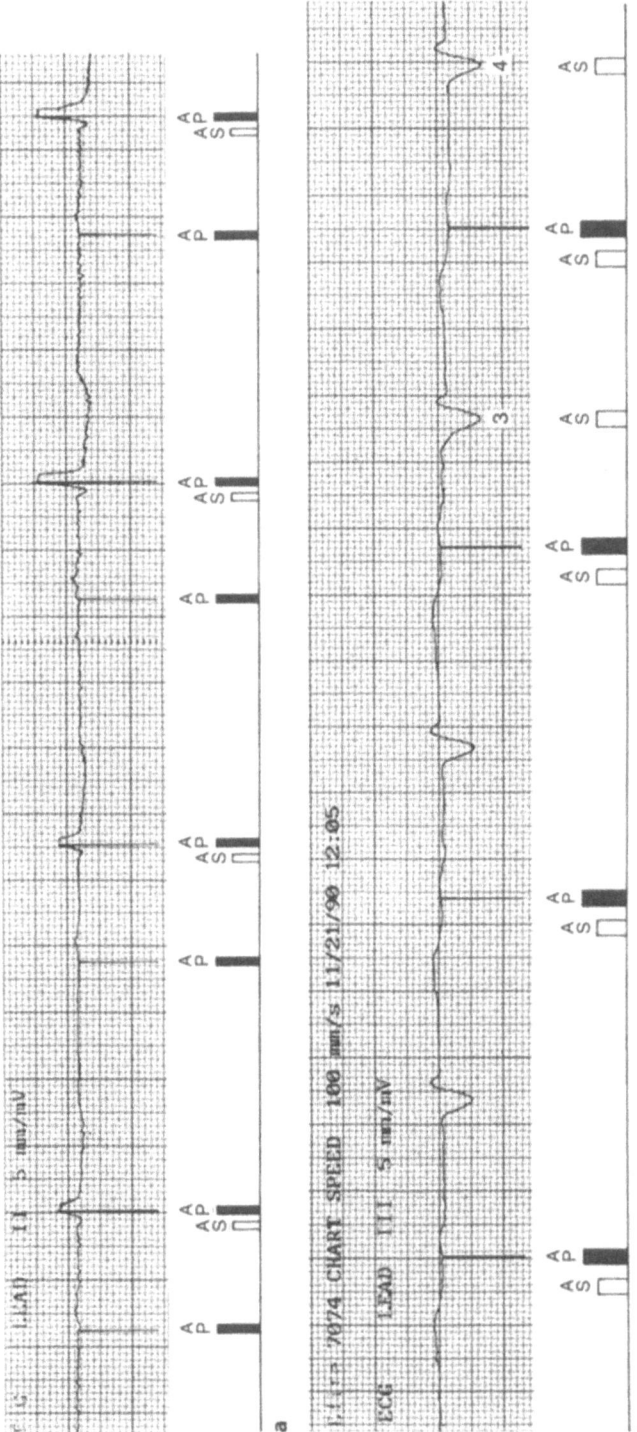

**Fig. 8.19. a** R wave sensing by a pacemaker in AAT mode, confirmed by the presence of spikes in the R wave and by the event markers **b** In this case, the third and fourth QRS complexes are sensed in the atrium but do not trigger pacing which is inhibited by the protection circuit against run-away pacing. The PR interval is short and the pacemaker cannot pace at a rate above 200 BPM

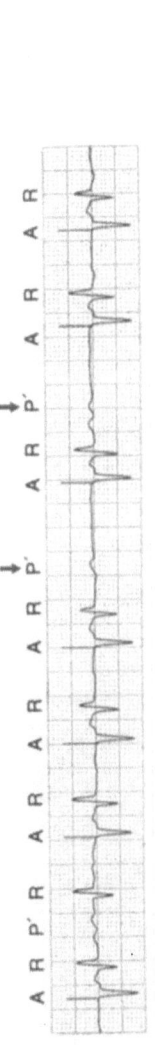

**Fig. 8.20.** Sensing of blocked atrial extrasystoles outside of the refractory period resets this AAI pacemaker and causes a decrease in heart rate below the programmed lower rate. This behavior is normal in AAI mode. *A* paced P wave; *P* sensed P wave; *P'* premature P wave; *R* R wave

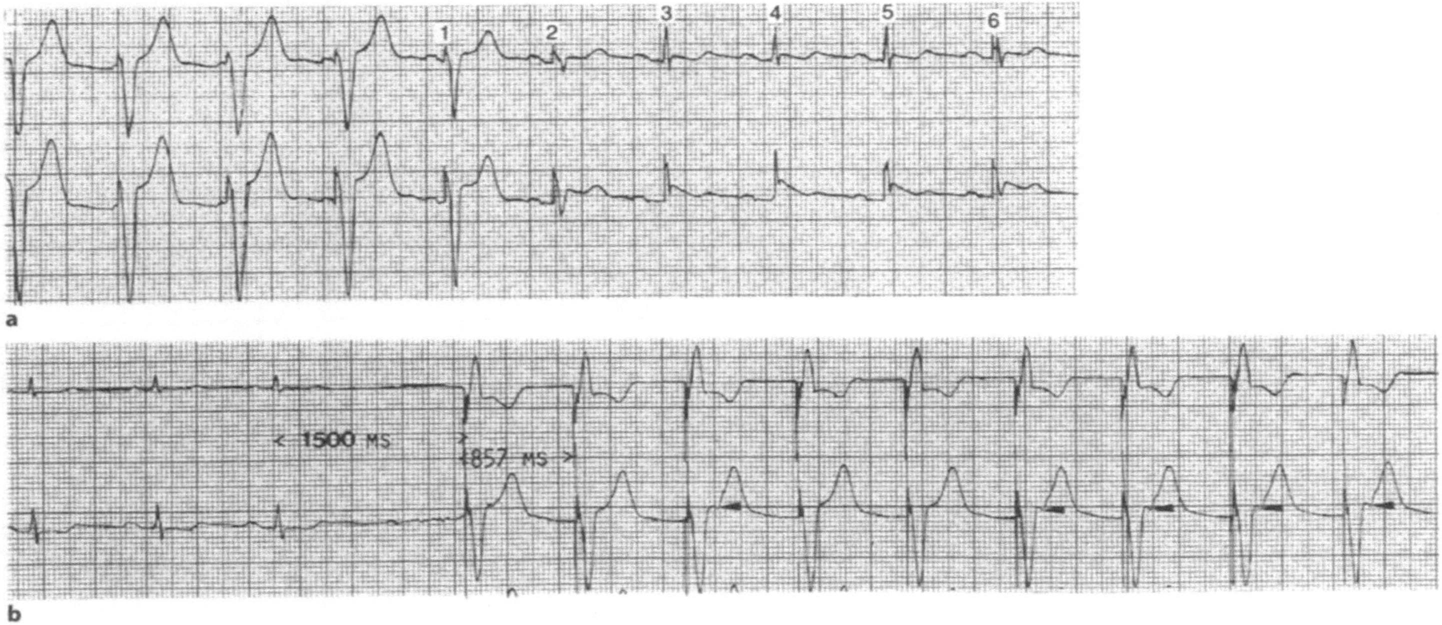

**Fig. 8.21.** Mode VVI, 70 BPM, hysteresis = 40 BPM. **a** The pacemaker is set at 70 BPM. There is no ventricular sensing. The rate is not slow enough to allow the sensing of spontaneous narrow QRS complexes by the pacemaker. All complexes are fusions (*1*) or pseudofusions (*2 – 6*). **b** Following carotid sinus massage, the pacemaker is activated at the rate hysteresis (40 BPM) with retrograde conduction (*horizontal arrow*)

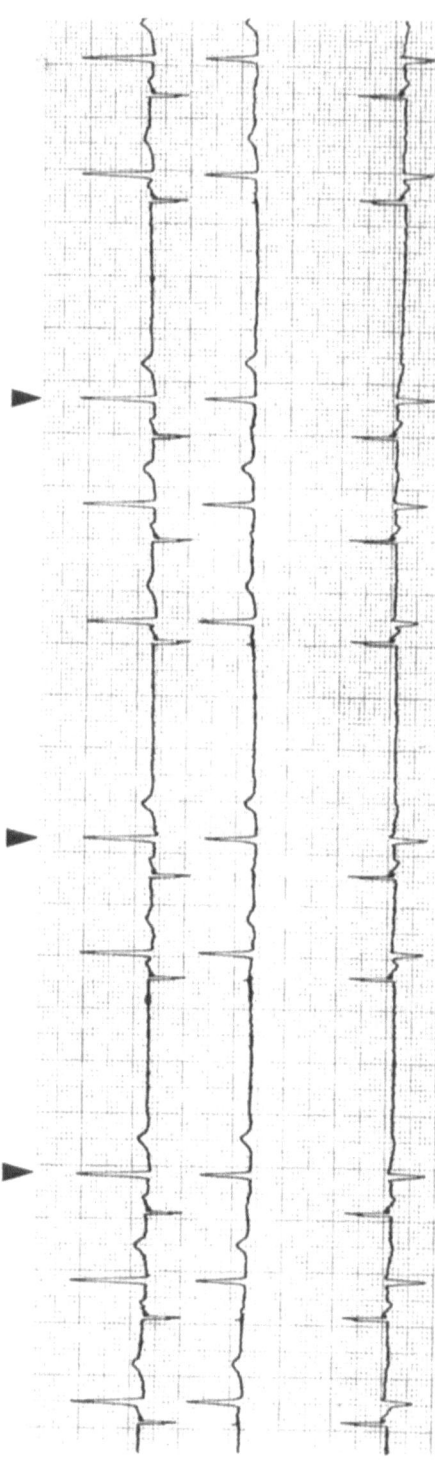

**Fig. 8.22.** AAI mode, 75 BPM, hysteresis = 40 BPM, refractory period = 400 ms, unipolar sensing. Resetting of the pacemaker at the end of the R wave, with escape at the hysteresis rate (40 BPM) when the PR lengthens. The spontaneous lengthening of the PR interval due to Wenckebach phenomenon causes the QRS to emerge from the refractory period of the pacemaker (*downward arrows*)

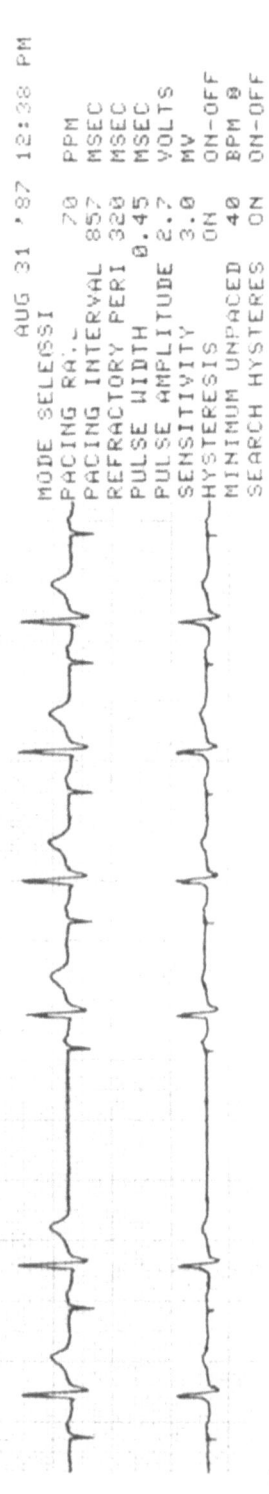

**Fig. 8.23.** AAI mode; 70 BPM; hysteresis = 40 BPM. „Search hysteresis" function by the Intermedics Nova II pacemaker. After each 255 paced cycles, the pacemaker lengthens its escape interval in search of an emerging spontaneous rhythm

## 8.2
# Programming of a Dual Chamber Pacemaker

This programming is more delicate because of the greater complexity of the pacemaker. One should follow some sort of check list that might be composed as follows.

## Identification of the Atrial and Ventricular Pacing Spikes

The proper interpretation of ECG tracings from paced patients requires the identification of pacing spikes of atrial and ventricular origin. A stimulus that just precedes a QRS complex may not be a ventricular spike if the preceding P wave was not sensed. Pacing function abnormalities, as well as competition between spontaneous and paced rhythm may cause fusions, pseudofusions and pseudo-pseudo-fusions (see Figs. 8.6, 8.7).

## Atrial Sensing

The lower rate should be programmed below the sinus rate, and the AVD should be short in order to obtain a ventricular spike indicative of proper atrial sensing. Atrial sensitivity is then decreased in successive steps (increase in the programmed setting). When AV conduction is preserved, loss atrial sensing has occurred when the ventricular spikes disappear and the spontaneous QRSs return (Fig. 8.24). Event markers may be helpful (Figs. 8.25, 8.26). Conversely, patterns of pseudofusion may develop (Fig. 8.27). The AAI or AAT modes may also be used as described.

If presence of complete AV block, loss of atrial sensing results in AV dissociation with asynchronous AV sequential pacing (Fig. 8.28).

Resetting of the pacemaker by an event sensed in the ventricle, for instance the T wave, must be looked for (Fig. 8.29). ECG markers and intracardiac electrograms are helpful adjuncts to the diagnosis. The same solutions as those described for AAI systems are applicable (adjustments of atrial sensing, of PVARP, of sensing polarity).

In presence of myosignals, the pacemaker may have two different responses: the myosignals are sensed in the atrium only, causing run-away ventricular pacing (see Fig. 3.41); or they are sensed in both chambers or in the ventricle only (Fig. 8.30, see also Fig. 3.12), causing inhibition of the pacemaker with emergence of a spontaneous rhythm or asystole, cause of syncope. In the latter case, the problem can be resolved as described for single chamber systems, or by the use of unconventional pacing modes such as DAD, DDT or DAT, which are infrequently available.

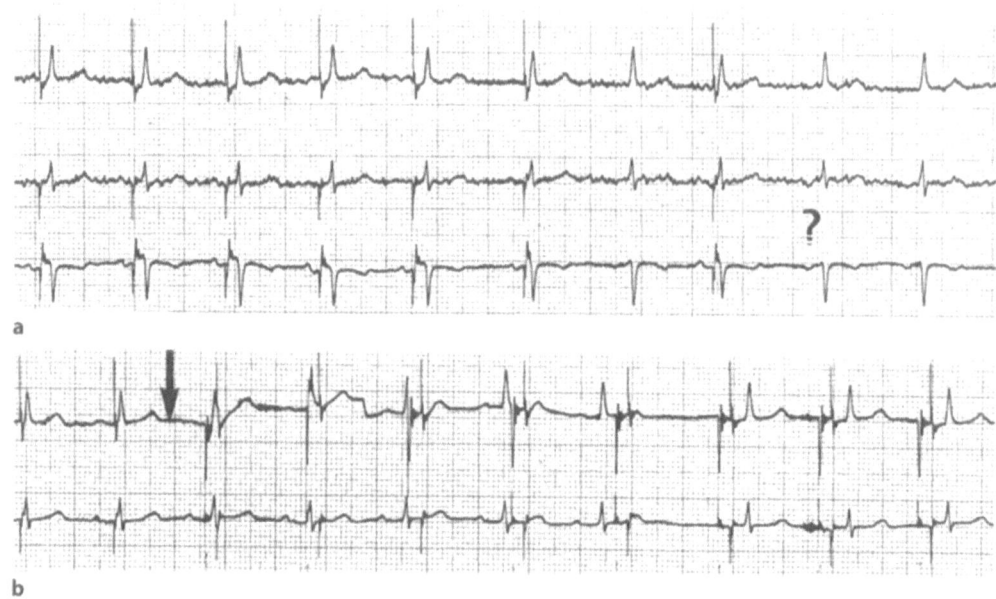

**Fig. 8.24.** DDD mode, 65 BPM, AVD = 90 ms, atrial sensitivity = 1 mV, ventricular sensitivity = 1.5 mV

**a** Are the spikes atrial or ventricular? Why are the spikes missing after a few cycles? (?) If the spikes are ventricular, they are ineffective since the QRS is narrow and there is a space between the spike and the QRS. If they are atrial, atrial sensing must be failing. Given the programmed AVD, the spikes seem more likely to be ventricular with failure to capture. The later disappearance of the spike would mean that the QRS is at least properly sensed, but that there is loss of atrial sensing since no ventricular stimulus was delivered. The very short programmed AVD would have preempted sensing of the QRS. The P waves have changed configuration and are no longer sensed

**b** The spike has been confirmed to be ventricular since, upon magnet application (*downward arrow*), the appearance of the spike is identical to that in **a**. Final diagnosis: loss of ventricular capture and intermittent atrial sensing failure from wandering atrial pacemaker. Correction would consist of increasing the ventricular pacing output and the atrial sensitivity

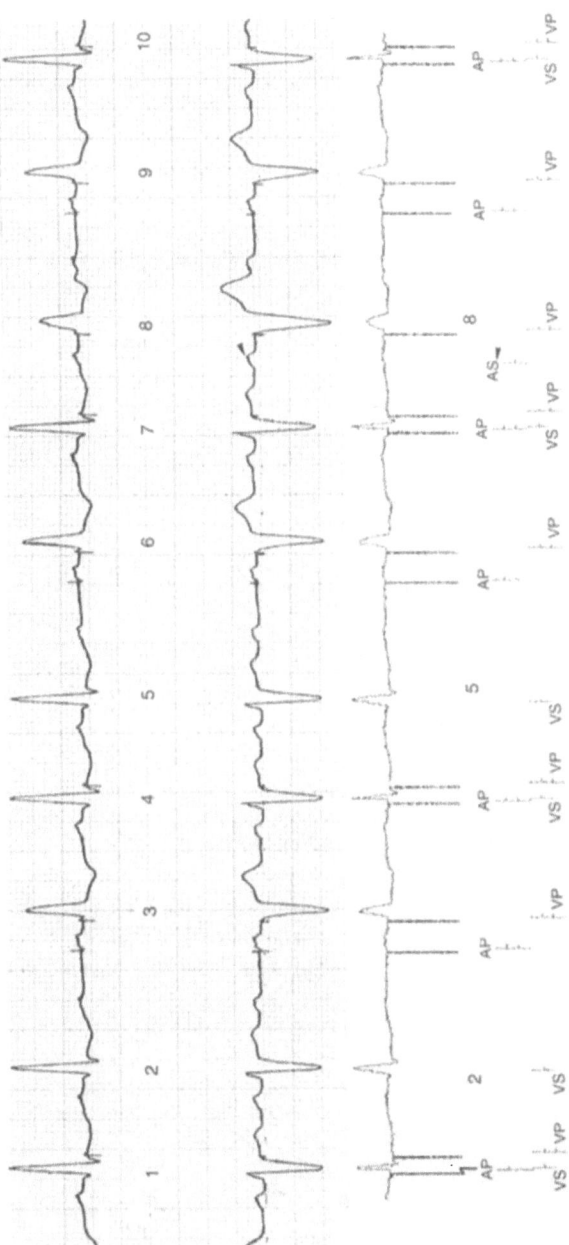

**Fig. 8.25. a** DDD mode, atrial sensitivity = 2.5 mV, AVD = 200 ms. Atrial pacing (*AP*), delivered at the end of the escape interval, is preserved (complexes *3, 6, 9*); atrial sensing (*AS*) is defective in complexes *2, 4, 5, 7, 10*, but effective in complex *8*. Ventricular pacing (*VP*) is effective throughout except when delivered in the safety window (complexes *1, 4, 7, 10*). The QRS complex is sensed after the blanking period, and a ventricular stimulus is delivered at the end of the safety window. The event markers help in making the diagnosis

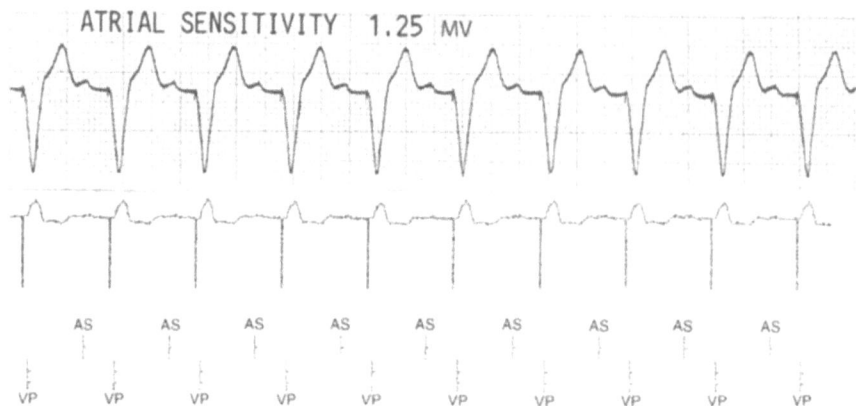

**Fig. 8.25. b** An increase in sensitivity to 1.25 mV restores normal function
*AP* atrial pacing; *AS* atrial sensing; *VP* ventricular pacing; *VS* ventricular sensing

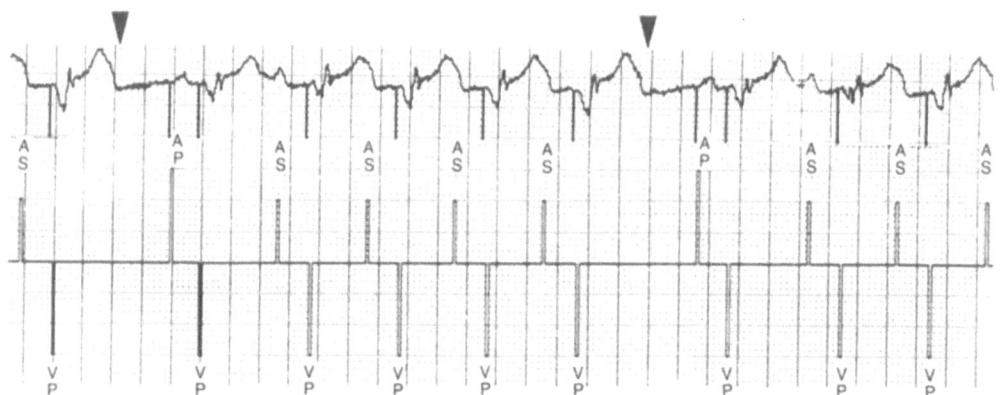

**Fig. 8.26.** DDD mode, upper rate 125 BPM, PVARP = 325 ms, AVD = 200 ms. Intermittent atrial sensing failure due to P waves occurring during PVARP (*arrows*). They are not displayed on the marker channel of this older generation pacemaker model. This situation can be rectified by shortening AVD and/or PVARP

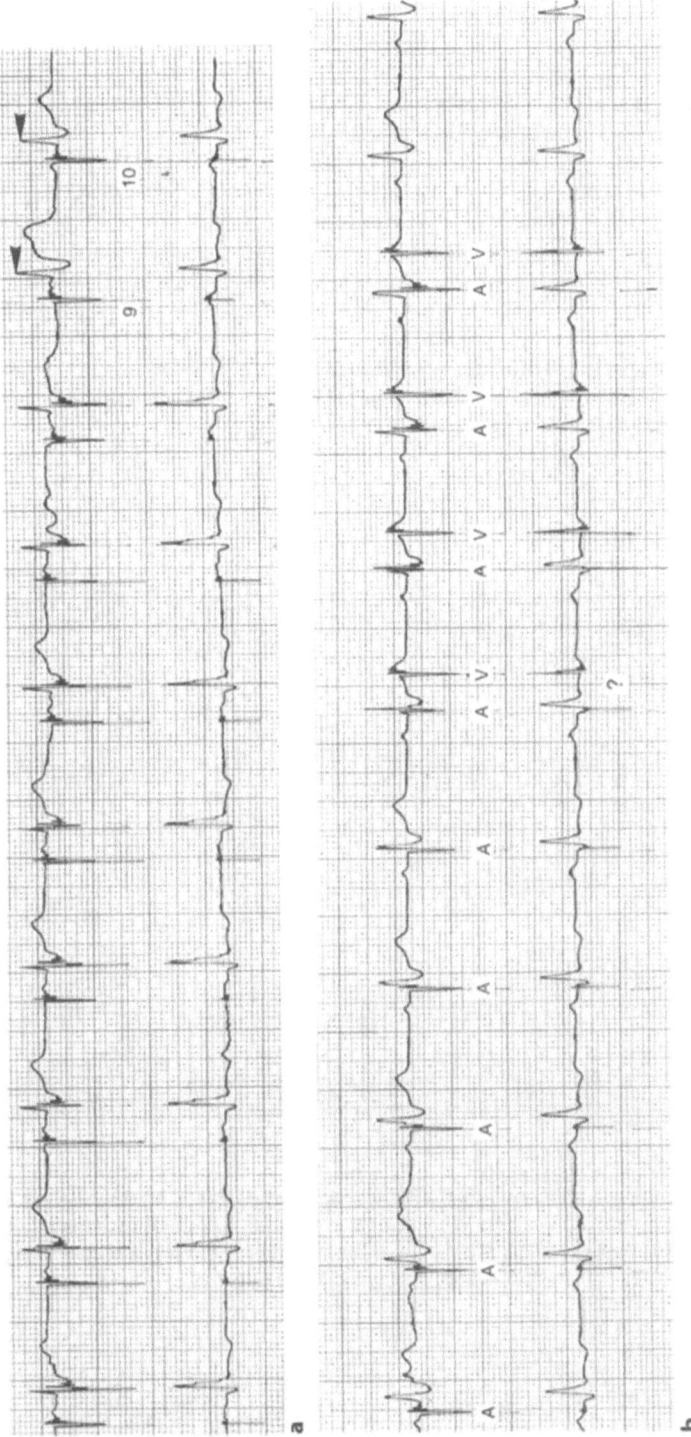

**Fig. 8.27a,b.** DDD mode, 62 BPM, AVD = 250 ms, atrial sensitivity = 1.2 mV

**a** Effective atrial pacing with normal AV conduction followed by pseudofusions from late ventricular sensing because of right bundle branch block. The R waves of complexes *9* and *10* are properly sensed since they fall within AVD, but the corresponding P waves were not sensed (additionally atrial sensing failure)

**b** Pseudo-pseudofusion. Pacing is atrial until an atrial stimulus falls on an R wave which was not sensed because it occurred in the blanking period; this is followed by ventricular pacing at the end of AVD (?) on four occasions. In the end, the last two R waves occur before the end of the atrial escape interval, which completely inhibits the pacemaker

*A* atrial stimulus; *V* ventricular stimulus

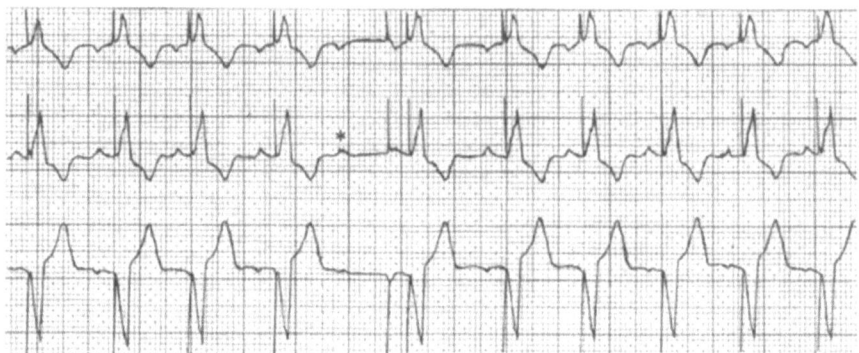

**Fig. 8.28.** DDD mode, 60/154 BPM, automatic AVD adjustment between 156 and 47 ms. Atrial sensing failure (*) in a pacemaker dependent patient. The solution of this problem consists of increasing the atrial sensitivity

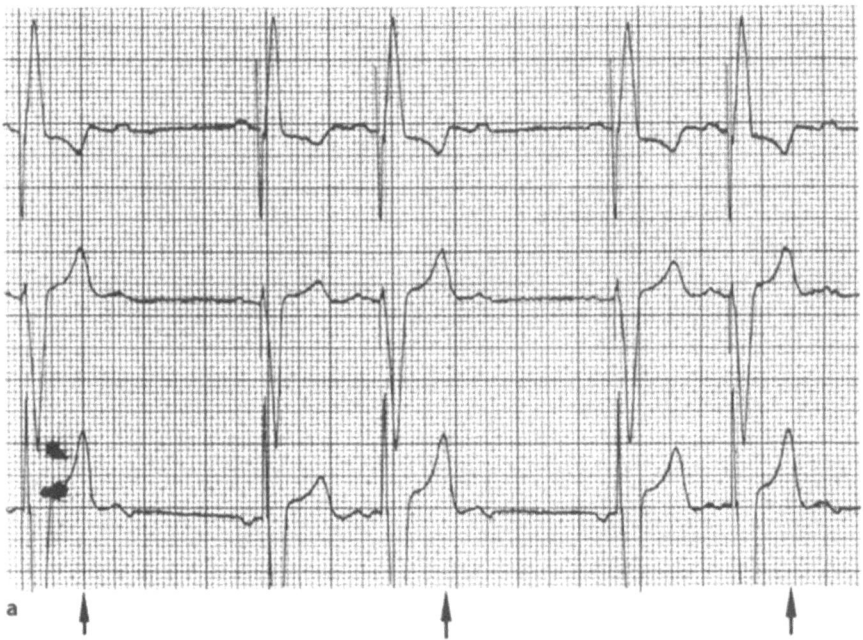

**Fig. 8.29.a** T wave sensing. VDD mode 50/110 BPM, atrial sensitivity = 0.25 mV; ventricular sensitivity = 2 mV, ventricular refractory period = 300 ms. Apparent atrial sensing defects in a pacemaker dependent patient. In fact, the pacemaker is recycling its escape interval from the T waves (*arrows*), preventing sensing of the following P waves

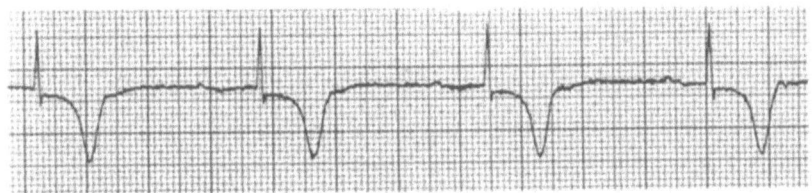

**Fig. 8.29.b** Confirmation of the phenomenon by reprogramming to VVI mode at 60 BPM, with fixed T wave inhibition and slow heart rate. The problem can be corrected by decreasing the ventricular sensitivity or increasing the ventricular refractory period

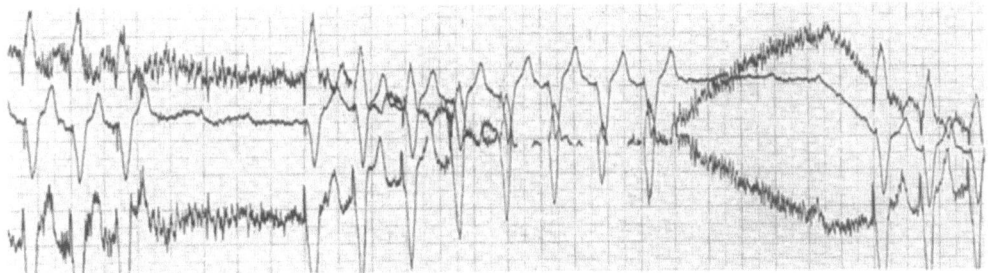

**Fig. 8.30.** Complete inhibition of DDD pacemaker by myosignal sensing in the ventricle

## Ventricular Pacing

With the AVD programmed short to test the atrial sensing threshold, one may also determine the ventricular capture threshold (Fig. 8.31), and the same principles apply as those described for single chamber testing, including safety precautions in the pacemaker dependent patient. Ideally, the automatic mode offered by the manufacturer is used, with the same reservation pertaining to the Wedensky effect. If the patient has preserved AV conduction, loss of ventricular pacing has occurred when native QRS complexes reappear (Figs. 8.31, 8.32). If the patient has complete AV block, loss of ventricular capture causes asystole (Fig. 8.33). The ventricular capture pacing threshold can also be tested by changing to VVI or VVT mode.

## Atrial Pacing

The lower rate is programmed faster than the spontaneous rate, with a longer AVD to better distinguish the paced P wave and, perhaps, the emergence of spontaneous QRS complexes. The automatic pacing threshold measurement programs may also be helpful (Fig. 8.34). If AV conduction is preserved, loss of capture is identified by the absence of a paced P wave and a QRS completely paced, sometimes followed by retrograde conduction (Fig. 8.35). One can also use the

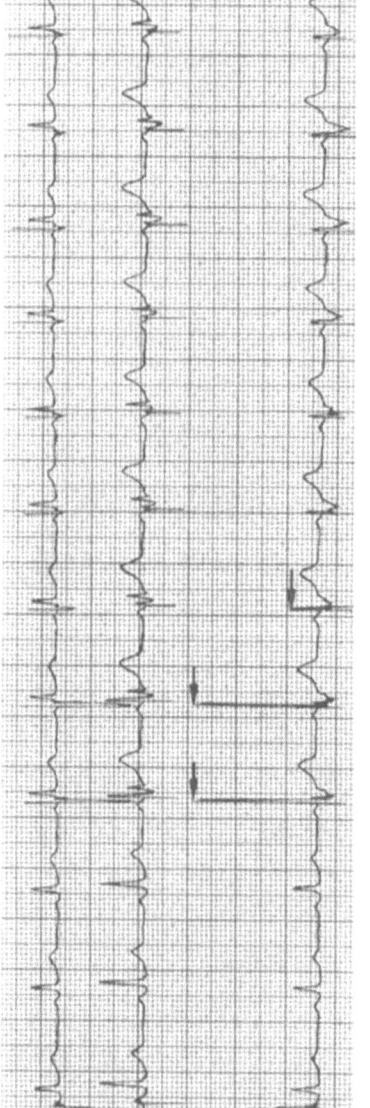

**Fig. 8.31.** Testing methodology of DDD pacemaker

**a** The quality of atrial sensing is examined with a short programmed AVD and slow lower rate; under these conditions, all sensed P waves should be followed by ventricular pacing. This allows also to test ventricular pacing causing a QRS and ST–T of a different morphology than the spontaneous complex. Atrial sensing and ventricular pacing thresholds can both be quickly tested by this method. *Arrows: Reprogramming to a short AVD* of 78 ms, low ventricular pacing output (2.5 V, 0.12 ms) and relatively low atrial sensitivity (2.2 mV)

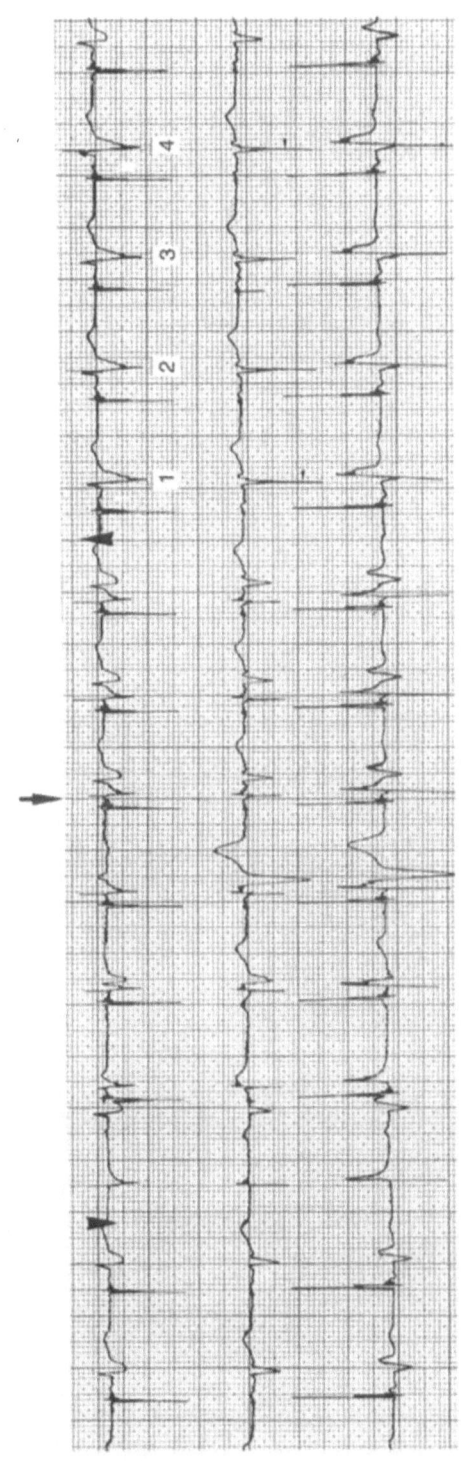

**Fig. 8.31. b** The magnet test (*between the arrowheads*) allows to verify (provided the magnet mode is D00) the effectiveness of atrial and ventricular pacing. In this example, atrial pacing is effective (being followed by a spontaneous QRS in presence of preserved AV conduction), but not ventricular pacing since the QRS remains unchanged and a space is visible between spike and QRS complex in all leads recorded. The *downward arrow* indicates first ventricular capture failure. When performing a magnet test, attention should be paid to the specific features of each model. In this case, after removal of the magnet, four AV sequential paced sequences are delivered at the programmed rate and AVD (complexes *1 – 4*)

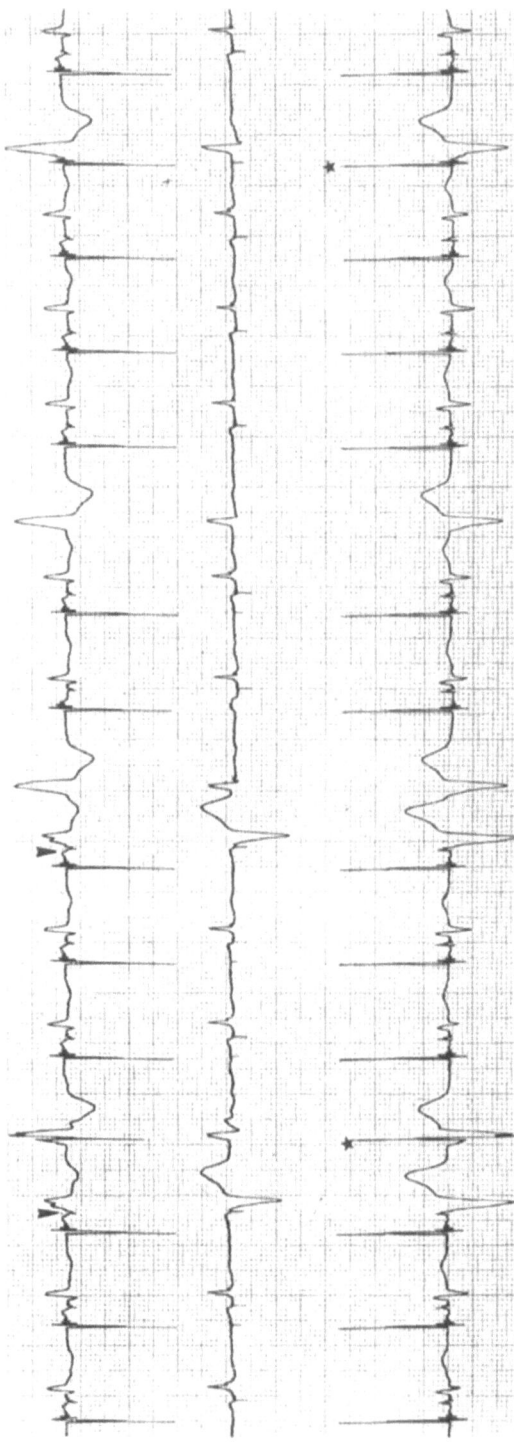

**Fig. 8.32.** Intermittent ventricular pacing failure in a pacemaker non dependent patient; there is absence of QRS modification, and presence of a space between pacing spike and QRS complex, except on two occasions (*arrows*). Ventricular sensing is preserved and atrial pacing is effective. The pacing spikes that are present at the onset of premature ventricular complexes (*) are atrial. The ventricular pacing output should be increased

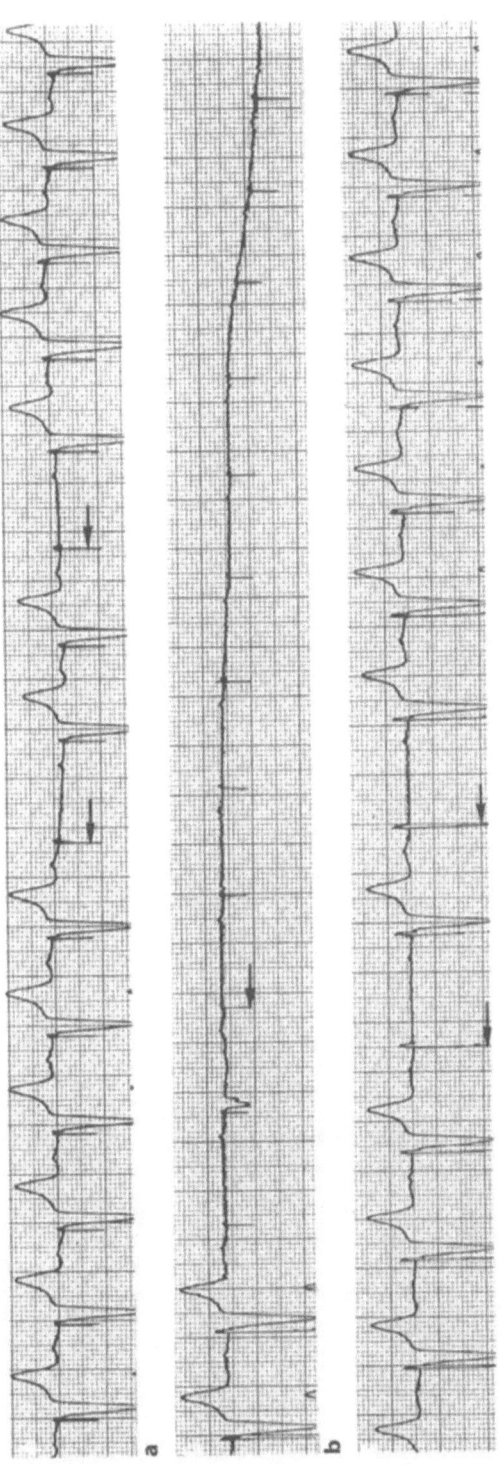

**Fig. 8.33a – c.** Importance of breathing maneuvers to test function abnormalities; all three tracings obtained in the same pacemaker dependent patient

**a** Occasional ventricular pacing failure at an output of 2.5 V/0.12 ms
**b** Development of ventricular asystole with deep breathing at the same pacing output
**c** Persistence of two instances of pacing failure (*arrows*) despite the increase in pacing output to 7.5 V. The lead is unstable; pacing threshold cannot be precisely measured. A reintervention is necessary

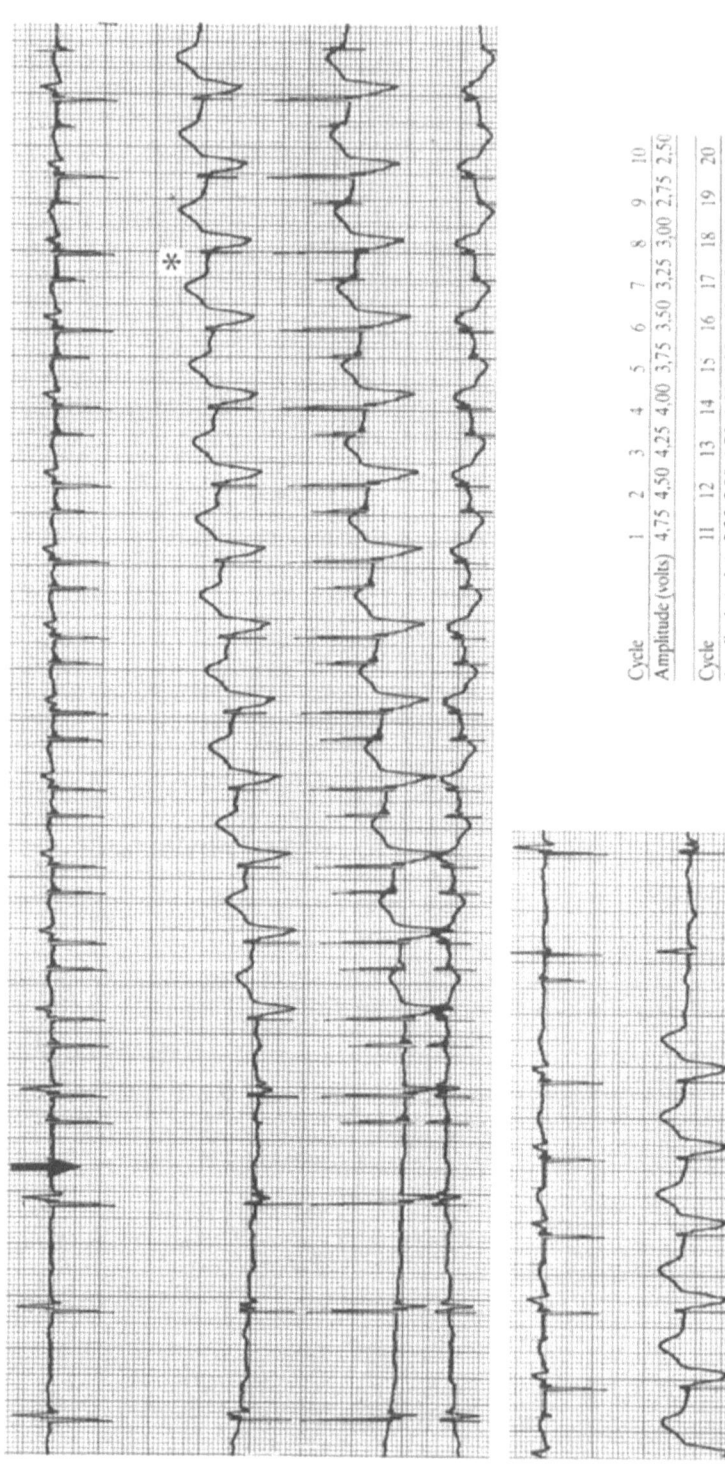

| Cycle | 1 | 2 | 3 | 4 | 5 | 6 | 7 | 8 | 9 | 10 |
|---|---|---|---|---|---|---|---|---|---|---|
| Amplitude (volts) | 4.75 | 4.50 | 4.25 | 4.00 | 3.75 | 3.50 | 3.25 | 3.00 | 2.75 | 2.50 |

| Cycle | 11 | 12 | 13 | 14 | 15 | 16 | 17 | 18 | 19 | 20 |
|---|---|---|---|---|---|---|---|---|---|---|
| Amplitude (volts) | 2.25 | 2.00 | 1.75 | 1.50 | 1.25 | 1.00 | 0.75 | 0.50 | 0.25 | 0.00 |

**Fig. 8.34.** Automatic atrial pacing threshold measurement by decrease in the pacing output from 4.75 to 0 V in steps of 0.25 V in D00 mode. Capture is lost (*) at the 12th spike (2 V)

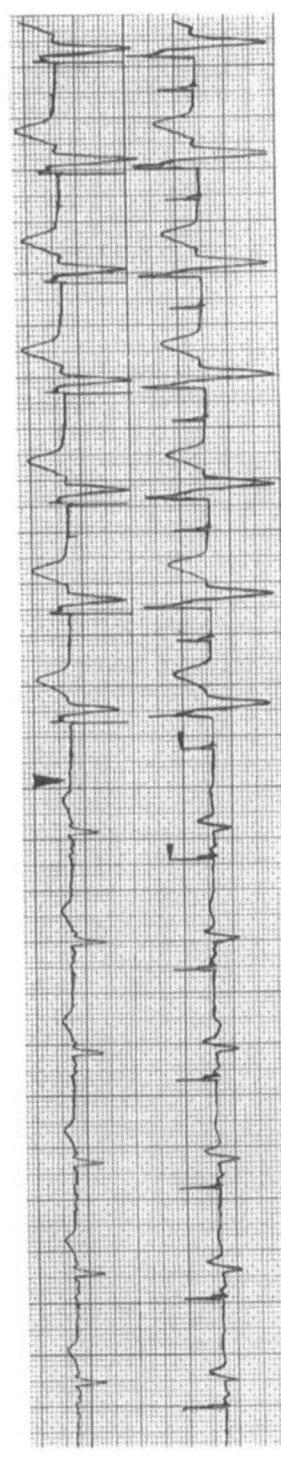

**Fig. 8.35.** With an inordinately long AVD and a lower rate above the spontaneous rate, the quality of atrial pacing and ventricular sensing can be evaluated if the PR interval is shorter than the programmed AVD. Thresholds may then be measured. At the time of loss of atrial pacing (*second horizontal arrow*) one may observe the development of retrograde conduction. *Downward arrow*, reduction of the atrial pacing output

AAI mode. In presence of AV block, loss of atrial capture can only be identified by the loss of P wave following the atrial pacing spike and, sometimes, the development of retrograde conduction after ventricular pacing (Fig. 8.36, 8.37). It is unusual not to be able to analyze paced P waves on a 12 lead ECG. If that were the case, the atrial pacing threshold should be tested with the assistance of echo-doppler to measure transmitral flow and examine the synchronization of the P wave relative to the paced QRS on the surface ECG. When pacing in the atrium is lost, the A wave is desynchronized.

In this case, also a transesophageal ECG may show the depolarization of the atrium.

## Ventricular Sensing

In VDD/DDD mode with a long AVD, if AV conduction is spontaneous without ventricular pacing, ventricular sensing can be measured by successive programming steps. Sensing has been lost when a ventricular pacing spike appears after the spontaneous QRS which, up to that point, was sensed during the AVD (Fig. 8.38).

The Biotronik Physios, Dromos and Eikos, and ELA Medical Chorum and Talent pacemaker models offer a DDT mode, the pacing spikes representing markers of atrial and ventricular sensing. The A and V sensitivity levels are programmed as in the AAT and VVT modes to determine the sensitivity thresholds. One must simply ascertain that the AV delay has been programmed long enough to avoid pseudofusion.

In patients with complete AV block, ventricular extrasystoles must reset the pacemaker if they are properly sensed (see Fig. 8.11) and fall outside the refractory periods. One may also program the VVI or VVT modes at slow rates. However, in the totally pacemaker dependent patient, the measure of the ventricular sensing threshold is impossible.

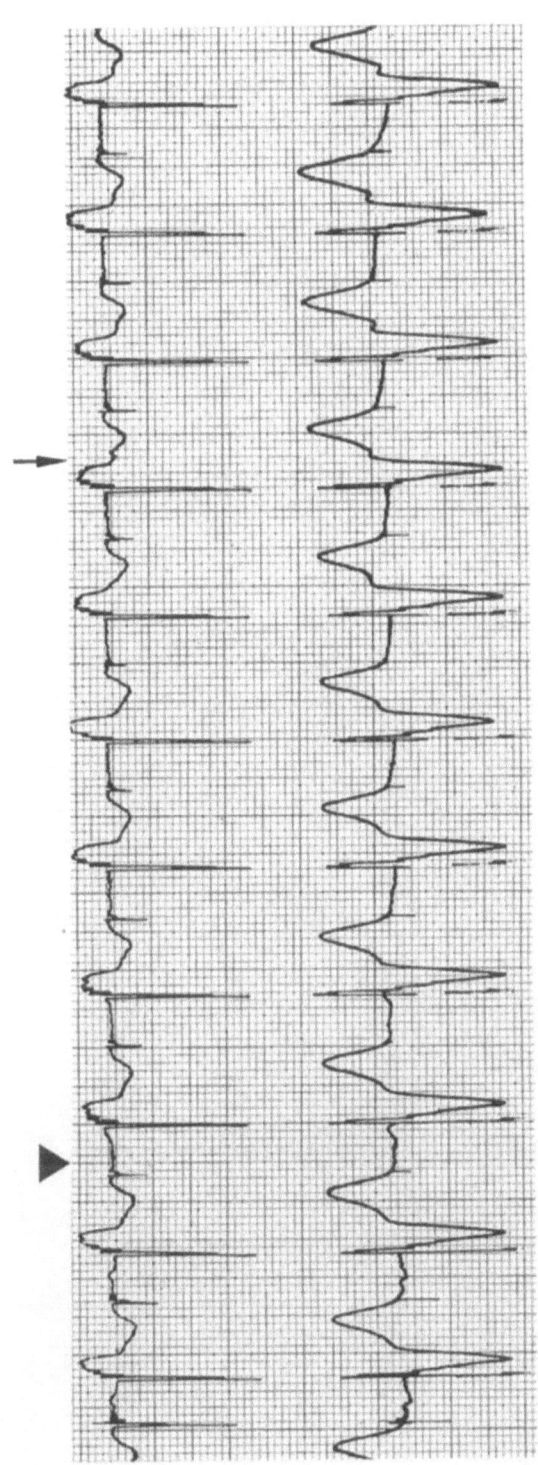

**Fig. 8.36.** Manual measurement of atrial pacing threshold by reprogramming. *Left:* effective pacing. *Right:* loss of atrial pacing (*large arrow*) and development of retrograde conduction (*thin arrow*)

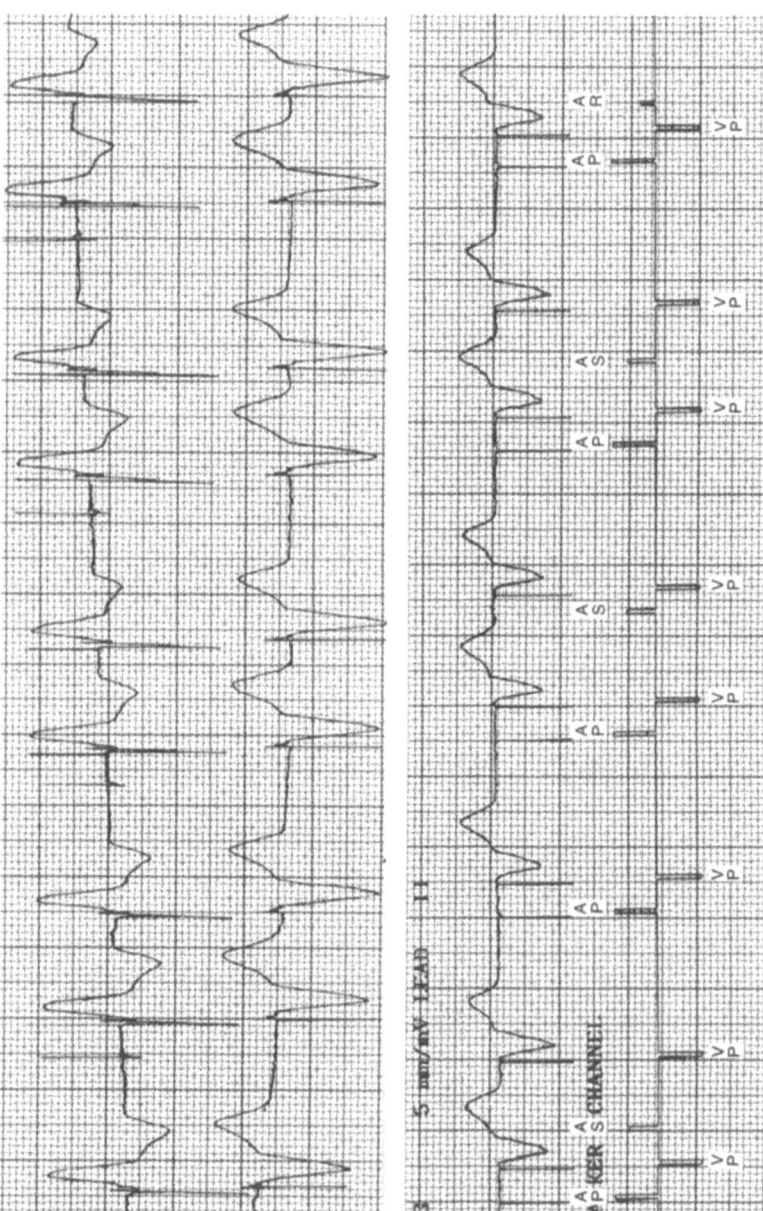

**Fig. 8.37. a** Manual measurement of the atrial pacing threshold by reprogramming in presence of poorly visible P waves. Event markers are helpful in this determination. Some P waves are sensed in the atrial refractory period (*AR*), just after ventricular pacing (*VP*), which indicates loss of atrial pacing (*AP*). *AS* atrial sensing outside the refractory periods.

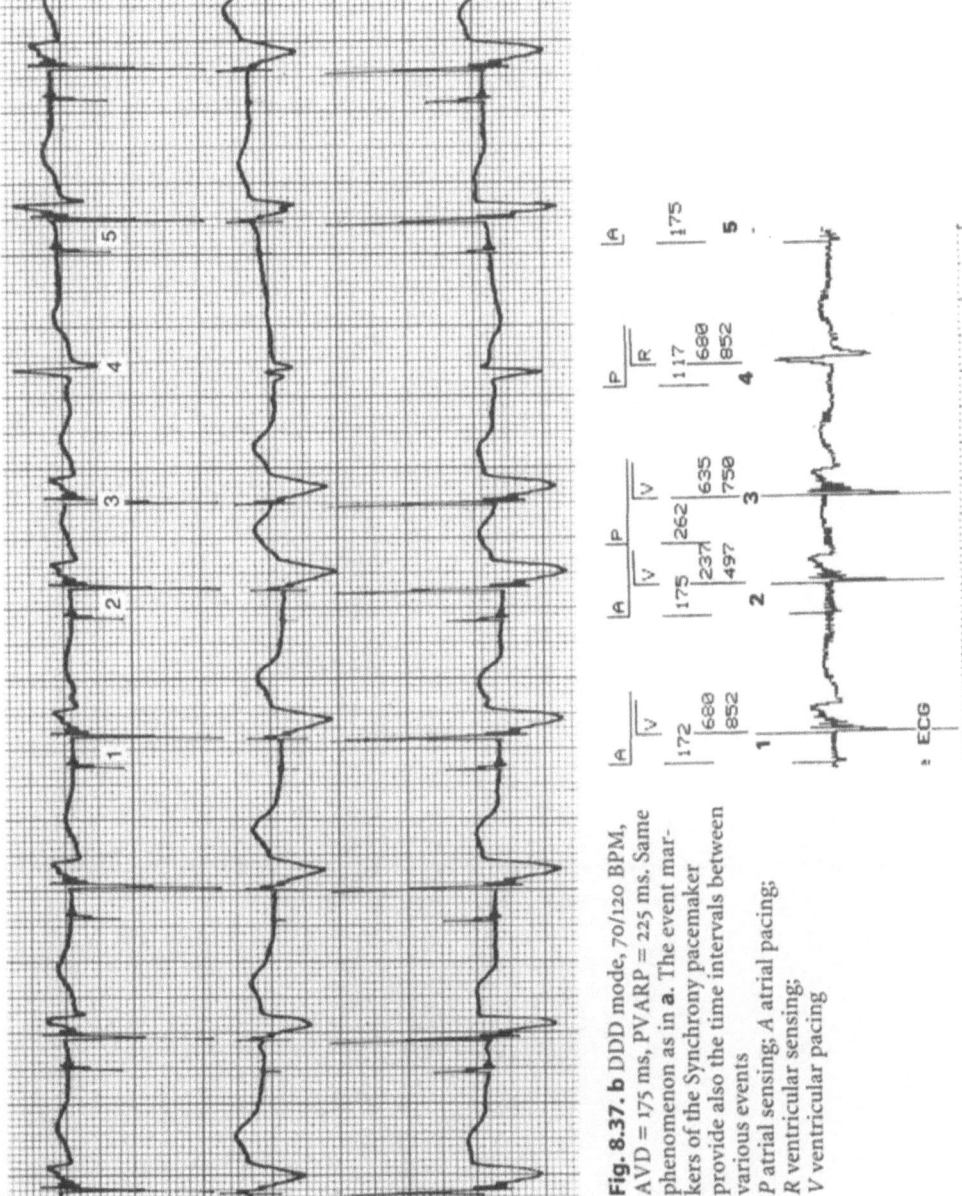

**Fig. 8.37. b** DDD mode, 70/120 BPM, AVD = 175 ms, PVARP = 225 ms. Same phenomenon as in **a**. The event markers of the Synchrony pacemaker provide also the time intervals between various events

*P* atrial sensing; *A* atrial pacing; *R* ventricular sensing; *V* ventricular pacing

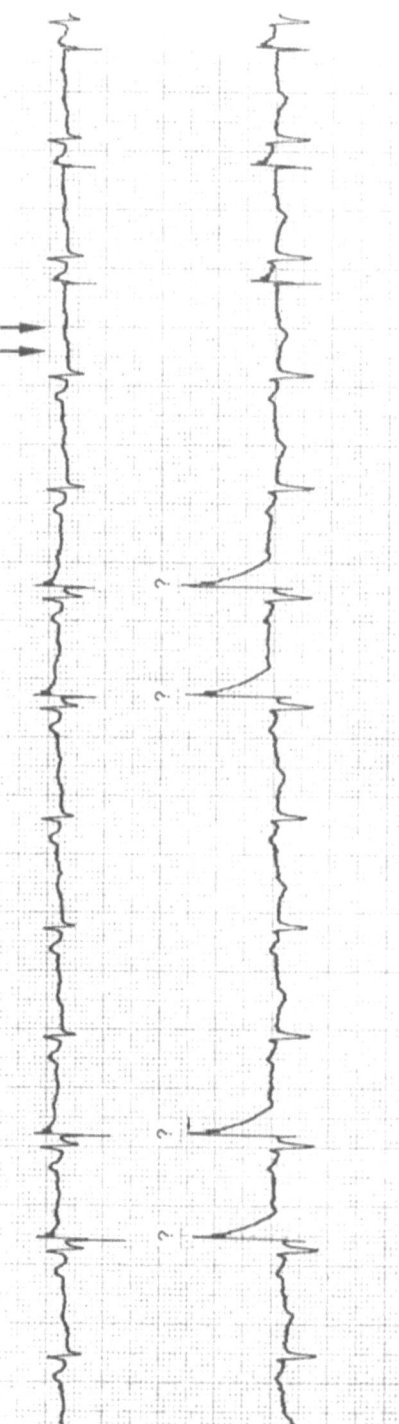

**Fig. 8.38.** DDD mode, 70/100 BPM; AVD = 260 ms; PVARP = 370 ms; atrial sensitivity = 0.6 mV; ventricular sensitivity = 4 mV. The pacing spikes marked with interrogation points and of similar appearance are ventricular. When the atrium is paced (*end of tracing*) during carotid sinus massage (*double arrow*), the atrial pacing spikes have an entirely different appearance. The ventricular pacing spikes appear at the end of a long AVD because the corresponding QRS complexes are not sensed. Thus, sensing failure is intermittent and can be corrected by increasing the sensitivity

## Atrioventricular Crosstalk

This is a common complication in dual chamber pacing, probably much more frequent than generally believed. Crosstalk consists of sensing of atrial pacing in the ventricle, which may cause two distinct behaviors: either inhibition of the pacemaker with risk of ventricular asystole and syncope in a pacemaker dependent patient and in absence of a safety window (Figs. 8.39, 8.40), or ventricular pacing at the end of the safety window (Figs. 8.41, 8.42).

Crosstalk is facilitated by the following factors, particularly when combined:

- High lower rate (Fig. 8.43)
- High atrial pacing output
- High ventricular sensitivity
- Unipolar atrial pacing and ventricular sensing configuration
- Short blanking period

Elimination of crosstalk requires the reprogramming of one or several of the parameters listed above, preferably the ventricular blanking period, knowing that some pacemakers are more susceptible than others. Caution must be exercised when programming a long ventricular blanking period since some late-coupled premature ventricular complex may not be sensed when falling during this period, resulting in the delivery of ventricular pacing at the end of AVD, usually in the vulnerable period of the ventricle (Fig. 8.44), which may be arrhythmogenic. The risk increases with longer AVDs. The same risk may be present in case of atrial sensing failure, as the spontaneous QRS which follows the P wave may fall in the blanking period, at the very moment of delivery of the atrial pulse, at the end of the escape interval, creating the same phenomenon.

## Ventriculo-Atrial Crosstalk

This consists of sensing of the far-field R wave in the atrium. This phenomenon remains usually unnoticed as a result of programming of sufficiently long PVARP. However, with modern pacemakers which provide very short absolute atrial refractory periods (atrial blanking), it is more likely to occur after programming of fall-back function or mode switch. Mode switch may be induced by double counting of the atrial activity, one linked to the normal P wave, and the other to the crosstalk (sensing of the far-field R wave; see p. 105, Fig. 3.51d,e)

## AVD After Paced Versus Sensed P Wave (AV Hysteresis)

This is an important difference (see Fig. 3.26) to take in consideration to optimize hemodynamics or, when AV conduction is preserved, to decrease the number of ventricular fusions.

If AV conduction is preserved, the following procedure can be followed: In VDD mode, with a lower rate below the sinus rate, the AVD is programmed such

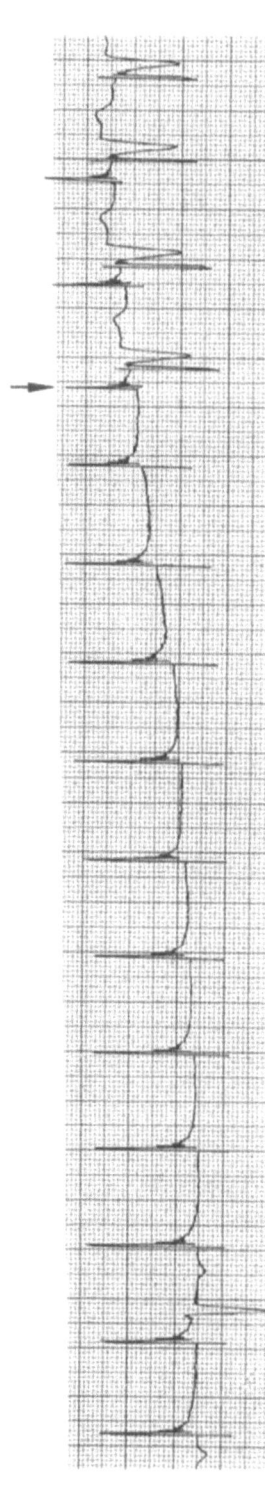

**Fig. 8.39.** DDD mode, AVD = 165 ms, atrial pacing output = 0.5 mV, blanking period = 13 ms. Experimental atrioventricular crosstalk illustrating the danger of pacing without safety window feature
**a** Pure atrial pacing with ventricular asystole; the phenomenon subsides only after emergency reprogramming (*arrow*) by activation of the red key on the programmer

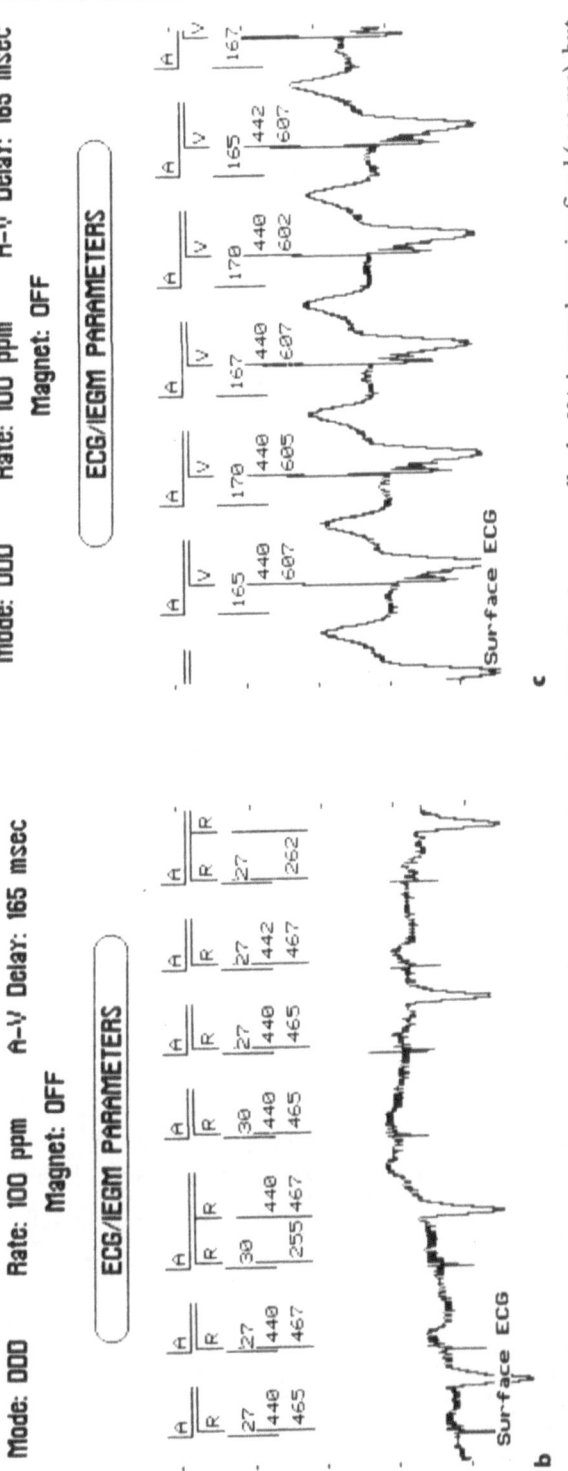

**Fig. 8.39. b** Event markers indicating crosstalk. The programmed rate is 100 BPM. During crosstalk, the VA interval remains fixed (440 ms), but the AVD is replaced by an interval A"R" of 27–30 ms. During crosstalk the pacing rate is approximately 128 BPM because of the AA intervals have shortened to 470 ms (as a consequence of the shortened AVD)
**c** Event markers showing return to normal function. AA has lengthened as the result of return of normal ventricular pacing at the end of the programmed AVD. The AA interval = 607 ms, and DAV = 165 ms, as programmed. Timing of this pacemaker is based on ventricular events

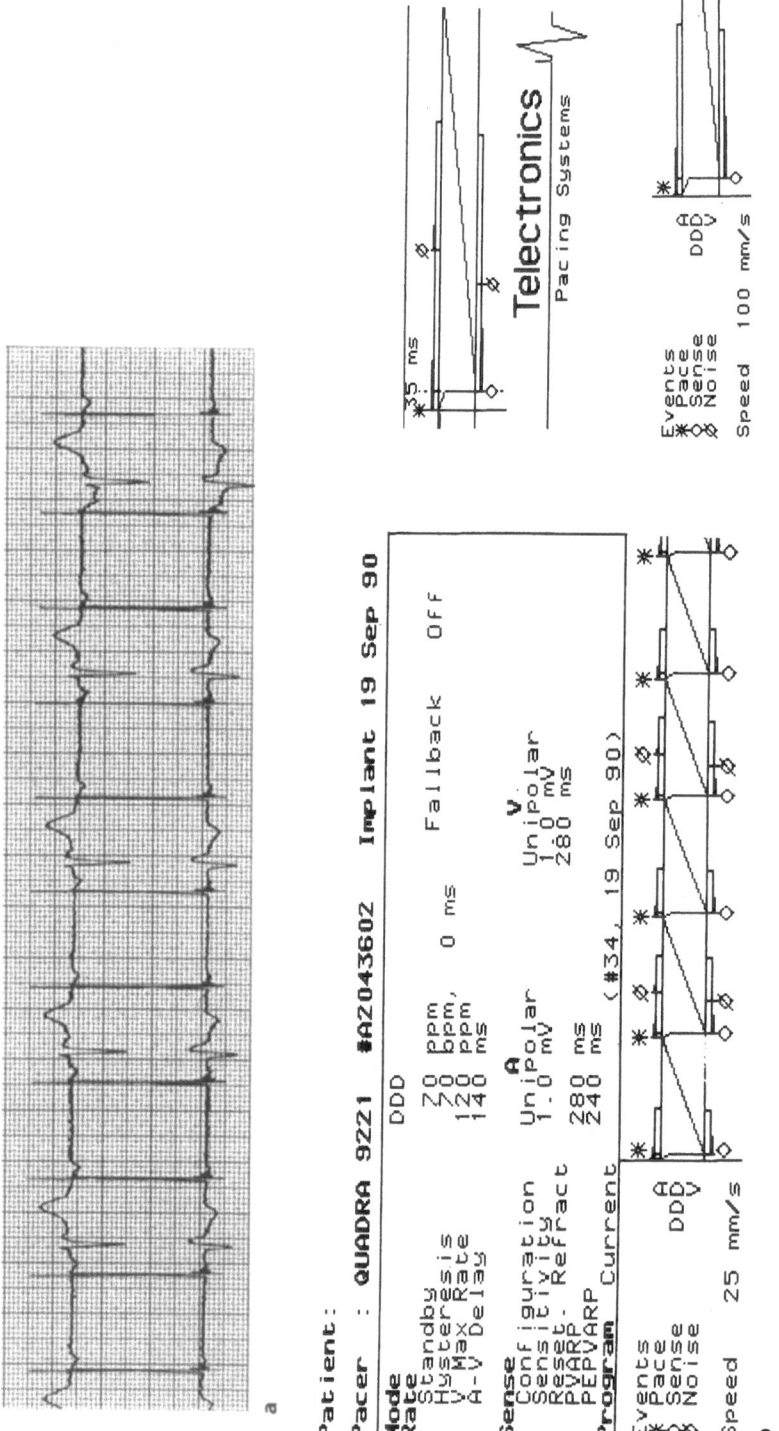

**Fig. 8.40. a** Atrioventricular crosstalk with acceleration of the atrial pacing rate. the A "R" interval is 35 ms
**b** The spontaneous R waves (2 : 1 AV block) are noted by the system, but fall within the ventricular refractory period. The end of the R wave is noted in the atrial channel as noise during the atrial refractory period

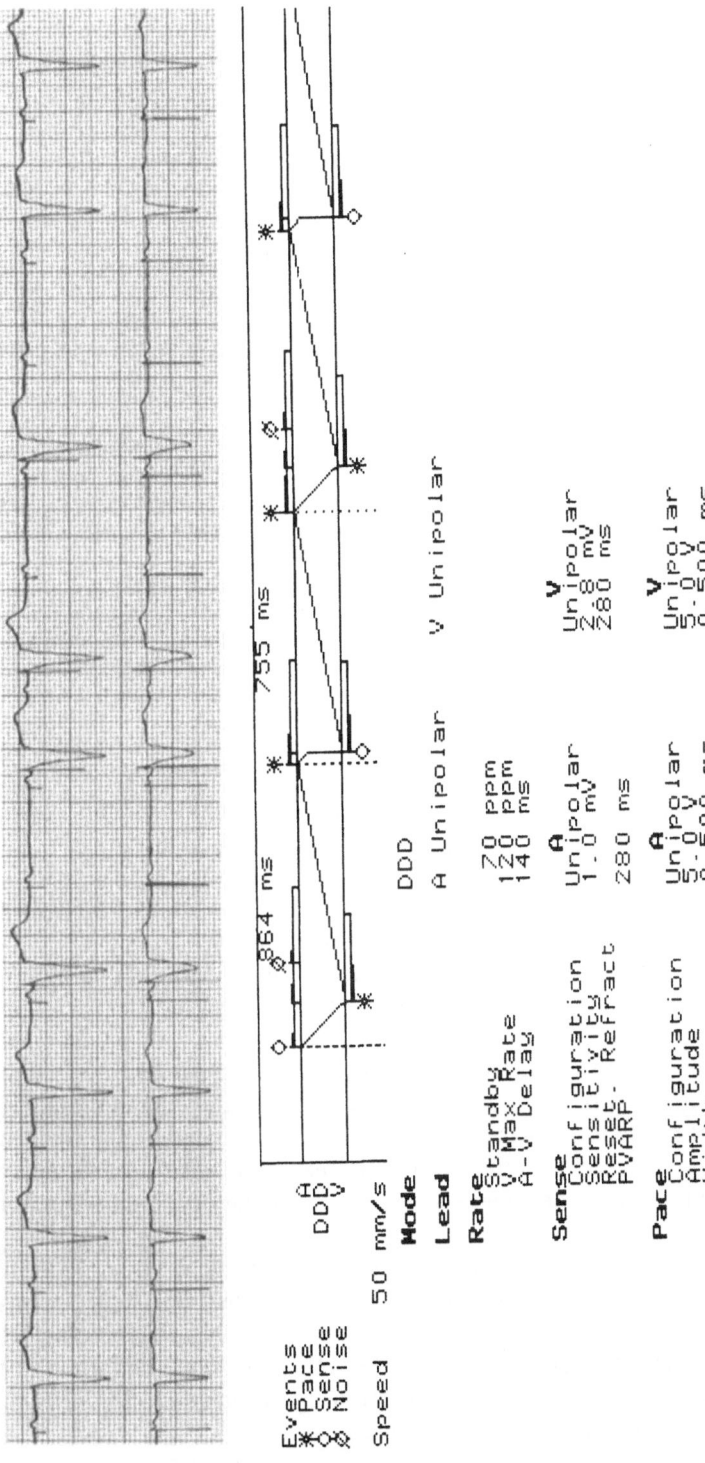

**Fig. 8.41.** 2 : 1 Crosstalk. The event markers printed at a 50 mm/s paper speed confirm the diagnosis: every other atrial stimulus is sensed by the ventricular channel. When two consecutive atrial paced events are not separated by R waves, the AA interval is shorter, excluding the diagnosis of poor ventricular connection

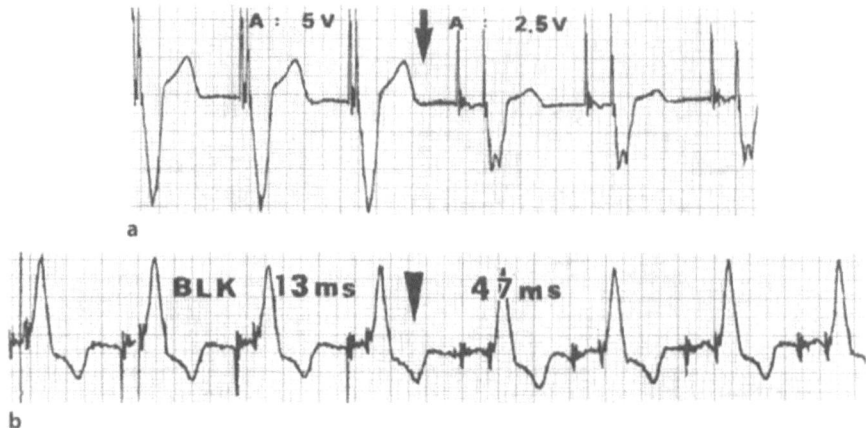

**Fig. 8.42. a** Ventricular based timing of paced events. Lower rate = 70 BPM; AVD = 205 ms. The VA interval is fixed. When the atrial pacing output is set at 5 V instead of 2.5 V, AV crosstalk with safety pacing occours with shortening of the AVD, which explains the faster pacing rate during crosstalk. *Arrow,* reprogramming of the atrial pacing output from 5 to 2.5 V
**b** Lower rate = 90 BPM; AVD = 200 ms. The AA interval is fixed, regardless of the AVD duration. The AVD is 94 ms during crosstalk (blanking period = 13 ms) and ventricular safety pacing. The AVD is 200 ms in absence of crosstalk (blanking period = 47 ms). *Arrow,* reprogramming of the ventricular blanking period from 13 ms to 47 ms

that the ventricular stimulus falls at a predictable time within the QRS to serve as a temporary marker. The lower rate is then programmed just above the sinus rate; next by programming in a stepwise fashion the AVD after a paced P wave, an attempt is made to reproduce the same relationship between the ventricular spike and the spontaneous QRS as was measured during VDD pacing.

In presence of complete AV block, Doppler echocardiography may be helpful. After a sensed P wave, with a DAV on the order of 150 ms, the time interval between the ventricular pacing spike and the peak of the A wave on the ventricular filling phase is measured. The same interval is then measured after a paced P wave. The difference between the two measurements is the value of the difference in AVD that needs to be programmed. After having programmed the nearest value, one should verify that the interval between ventricular stimulus and peak of the A wave is indeed the same as that measured in the VDD mode. The average value is 50–75 ms.

This difference in programmed AVD enters in the calculation of TARP if the pacemaker operates in DDDR, and if the ongoing rhythm is rate responsive. Therefore, the 2:1 pacemaker AV block rate is lower with atrial pacing, which decreases the atrial sensitivity of the system. It is, therefore, important to program a short PVARP and to use the protection algorithm against ELT after verification of its proper operation (see p. 101 ff.).

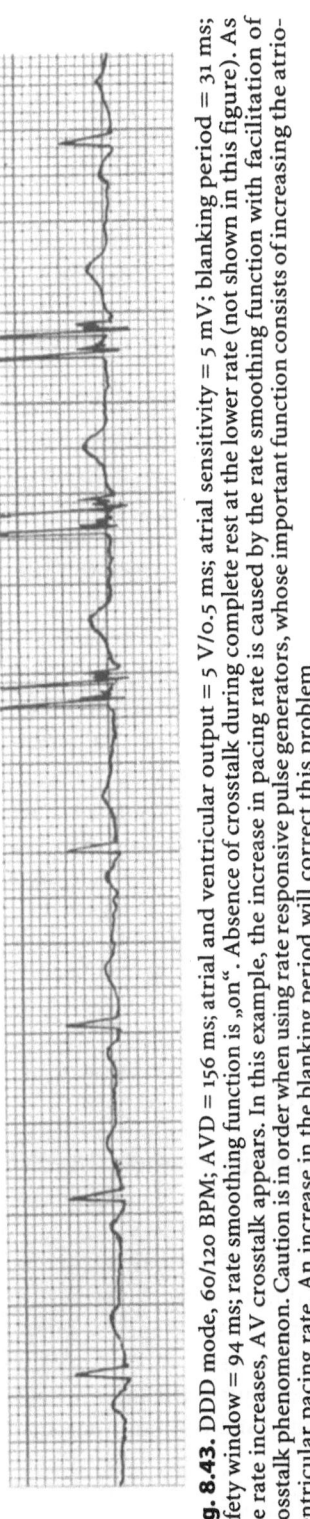

**Fig. 8.43.** DDD mode, 60/120 BPM; AVD = 156 ms; atrial and ventricular output = 5 V/0.5 ms; atrial sensitivity = 5 mV; blanking period = 31 ms; safety window = 94 ms; rate smoothing function is „on". Absence of crosstalk during complete rest at the lower rate (not shown in this figure). As the rate increases, the increase in pacing rate is caused by the rate smoothing function with facilitation of crosstalk phenomenon. In this example, AV crosstalk appears. Caution is in order when using rate responsive pulse generators, whose important function consists of increasing the atrio-ventricular pacing rate. An increase in the blanking period will correct this problem

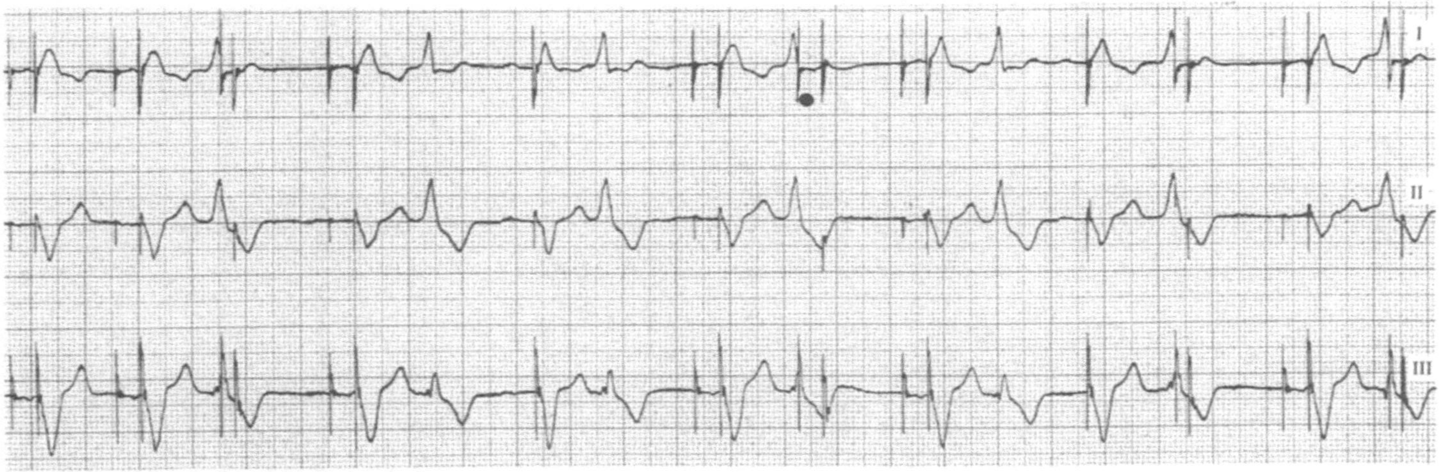

**Fig. 8.44.** DDD mode, 75/142 BPM; AVD = 200 ms; atrial and ventricular pacing output = 5 V/0.5 ms; ventricular sensitivity = 2.5 mV; blanking period = 47 ms; safety window = 94 ms. Late-coupled ventricular extrasystoles overlapped by atrial pacing and, consequently falling inside or outside of the blanking period. When the extrasystole falls past the blanking period, it is sensed and a ventricular pulse is delivered at the end of the safety window, 94 ms after the atrial spike (3rd, 10th and 12th paced events). If falling within the blanking period, they are not sensed and the pacemaker delivers a ventricular pulse at the end of AVD, 200 ms after the atrial spike (*dot*) and may fall in the vulnerable period. This may cause dangerous ventricular tachyarrhythmias

## Atrioventricular Delay (AVD)

The AVD is an important component of the preservation of normal physiology (see p. 186). If the AV conduction time is normal, and neither obstructive cardiomyopathy nor exercise-induced atrioventricular block is present, one may program a longer AVD than the patient's native PR interval; otherwise, the 2 : 1 pacemaker AV block rate is considerably lowered which increases the risk of induction of ELT (see p. 96). This is practical only when AV block is paroxysmal and infrequent. In these same circumstances, one may also use the AVD hysteresis function (Vitatron, Pacesetter) or the automatic mode switch from AAI to DDD (ELA Medical Chorus II, Chorum and Talent).

In a patient suffering from obstructive cardiomyopathy, the AVD must be programmed 80–100 ms shorter than the spontaneous PR interval to impose ventricular pacing, which is beneficial in this disorder (see p. 184). The PR interval may change over time either from the evolution of the underlying heart disease, or, more likely, as a result of changes in drug therapy. To guarantee stable ventricular capture in patients with obstructive hypertrophic cardiomyopathy, the Trilogy (Pacesetter) pacemaker offers a programmable negative AV search hysteresis as a function of the measured PR interval. However, this may mean an excessively short AVD in a patient suffering from poor left ventricular compliance and who is no longer taking full advantage of AV synchrony. Consideration should, then, be given to higher doses of negatively dromotropic drugs, to biatrial resynchronization, or to ablation of the AV junction.

In contrast, in absence of obstructive cardiomyopathy, but in presence of 1st degree AV block, it has been shown that the AVD should preferably be adjusted according to the rules prescribed for complete AV block. In such cases, an algorithm of automatic rate-related AVD shortening is desirable (Fig. 8.45; see also Chap. 4). As discussed before, the optimal AVD duration in the VDD mode is between 80 and 120 ms at rest, and between 50 and 100 ms during exercise. Its optimal individual setting (at least at rest) may require Doppler echocardiography.

A simple echocardiographic technique is available to set the AVD at an optimal value. As stated earlier, if the AVD is too short, the A wave is truncated by the beginning of ventricular systole. If it is too long, the atrioventricular valve closes and remains closed up to the time of onset of ventricular systole. The difference between programmed AVDs is longer than the difference between the ventricular spike-to-end-of-A wave intervals (since when the AVD is programmed short, the A wave is truncated). The part of the A wave that is truncated when the AVD is programmed too short has a duration which, in theory, should be equal to the difference between the programmed AVDs and the intervals from ventricular spike to the end of A wave. Consequently, this calculated difference added to the short tested AVD should coincide with the optimal AVD, i.e. the AVD which guarantees the longest filling time without interruption of the A wave.

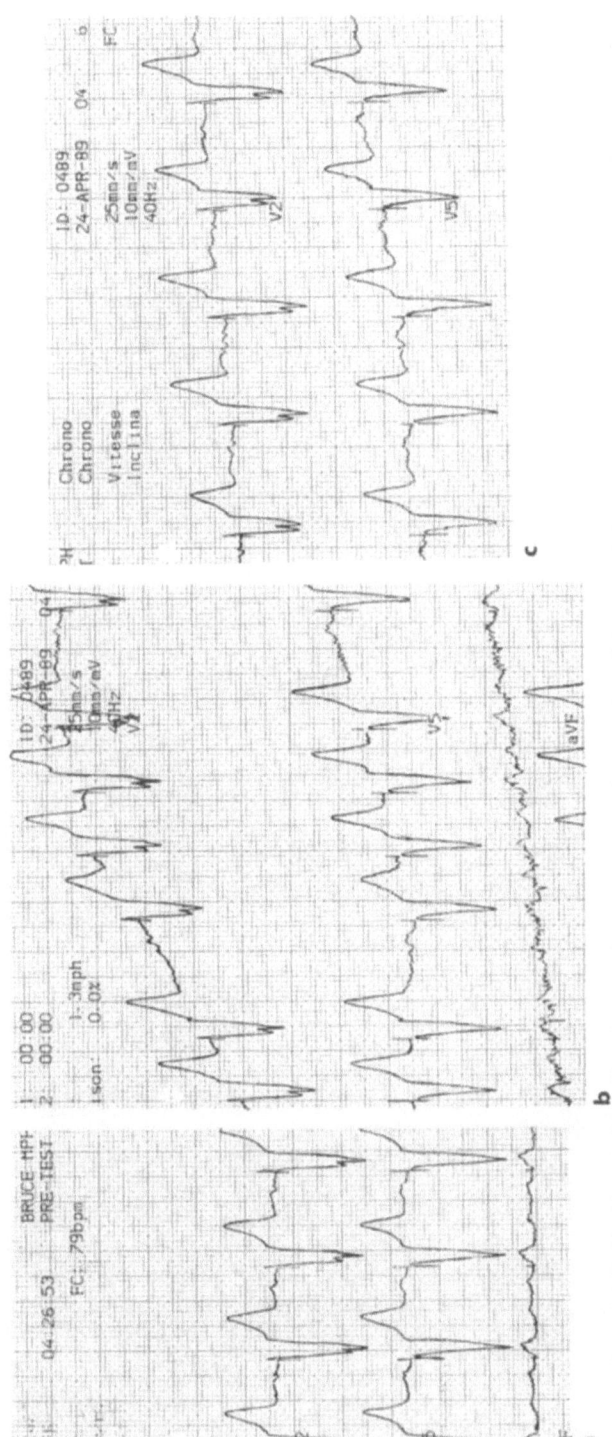

**Fig. 8.45a–d.** DDD mode 50/120 BPM; fixed AVD = 156 ms; PVARP = 297 ms

**a** Proper atrioventricular synchronization at rest

**b** Shift to Wenckebach phenomenon at the onset of exercise, when the sinus rate has crossed the programmed upper rate

**c** When the sinus rate has crossed the maximal atrial sensing rate (AVD + PVARP = 156 + 297 ms = 132 BPM) every other P wave falls in PVARP, and the AV association is 2 : 1; i.e. the ventricular pacing rate falls down to the half of the spontaneous atrial rate

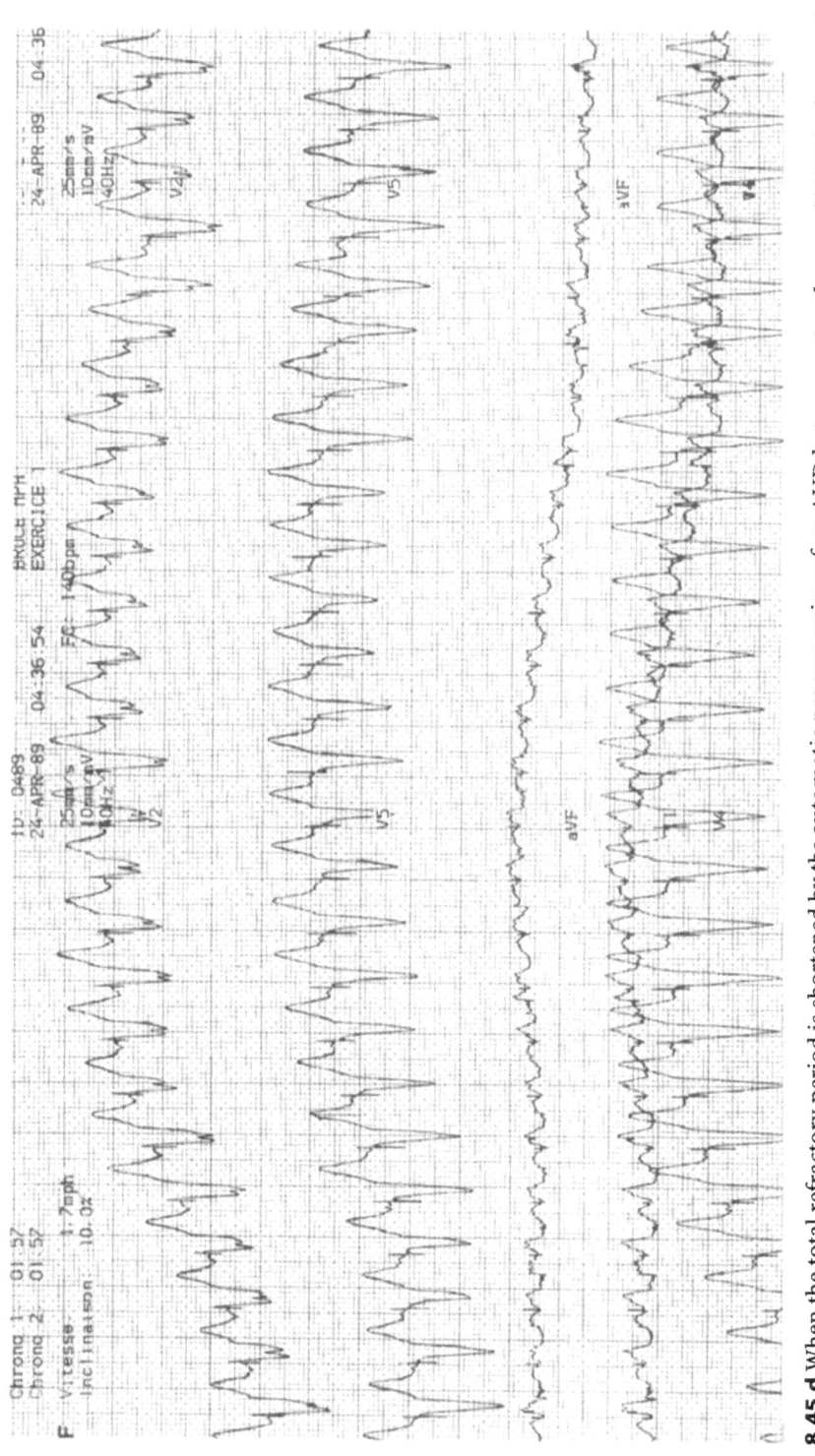

**Fig. 8.45.d** When the total refractory period is shortened by the automatic programming of an AVD between 156 and 47 ms, TARP is shortened (AVD + PVARP = 47 + 297 ms = 174 BPM), and the upper rate may be increased to 154 BPM to maintain 1 : 1 AV association during exercise

The following formula:

{[Long AVD - short AVD] - [(ventricular spike-mitral valve closure)short AVD - (ventricular spike-mitral valve closure)long AVD]} + short AVD = optimal AVD

has been tested is dozens of patients and, when compared with more classical methods, has yielded satisfactory results (see also p. 191, Chap. 4).

An automatic system computing the optimal AVD would be ideal. Sorin has suggested a measure of the Peak Endocardial Acceleration as a function of the programmed AVD to optimize its value, which would allow its automatic programming. Indeed, when a short AVD has been programmed, the mitral valve closes abruptly, interrupting the atrial systolic flow, generating additional vibrations. The PEA amplitude, thus, correlates with the lowest PEA amplitude, just before its increase, when further shortening of the AVD causes enhanced mitral valvular vibrations. However, this concept is still being examined experimentally.

## The Postventricular Atrial Refractory Period (PVARP)

Setting of the PVARP depends on the availability and effectiveness of an anti ELT algorithm. If the algorithm is not available, or ineffective, programming of PVARP must be longer than the retrograde conduction time, at the cost of lowering the 2 : 1 pacemaker AV block rate. Indeed, the discrimination of sinus P waves versus retrograde P waves by the programmed atrial sensitivity is rarely possible (Fig. 8.46). The retrograde conduction time may be measured by the event markers or with the help of electrograms while pacing in the VVI mode at a rate above the sinus rate. Testing of protection algorithms against ELT requires the induction of the tachycardia by pacing at a rate above the sinus rate, with the highest atrial sensitivity, a very short PVARP, and a subthreshold atrial pacing output. In presence of retrograde conduction, the tachycardia will be induced, and the efficacy of the algorithm can be tested. If the rate of ELT is equal to the programmed upper rate, the algorithm can be used and programming of PVARP should be short to enhance atrial sensing. If the rate of ELT is slower than the upper pacing rate and if the pacemaker is unable to recognize it, it is advised to program a PVARP longer than the retrograde conduction time (Fig. 8.47). In a patient who has no retrograde conduction at rest, we prefer short PVARPs as long as the system offers some kind of protection against ELT.

These considerations must be reviewed each time the programming of a high 2 : 1 pacemaker AV block rate is needed to sense rapid atrial rhythms or to achieve a fast upper rate, as discussed on p. 88 f.

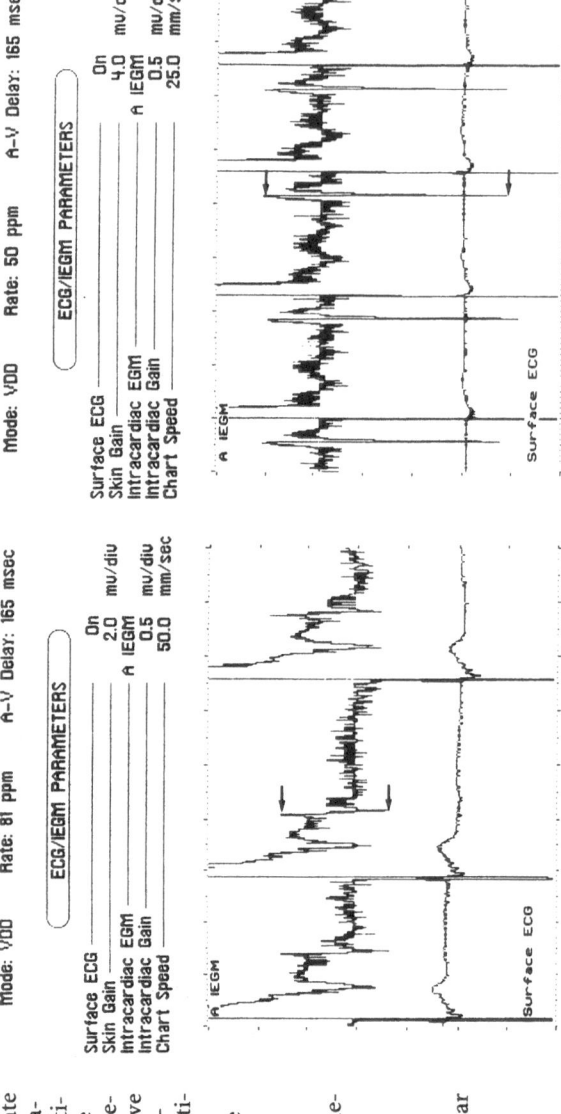

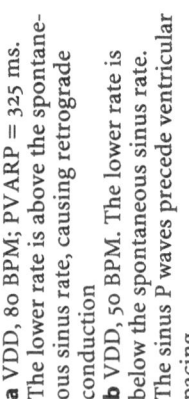

**Fig. 8.46a,b.** Attempt to differentiate retrograde P waves from sinus P waves by programming of atrial sensitivity. In this example, the amplitude of retrograde P wave is approximately one half of that of the sinus P wave (see *horizontal arrows*). It is recommended to program the atrial sensitivity in this way so that the sinus P waves are securely detected and the retrograde P waves are not seen by the pacemaker
**a** VDD, 80 BPM; PVARP = 325 ms. The lower rate is above the spontaneous sinus rate, causing retrograde conduction
**b** VDD, 50 BPM. The lower rate is below the spontaneous sinus rate. The sinus P waves precede ventricular pacing

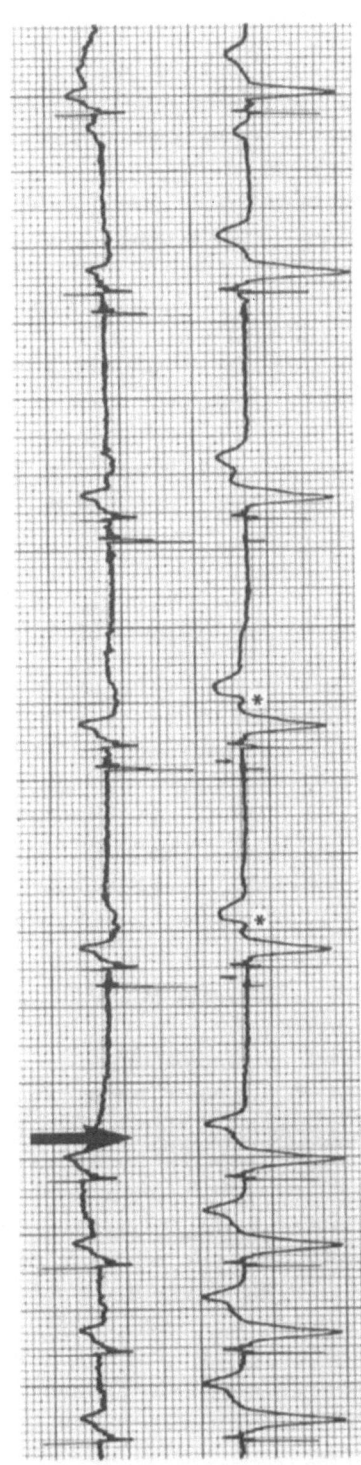

**Fig. 8.47.** Typical mode of interruption of ELT, here at the upper rate (130 BPM): PVARP was increased from 250 to 325 ms (*arrow*). Note the persistence of retrograde conduction behind the three post tachycardia QRS complexes. This is made possible by the ineffective atrial stimulation. However, ELT is not reinduced because each retrograde P wave (*) falls in PVARP

## Other Parameters

The *upper rate* is usually programmed faster than the patient's peak exercise heart rate, but should be programmed at a slower rate in presence of known coronary heart disease, aortic stenosis, or atrial arrhythmias without effective protective algorithm.

No strict rule has been formulated for the programming of the *lower rate*. We prefer to program it slow in a patient with coronary heart disease, and faster in presence of paroxysmal atrial arrhythmias (as a preventive measure).

The *protection function against atrial arrhythmias* should be chosen systematically, if available (see p. 146 ff.).

The indications for *rate responsiveness* have been discussed on p. 186. Each sensor must be tested during exercise, according to the usual practice, equipment and experience of individual implanting centers, and to the patient's functional capacity and underlying disease. Because of the constraints on the operation of the pacemaker represented by rate responsive pacing, the latter should only be used when clearly indicated (see p. 200). One should simply remember to minimize the competition between rate responsiveness and spontaneous rate to lower the risk of proarrhythmia (see Fig. 8.50).

Rate responsiveness should preferably be used only:

- In cases of symptomatic chronotropic incompetence.
- In cases of sudden variations in sinus rate due to sinus arrest, rate responsiveness acting as a smoothing function; however, in this situation, rate responsiveness should remain in the background with respect to the spontaneous rate, ideally in conjunction with rate hysteresis.
- As an element controlling the ventricular rate in patients with high degree AV block at the time of mode switch due to paroxysmal atrial arrhythmias. In all cases, the upper responsive rate should be kept in a range low enough to avoid adverse effects.

Programming of complex functions will not be discussed here. Instead, the reader is referred to the written recommendations found in the physician's manual printed by each manufacturer.

The exercise test, which we recommend as a routine procedure in the 3 months after implantation for all dual chamber and rate responsive systems, may reveal unusual behavior. The main goals of the test consist of verifying the integrity of atrial sensing, the absence of crosstalk and myosignal inhibition, and of rhythm disturbances that might interfere with pacing, as well as the proper programming of AVD, of rate responsiveness, and of the upper rate. In our experience, revision of the programming of one or more parameters is necessary in nearly 60% of cases (Figs. 8.48 – 8.53).

The description of this follow-up procedure cannot be comprehensive since it depends partially on the device model and on each patient and underlying pathology. This is particularly applicable to the special functions, while the basic parameters are typically examined according to the check list suggested in this chapter.

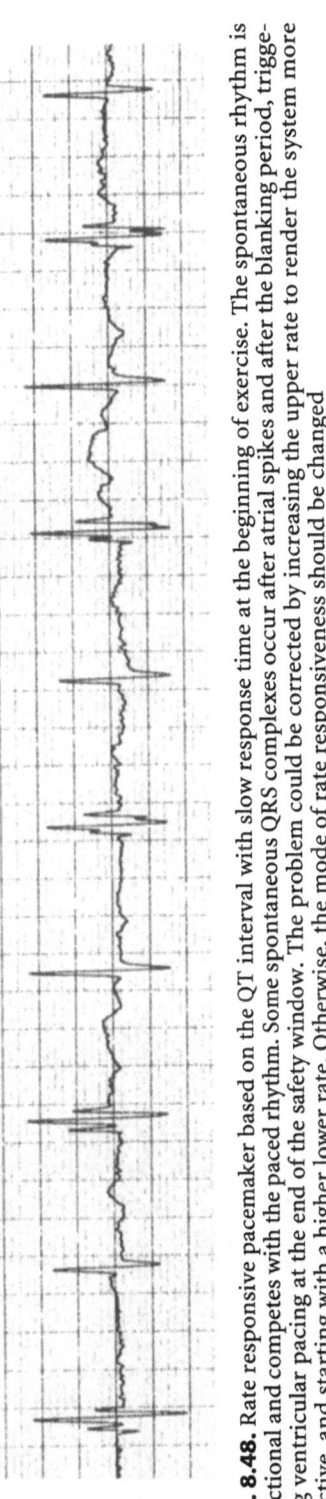

**Fig. 8.48.** Rate responsive pacemaker based on the QT interval with slow response time at the beginning of exercise. The spontaneous rhythm is junctional and competes with the paced rhythm. Some spontaneous QRS complexes occur after atrial spikes and after the blanking period, triggering ventricular pacing at the end of the safety window. The problem could be corrected by increasing the upper rate to render the system more reactive, and starting with a higher lower rate. Otherwise, the mode of rate responsiveness should be changed

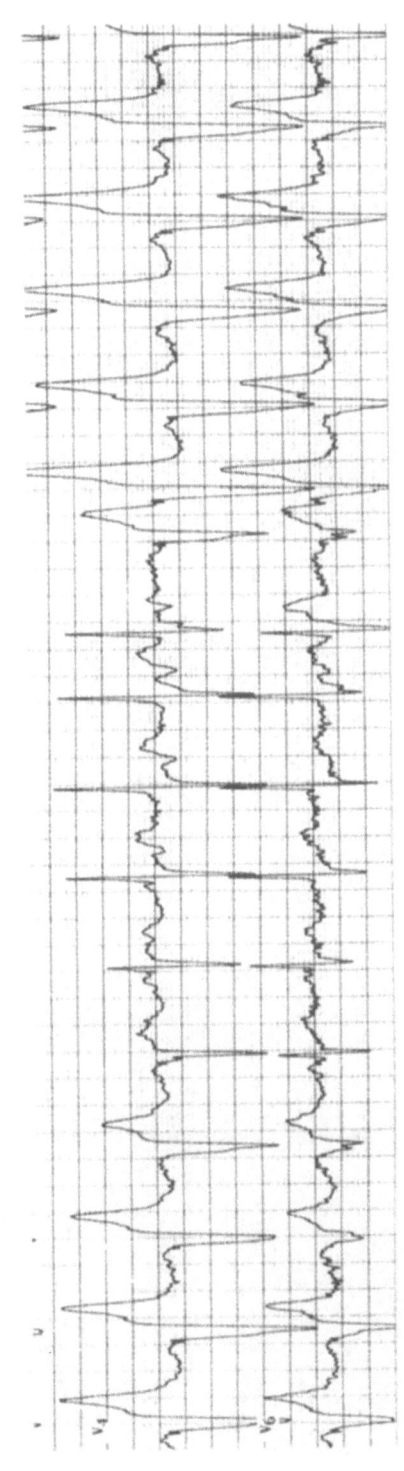

**Fig. 8.49.** DDD pacemaker implanted in a patient with 2 : 1, second degree AV block. The atrial rate has crossed the maximal atrial tracking rate ( 2 : 1 pacemaker AV block rate), inducing 2 : 1 response. In addition, some P waves are no longer sensed, allowing the appearance of spontaneous QRS complexes

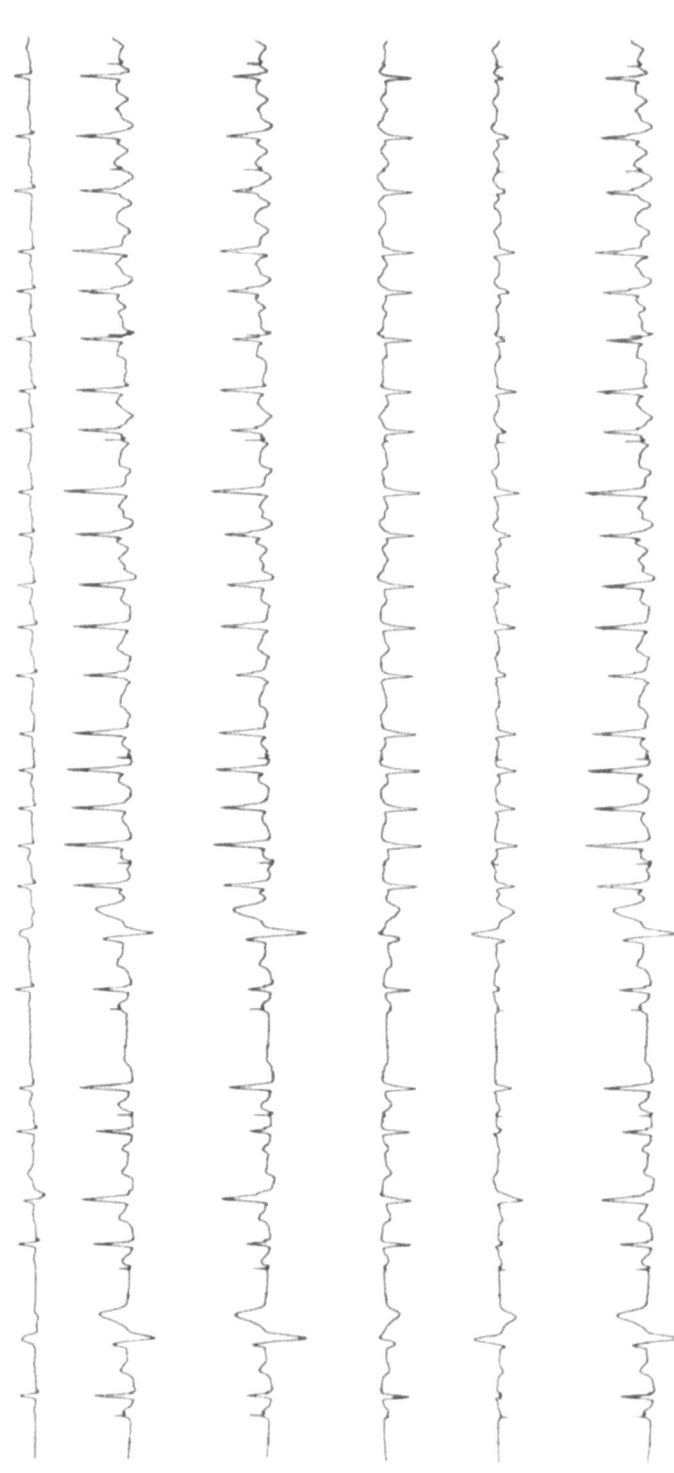

**Fig. 8.50.** Sensing failure of an AAI pacemaker with triggering of an atrial arrhythmia during exercise

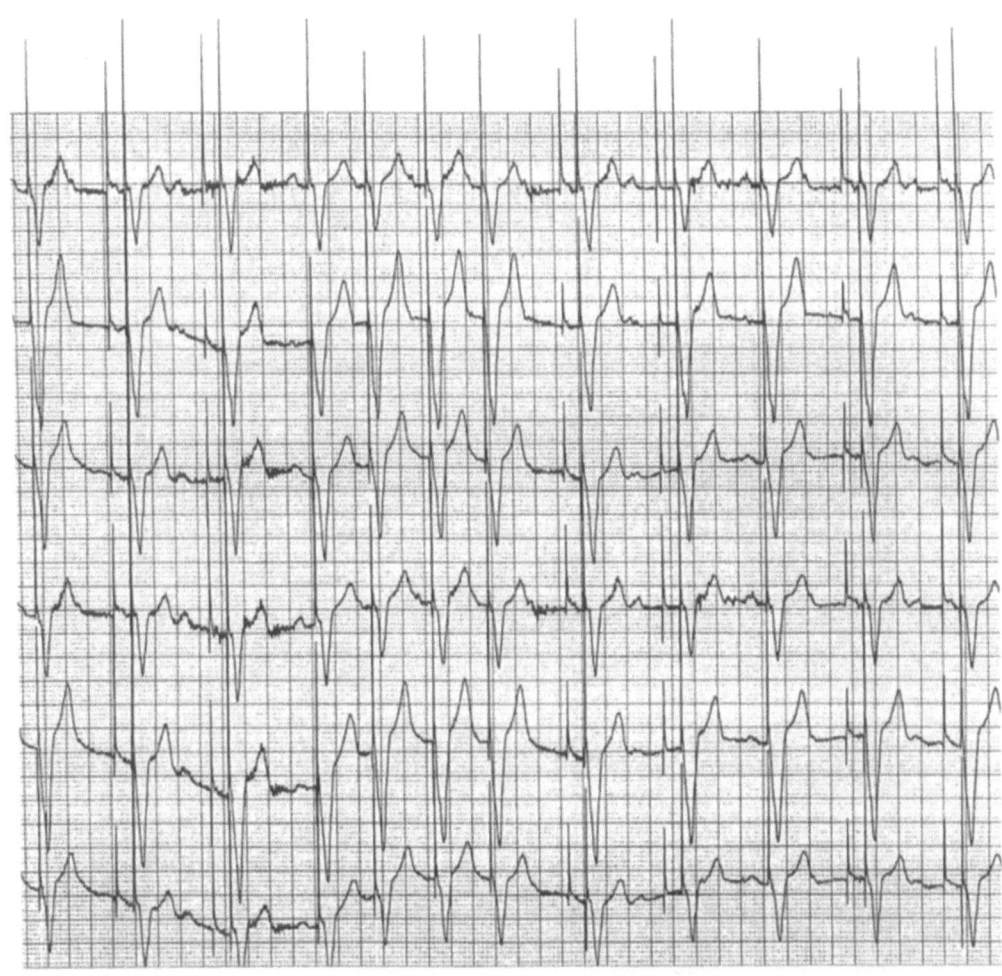

**Fig. 8.51.** Intermittent atrial sensing failure during exercise at an atrial sensitivity of 0.5 mV, whereas sensing was flawless at 3.5 mV at rest

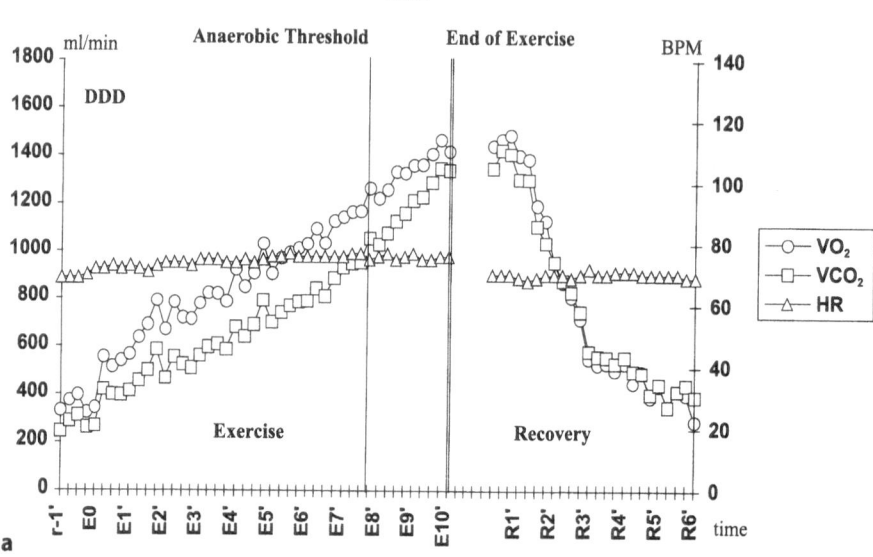

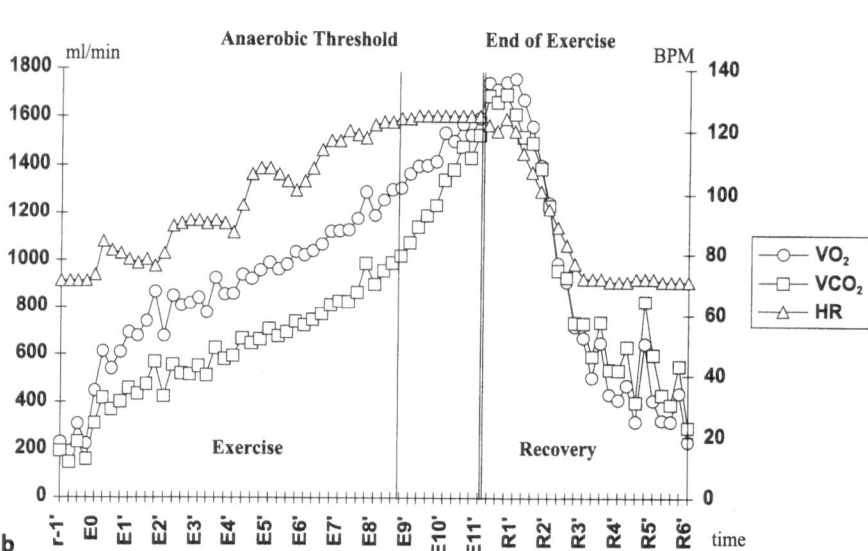

**Fig. 8.52. a** DDD mode cardiorespiratory stress test in a patient with severe chronotropic incompetence. The atrial rate did not exceed 75 BPM. The exercise lasted 10 min 15 s with a maximum $VO_2$ of 1480 ml/min. The anaerobic threshold was obtained after 8 min of exercise for a $VO_2$ of 1180 ml/min

**b** DDDR mode cardiorespiratory stress test in the same patient with a maximal programmed sensor rate of 130 BPM and with the same exercise profile. The exercise lasted 11 min with a maximum $VO_2$ of 1650 ml/min. The anaerobic threshold was obtained after 8 min 45 s of exercise for a $VO_2$ of 1350 ml/min and a heart rate of 120 BPM. The DDDR mode has thus brought a significant benefit in terms of exercise duration and of metabolic performance compared to the DDD mode stress test

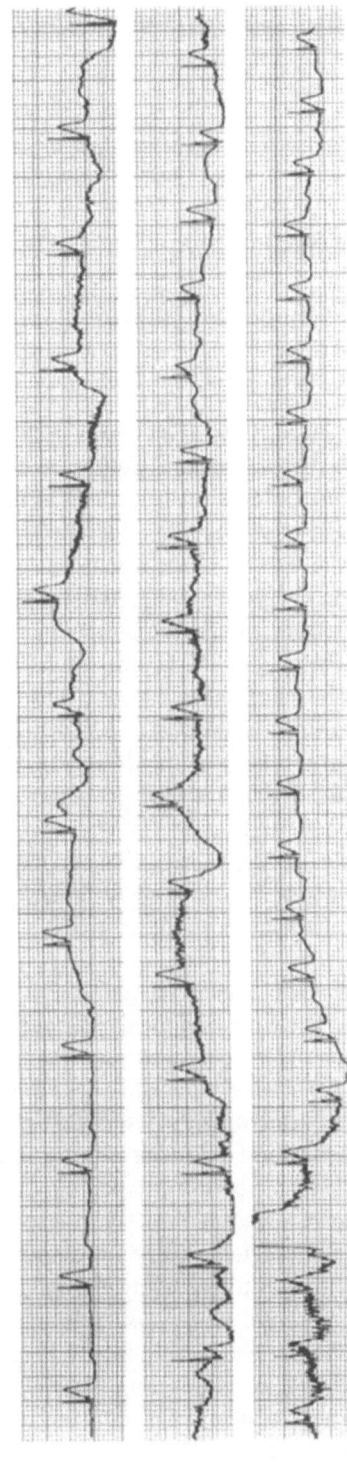

**Fig. 8.53.** Excessive rate response in a patient with activity driven (activity sensor) pacemaker, causing palpitation during moderate effort

# CHAPTER 9

# Pulse Generator and/or Lead Replacement

## 9.1
## Reasons for Replacement of the Implanted Material

### Indications for Replacement of the Pulse Generator

The pulse generator needs to be replaced for the following reasons:

- The elective replacement indicator has been reached, according to the manufacturer's prescriptions, and on the basis of magnet rate, and/or pulse duration, and/or measurement of internal impedance of the battery (see p. 272).
- The pacemaker had suffered form severe interference which has destroyed or altered one of its functions (beware of transient dysfunctions). A depleted pulse generator should never be left in place because of its possible interaction with the newly implanted material.
- The pacemaker can no longer be interrogated or programmed.
- The pacemaker causes a different behavior than that which has been programmed, even after having explored all possible solutions by modifying the program. One should refrain from incriminating the device since, a priori, most programming problems can be solved provided a precise diagnosis has been made.
- The device has been recalled by the manufacturer. In a pacemaker dependent patient, we proceed systematically with replacement of the device when the manufacturer advises closer surveillance because of an unusually high incidence of failure.
- An infection or erosion of the system has developed.
- At the time of a local intervention (lead exchange, revision of the pocket), if the pulse generator has already been in place for several years and has a life expectancy reduced to less that 50%. The life expectancy can be calculated with the formula described on p. 39.
- As the end of life of the pulse generator is approaching, and it becomes necessary to reprogram pacing output such that the energy consumption is increased, one runs the risk to shorten the end of life from overconsumption of a depleted battery. In pacemaker-dependent patients, consideration should be given to replacing the pulse generator as the end of life is approaching, before the actual onset of the indicator.
- The patient is disabled by pectoral muscle stimulation and a conversion to bipolar pacing is not possible.
- The pacing mode is modified (addition of a second lead, need for rate responsiveness).

## Indications for Lead Replacement

The pacing lead needs to be replaced for the following reasons:

- Conductor fracture or insulation failure.
- Infection or erosion.
- The lead is bipolar but functions only in a unipolar configuration.
- The lead is old and made of polyurethane, belonging to a defective series (examples: Medtronic lead models 6972, 4012, 4004, 4082).
- The lead has been damaged at the time of pulse generator replacement, and is bipolar or made of polyurethane.
- Poor electrical characteristics measured at the time of pulse generator replacement from chronic rise in threshold or intercurrent infarction at the site of electrode implantation (pacing threshold current $> 3$ mA/0.5 ms), unacceptably high sensing threshold, inordinately low ($< 300$ $\Omega$) or high ($> 1500$ $\Omega$, except in „high Ohm leads") impedance.
- A bipolar configuration is obligatory and the existing lead is unipolar.
- The lead is epicardial and older than 10 years, beyond which the failure rate is approximately 2% per year.
- A specific type of rate responsiveness is needed, requiring the use of a special lead.

## Grounds for Changing the Pacing Mode

Changes in the pacing mode are made in the following situations:

- From VVI/VVIR to DDD/DDDR, systematically if the patient has remained in sinus rhythm at the time of replacement of a depleted VVI pacemaker, observing the indications that were listed in Chap. 4. The conversion should be made earlier in presence of VVI/VVIR pacemaker syndrome, or in case of recurrent syncope or near syncope in carotid sinus hypersensitivity or vaso-vagal syndrome.
- From VVI to VVIR when the patient with atrial fibrillation has developed slow ventricular response without appropriate rate acceleration during exercise.
- From AAI to DDD/DDDR when AV conduction abnormalities appear. The conversion is made selectively at the time of pulse generator replacement for bundle branch block or PR prolongation, and earlier in case of higher degree AV block or significant prolongation of the Wenckebach cycle.
- From AAIR to DDDR for the same indications and in the case of AAIR pacemaker syndrome (see p. 197).
- From DDD to VVI/VVIR if a permanent atrial tachyarrhythmia has developed despite therapeutic efforts to suppress it.
- From AAI/AAIR to VVI/VVIR for the same indications and if AV block is present. VVIR will be chosen in case of chronotropic incompetence.

## 9.2
## Reintervention Techniques

A reintervention results from a logical decision process based on notions that have been described in Chap. 5. Emergency reinterventions to be performed before an accurate diagnosis has been posed are rare. In emergency cases, temporary reprogramming or temporary pacing, usually provide enough time to prepare for a reintervention under the best possible conditions.

The expertise of the operator is even more important than in an original implant because of considerations of connectors' compatibility which will be thoroughly discussed.

### Preparation

One must know precisely what type of lead and pulse generator was implanted and have available the appropriate screw drivers, repair kits, stylets of several sizes from the various manufacturers, adapters, silicone rubber, and mineral oil. The reintervention must have been planned, and the necessary tools selected, in advance. Otherwise, the procedure may be complicated. As in the case of a primary implant, an external pacing system or an infusion of isoproterenol should be ready for pacemaker dependent patients.

### The Procedure

The local anesthesia must be more extensive than in the original procedure because it is less effective in scar tissue where it diffuses poorly. Care should be taken not to puncture a previously implanted lead since it may damage the insulation and cause a subsequent current leak. If the pulse generator has not migrated, the same incision is used; otherwise, a different incision will need to be performed at the superior edge of the pulse generator.

The approach to the pacemaker must be careful, without electrocautery in pacing dependent patients because of the risk of damage to the device complicated by asystole. The leads must be spared as the can is being approached; failure to do so means repair, or even replacement of an irreparable lead. Dissection, instead of cutting, proceeds plane by plane, down to the pulse generator which can be palpated and becomes finally visible through the thinned, transparent wall of the pocket.

A small opening of the pocket is made over the can, and with the assistance of a retractor, extended with the tip of the scissors under visual control, perhaps guided by palpation to locate the leads, until wide enough to proceed with extraction of the device. A heavy, blunt, atraumatic clamp is used to grasp the pulse generator without crushing the implanted electrode(s).

When a unipolar pacemaker is being extracted, one watches the oscilloscope to determine the pacemaker dependency of the patient, knowing that the reinsertion of a corner of the device is enough to reestablish electrical continuity. The can must be extractable without difficulty. Scar tissue obliterating the connector is dissected away. If the lead is encased in fibrotic tissue, it can be freed with electrocautery along its tract, as long as it is made of silicone. If it is made of polyurethane, the lead must be dissected with great care, since the electrical scalpel can damage its insulation. One must avoid pulling on the lead in an attempt to widen the workable surface; this maneuver, as any other coarse maneuver, may damage the insulation, the conductor and/or the lead connector.

Sterile cables are needed to test thresholds and are prepared and connected to an external pacing system set at a high output and at a rate adjusted according to the patient's sinus rate. At the implant site, the positive pole (red) is connected to a self retractor in contact with the tissues. The lead is disconnected with the tools appropriate for the implanted model. Disconnection may be tedious, either because the Allen screw is locked, or because the connector are coated with silicone which has to be removed with fine forceps. The disconnection must be atraumatic, by pulling on the lead as close as possible to the pacemaker header, holding it where it has been reinforced, never along its body. Before disconnecting, the patient's pacemaker dependency should be examined by separating the can from the tissues for a few seconds. If the patient is indeed pacemaker dependent, and no external pacing system has been prepared, isoproterenol is administered and the same maneuver is repeated. If the patient remains pacemaker dependent, the interface with the external pacing system must be checked and the disconnection performed while the pulse generator is kept in contact with the tissues. As soon as the lead connector has been freed, it must be interfaced with the negative pole (black) of the pacing system analyzer. Should the external system fail, one can always reconnect the lead to the can. If the disconnection cannot be completed, or if the lead connector has been damaged, a repair is attempted or, after having cut the lead, a connector kit is put in place, scrupulously following the instructions of the adapter's manufacturer.

Finally, if one knows that the lead connector needs to be replaced in a pacemaker dependent patient, that the lead will need to be cut and repaired, and that the lead is made of silicone, one can isolate the conductor a few centimeters away from the connector and interface the negative pole of the pacing system analyzer before cutting the lead. The same procedure can be followed in case of insulation failure or conductor fracture, as long as it is extravascular, can be repaired, and as long as the rest of the lead is intact. In doubt, one proceeds with replacement of the lead.

To disclose an intermittent pacing failure, dynamic maneuvers may be helpful, such as gentle traction on the lead, coughing, deep breathing, while looking for changes in the electrical characteristics of the lead.

After achievement of hemostasis, thresholds are measured according to the same guidelines as during a primary implant (see p. 218 ff.). If the connector of the previously implanted lead is not compatible with the new pulse generator, adapters are available. One should choose the shortest possible kind to minimize the amount of implanted material. Thresholds are retested after the adapter has been connected. Connection problems will be discussed in upcoming pages.

If, in the course of these various maneuvers, the insulation has been cut or damaged, it still can be repaired as long as it is made of silicone and the conductor is intact. This requires to cover the traumatized area with a silicone sleeve, sealed with silicone rubber, and ligated at each end.

If the lead needs to be exchanged for whatever reason, except infection, we prefer to abandon it, unless it has been in place for less than 1 year. If it is abandoned, the least material should be left in place by freeing the lead from the surrounding fibrosis down to a few centimeters from its site of introduction, where it should be cut. The stump must be insulated with a silicone cap tied to the lead body and further sealed with silicone rubber, before burying it in the deep subcutaneous tissues to prevent their erosion.

It the lead must be removed, because of an infection, for instance, it should be freed up to its point of fixation, and handled as described on p. 377 f.

If a new lead is implanted (addition of an atrial lead to convert from VVI to DDD mode, or addition of a ventricular lead to convert from AAI to DDD mode), exclusive of the cases of infection discussed on p. 375 f., another venous approach should be sought as described in chapter 5. One should avoid as much as possible the use of the contralateral side, unless absolutely necessary, since venous accesses must be spared for possible subsequent procedures. An additional incision to gain access to the vein should be made only if the original incision over the pulse generator is distant from it. The procedure, otherwise, is as that of a primary implant. The new lead is fixed to the deep layer and tunneled to the pulse generator.

A new pocket should be prepared for the pulse generator:

- If the wall of the original one is calcified, since a breakdown of electrical communications may occur with a unipolar system, and because calcifications promote infectious complications
- If the device is so superficial as to threaten the skin integrity
- If the can has migrated toward the axilla or to a distant caudal position

The new pocket should be prepared in a usual location, or placed subpectorally if erosion is a concern, as long as the system can be used in a bipolar configuration; the can should be anchored if loose cutaneous tissues mandate it. If the original pocket is preserved, it should be widened to accomodate a larger device, a rare situation nowadays, or partially obliterated if the can is noticeably smaller than the previous one, to prevent the twiddler syndrome. The pulse generator is then connected and placed in the pocket which is closed in layers after it has been rinsed with an antiseptic solution, and after blood and air have been evacuated.

The postoperative surveillance is the same as that described for an original implantation. If no lead was replaced, the patient may be discharged from the hospital the next day; otherwise, the recovery will be as recommended for a primary implant.

## Connection Problems

Until approximately 1976, connection problems were due mostly to the multiplicity of interfaces manufactured, including the mere introduction of the bare conductor wire inside the header, secured by an Allen screw, or the insertion of a fully insulated lead with the contact established by a sharp needle perforating the insulation, or various solutions borrowed from the standard electric industry such as bipolar plugs or unipolar pin connectors.

From 1976 on, a choice was offered between two unipolar pin connectors, 4.75 and 6 mm in size, respectively; in a bipolar system, the connector was bifurcated, 4.75 mm in size. In March 1984, a group of manufacturers introduced a voluntary standard 1, designated as VS-1. In June 1986, the task force ISO/IEC defined the objectives and goals of the project which lead to the establishment of an international norm. Between January and October 1987, a project of official international standard (Draft International Standard) was developed under the auspices of the International Standard Organization (ISO) under the label IS-1.

In January 1989, the last modifications were reviewed by ISO followed by publications of the IS-1 standard which should be used by all manufacturers. To no avail, however, since some companies continue to manufacture VS-1 connections which do not simplify the task of implanters. This diversity of connections currently complicates the pulse generator-lead interface.

When replacing a pacemaker, the connection problems are the same as at a primary implant when the lead(s) are of the 3.2 mm variety. Difficulties, currently, involve patients who have unipolar or bipolar leads of the old 4.75 or 6 mm standards, in whom a 3.2 mm pulse generator needs to be implanted.

In presence of a bipolar lead, whether 4.75 mm bifurcated, or in-line 4.75 or 6 mm, one has the choice between a conversion to a unipolar system with an appropriate unipolar adapter, interfaced with the cathodal/negative pole, if bipolar pacing and/or sensing are not absolutely necessary, or the use of an adapter to preserve bipolarity. Depending on the characteristics of the case one will choose the following adapter:

- A bifurcated bipolar 4.75 mm model
- Cordis bipolar in-line 6 mm model
- An Intermedics bipolar in-line 6 mm model
- A Medtronic bipolar in-line 3.2 mm former generation model

To avoid any surprise, one should have these various items available in stock, and know precisely in advance what type of lead has been previously implanted (Fig. 9.1).

In a patient who has a unipolar 4.75 or 6 mm lead, one uses a unipolar 4.75 or 6 mm adapter, or one cuts the lead distal to the reinforced insulation, removing the insulation over the length necessary to insert it into a 3.2 mm adapter. Depending on the case, one of the following adapters may be chosen:

- A short adapter of the Sorin type, carefully choosing a dextro- or levorotating model according to the orientation of the conductor coil of the cut lead

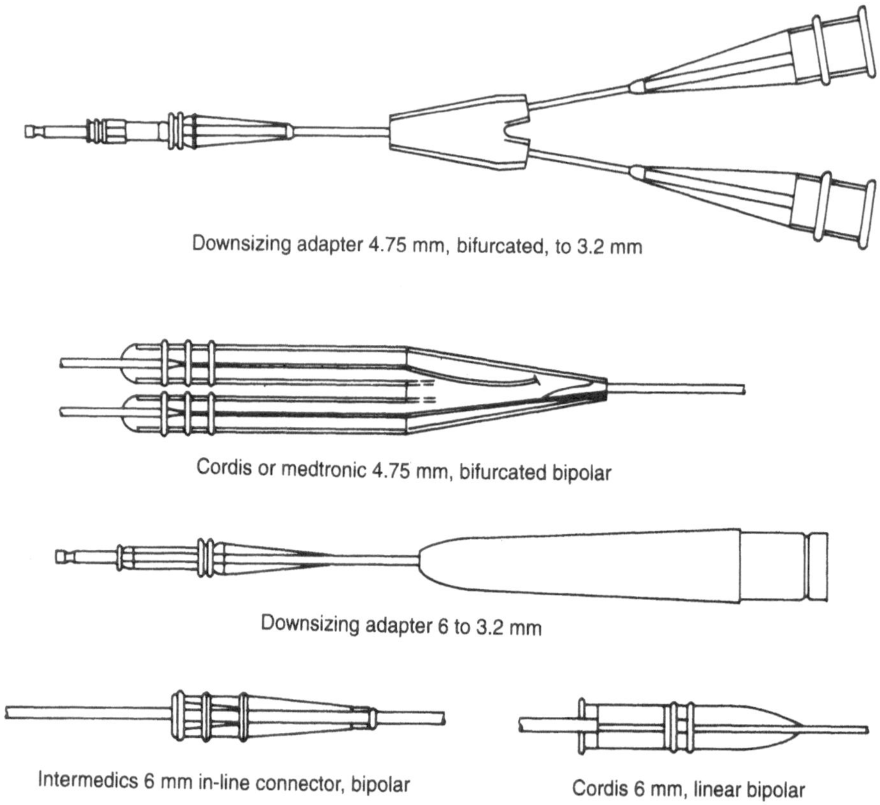

Downsizing adapter 4.75 mm, bifurcated, to 3.2 mm

Cordis or medtronic 4.75 mm, bifurcated bipolar

Downsizing adapter 6 to 3.2 mm

Intermedics 6 mm in-line connector, bipolar

Cordis 6 mm, linear bipolar

**Fig. 9.1.** Selected examples of connection adapters

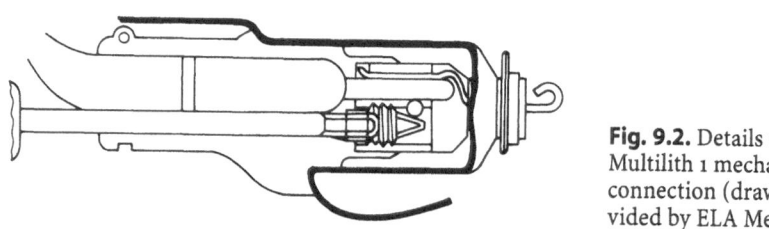

**Fig. 9.2.** Details of the Multilith 1 mechanical connection (drawing provided by ELA Medical)

- A somewhat longer adapter, of the Osypka VKU 17 type, although difficulties may be encountered in its insertion if the lead has a somewhat oversized external diameter

One of these two models may be needed when disconnecting the lead from the depleted pulse generator is impossible, or if the connector is damaged upon its disconnection.

Impossibility of disconnecting a previously implanted pulse generator may be due to:

- Locked or rusted Allen screw
- Too tight a screw resulting in stripping of the slot that accommodates the wrench; this problem should no longer be seen with ratcheting screw drivers
- A locked sub-connection despite a loosened Allen screw, which may occur with the former generation ELA Medical Multilith 1140 connections (Fig. 9.2)

Whatever the procedure chosen to adapt a 4.75 or 6 mm unipolar lead, all have potential shortcomings:

Adapters which closely accomodate a previously implanted lead interrupt pacing only briefly, as in the case of a straight forward replacement, as long as it has been connected to the pulse generator inserted in the pocket. However, their non negligible size may be a problem in emaciated patients, although the excess material can be buried behind muscle, reserving the pocket for the pulse generator. In addition, some adapters are connected to the lead by simple fit (without Allen screw), which may be a cause of poor electrical contact.

As mentioned earlier, adapters which are connected to the bare conductor after removal of the insulation require longer cessation of pacing, which may force temporary external pacing. In addition, short adapters may dislodge over time from excessive stress at their outlet from the pacemaker header by a mechanism similar to that described in insulation failure due to a short header receptacle which does not properly cover the junction between the stiff pin and the soft lead body (see p. 44 f.).

## Reinterventions in Presence of Infection

### General Strategy

The management of this complication is always delicate and must be considered on a case-by-case basis, given the advanced average age of paced patients. Morbidity and mortality are high, particularly since most infections are due to Staphylococcus species.

The general strategy of reintervention is based on the patient's history and dependency on pacing, though above all on the microorganism involved and the presence of vegetations which should be looked for with transesophageal echocardiography.

In case of infection due to another organism than Staphylococcus such as Serratia, Pseudomonas aeruginosa, Proteus or Candida, whose source has been clearly identified and treated as unrelated to the pacemaker pocket, management can be limited to antimicrobial therapy guided by the usual recommendations, and verifications of the eradication of the infection after discontinuation of treatment.

In all other cases, all pacing material must be removed, which may pose sometimes major technical problems (see p. 377 f.). This may be true even when the infection is limited to the pocket, because the microorganisms colonize the insulating material and reach the circulation by contiguous propagation. It is therefore futile to attempt treating the complication by approaching the lead(s) at a site remote from the infected pocket, in apparently uninfected territory, and to abandon its distal portion.

The strategy depends next on the presence or absence of vegetations:

- If present, and with a diameter greater than 1 cm, treatment should consist of their removal under extracorporeal circulation to prevent septic pulmonary emboli. A recent technique of thrombo-suction under echocardiographic guidance has been described which may help avoiding the complexity of the surgical approach.
- If the vegetations are less than 1 cm in diameter, one may proceed with endovascular lead extraction as described below.

Timing of the reintervention depends on the degree of pacemaker dependency:

- If the patient is not pacemaker dependent and the risk of major conduction disturbance is low, the entire system is explanted in the same conditions as described earlier. At the pocket site, all necrotic, fibrotic and calcified tissues are excised, and the infected area, after extensive rinsing and cleansing, is left exposed, filled with gauze, and covered with an occlusive dressing. Gauze and dressing are changed daily initially, then at longer intervals until healing of the wound. When dressings have remained clean for several days, and after meticulous preparation of the new implant site, the new system is implanted as for a primary implant, under antimicrobial therapy guided by microbiologic cultures and sensitivity testing, which should have been instituted from the very beginning. In the case of major initial infectious manifestations with systemic symptoms or septicemia, several days of apyrexia should elapse before proceeding with reimplantation.
- If the patient is pacemaker dependent, pacing must remain available until the reintervention. Several techniques may be considered. Except in the case of septicemia, the pacemaker, in unipolar configuration, may remain connected to the ventricular electrode left in place, with its active side held against the skin by an occlusive dressing away from the wound. Or, though we view this as risky, a temporary lead may be placed while closely watching the venous insertion point and changing site regularly. The wound is kept open and handled as described earlier; the new active fixation system is inserted, and the original ventricular lead is finally removed.

In this situation of pacemaker dependency, if the infection is under poor control, the epicardial approach should be considered to remove the system rapidly while excluding the circulatory system.

## Lead Extraction

Removal of the infected lead(s) represents the main challenge of this complication. Lead extraction may be simple or quite complicated. Whichever technique is used, all efforts must be made to avoid complications, including lead rupture or migration, valvular damage, venous tear, cardiac tamponnade, and death. Several techniques are available.

Direct traction on the lead is effective, but one must avoid tearing the insulation or stretching the conductor which may jeopardize the use of other approaches. A traditional method consists of continuous traction by weights suspended to a cable maintained in the axis of the lead over a pulley. Initial weights of 200 – 300 g are gradually increased by 50 g daily, up to a maximum of 500 g. In our experience, this method has reliably allowed the removal of the lead from the heart. On rare occasions, the lead is severed and must be retrieved by femoral approach, and may remain trapped in the peripheral venous system requiring surgical liberation. This technique mandates close, continuous surveillance of the patient, including hemodynamic and electrophysiologic status.

Consequently, techniques of endocavitary extraction are currently favored. The technique described by Byrd, requiring instrumentation manufactured by Cook, consists of introducing inside the lead conductor a calibrated stylet equipped at its end with a metal wire coiled in a clockwise fashion. By rotating the stylet in the reverse direction, the wire is locked in the conductor's spirals. The locking stylet must, therefore, be advanced into the lead as close as possible to the distal electrode. This allows to exert vigorous traction at that level without risking to stretch or rupture the conductor or insulation. This maneuver may be complemented by countertraction applied on the endocardium by a rigid or semi-rigid sheath advanced, from the venous entrance point, over the lead to be extracted, allowing its separation from endovenous or endocardial fibrotic processes. The lead is extended using the locking stylet to allow the sheath to glide along the lead. Applying too much traction incurs the same risks as simple traction. Two approaches are available:

- The superior approach which allows to intervene from the proximal end of the lead. If too much traction needs to be applied, or if passage through occluded veins is overly difficult, this approach must be abandoned.
- The inferior approach, used when the superior approach has been unsuccessful, or when the lead has been severed and is floating within the central circulation. Performed from a femoral puncture, the technique requires the use of basket catheter which snares the lead, and a countertraction sheath.

One other technique (Vasco Extor) can be used. The locking stylet is equipped at its end with two externally controlled wings which are locked in the spirals of the conductor. This device offers the advantage of not needing to calibrate the internal lumen of the lead exactly before its use, and makes it possible to remove the stylet with an external rotating motor (Fig. 9.3).

These various lead extraction techniques include risks of hemothorax and tamponnade from myocardial perforation or tear. Therefore, they must be performed

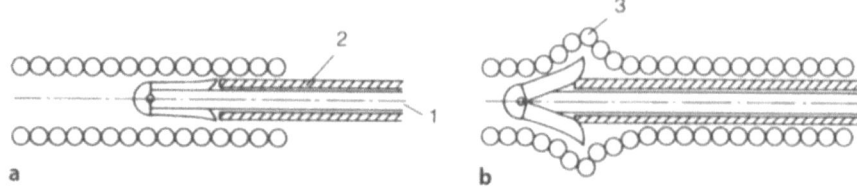

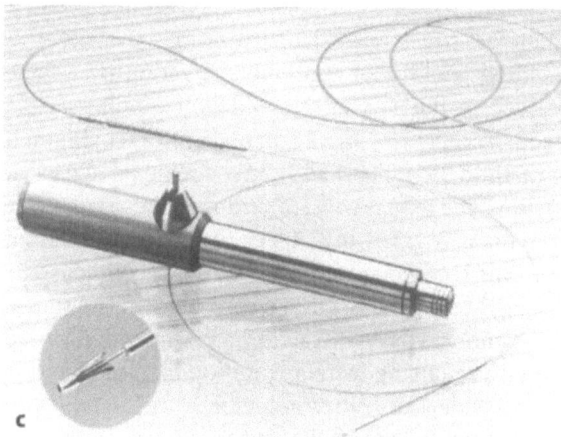

**Fig. 9.3.** Lead extraction system, catching the lead from inside, as close as possible to its tip. Figure provided by Vascomed
**a** The stylet is introduced (*1*, wire with anchors; *2*, plastic tube)
**b** The two externally controlled anchors are locked in the spirals of the conductor (*3*)
**c** Lead extraction equipment

in specialized centers with access to cardiothoracic surgery. Overall, these extraction techniques are successfully applied when the leads to be extracted have been implanted for 6–8 years. Past that period, fibrotic adhesions become so prominent as to make the success of the procedure considerably less certain.

Surgical extraction under extracorporeal circulation is no longer indicated except in cases of failure or unfeasibility of these endovascular techniques, or in a few special cases, for instance in presence of large vegetations adhering to the lead. However, a thrombosuction method has been described to avoid open heart surgery in presence of vegetations. An echocardiographically guided sheath is introduced via the femoral approach toward the vegetations which are aspirated, allowing the culture of the collected specimen for confirmation of the infectious process. The removal of large vegetations, whose presence at the time of lead extraction may be dangerous, is the other advantage offered by this procedure.

These considerations should not distract from remembering that management of pacing system infections remains above all preventive. At implantation, the rigorous sterile precautions are those typically taken in surgical prosthetic implants. The procedures must be performed in an environment prohibited to infected cases. Finally, all patients who have received a pacing system should benefit from the same prophylactic measures as those recommended in patients who have received artificial valves.

# CHAPTER 10

# Conclusions

It was a considerable challenge, 15 years ago, to predict the future of cardiac pacing. It seems just as difficult to imagine what will be implanted in 10 years. Some advances, however, are particularly desirable, and are awaited.

In our opinion, the most pressing improvements pertain to pacing leads. Atrial pacing threshold rises remain all too common and too troublesome, even with the combined use of carbon and steroids, currently the most effective methods of prevention. Ongoing research is aiming at amplifying the atrial electrogram far beyond what is conceivable nowadays. The design of new electrodes requires a level of technology well above the capabilities of industrial production, and remains in the realm of research laboratories. The overall reliability of pacing leads has become quite acceptable, with life expectancies of 15 – 20 years for the current models. On the other hand, manufacturers have not reached a consensus with respect to the design of a universal connector, which complicates considerably the task of implanting physicians. Finally, progress in needed in the area of lead extraction methods.

The evolution of pulse generators is directly related to the size of microprocessors. With the expectancy of memory sizes of several hundreds of kilobytes, one can imagine the development of devices the functions of which will be loaded „à la carte," namely according to the individual needs of each patient. The use of various sensors of biologic signals should continue to grow, not only for rate responsive pacing, but also to assist in the control of antitachycardia protection algorithms, or as an electrophysiologic or hemodynamic surveillance tool. As an example, Medtronic has oriented its research efforts toward the monitoring of blood oxygen saturation combined with pulmonary arterial pressure. Sorin has included an accelerometer at the tip of a traditional pacing lead, which allows to measure cardiac motion, the application of which goes well beyond cardiac pacing. ELA Medical offers the continuous recording of the minute ventilation profile, and of important bradycardic or tachycardic events. These examples illustrate the possibilities offered by microcomputers at the service of diagnostic tools, a fundamental concept put forth by Mugica in the early 1980s. Progress in software development should also allow the automatization of most functions which, nowadays, need to be programmed. Several examples may already be cited, such as automatic pacing and sensing threshold determinations, mode switching, protection against pacemaker mediated reentrant tachycardia, autocalibration of the slope of rate responsiveness, etc.

Will the day come of implantable diagnostic centers capable of directing complex therapies (antibradycardia and antitachycardia pacing, defibrillation), including pump delivery of antiarrhythmic, inotropic, or vasodilatating agents? Difficult to conceive today, progress in microengineering may, one day, offer the technical solutions required to successfully complete such projects.

In 10 years, the face of this medical specialty will likely be completely changed, and the approach to patients suffering from conduction disorders certainly much different.

# General

## The Magnet Modes

All pacemakers from a given manufacturer, if not each model, have their own response to the application of a magnet. Catalogs of the various pacemaker brands and models, old and current, describing the magnet mode response at the beginning and the end of the devices' lives, have been published by several companies, e.g. by Medtronic and Pacesetter.

## Medical Emergencies in Paced Patients

All paced patients can be given, as any ordinary patient, urgent medical care including cardiopulmonary resuscitation.

- External cardiac massage can be performed as usual. The only concern pertains to dislodgment of the lead if it has been implanted recently.
- Transthoracic DC shocks may be delivered and should be directed along the antero-posterior axis, perpendicular to the lead-pulse generator axis to minimize the currents passing through the pacing lead which may cause exit block. The pacing system may be damaged and should be controlled afterwards.
- All metabolic disorders and/or hypoxia may cause loss of pacing capture.
- The use of a magnet allows sometimes to induce asynchronous pacing at a higher output than programmed; however, caution is advised since the magnet mode is most often asynchronous.
- The magnet may also be able to interrupt a pacemaker mediated tachycardia, or limit the ventricular rate of a dual chamber pacemaker accelerated by an atrial arrhythmia.
- The emergency may be due to a device dysfunction, a depleted battery, or a lead failure, forcing an immediate intervention to reestablish pacing.
- The appearance of fever in a paced patient may be considered an emergency since it suggests the systemic dissemination of a microorganism, and perhaps its seeding onto the prosthetic material.

## Questions Asked by Paced Patients

Physicians exposed to patients who have received pacemakers are often asked various questions, most of which are quite legitimate. It may, however, be difficult to provide rapid and clear answers. Most questions are straightforward, or consist of inquiries relative to environmental interferences.

### The Simple Questions

### Do I Really Need a Pacemaker?

When the formation or propagation of the impulse that makes your heart contract is disturbed, the cardiac rhythm becomes abnormal. This reduces the oxygen carried to your body, decreases the work and efficiency of your brain, which you perceive as general fatigue, lightheadedness, even loss of consciousness and falling spells. A regulator of the rhythm (the pacemaker) can greatly improve the situation, or even eliminate the symptoms, more effectively than any medication.

### What Does a Pacemaker Look Like and How Does It Work?

Thanks to microeengineering, new pacemakers are no larger than a matchbox. The flat can contains the pulse generator and the power supply. One or two flexible leads link the can to the heart trough a vein. The tip of the lead emits small electrical pulses which cause a heart beat only when necessary, that is when your heart beats at a rate below 60 – 70 beats per minute (BPM), or when the beat is irregular.

### How Long Does a Pacemaker Last?

In past years, pacemakers lasted 10 years or longer. Today, as a result of the reduction in their size, hence of the battery, and depending on the complexity of the device, their life expectancy has decreased considerably, down to an average of 5 years. At the end of this period, the generator is replaced and the lead is checked. If the latter is functioning well, only the can will be exchanged; otherwise, both will be replaced.

### How Does One Implant a Pacemaker?

An approximately 5-cm (2-in.) incision is performed under local anesthesia below the clavicle to reach the vein through which one or two leads are introduced and advanced to the heart. The proper placement and stability of the lead(s) is then checked by somewhat lengthy measurements, after which it is fixed to the heart. A pocket is then prepared between skin and muscle. The pulse generator and the lead are connected together and placed in the pocket which is then carefully closed. The procedure is mostly painless. The two moments during which some pain may be expected are during infiltration of the anesthetic, and when the pocket is being created. You will remain awake throughout the procedure, and rarely is another form of anesthesia necessary. This operation is, therefore, well tolerated by patients and you will be rapidly on your feet thereafter.

### How Long Does the Procedure Last?

It depends on whether one or two leads need to be implanted, on the ease of accessing the vein and the heart chamber(s), and of the quality of the measurements which need to be made. Consequently, the procedure typically lasts between 45 and 90 min.

### How Long Will I Need to Be in the Hospital?

The length of stay in the hospital depends on associated illnesses and on the proper function of the system after its implantation. We consider 3 to 5 days to be sufficient to confirm that the lead(s) is (are) staying in place, to monitor the early changes that may occur in the pacing measurements, and to finely tune the programming of your pacemaker according to your needs. You will be able to get out of bed the day after the implant, and you probably will feel quickly better as a result of a better heart function and blood supply to your brain.

### When Will I be Allowed to Take a Bath or Shower?

You must wait until the wound is properly closed; showering is allowed after the stitch(es) has been removed, and bathing 2 weeks thereafter.

### What Should I Watch for Now that I have a Pacemaker?

- Check your pulse every morning. Ask your doctor to let you know the slowest heart rate that you should be measuring, according to the way your pacemaker has been set. If the heart rate that you have counted is below that, notify your doctor.
- Watch the pacemaker pocket daily; if it becomes swollen, red and hot, particularly if it is also tender, get in touch with the hospital where it has been implanted immediately. Do not try to use ointments; it is simply a waste of time.
- Do not expose the pocket area to sunlight for extended periods of time. The titanium can absorb large quantities of heat that, when returned to the surrounding tissues, may burn them. Protect that area with white garment.
- When you see a physician or dentist who does not already know you, inform them that you have a pacemaker.
- Always keep you pacemaker identification card with you, together with your personal identification papers.
- Present regularly for follow-up visits.

- Before engaging in long travel, ask you physician to give you names and addresses of centers where you could turn to in case of problems.
- Do not twiddle the pacemaker can.
- Avoid suspenders which may irritate the skin over the pacemaker. If you must wear them, use some sort of cushioning protection under the suspender.
- Stay away from powerful electromagnetic fields such as radiotransmitters, rotating electrical motors, antitheft devices in department stores, etc.

### What I Am Allowed to Do as a Patient Who Has a Pacemaker?

In general, you can live normally and do whatever you wish. In doubt, ask your implanting physician or medical center. If you have no associated illness or underlying heart disease, you may engage again in all sports, without restriction. You may bathe, swim, take showers and enter a sauna. You may go about your domestic chores or recreational activities without fear. You may have a perfectly normal sex life. You may travel by car, train, boat or airplane. After having consulted with your personal physician, or the physician at your work place, you may return to your professional occupation. Ask your physician, however, to let you know about problems that may occur as a result of certain activities (in your private or professional life), which is unusual.

### Do I Have to Rest More Often? Am I Now a Cardiac Cripple?

Your exercise capacity is not limited because you have a pacemaker. On the contrary, you are probably in better health than before its implantation.

### Which Medications Should I, and May I Take from Now on?

You may continue taking most medications, particularly in case of heart or circulatory disorder. Taking medications does not usually modify the behavior of a pacemaker, though you want to confirm this with your physician. The regulating action of your pacemaker may allow to stop some of your medications, or reduce their dosages. Conversely, the presence of your pacemaker may allow to give you some medications which you need, or increase the doses of those you are already taking.

### How Does One Die with a Pacemaker?

When your heart is no longer able to contract in response to the electrical pulse delivered by the pacemaker, you will die naturally. The pacemaker will continue to function, and could be compared to a conductor giving a concert without an orchestra.

## What Breakdowns Can One Expect from a Pacemaker?

As any other instrument, a pacemaker may fail, which is rare. The lead may be damaged or get out of position. The tissue around its tip may become so irritated as to prevent proper pacing. These are reasons why your pacemaker must be checked regularly, daily by yourself, infrequently by the implanting center, and in-between by your regular physician.

## Should I Wear the Seat Belt in a Car?

As any other occupant of a car, you must wear your seat belt. The risk of sustaining an injury without seat belt is much greater than that of damage to the device by the belt. One may consider placing a small cushion between belt and pacemaker. Any serious accident should be followed by a pacemaker check. Having a pacemaker does not prohibit you from driving a car.

### Environmental Interference

Questions asked by pacemaker patients often involve fear of environmental disturbance of the function of the device. The effects of interference on pacemakers have been studied, though it is impossible to take all situations into account. Protections against interference vary from one model and manufacturer to the other, such that some environmental signals may have different effects on different pacemakers. When purchasing an electric appliance, care should be taken to verify the manufacturing safety label. Regular controls of their proper operation is also advised.

The following electrical instruments, though often suspected of causing interferences, have no effects on pacemakers, provided they (the instruments) are in good working condition:

- Typewriters, computers, pocket calculators
- Vacuum cleaners
- Elevators, escalators
- TV sets, radios
- Toasters
- TV or stereo-system earphones
- Quartz watches
- Washing machines
- Modern microwave ovens
- Lawn mowers
- Ultrasonic devices as used in dental offices

On the other hand, interference induced by the following instruments or machines may affect pacemaker function (see Table A1).

**Table A1.** External sources of interference and their possible effect on the pacemaker. [Modified from Irnich W (1992) Deutsches Ärzteblatt 89 (37A1): 2957 and Irnich W, Batz L (1994) Herzschrittmacher 14 (6): 239]

| Interference factor | Intensity | Precondition | Remedy |
| --- | --- | --- | --- |
| **Home** | | | |
| Television operation/ sensor keys | Strong | Switching every second (improbable) | Switch more slowly |
| Electric blanket, cushion | Weak | Immediate vicinity | More distance from pacemaker |
| Electric heater | Minimal | | Unnecessary |
| Coffee-mill | Minimal | | Unnecessary |
| Microwave oven | Minimal | See text, p. 258 | See text, p. 258 |
| Electric razor | Weak | Immediate vicinity | Change to storage battery or to razor without oscillating armature |
| Electric toothbrush | Medium | Immediate vicinity | Normal toothbrush |
| **At work** | | | |
| Lathe | Minimal | | Unnecessary |
| Three-phase/A.C. motors | Weak | Immediate vicinity | If necessary, keep more distance |
| Electro-steel oven (blast furnace) | Very strong | Vicinity | No work near such furnaces, distance at least 25 m |
| D.C. motors | Medium/strong | Immediate vicinity | Keep a distance to motor depending on current strength |
| Hand drill | Strong | Drilling before chest | Keep more distance to drill |
| Welding set | Strong | Vicinity | Keep more distance |
| **Environment** | | | |
| Car-ignition vicinity | Strong | Direct vicinity(e.g. During repairs) | Keep more distance |
| Theft-protection | See text, p. 258, 387 | See text, p. 258, 387 | Handles or go through quickly |
| E locomotive | Strong | Relative vicinity | Keep a distance |
| Electric steel furnace | Very strong | Vicinity | Do not visit steel factories |
| Airport controls (gate and hand detector) | Generally minimal | Usually weak magnetic field | Show pacemaker card; (metal detector might trigger alarm |

**Table A1.** (continued)

| Interference factor | Intensity | Precondition | Remedy |
|---|---|---|---|
| Police-radar | Minimal | | Unnecessary |
| Radio and amateur transmitters, not TV transmitters | Medium/strong | Vicinity | Keep away |
| Streetcar | Weak | Possibly vicinity to motor | Keep away from motor |
| Some cellular phones analog or digital (see text) | Weak | Certain pacemaker models, spacing < 25 cm | Look at the pacemaker list, spacing > 25 cm |
| Some portable phones analog or digital (see text) | Weak | Certain pacemaker models, spacing < 40 cm | Look at the pacemaker list, spacing > 40 cm |
| Cordless phones | | No influence | |

For risks of interference in a *medical environment*, see p. 259–261.

## Mobile Telephone

Mobile telephone (cellular phone) can interfere with some pacemaker models. It is recommended to consult the appropriate listings and manuals. All pacemakers seem safe as long as the hand held device (handy) remains at least 25 cm (1 ft) away from the pulse generator during use (dialing and transmission up to 2 $\Omega$ power) whereas the antenna of portable systems, which may have a transmission power close to 7 $\Omega$, should be kept at least 40 cm (1.5 ft) away from the pacemaker area. Garments containing fine metallic threads, which are sold commercially, may have a protecting effect against electrical interference.

Cordless telephones, with a range of approximately 300 m (1000 ft) from the base station, do not interfere with pacemakers (according to our present knowledge).

## Bipolar Versus Unipolar Pacing Systems

Bipolar pacing systems are generally less susceptible to electromagnetic interferences than unipolar systems. On the other hand, unipolar and bipolar systems are equally susceptible to interferences by high frequency electrical fields. A particular mention should be made of the antitheft systems installed in department stores in recent years, which are different from the earlier. These systems use now higher energy and low frequencies that were quite safe for patients with bipolar systems. In this instance, bipolar systems offer a distinct advantage.

## Additional Theoretical Notions of Electricity

Electromotive force, measured in volts (V) is expressed as: V=I (current, the quantity of electrons flowing per second through the conductor, expressed in milliamperes) R (resistance in KΩ). This relationship is known as Ohm's law (Figs. A1 – A3).

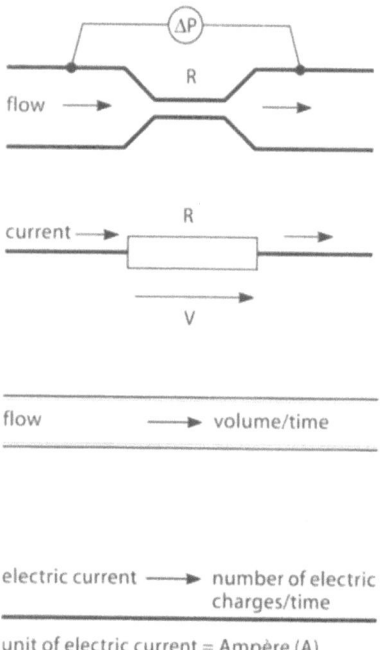

**Fig. A1.** An electrical resistance (R) impedes the passage of electrical current. The unit of measurement is the Ohm (Ω). This phenomenon creates a voltage (V), according to a pressure difference (ΔP) at the poles of the resistance (R) in water tube systems
*Above*, water tube system with flow
*Below*, electrical system

**Fig. A2.** The electrical current is likened to a flow of electrical charges. The intensity of current is the number of charges put out per second. A flow of electrons (negative charges) moves from the negative to the positive pole. By convention, electrical current flows in the other direction. Current is present only if there is a potential difference and if the circuit is closed. The unit of current measurement is the ampere (A). *Above*, water tube system. *Below*, electrical system

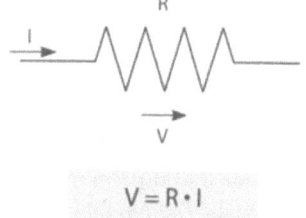

**Fig. A3.** 1 Ohm is the resistance (R) present between 2 points on a conductor when a constant voltage (V) of 1 V applied between these 2 points creates a current (I) of 1 Ampere. This fundamental law is known as Ohm's law

At constant voltage, the current is inversely proportional to the resistance of the system. As resistance increases, current decreases and pacing may no longer be effective. As resistance decreases, current increases at the cost of a waste of power of the pacemaker.

The charge delivered, (in microcoulombs) is equal to the current multiplied by the pulse duration (in ms). It is proportional to the pulse duration.

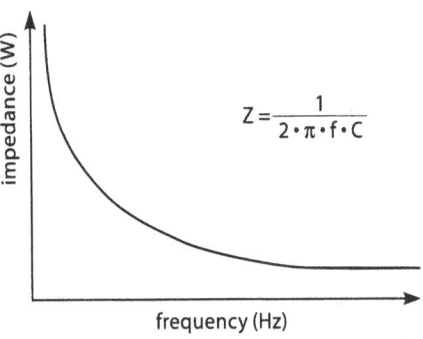

**Fig. A4.** The curve of variations in impedance of a capacitor as a function of the frequency of the applied current is a curve of the 1/X type. The higher the frequency, the lower the impedance (and vice versa). If frequency is = 0 (direct current), impedance becomes infinite (a capacitor offers an infinite impedance to direct current)

Energy is determined by the following formula:

Energy (in microjoules) delivered with each pulse
= volts × current × pulse duration
= volts² × pulse duration/resistance

For a constant delivered voltage over time, energy increases as the square of voltage and proportionally to pulse duration. However, as a result of polarization of the pacing electrode, voltage decreases over time, a phenomenon that has very important practical consequences.

The terms „resistance" and „impedance" are often used interchangeably, though they have slightly different meanings. Impedance (Z, expressed in ohms) is for alternating current the equivalent of resistance for direct current. It is, in other words, a dynamic resistance, a function of the alternating signal frequency (Fig. A4). The term impedance is, therefore, more accurate.

A resistor impedes the electrical flow by the nature and dimensions of the conductor material. Metals are good conductors and offer weak resistance to the flow of electrons. Their physical characteristics determine resistance: two conductors made of the same metal, and with the same cross section, have resistances proportional to their lengths; if one is twice as long as the other, its resistance will be twice as high. If their lengths are the same, but the cross section of one is one half that of the other, the latter will have a resistance twice as low since resistance is inversely proportional to the cross section.

In cardiac pacing, impedance of electrical current is both resistive and capacitive. The lead, which transfers the electrons, offers some resistance. The tissues have their own resistance, though the electrical charges that flow through them are ionic in nature. The cathode in contact with the endocardium is negatively charged by electrons, such that the electrode is rapidly surrounded by positive ions, themselves layered with negative ions. Consequently, the two ionic layers act as a capacitor opposing the transfer of electrical charges from the electrode, a phenomenon known as polarization (Fig. A5). The capacitive effect of polarization increases over time for as long as the stimulus is applied, reaching its peak at the end of pulse delivery, and slowly decaying thereafter. As a consequence, the voltage actually applied to the myocardium decreases during delivery of the

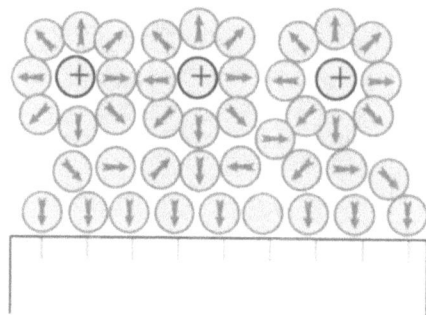

**Fig. A5.** When an electrode is placed in an electrolyte solution, electric charges are formed until an equalization of electrochemical potentials has been reached. The voltage of this polarization depends on the material used and on the type of electrolyte solution. In absence of pacing, there is, in permanence, a thin layer of charges on the surface of the electrode. This layer is itself separated from the electrode by a layer of water molecules adsorbed on its surface. This structure is known as „Helmholtz' double layer", and corresponds electrically to a high capacitance (5–50 µF/cm$^2$)

stimulus; the energy wasted in the phenomenon of polarization contributes to the depletion of the pacemaker battery.

The phenomenon of polarization is a function of the pulse duration and should be minimized by the programming of relatively short pacing pulse durations.

## Additional Facts on Stimulating the Heart

Two types of pacing pulses may be generated from the power delivered by the pacemaker battery: constant current versus constant voltage pulses.

The strength of a constant current pulse remains unchanged regardless of the pulse duration and the circuit resistance (no matter how high). Its effect is to mobilize a predetermined number of electrical charges across cellular membranes, whatever the necessary voltage to be applied may be. The modification of the local electrical field depends on the local current density (amount of current per unit of surface of the traversed structure), and on the local resistance of the tissues (according to Ohm's law). The system is comparable to a pump guaranteeing a constant flow through a tube, even if its caliber decreases (see Fig. A1).

A constant voltage pulse maintains its strength by adjusting its duration whatever the circuit resistance may be (no matter how low). The local electrical field is modified by maintenance of a flow of charges sufficient to keep the voltage between the two poles of the circuit constant, at the desired value. This system resembles a tank which maintains its water level, hence its pressure, constant, irrespective of the quantity of its run off. Today's pacemakers are of a constant voltage type.

The battery charges a capacitor through a resistance (Figs. A6–A9). The duration of the charge depends on the value of the resistance. The discharge of the capacitor occurs only if the clock of the pulse generator allows the closure of a switch for a duration equal to the programmed pulse duration, with a constant negative voltage toward the myocardium. In the beginning of the pacing pulse, the voltage is equal to the voltage delivered by the pacemaker battery. The current strength depends on the circuit impedance, equal to the sum of the resistances of the pacing lead (approximately 10 Ω), the electrode-heart interface (200–500 Ω if the electrode is in close contact with the endocardium, approximately 100 Ω if it is surrounded by blood, i.e. a poor electrode-tissue interface is associated with low impedance), surrounding tissues (10–30 Ω), and a resistance due to lead polarization of a capacitive type, as was just described, at the electrode-heart interface. Over time, this polarization increases while delivered current intensity decreases. This means that the wider the pulse, the greater the decay in delivered voltage over time. When the switch reopens, the current goes in the opposite direction, creating a positive pulse of sufficient strength to stimulate the myocardium, occurring during the latter's refractory period, and decaying exponentially over several hundreds of milliseconds. To accelerate the recharge of the capacitor some devices are equipped with a recharge circuit which operates a few milliseconds after the pacing stimulus, thus creating a biphasic pulse (negative/positive). The advantage of this system is the ability to pace at high rates and, especially, to shorten the duration of the pacemaker's refractory periods.

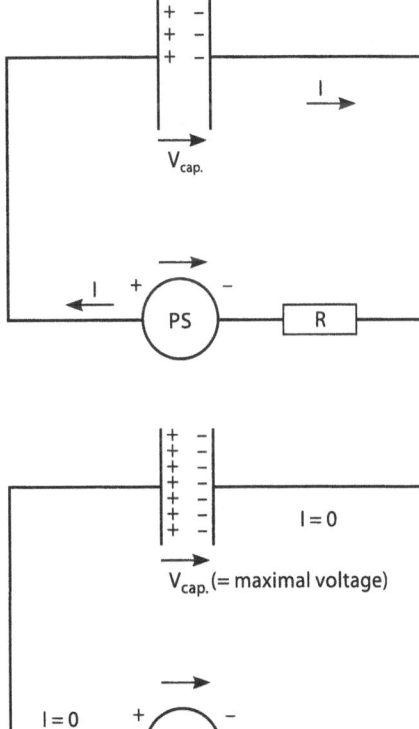

**Fig. A6.** The electrical capacitor is an element which acts as a reservoir accumulating electrical charges. It consists of two conductive surfaces separated by dielectric material which bars the passage of electrical charges from one surface to the other. If the two surfaces are connected to a battery, electrons are attracted by the plate which is interfaced with the negative pole, while the positive charges are attracted by the other plate. This gradually creates a voltage between the two plates of the capacitor which becomes charged
$V_{cap}$ voltage of capacitor; $I$ current; PS power source; $R$ resistance

**Fig. A7.** A state of equilibrium takes place when the voltage between the two plates is equal to that of the battery. At that moment, no further current is flowing: the capacitor is saturated, or charged
$V_{cap}$ maximal voltage of capacitor; $I$ current; PS power source; $R$ resistance

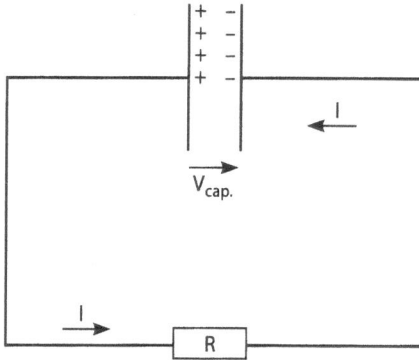

**Fig. A8.** If polarity is changed, the electrical charges will flow in the direction opposite to the process of charge: the capacitor will discharge until it has reached zero voltage. Direct current does not pass through a capacitor
$V_{cap}$ voltage of capacitor; $I$ current; $R$ resistance

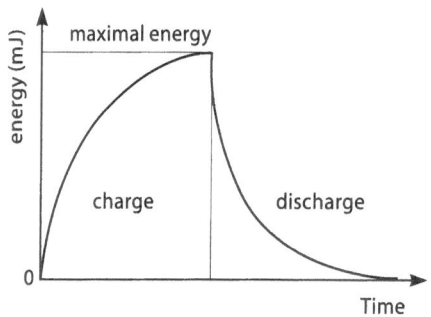

**Fig. A9.** When a capacitor is charged through a resistance, the latter limits the charge current. The voltage at the poles of the capacitor increases gradually. The voltage between the source and the capacitor decreases, reducing further the available charge current. The voltage at the poles of the capacitor assumes an exponential shape. Upon discharge, the same phenomenon is observed, however in the reverse direction. The energy stored in the capacitor depends on the applied voltage, as well as on the value of the capacitor. Some materials, such as tantalum, allow a considerable increase in the capacitance while maintaining a reasonable size of the capacitor. The unity of measurement of a capacitor is the Farad (F).

# Special Non-Responsive SSI Mode Functions that Control the Escape Rate

## Bradycardia Diagnostic Functions

The Sorin Theorema 90 pacemaker model offers a bradycardia diagnostic function. It is a form of hysteresis which allows the emergence of a slow spontaneous rhythm (to a minimum of 30 BPM); however, instead of immediately returning to the programmed lower rate following a first paced beat, pacing continues at the slow rate for several programmable cycles. When the pacemaker has effectively paced at the slow rate for the programmed number of cycles, the device logs a bradycardia episode into its statistics (Fig. B1). This function may serve as a diagnostic tool; however, since the device is single chamber, it cannot distinguish ventricular pauses due to sino-atrial block, versus those due to atrioventricular block, versus postextrasystolic compensatory pauses.

The ELA Medical Chorus series models provide a surveillance of atrial and ventricular events during pauses and bradycardic events by memorizing the event markers via a program specially loaded into the device's RAM. Date and time of the various episodes are also memorized (see p. 305 ff.).

## Rate Smoothing

In Vitatron models, this function is called Flywheel. The DPG was the first to offer this type of algorithm. In the ELA Medical Opus model, a programmed slope of acceleration defines the way the pacemaker determines the escape rate as a function of the accelerations in the spontaneous rate. Every eight cycles, the pacemaker analyzes the spontaneous acceleration and readjusts the value of the escape interval according to the measured acceleration and to the value of the programmed slope of acceleration. The higher the programmed value, the closer will the pacemaker be able to follow the acceleration of the spontaneous rhythm. The slope of deceleration, which is programmable, defines the speed of rate smoothing, in effect every eight cycles. The function may be disturbed by extrasystoles falling at the time when the pacemaker calculates the escape interval. A short cycle may, indeed, artificially accelerate the pacing rate, up to a program-

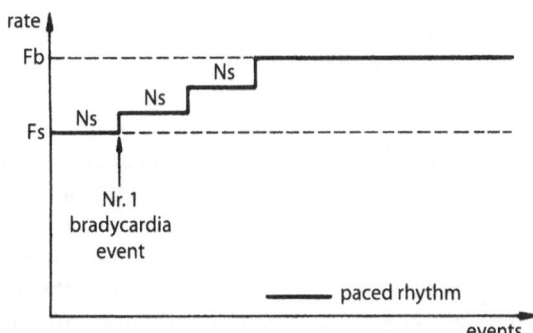

**Fig. B1.** Bradycardia search function by the Sorin Theorema 90 pacemaker. When the device has paced at the bradycardia rate (*Fs*) for the programmed number of cycles (*Ns*), a bradycardia episode is logged in, and the pacemaker returns to the programmed lower rate (*Fb*). Illustration by Sorin

mable level. If programmed appropriately, these functions may, nevertheless, help patients who perceive adversely marked variations in rhythm due to intermittent conduction block.

### Dynamic Overdrive

The purpose of this function, included in the Vitatron models, is to offer a reacceleration of the pacing rate as soon as a spontaneous complex has been sensed. The ultimate goal is to prevent the development of arrhythmias facilitated by spontaneous pauses. The disadvantage is a tendency to a systematic acceleration of the system, which consumes power and may cause symptoms. No large scale evaluation has been performed to confirm the validity of this function.

### Sleep Rate

This function, offered by several pacemaker models, allows a decrease in the lower rate to a programmable level, below the diurnal lower rate, during nighttime, when a rapid pacing rate is unnecessary and power consuming. It may be a problem when the patient's routine is variable, for example when changing time zone. A recent improvement consists of the detection, by the pulse generator's rate responsive sensor, of prolonged resting periods, which causes the self reprogramming of the lower rate (Sorin, Swing model).

### Special Non-Responsive DDD Mode Functions that Control the Escape Rate

Among the special functions which control the AV pacing rate, mention should be made of the Vitatron Diamond and Ruby models, which include a Flywheel, the Intermedics Cosmos II, the Pacesetter Trilogy, and the Medtronic Thera which offer sleep rates, and the CPI Vigor and ELA Medical Chorus, which offer rate smoothing functions. These algorithms operate according to principles described in the appendix with respect to single chamber devices, with the control of heart rate being based primarily on the atrium (Fig. B2). However, the function of the CPI models is slightly different, with the rate smoothing being based on the ventricle. When the atrial rate accelerates beyond the value allowed by a programmed acceleration percentage, AV dissociation occurs, with the goal of limiting the acceleration of the ventricular rate and, consequently, the perception of palpitation by the patient (Fig. B3). During slowing, AV synchrony is guaranteed.

The ELA Medical Chorus II and Chorum models offer a different type of rate smoothing. The slowing of the pacing rate is accomplished according to a programmable slope as a function of an average of the eight preceding cycles, excluding atrial extrasystoles defined by their prematurity relative to the ongoing sinus cycle. This algorithm has eliminated the undesirable accelerations that were observed by earlier generation models from the same manufacturer.

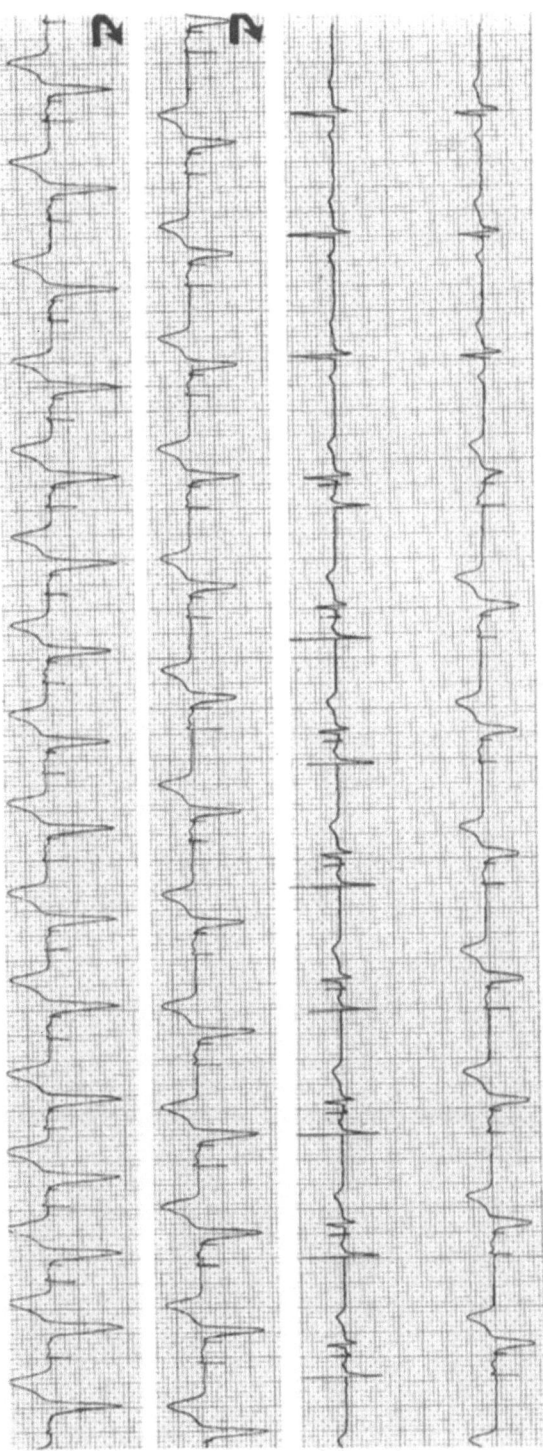

**Fig. B2.** The ELA Medical Chorus rate smoothing algorithm is intended to prevent abrupt falls in heart rate due to sinus arrest. In case of sinus arrest, atrial pacing begins with an escape cycle slightly longer than the memorized PP interval, after which the pacemaker decreases the pacing rate after every eight cycles. In this example, the algorithm of automatic adaptation of the AVD as a function of the heart rate has also been activated. Consequently, the AVD is short at rapid rates and longer at slower rates

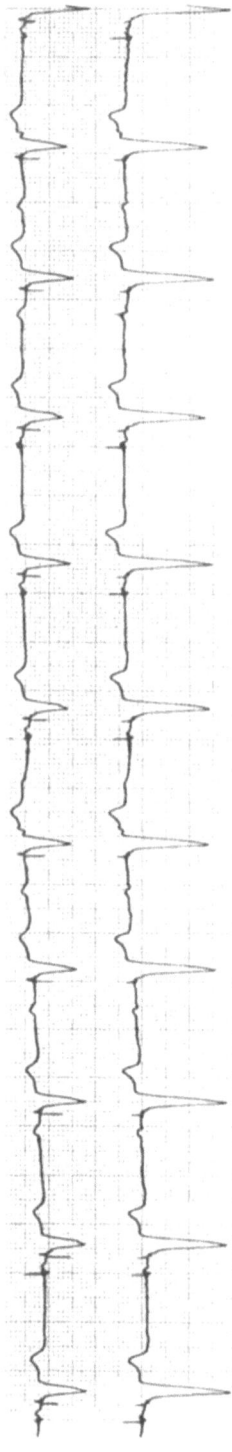

**Fig. B3.** The rate smoothing algorithm included in the CPI DDD pacemakers is intended to prevent abrupt variations in ventricular rate when accelerating as well as when slowing. In this example, the atrial rate accelerates faster than allowed by the programmed slope of acceleration (6%). The ventricular rate accelerates by 6% with AV dissociation

# Automatic Search of Spontaneous QRS

## The Vitatron and Pacesetter Systems (AV Search Hysteresis, AVD Scanning)

In the Vitatron system, a 64 ms window is added to the AV interval, when a QRS complex is sensed during that interval. If AV conduction deteriorates, a ventricular stimulus is delivered at the end of this window; this is followed by 31 cycles (nominal value) with the programmed AVD. At the 32nd cycle, in absence of spontaneous QRS complex falling during the AVD, which would reinstore the search window, the AVD is again lengthened by 64 ms to allow the sensing of a spontaneous QRS complex. If none is sensed, a new 32-cycle sequence is initiated (Fig. B4a). A similar algorithm is included in the Pacesetter Trilogy pacemaker (B4b).

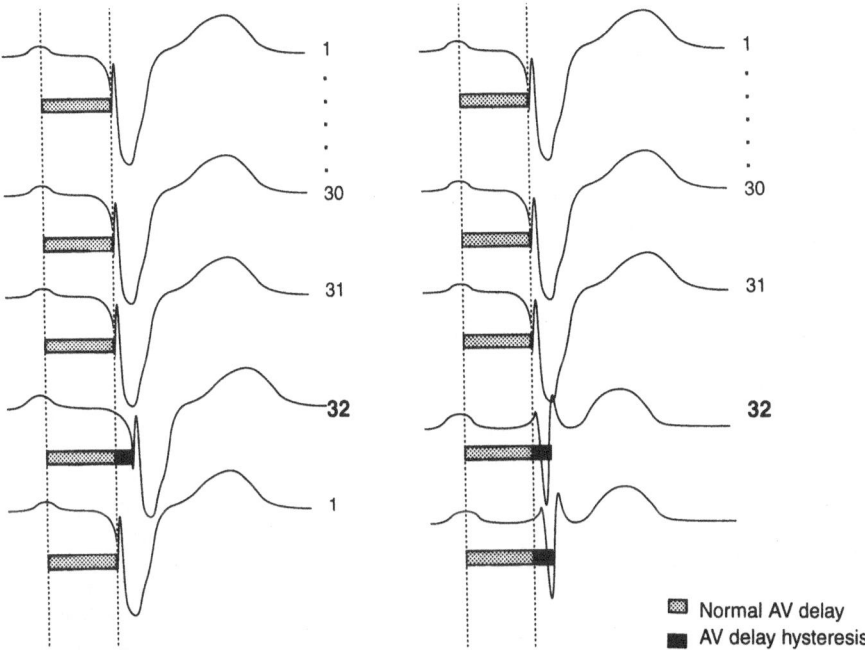

▩ Normal AV delay
■ AV delay hysteresis

**Fig. B4. a** Details of the automatic AV search hysteresis function (AVD scanning) of the Vitatron Ruby and Diamond models. Every 32 cycles, the programmed AVD lengthens by 64 ms. In absence of ventricular sensing, the next AVD returns to the original programmed value. In presence of a sensed ventricular event, the AVD remains lengthened by the amount of hysteresis as long as a ventricular event is sensed after each atrial event

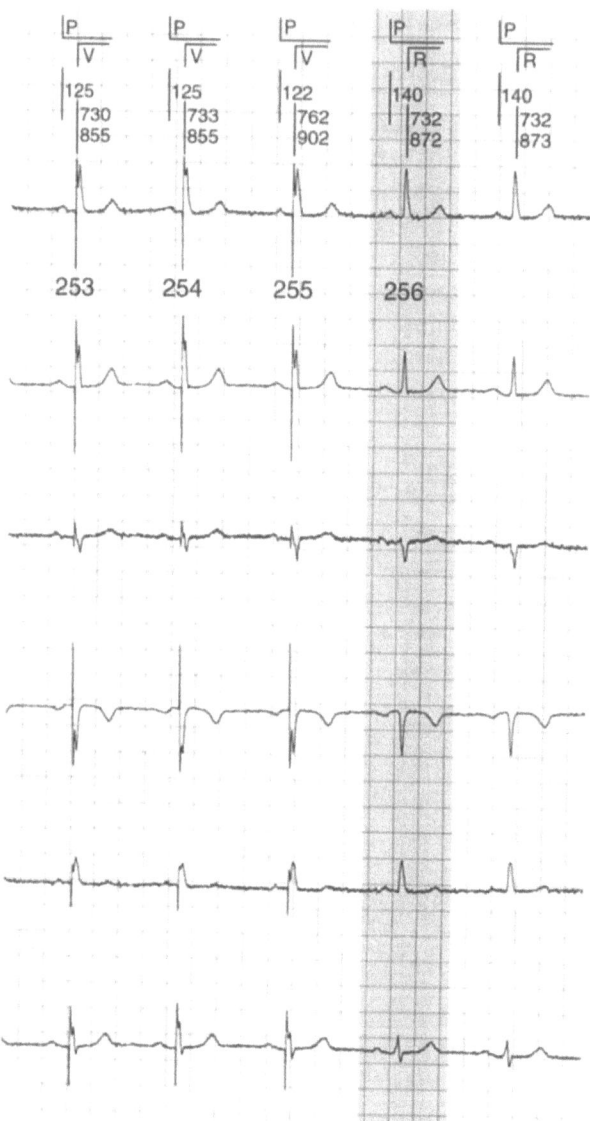

**Fig. B4. b** Details of the automatic AVD hysteresis function of the Pacesetter Trilogy model similar to **a**: Every 256 cycles, the AVD lengthens by a programmed interval (AV search hysteresis, AVD scanning)

### Automatic Switching from AAI to DDD; the ELA System

An average of eight PR intervals is calculated, increased by 31 ms, and applied after each sinus P wave, without initiation of ventricular refractory period following the QRS. The physiologic shortening of the PR interval with exercise is also taken into consideration. If no spontaneous QRS occurs during the average PR interval + 31 ms, the system switches to DDD mode, with an AVD corresponding to the value of the PR interval measured during its operation in the ADI mode. At the same time, the protection algorithms against ELT and atrial arrhythmias are activated, and the mode switch is logged into the statistics. After 100 cycles, the AVD is lengthened by 31 ms to allow a return of spontaneous QRS complexes, and a switch back to the ADI mode if eight consecutive P waves have been followed by spontaneous QRS complexes.

## Separate Programming of the Upper P Wave Synchronous Rate and of the Maximal Sensor Rate in DDDR Pacemakers

In some currently available DDDR pacemakers, one can program two distinct upper rates:

1. A typical upper rate which corresponds to that usually found in typical DDD pacing
2. An upper AV pacing rate linked to the rate responsive function (maximal sensor rate)

The challenge consists of knowing when to program a maximal sensor rate below, at, or above the upper P wave synchronous rate, and the meaning of these various choices.

### The Maximal Sensor Rate (MSR) is Programmed Below the Upper P Wave Synchronous Rate (UR)

There is no operational conflict, at least in the range of sinus rates between the lower rate and the upper P wave synchronous rate. Indeed, even if the rate responsive function drives the atrial rate to its programmed upper limit, the pacemaker remains free to track the atrial rate, when the latter rises above the maximal sensor responsive rate, up to the programmed upper P wave synchronous rate (Fig. B5). However, the usefulness of the rate responsive function is unclear, and the indication for such programming, or even such pacemaker, seems questionable. Indeed, if the patient is able to increase the sinus rate spontaneously, what is the purpose of the rate responsive function? The only apparent reason may be the avoidance of too abrupt a decrease in the sinus rate upon cessation of exercise; however, in such case, smoothing of the atrial rate would be sufficient or the sensor rate is used as rate smoothing function (see p. 297, Fig. 7.11cIII).

### The Maximal Sensor Rate Is Programmed at the Upper P Wave Synchronous Rate

With the proper indication, which should at least include chronotropic incompetence, the behavior of the pacemaker should be *a priori* appropriate. Sensor responsive rate and sinus rate may compete in the range between lower rate and upper rate, though the latter case should be exceptional. If the indication is proper, the atrial rate should be driven only by the rate responsive function. Otherwise, when the sinus rate rises above the upper P wave synchronous rate, Wen-

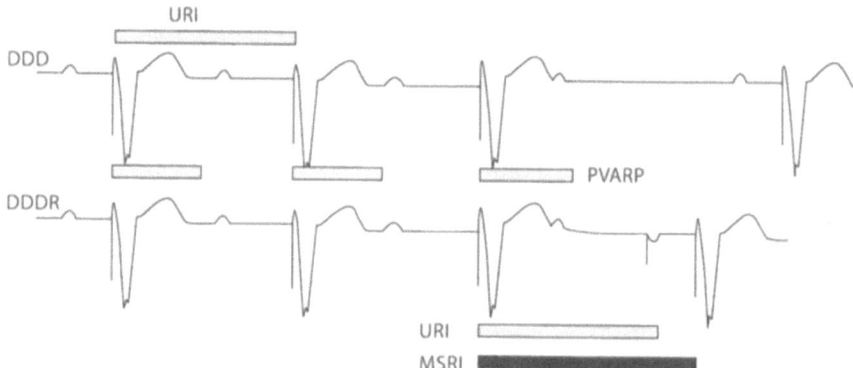

**Fig. B5.** Maximal sensor rate (MSR) < upper rate (UR); minimal sensor rate interval (MSRI) > upper rate interval (URI). Absence of competition between spontaneous and paced P waves. Even if the sensor drives the atrial rate to the maximal sensor rate (corresponding to the minimal sensor rate interval (MSRI)), it does not prevent the spontaneous atrial rate to be tracked up to the programmed upper P wave synchronous rate (corresponding to the upper rate interval). The advantage of this programming consists of the attenuation of long cycles, during Wenckebach behavior, when the P wave falls in PVARP (upper tracing). The sensor forces AV pacing at an escape interval which, theoretically, avoids competition between the P wave blocked in PVARP and the paced A wave (lower tracing)

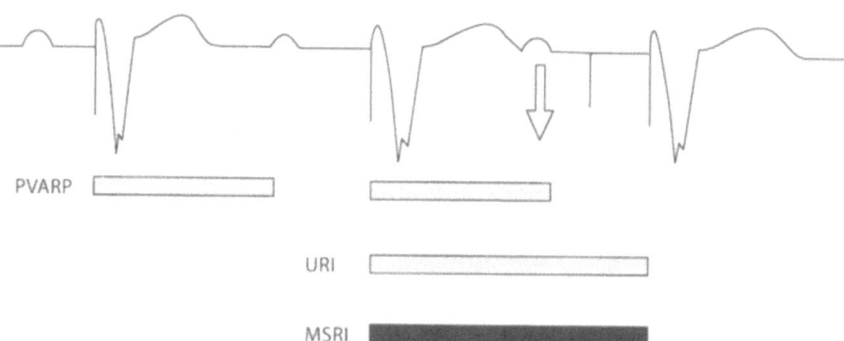

**Fig. B6.** Maximal sensor rate (MSR) = upper rate (UR); minimal sensor rate interval (MSRI) = upper rate interval (URI). AV pacing is driven solely by the sensor between the lower rate and the maximal sensor rate (corresponding to the minimal sensor rate interval (MSRI)). In contrast, if the atrial rate rises above the programmed upper P wave synchronous rate, the behavior becomes Wenckebach like, as in typical DDD mode. The difference between the DDDR and the DDD modes consists of the interruption of the pause by the sensor, forcing AV pacing after the blocked P wave which fell in PVARP. However, the atrial stimulus induced by the sensor, very near the P wave blocked in PVARP, may be either ineffective or arrhythmogenic

ckebach behavior is induced, and some of the P waves fall in PVARP at the end of each period. The result is usually, in typical DDD mode, a ventricular pause until the next P wave. In such case, the duty of the rate responsive function consists of limiting this ventricular pause caused by Wenckebach behavior. Some authors have described this behavior as satisfactory. However, by happening during the atrial escape interval, usually very short since exercise has brought the sinus rate beyond the programmed upper rate, the atrial stimulus forced by the rate responsive function is likely to fall very near the P wave that was blocked in PVARP, at the end of the Wenckebach cycle. This atrial stimulus may be either ineffective, which is of no particular concern, or, since it often falls in the atrial vulnerable period, it may induce an atrial arrhythmia (Fig. B6). However, we wish to underscore that, in presence of a proper indication for rate responsiveness, because of the underlying chronotropic incompetence, the risk of this complication is low. To eliminate it, the Medtronic Thera pacemakers impose a lower limit to an atrial stimulus delivered after a spontaneous P wave falling in PVARP.

### The Maximal Sensor Rate Is Programmed Above the Upper P Wave Synchronous Rate

This programming is more complex. There should be no particular problem between the lower rate and the upper P wave synchronous rate. When the maximal sensor rate rises above the upper P wave synchronous rate, the rate responsive function drives AV pacing up to the programmed maximal sensor rate. If the indication was poor, that is in absence of significant chronotropic incompetence, or if the slope of rate responsiveness was programmed too shallow, in the range of atrial rates included between the programmed upper P wave synchronous rate and the maximal sensor rate, the atrial rate is likely to surpass the sensor driven rate with the following consequences: the spontaneous P wave inhibits atrial pacing which, otherwise, would have been induced by the rate responsive function; this initiates an AVD. Since, in this range of heart rates, the pacing cycle is solely controlled by the rate responsive function, ventricular pacing is not allowed at the end of the AVD because the shortest AV synchronized cycle dictated by the sensor has not elapsed; consequently, the AVD must be lengthened. A true Wenckebach behavior is induced between the programmed upper P wave synchronous rate and the maximal sensor rate. As in any other Wenckebach structure, a P wave falls in PVARP and is not followed by ventricular pacing. However, since the escape interval, dictated by the sensor, is short, the next atrial event is paced, and likely to be either ineffective or arrhythmogenic (Fig. B7), except if the pacemaker imposes a lower limit to the cycle between a spontaneous P wave sensed in PVARP and the next atrial paced event, as in the case of the Medtronic Thera pacemaker.

This problem is also likely in the event of a short burst of atrial extrasystoles at rates between the upper P wave synchronous rate and the maximal sensor rate. When a patient with sinus node dysfunction and/or chronotropic incompetence is known to have atrial tachyarrhythmias, we consider this behav-

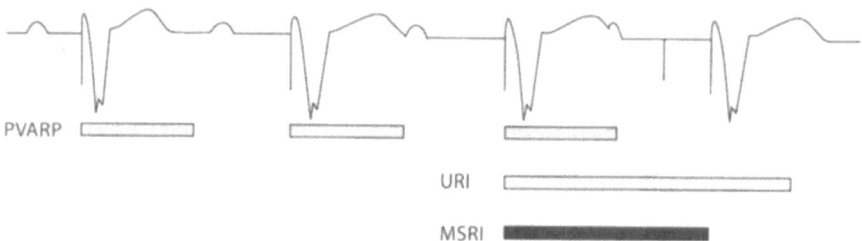

**Fig. B7.** Maximal sensor rate (MSR) > upper rate (UR); minimal sensor rate interval (MSRI) < upper rate interval (URI). No conflict is expected in presence of a proper indication. Conversely, in absence of chronotropic incompetence and if the atrial rate is capable of rising above the sensor rate, the P waves inhibit atrial pacing while the V-V intervals are dictated by the maximal sensor rate (corresponding to the minimal sensor rate interval (MSRI)); the behavior is Wenckebach-like (between URI and MSRI). If a P wave falls regularly in PVARP, the following paced atrial event occurs very early because the atrial escape interval, dictated by the sensor, is very short. Consequently, that atrial spike is likely to be either ineffective or arrhythmogenic

ior as undesirable. Consequently, in patients at risk of atrial tachyarrhythmias, one must:

- Program a slow upper P wave synchronous rate since, if an atrial tachyarrhythmia develops, it will cause a modest acceleration of the ventricular rate, without much hemodynamic consequence
- Program a rapid maximal sensor rate to allow enough effort, at the risk of converting the pacemaker's behavior from DDDR to pseudo-VVIR (Wenckebach-like association, competition between spontaneous and paced rhythm) when the sinus rate is between the upper P wave synchronous rate and the maximal sensor rate.

The reasons for this mandatory programming may be several:

- Absence of effective and rapid protection against ELT, hence an obligation to program a long PVARP; this results in a low 2 : 1 point, and a risk of poor sensing of rapid atrial rhythms
- Even in presence of proper sensing of these rapid atrial rhythms, absence of protection against pacemaker induced ventricular tachycardia, such as fallback function, or automatic mode switch to a VVIR or DDIR mode

## Protection Algorithms Against Atrial Arrhythmias

The first system, known as dual demand was introduced in the Siemens 674 model, still in use in the Biotronik Physios and Dromos pacemakers (Fig. B8). The atrial refractory period is renewable in case of sensing of an atrial event during that period, resulting in a DVI-like behavior at the lower rate.

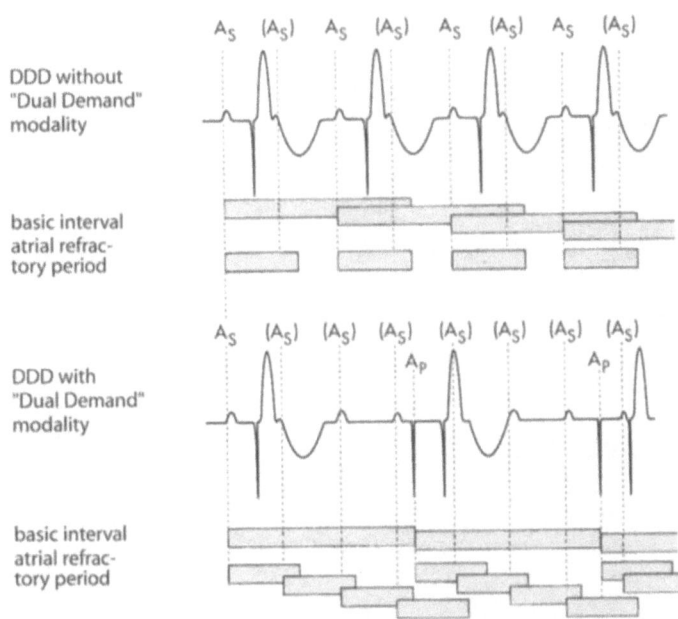

**Fig. B8.** Dual demand function of the Biotronik Physios pacemaker. Any atrial event sensed during the refractory period recycles that refractory period. The pacemaker behavior becomes DVI-like, guaranteeing a protection against the atrial arrhythmias sensed by the pacemaker. Illustration provided by Biotronik

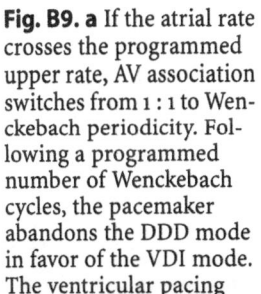

**Fig. B9. a** If the atrial rate crosses the programmed upper rate, AV association switches from 1 : 1 to Wenckebach periodicity. Following a programmed number of Wenckebach cycles, the pacemaker abandons the DDD mode in favor of the VDI mode. The ventricular pacing rate decreases gradually to the fallback rate. When the atrial rate returns to a value below the programmed upper rate, the pacemaker switches back to DDD mode with gradual reassociation of ventricular pacing and atrial sensing

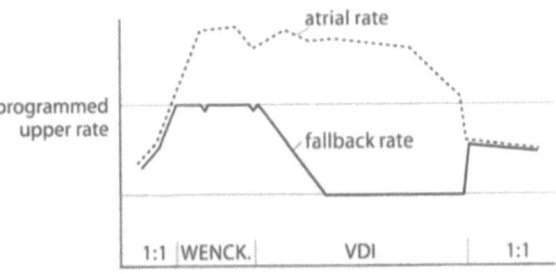

The next system developed consisted of fallback (CPI 925). In case of atrial tachyarrhythmia, the pacemaker operates in a Wenckebach mode over a usually programmable number of cycles, then switches to a slow VVI mode, while continuing to monitor the atrial rate, thus behaving in a VDI-like mode. In DDDR pacemakers and the Chorus RM in DDD(R) mode, the switch is to VDIR. When the atrial rate returns to within the normal range, the pacemaker switches back

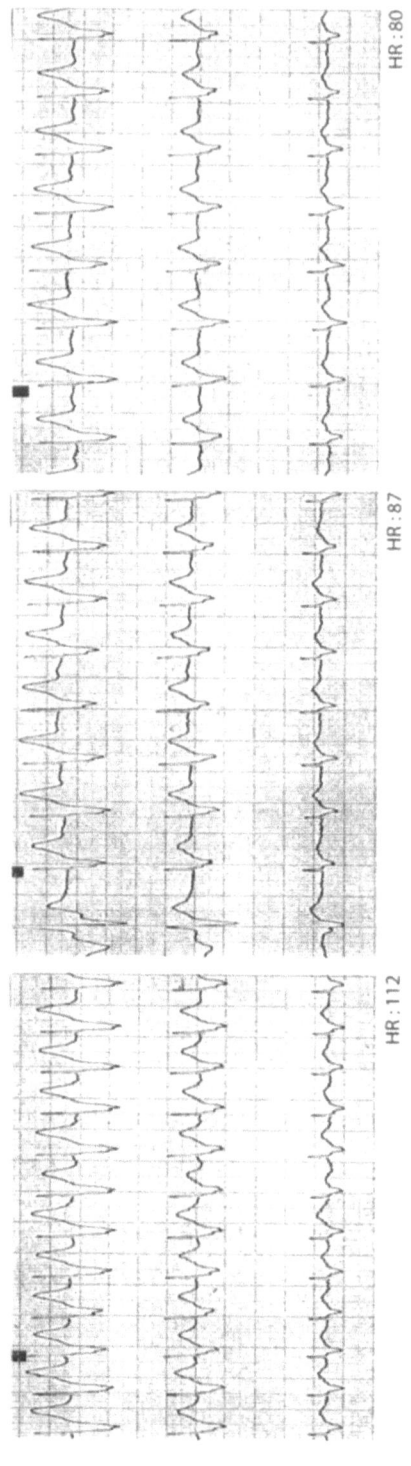

**Fig. B9. b** Example of fallback in response to atrial tachyarrhythmia
*HR* heart rate

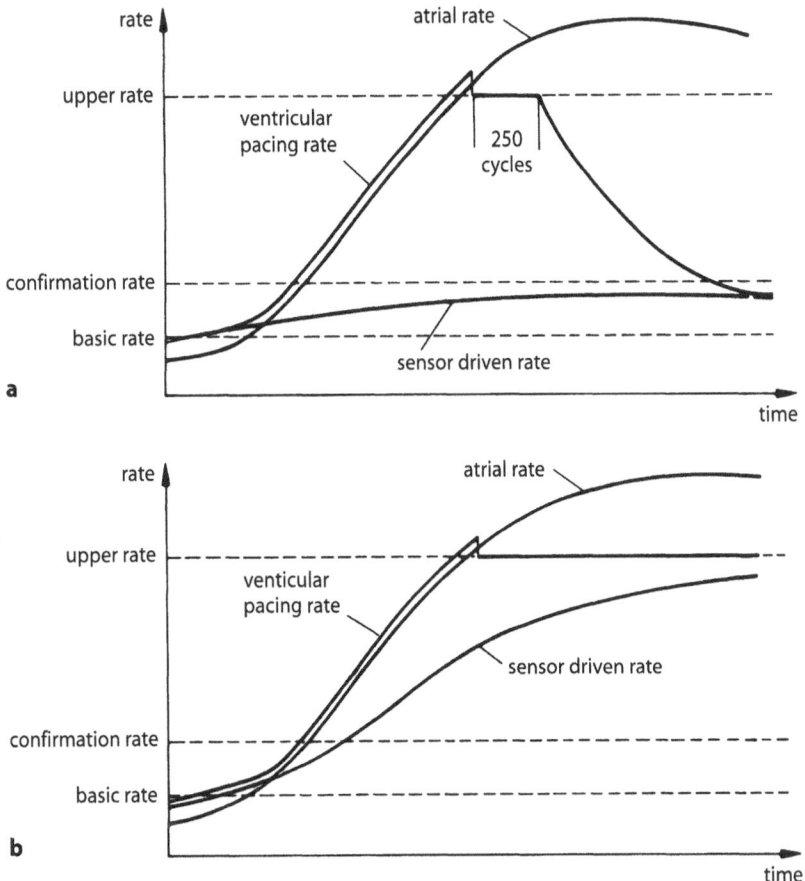

**Fig. B10. a** The Sorin Swing DR pacemaker incorporates the information provided by its sensor. If the sensor indicates no activity at the time of rapid atrial rhythm, the pacemaker switches to fallback
**b** If the sensor indicates presence of activity, the rate remains continuously near the upper rate. Illustrations provided by Sorin

to the DDD mode (Fig. B9). The disadvantage of this type of algorithm is that, before the automatic switch to DDD or VDI mode, the maximal ventricular pacing rate must have been reached, and the Wenckebach mode induced, which constitutes an unnecessary acceleration of the ventricular rate with possible development of symptoms. Furthermore, the possible loss of sensing of pathologic atrial signals may cause the resetting of the Wenckebach counter to zero and prevent the initiation of fallback. The Sorin Swing DR1 are the only pacemakers which induce a VVI(R) mode at a pacing cycle, 100 ms longer than the shortest programmed cycle when the sensed atrial rate is above the programmed upper rate (see Fig. 3.89). After a number of ventricular cycles automatically determined by the Swing pacemaker according to the information provided by the sensor during DDDR mode, the pacing rate decreases (Fig. B10).

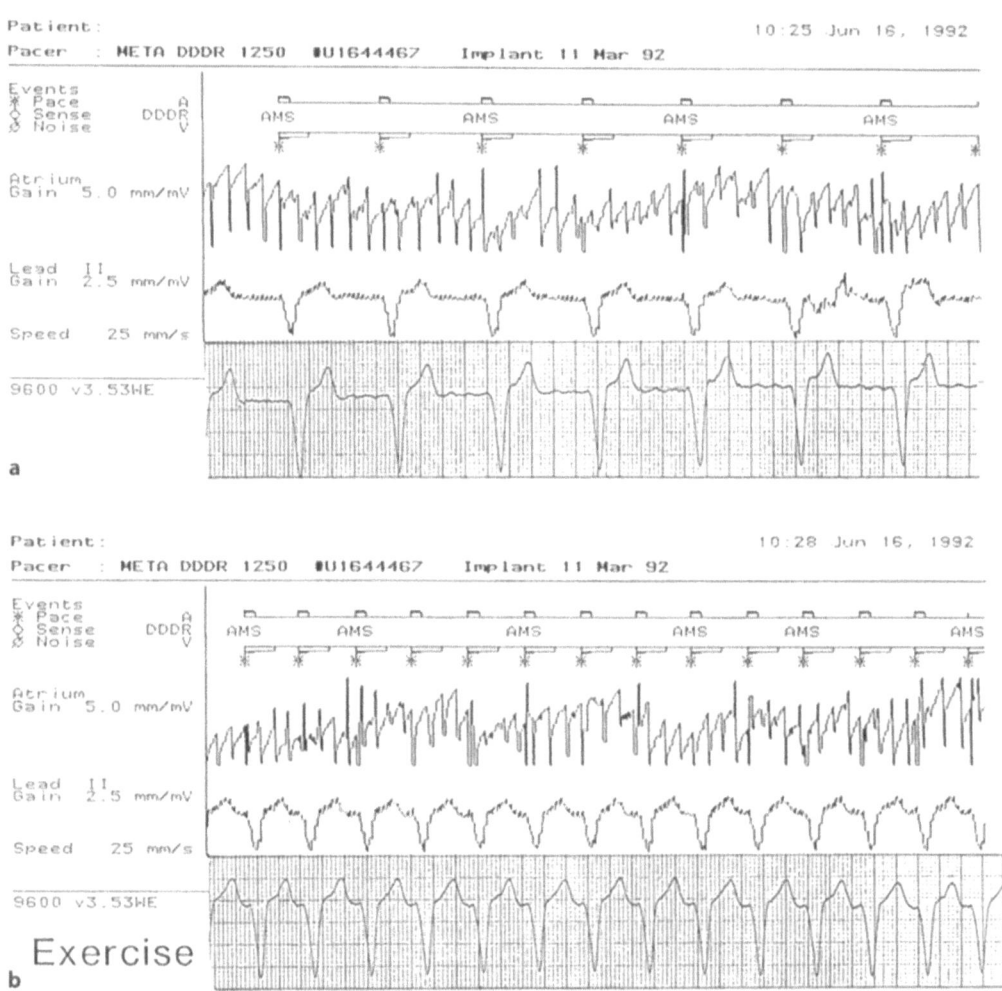

**Fig. B11. a** Atrial fibrillation properly sensed by the Telectronics META DDDR 1250, which switched automatically to the VVIR mode
**b** Confirmation of the VVIR mode by exercise. Illustration provided by S. Barold
*AMS* automatic mode switch

The CPI Vigor DR and ELA Medical Chorus systems memorize the number of fallback episodes. That information is of relative accuracy since the only element that distinguishes a pathologic rhythm from rapid sinus rhythm is the programmed value of the upper rate. By loading a special program into the ELA Medical pacemakers' RAM, one can obtain a marker channel and stored electrograms of the atrial rhythm during fallback. Some pacemakers have a somewhat different behavior to prevent unnecessary accelerations of the ventricular pacing rate before switch to fallback. The Vitatron Quintech DDD 931 and Harmony

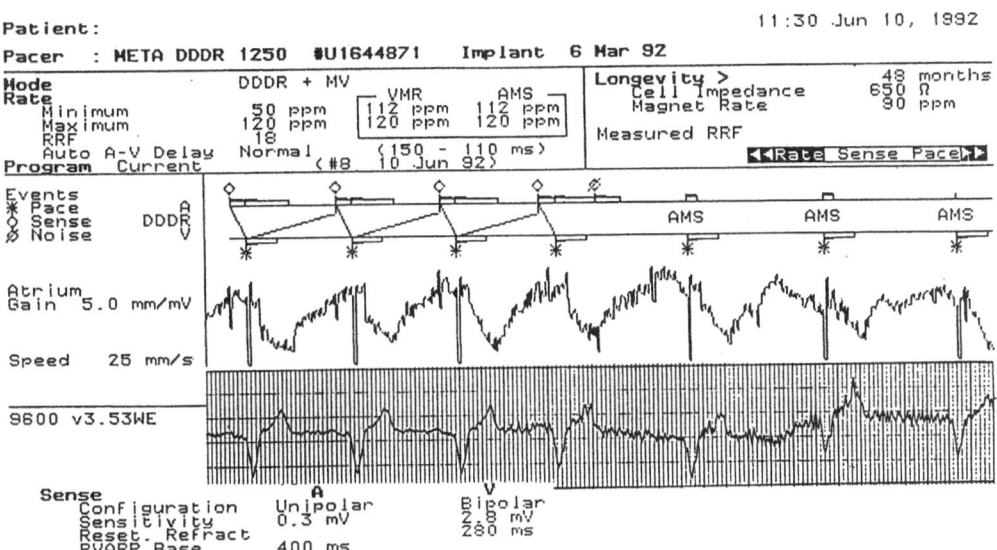

**Fig. B12.** Automatic mode switch of a Telectronics META DDDR 1250 pacemaker in response to single atrial premature event with persistence of the VVIR mode for eight cycles. Illustration provided by S. Barold
*AMS* automatic mode switch

models include an atrial monitoring window extending 100 ms past the PVARP. If a P wave falls within this window over five consecutive cycles, a 70 ms period is liberated at the end of PVARP which allows the following accelerating P waves to synchronize ventricular activity in a classic Wenckebach fashion, representing an improvement since it offers a higher 2 : 1 point. This involves a shortening of PVARP to maintain a ventricular pacing rate near the upper rate in response to a physiologic increase in the atrial rate. If fewer than five consecutive P waves have fallen in that 100 ms post-PVARP window, ventricular pacing is slowed, the pacemaker remaining in DDD mode with a 2 : 1 AV association.

The ELA Medical Chorus II measures the average ongoing sinus cycle, excluding premature atrial events occurring at coupling intervals at least 25% shorter than the preceding sinus cycles. If a P wave falls within this monitoring interval of atrial acceleration, equal to 75% of the preceding sinus cycles, (i.e. the P wave must be premature by at least 25%), it initiates neither AVD nor ventricular pacing, but recycles an escape interval equal to the monitoring interval. A phase of suspected arrhythmia is initiated which, if the arrhythmia is sustained, lasts 30 seconds, with n:1 AV association, depending on the atrial rate, on the upper rate now reduced to 120 BPM, with an AVD shortened to 31 ms to facilitate sensing of rapid atrial rhythms. At the end of this phase of arrhythmia suspicion, if the arrhythmia is persistent, the pacemaker switches to the VDI mode at a rate of 70 BPM for as long as the arrhythmia is present. In this case, sensing during PVARP participates in the diagnosis of atrial arrhythmia which is logged into the pacemaker statistics, while the atrial cycles are filed in the system Holter memory. In this model, PVARP might ultimately be useless, since the possible occurrence of retrograde conduction would most likely be interpreted as an atrial extrasystole, given its prematurity with respect to the preceding sinus cycles.

The Chorum follows the same algorithm, though using the concept of probable atrial arrhythmia to account for potential loss of atrial sensing during ongoing tachyarrhythmia. The mode switch is to DDIR. The Telectronics Meta DDDR 1250 and 1254 pacemakers take into account atrial events which fall in PVARP. The length of PVARP depends on the programmed value and on the sensor indicated rate. PVARP decreases as the rate measured by the sensor increases between back up and upper rates. Mode switch from DDDR to VVIR occurs when an atrial event (model 1250) is sensed in PVARP past the 100 ms of absolute refractory period (Fig. B11). Mode switch takes place over a single cycle such that isolated atrial extrasystoles or a retrograde P wave are sufficient to cause the switch (Fig. B12). This prompted the upgrade of the 1254 model in which mode switch takes place only after more than 5 or 11 atrial events have been sensed, at programmable rates faster than 150, 175 or 200 BPM. Three long atrial cycles, or an atrial pause longer than 1 second reinstate the DDDR mode (Fig. B13). Though its specificity is higher, this system continues to switch mode relatively easily in response to bursts of atrial extrasystoles. The Intermedics Marathon pacemaker utilizes a similar algorithm based on sensing of short, consecutive atrial cycles.

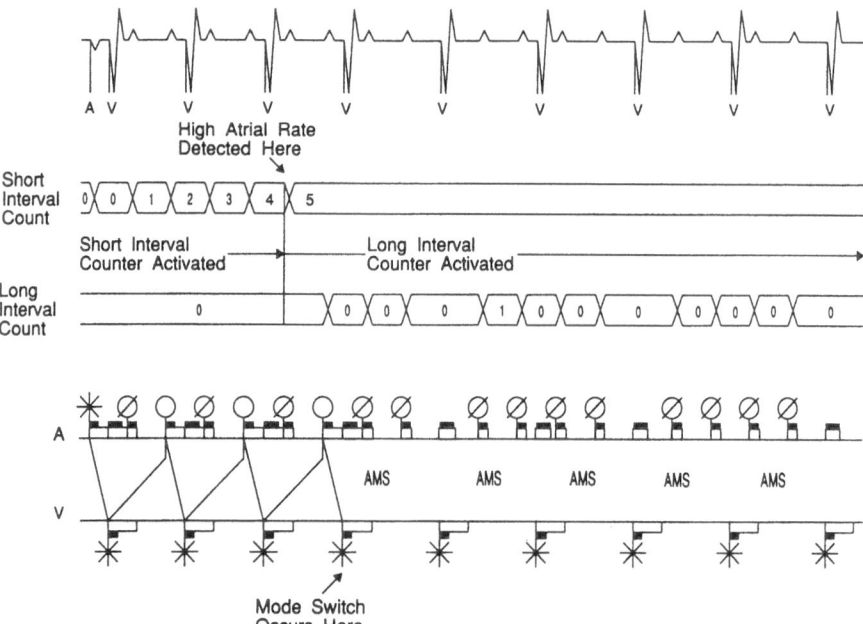

**Fig. B13. a** Improvement over the preceding system brought to the 1254 model which switches mode only after having sensed 5 or 11 (5 in this example) rapid atrial cycles Illustration provided by Telectronics

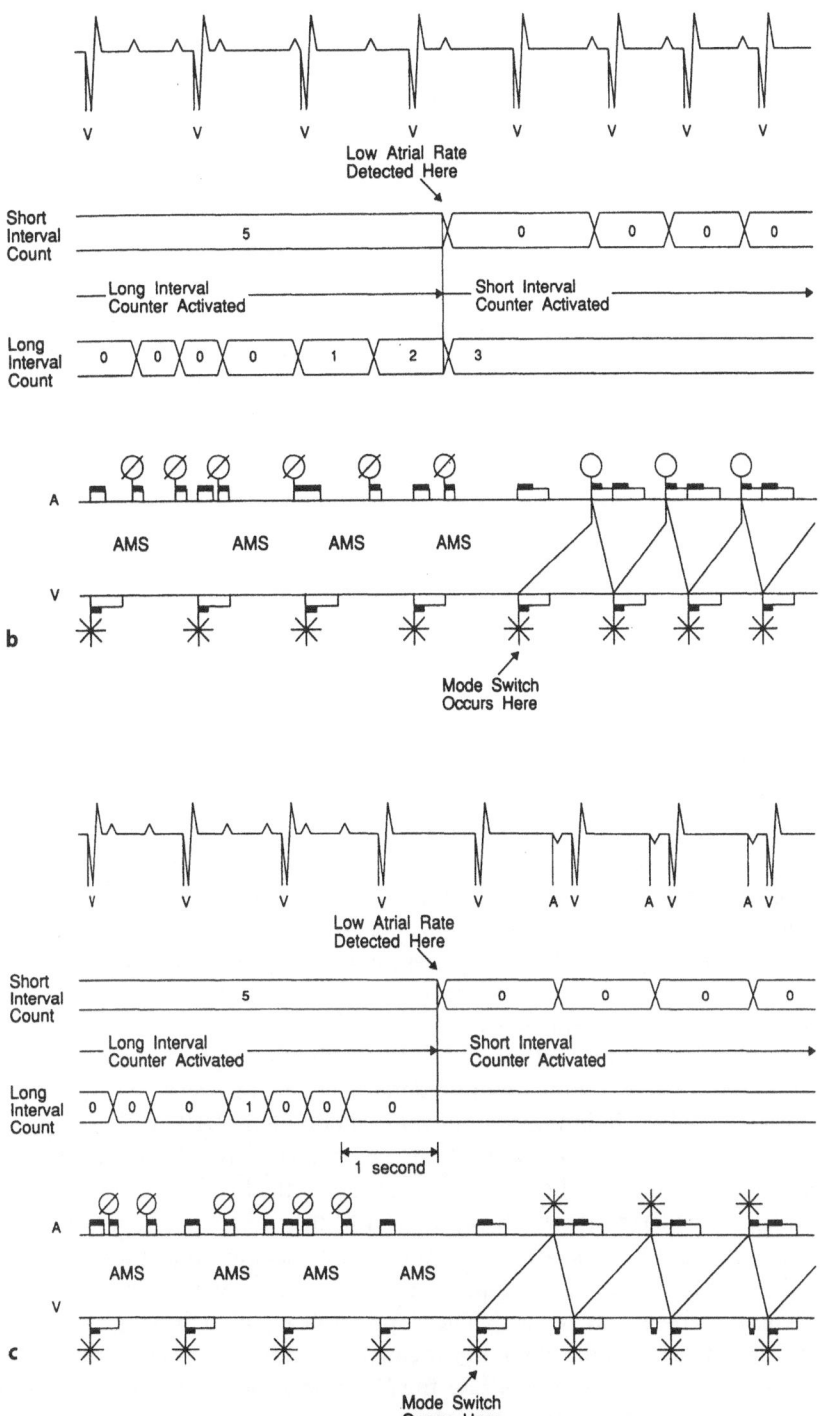

**Fig. B13. b** Exit out of VVIR mode after sensing of 3 long atrial cycles. Illustration provided by Telectronics
**c** Same behavior as in **b** after an atrial pause of 1 s. Illustration provided by Telectronics

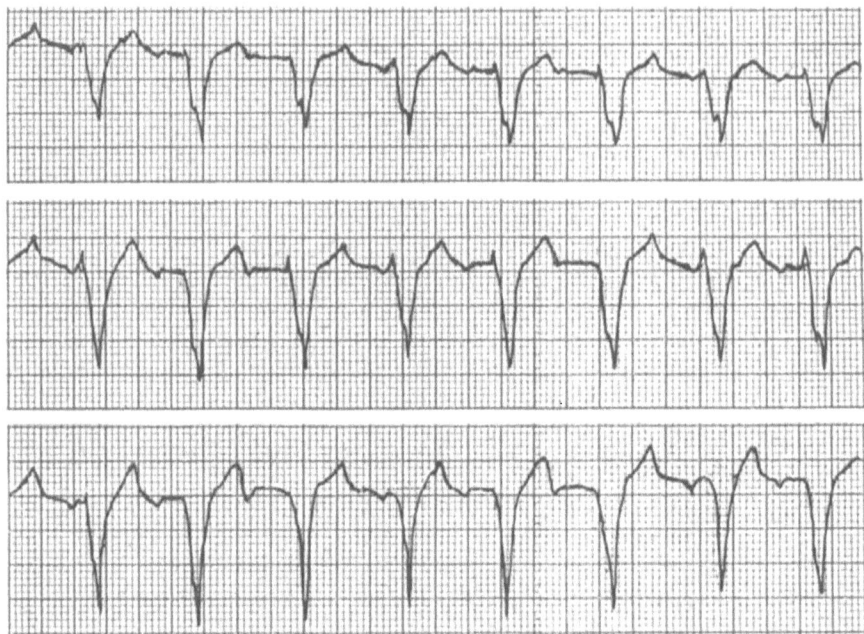

**Fig. B14. a** Protection offered by the conditional ventricular tracking limit of an Intermedics Relay 294–03 pacemaker. The underlying atrial rhythm is flutter

The Intermedics Relay and Unity pacemakers include a conditional ventricular tracking limit (CVTL), the value of which is equal to the lower rate + 35 BPM; the information provided by the rate responsive sensor is also utilized. When an arrhythmia develops while the patient is at rest, the ventricular pacing rate is limited by the CVTL (Fig. B14a). However, as soon as the sensor signals the need to increase the heart rate beyond 20 BPM above the lower rate, the protection algorithm is no longer activated (Fig. B14b). Furthermore, if the sinus rate rises above CVTL at rest, at the onset of exercise, during recovery, or from emotional causes, AV dissociation may appear, the mode being DDD with an upper rate slowed down to the conditional tracking rate (Fig. B14c). The Vitatron Ruby pacemaker compares the ongoing atrial rate with the physiological sinus rate, (PSR), a calculated rate which cannot vary by more than 2 BPM per cardiac cycle and tracking the sinus rate. If the atrial rate rises above the upper rate, and the PSR is situated between the upper rate and the upper rate minus 25 BPM, a Wenckebach mode is initiated with a new upper rate equal to the original upper rate multiplied by 1.25. If the PSR is not situated within this range at the time the atrial rate has risen above the upper rate, the AV association is n:1 with a maximal ventricular rate equal to the lower rate multiplied by 1.5 (minimum = 100 BPM). Each activation of the protection algorithm is logged into the statistics.

One other original system can be found in the Vitatron Diamond and Saphir in a function designated as physiological rate. A band 15 BPM above and 15 BPM

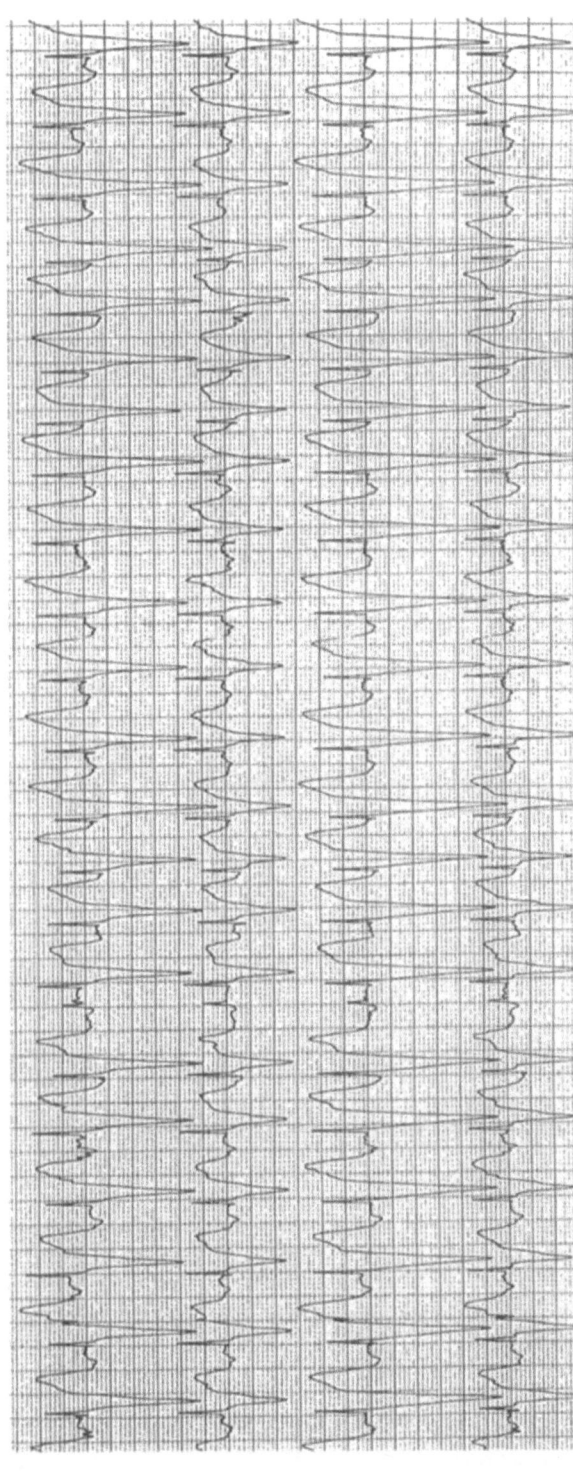

**Fig. B14.b** Upon exercise, the conditional ventricular tracking limit is no longer in effect and the patient no longer protected

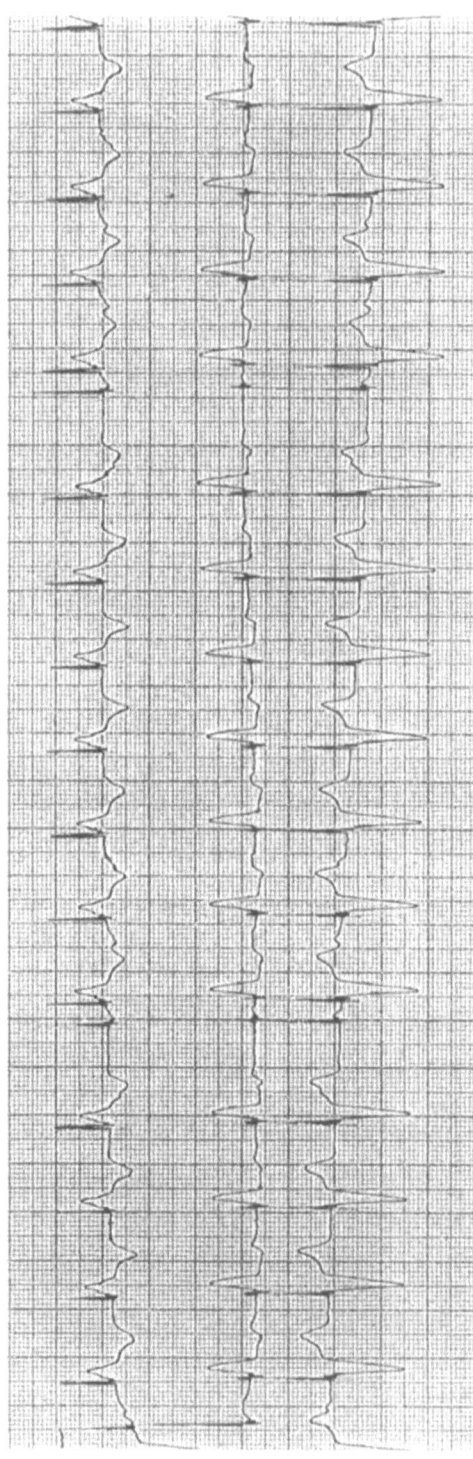

**Fig. B14.c** Two minutes 30 s into recovery, as the sensor registers no further acceleration, the conditional ventricular tracking limit is reinstated with AV dissociation since the atrial rate is faster than the conditional ventricular rate

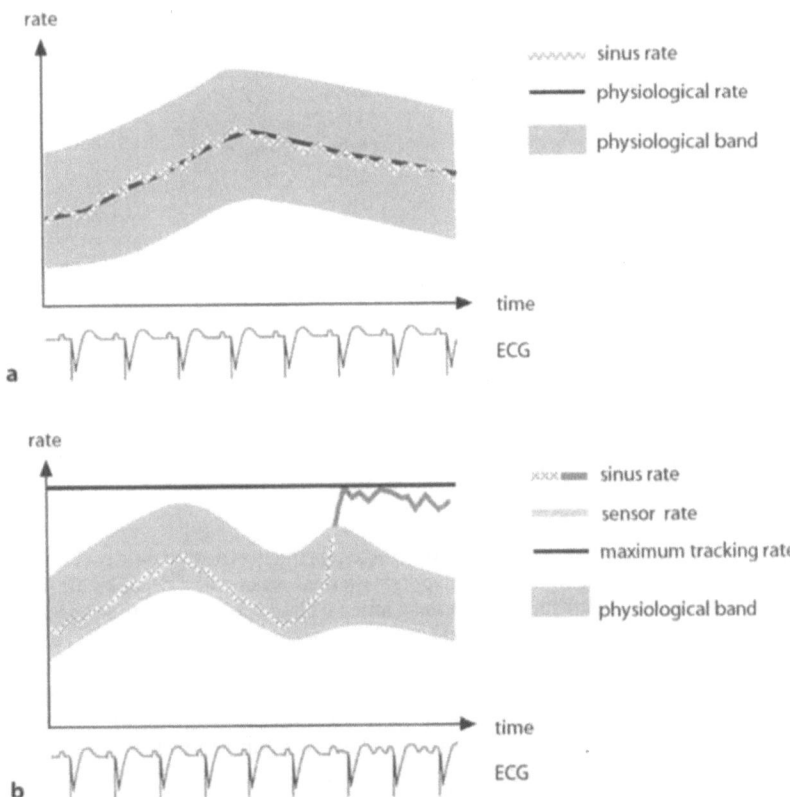

**Fig. B15. .a** The Vitatron Diamond pacemaker calculates a physiologic rate with a maximal variation of 2 BPM per cardiac cycle. A physiologic range is also defined which spans between 15 BPM above and 15 BPM below the physiologic rate. Any atrial event falling outside this range is interpreted as pathologic. When the atrial rate rises abruptly above the physiologic range, the pacemaker switches to the DDIR mode from one cycle to the next. Illustrations provided by Vitatron

below the ongoing sinus rate (or rate responsive rate if the device has been programmed in the DDDR mode) follows the PSR, a physiologic rhythm at a calculated rate varying by no more than 2 BPM per cycle (Fig. B15a). As soon as an atrial event rises above this rate by 15 BPM, at a coupling interval no longer than 600 ms, the mode switches to DDI (or DDIR if the programmed mode is DDDR) which keeps the pacemaker from running away in response to an atrial tachyarrhythmia. The escape interval will be either that determined by the lower rate, or by the smoothing algorithm (if Flywheel is activated, with an onset at a rate equal to the ongoing atrial rate just before switch to DDI minus 15 BPM), or that determined by the sensor if the programmed mode is DDDR (Fig. B15b). If the event is an isolated atrial extrasystole, the escape interval is no longer than 325 ms to allow return to the DDD mode and prevent the onset of ELT.

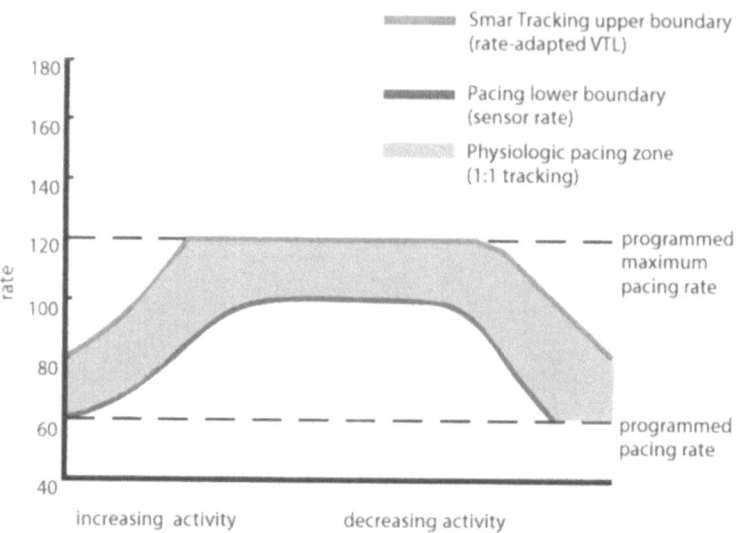

**Fig. B16.** The pacemaker (Marathon, Intermedics) triggers the dynamic fallback when the atrial rate exceeds a rate limit which depends on the sensor one. The lower limit rate is the lowest value of the Ventricular Tracking Limit (VTL) applied when the sensor indicates rest. As soon as the sensor detects exercise, VTL increases with the sensor rate according to a programmed „response." On the other hand, as soon as the sensor decreases the driven rate, VTL decreases according to a programmed „decay." To this dynamic fallback can be added an optional mode switch. The mode switch is triggered when the atrial rate exceeds a programmable „tachycardia" rate with a programmable number of short atrial cycles. Illustration provided by Intermedics

The Intermedics Marathon can also utilize a physiologic band of programmable width to distinguish rhythms, combined or not with another option (Fig. B16). SmarTracking means a „Ventricular Tracking Limit" (VTL) that pays attention to the Sensor. The management of high atrial rates requires the pacing system to differentiate adequately between pathological atrial tachyarrhythmias and high atrial rates which may be appropriate during exertion. By continuously monitoring sensor input, SmarTracking – gives the patient a „floating" ventricular tracking limit based on activity.

The Medtronic Thera has yet another behavior (Fig. B17). To ensure reliable detection, the Thera i DR and Kappa 400 DR (Medtronic) pacemakers employ a new parameter called „mean atrial interval" (MAI). MAI is not an arithmetic mean, but rather an index that tracks the beat-to-beat atrial cycle length: if PP interval is less than the MAI, MAI is decreased by 23 ms; if PP interval is greater than the MAI, MAI is increased by 8 ms. Mode switching in DDIR occurs when the mean atrial rate (MAR) has reached the programmed Switch Rate. MAI decreases more for short cycles than it increases for long cycles, so Mode Switch will occur even in case of temporary atrial loss of sensing during supraventricular tachycardias. MAI is also little affected by isolated events such as PACs or short runs of supraventricular tachycardias.

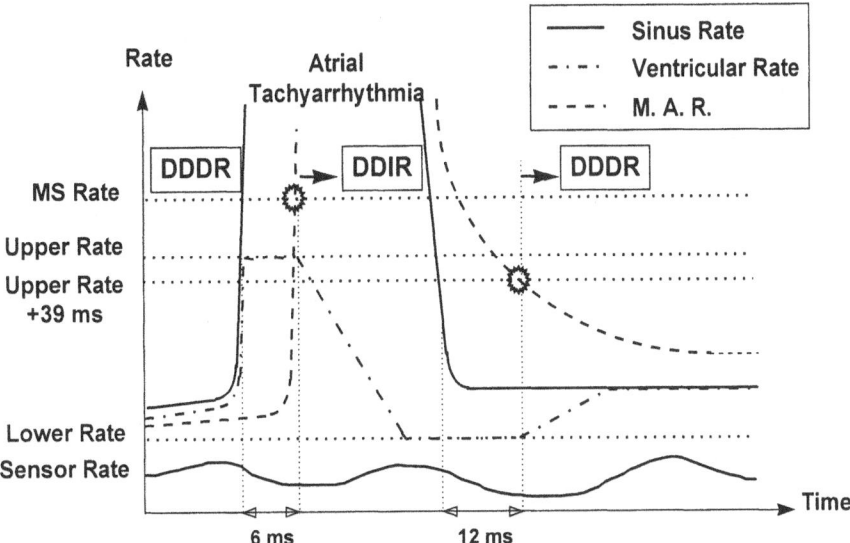

**Fig. B17.** The Thera and Kappa (Medtronic) mode switching: Mean Atrial Interval (MAI) corresponding to Mean Atrial Rate (MAR), is limited in the rate at which it can track the detected atrial rate. Isolated events such as PACs leave the MAI (or MAR) essentially unaffected. The precipitous onset of atrial tachycardia results in a rapid rise of MAR. When it reaches the tachycardia detection rate mode switching occurs
*MS Rate,* mode switch rate

Finally, the Pacesetter Trilogy pacemaker includes a similar protection algorithm, counts all episodes of rapid atrial rhythms, indicates their duration, and classifies them according to the mean atrial rate during the arrhythmia.

## Lower Rate Timing of the Pacemaker

Modern pacemakers operate from a time base whose reference may be strictly atrial (Fig. B18a), strictly ventricular (Fig. B18b), or mixed, depending on the circumstances. Pacemakers with ventricular-based lower rate timing initiate the atrial escape interval from a ventricular event, whether naturally conducted, premature, or paced at the end of the AV delay. This causes variations in the interatrial events depending on the origin of the QRS. The VR or VV interval is constant. Similarly, pacemakers with atrial-based lower rate timing initiate the pacing interval solely on the basis of atrial events. This causes variations in the ventricular events depending on whether the QRS is naturally generated or paced. The AA interval is constant.

Other pacemakers have a mixed behavior, for example using an atrial-based lower rate timing; except after ventricular extrasystoles where a ventricular-based lower rate timing is applied. A detailed description of these behaviors is beyond the scope of this treatise, though they explain the surprising fluctuations of the atrial or ventricular (depending on the pacemaker model) escape intervals observed on the surface electrocardiogram.

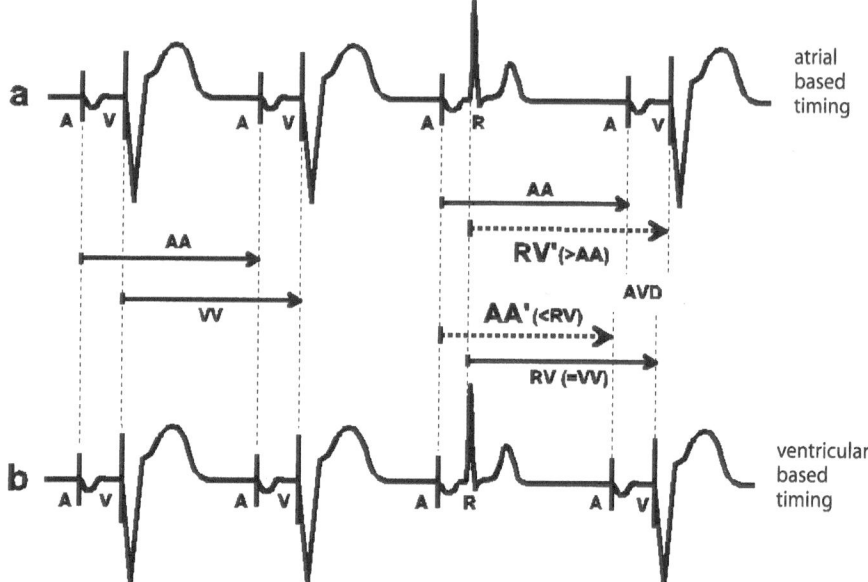

**Fig. B18. a** In pacemakers with atrial-based lower rate timing, the system maintains a constant atrial escape interval, no matter the value of the PR interval when an atrial event is conducted to the ventricle. After a PR interval, shorter than the programmed AV delay, and in the absence of a ventricular sensing during the AVD of the following cycle, the RV interval is longer than the AA one

**b** In pacemakers with ventricular-based lower rate timing, the system maintains a constant ventricular escape interval, no matter the value of the PR interval when an atrial event is conducted to the ventricle. After a PR interval, shorter than the programmed AV delay, and in the absence of a ventricular sensing during the AVD of the following cycle, the RV interval is shorter than the AA one

## The European Pacemaker Cards and Codes 1998

# CODE EXPLANATION FOR IMPLANTATION

## ① SYMPTOM

| CATEGORY-CODE | | SPECIFICATION |
|---|---|---|
| UNSPECIFIED | A1 | Unspecified |
| | A2 | Uncoded |
| SYNCOPE | B1 | Syncope |
| | B2 | Dizzy spells |
| | B3 | Bradycardia |
| TACHYCARDIA | C1 | Tachycardia |
| OTHER | D1 | Prophylactic |
| | D2 | Heart Failure |
| | D3 | Cerebral dysfunction |

## ③ AETIOLOGY

| CATEGORY-CODE | | SPECIFICATION |
|---|---|---|
| UNSPECIFIED | A1 | Unspecified |
| | A2 | Uncoded |
| UNKNOWN | B1 | Unknown |
| | B2 | Conduction tissue fibrosis |
| ISCHAEMIC | C1 | Ischaemic |
| | C2 | Post infarction |
| CONGENITAL | D1 | Congenital |
| IATROGENIC | E1 | Surgical complication |
| | E2 | Surgical |
| | E3 | Ablation |
| C.S.S. | F1 | Carotid Sinus Syndrome |
| OTHER | G1 | Cardiomyopathy |
| | G2 | Myocarditis |
| | G3 | Valvular heart disease |

## ② ECG INDICATIONS

| CATEGORY-CODE | | SPECIFICATION |
|---|---|---|
| UNSPECIFIED | A 1 | Rhythm unspecified |
| | A 2 | Rhythm uncoded |
| SINUS RHYTHM | B 1 | Normal sinus rhythm |
| AV BLOCK | C 1 | 1° heart block |
| | C 2 | 2° heart block - unspecified |
| | C 3 | 2° heart block - Wenckebach |
| | C 4 | 2° heart block - Mobitz |
| | C 5 | CHB - QRS unspecified |
| | C 6 | CHB - narrow QRS |
| | C 7 | CHB - wide QRS |
| BUNDLE BRANCH BLOCK | D 1 | BBB – unspecified |
| | D 2 | RBBB - incomplete |
| | D 3 | RBBB - complete |
| | D 4 | LBBB - complete |
| | D 5 | LAHB |
| | D 6 | LPHB |
| | D 7 | RBBB + LAHB + normal PR |
| | D 8 | RBBB + LPHB + normal PR |
| | D 9 | RBBB + LAHB + long PR |
| | D10 | RBBB + LPHB + long PR |
| | D11 | LBBB + long PR |
| SICK SINUS SYNDROME | E 1 | SSS - unspecified |
| | E 2 | SSS - SA exit block |
| | E 3 | SSS - SA arrest |
| | E 4 | SSS - bradycardia |
| | E 5 | SSS - brady-tachy |
| | E 6 | A. Flutter/Fib. + bradycardia |
| ATRIAL TACHY | F 1 | Atrial tachycardia |
| | F 2 | Pre-excitation |
| VENTRICULAR TACHY | G 1 | Ventricular extrasystoles |
| | G 2 | Ventricular tachycardia |
| | G 3 | Paroxysmal VF |

# CODE EXPLANATION FOR EXPLANTATION

## ⑤ GENERATOR CHANGE

| CATEGORY-CODE | | SPECIFICATION |
|---|---|---|
| UNSPECIFIED | A1 | Unspecified |
| | A2 | Uncoded |
| ELECTIVE | B1 | Elective |
| | B2 | Recall |
| | B3 | System change - hemodynamic |
| | B4 | System change - pacer syndrome |
| | B5 | System change - palpitations |
| | B6 | System change - electrode problem |
| | B7 | EMG inhibition |
| | B8 | Extra cardiac stimulation |
| SURGICAL | C1 | Mechanical protrusion |
| | C2 | Erosion |
| | C3 | Infection |
| | C4 | Wound pain |
| FAILURE MINOR | D1 | Failure - unspecified |
| | D2 | Failure - undersensing |
| | D3 | Failure - oversensing |
| | D4 | Failure - magnetic switch |
| | D5 | Failure - programming |
| FAILURE MAJOR | E1 | Failure - unspecified |
| | E2 | Failure - no output |
| | E3 | Failure - low output |
| | E4 | Failure - slow rate |
| | E5 | Failure - fast rate |
| | E6 | Failure - connector |
| | E7 | Failure - encapsulation |
| FAILURE BATTERY | F1 | Normal E.O.L. |
| | F2 | Premature E.O.L. |

## ⑥ ELECTRODE CHANGE

| CATEGORY-CODE | | SPECIFICATION |
|---|---|---|
| UNSPECIFIED | A1 | Unspecified |
| | A2 | Uncoded |
| ELECTIVE | B1 | Elective |
| | B2 | Displacement |
| | B3 | Exit block |
| | B4 | EMG inhibition |
| | B5 | Extra cardiac stimulation |
| | B6 | Perforation |
| | B7 | Undersensing |
| SURGICAL | C1 | Infection - ulceration |
| FAILURE | D1 | Connector failure |
| | D2 | Insulation break |
| | D3 | Conductor break |

## ⑦ INDICATIONS FOR FILE CLOSURE

| CATEGORY-CODE | | SPECIFICATION |
|---|---|---|
| UNSPECIFIED | A1 | Unspecified |
| | A2 | Uncoded |
| DEATH | B1 | Death unrelated to pacemaker |
| | B2 | Death related to pacemaker |
| | B3 | Death - sudden |
| | B4 | Death - cause unknown |
| | B5 | Death - lead related |
| LOST TO FOLLOW-UP | C1 | Lost to follow-up |
| | C2 | Hospital transfer |
| | C3 | Pacemaker removed |

## Some Literature on Cardiac Pacing

### Works in English

Barold SS, Mugica J (1988) New perspectives in cardiac pacing. Futura, Mount Kisco, NY

Barold SS, Mugica J (1991) New perspectives in cardiac pacing 2. Futura, Mount Kisco, NY

Barold SS, Mugica J (1993) New perspectives in cardiac pacing 3. Futura, Mount Kisco, NY

Ellenbogen KA, Kay GN, Wilkoff BL (1995) Clinical cardiac pacing. Saunders, Philadelphia

Furman S, Hayes DL, Holmes DR Jr (1993) A practice of cardiac pacing. Futura, Mount Kisco, NY

Lau CP (1993) Rate adaptive cardiac pacing: single and dual chamber. Futura, Mount Kisco, NY

Sutton R, Bourgeois Y (1993) The foundations of cardiac pacing: an illustrated practical guide to basic pacing. Bakken Research Center Series. Futura, Mount Kisco, NY

Dreifus LS, Fisch C, Griffin JC, Gillette PC, Mason JW, Parsonnet V (1991) Guidelines for implantation of cardiac pacemakers and antiarrhythmia devices. A report of the American College of Cardiology/American Heart Association Task Force on Assessment of Diagnostic and Therapeutic Cardiovascular Procedures (Committee on Pacemaker Implantation). Circulation 84:455–467

Malcolm C, Ward D, Camm J, Rickards AF, Ingramm A, Perrins J, Charles R, Jones S, Cobbe S (1991) Recommendations for pacemaker prescription for symptomatic bradycardia. Br Heart J 66:185–191

### Works in French

Barold SS, Mugica J, Ripart A (1993) La Stimulation Cardiaque. (translation of: New perspectives in cardiac pacing 2). Masson, Paris

Daubert C, Ritter P, Cazeau S (1993) Actualités en Stimulation Cardiaque Définitive, Médicorama, distribué par Dausse-Synthelabo

Fontaine G, Grosgogeat Y, Welti J Jr (1985) Essentiel sur les Pacemakers. Collection Tardieu. Masson, Paris

Groupe Français de stimulation cardiaque (1984) La stimulation cardiaque physiologique. Maloine, Paris

Ritter Ph, Fischer W (1997) Pratique de la Stimulation Cardiaque. Springer, Paris

### Works in German

Alt E, Kogleck W (1998) Schrittmacher- imd Defibrillatortherapie des Herzens: Grundlagen und Anwendungen. perimed-spitta

Fischer W, Ritter Ph (1996) Praxis der Herzschrittmacher Therapie. Springer, Berlin

Lampadius MS (1997) Herzschrittmacher-Typenkartei. Lampadius, Munich

Lemke B, Fischer W, Schulten HK (1996) Guidelines for Cardiac Pacemaker Therapy of the „Kommission für Klinische Kardiologie," and the working groups on „Pacemakers" and „Arrythmia" of the Deutschen Gesellschaft für Kardiologie-, Herz- und Kreislaufforschung (in German). Z Kardiol 85:611–628

Markewitz A, Hemmer W (1988) Handbuch der Schrittmachertherapie. Medplan, Munich

### Works in Japanese

Kunisada K, Fischer W, Ritter Ph (1998) The Practice of Pacemaker Therapy (in Japanese). Springer, Tokyo

## Journals in English

European Journal of Cardiac Pacing and Electrophysiology (EJCPE): EBM Erdmann-Brenger GmbH, Medizinischer Verlag, Gleiwitzer Straße 43, D-München, Germany. Editor: *Sutton R*, London, UK

Pacing and Clinical Electrophysiology (PACE): Futura Publishing Company, P.O. Box 330, Mount Kisco NY 10549, USA. Editor: *Furman S*

## Journals in French

Stimucoeur – Stimulography. 1, rue Bel Air 54520 Nancy – Laxou, ou CHU Rangueil, 31054 Toulouse Cedex. Éditeur: *Dodinot B*

## Journals in German

Herzschrittmacher: EBM Erdmann-Brenger GmbH, Medizinischer Verlag, Gleiwitzer Straße 43, D-81929 Munich, Germany. Editor: *Saborowski F*

Herzschrittmachertherapie und Elektrophysiologie: Springer-Verlag GmbH und Co KG Heidelberger Platz 3, -D-14197, Berlin, Germany. Editor: *Klein H*

## Journals in Italian

Cardiostimulazione: Luigi Pozzi, Via Panama 68, 00198 Rome, Italy. Editore: *Santini M*

## Technical Information

Association Européenne de Stimulo – Vigilance, Stimarec, *Pioger G, Petitot JC, Godin JF,* Hôpital Jean Rostand, 39 rue Jean Le Galleu, 94206 Ivry-sur-Seine Cedex, France

# Sources of Figures

- 1.20, 2.4, 3.8, 3.15, 3.18, 3.19c, 3.27, 3.30, 3.31, 3.44a–c, 3.45, 3.48a–c, 3.50, 3.51a–c, 3.52d, 3.53a, b, e, f, 3.55c, 3.56c, 3.80a, b, 3.83, 3.84, 3.85a–c, 3.86, 3.87, 3.95, 4.15, 5.22, 6.2, 7.1a, b, 7.3a, b, 7.4, 7.5a, b, 7.10a, 8.1, 8.3, 8.4, 8.5a–c, 8.7a, b, 8.8, 8.9, 8.10, 8.11, 8.12a–c, 8.13, 8.14a, 8.15, 8.17, 8.18a–c, 8.19a, b, 8.21a, b, 8.22, 8.23, 8.24a, b, 8.25a, b, 8.26, 8.27a, b, 8.28, 8.29a, b, 8.30, 8.31a, b, 8.32, 8.33a–c, 8.34, 8.35, 8.36, 8.37a, b, 8.38, 8.39, 8.40, 8.41, 8.42a, b, 8.43, 8.44, 8.45a–d, 8.46a, b, 8.47, 8.53, B.2, B.3 *Stimulography*, B. Dodinot, Nancy, France
- 2.23b, 2.39b, 3.65 Pacesetter Inc., St. Paul, USA
- 2.23c, 3.76, 3.77, 3.78, B.4, B.15a u. b Vitatron Medical B.V., Dieren, Niederlande
- 2.40, 3.82a u. b, 3.90, 9.2 Ela Medical, Montrouge, Frankreich
- 3.9, 3.63, 3.68b, 7.11b Intermedics S.A., Le Locle, Schweiz
- 3.38, 3.53c, 6.5 Collège Français de Stimulation Cardiaque, Toulouse, France
- 3.58 Futura Publishingm Mount Kisco, USA
- 3.59b Dr. Hartung
- 3.62, 3.72b Cardiac Pacemakers Inc., St. Paul, USA
- 3.64, 3.75b, 3.89, B.1, B.10 u. b Sorin Biomedica S.p.A., Saluggia (VC), Italien
- 3.66e, B.13a–c Telectronics Inc., Denver, USA
- 3.68a, 3.75a, B.8 Biotronic, Berlin
- 4.4, 4.10 Laboratoires Synthelabo, Paris
- 5.21b Telectronics, Australia
- 6.10 Futura Publishing Company, Armonk, USA
- 7.19 Medtronic Inc. St. Paul, USA
- 9.3a–c VascoMed, Weil am Rhein, Deutschland
- B.11b S. Serge Barold

## Some Internet Addresses

### International Societies and Organizations

| | |
|---|---|
| European Society of Cardiology | http://www.escardio.org/ |
| European Working Group on Arrhythmias | http://www.sghms.ac.uk/cardiology/eurtop/arrh.htm |
| European Working Group on Cardiac Pacing | http://www.heart.org.uk/ewgcp2.nsf |
| International Society and Federation of Cardiology | http://www.isfc.org/ |
| World Health Organization | http:/www.who.org/ |

### National Societies and Organisations

| | |
|---|---|
| American College of Cardiology | http://www.acc.org/ |
| American Heart Association | http://www.amhrt.org/ |
| Argentine Society of Cardiology | http://www.sac.com.ar |
| Brazilian Society of Cardiology | http://www.cardiol.br |
| British Cardiac Society | http://www.cardiac.org.uk |
| Canadian Cardiovascular Society | http://www.hsf.ca & http://www.venuevest.com |
| Chilean Society of Cardiology & Cardio-vascular Surgery | http://www.reuna.cl/cardiologia |
| Finnish Cardiac Society | http://www2.fimnet.fi/fcs |
| French Society of Cardiology | http://www.webcardio.com/la_sfc.htm |
| Cardiostim | http://www.cardiostim.asso.fr/ |
| German Cardiac Society (GCS) | http://www.uni-duesseldorf.de/WWW/DGK |
| Hellenic Cardiological Society | http://www.eexi.gr/hcs/ |
| Hungarian Society of Cardiology | http://www.koranyi.hu/mkt/mkt.htm |
| Italian Society of Cardiology | http://www.medicnet.it/sic/ |
| Italian Society of Pediatric Cardiology | http://www.unich.it/sicpages.htm |
| Japanese Circulation Society | http://www.netjcs.or.jp/ |
| NASPE | http://www.naspe.org/ |
| Netherlands Society of Cardiology | http://www.icin.knaw.nl/ |
| Polish Cardiac Society | http://www.am.lodz.pl/PTK/index-e.htm |
| Portuguese Society of Cardiology | http://www.spc.pt/indice2.htm |
| Spanish Society of Cardiology | http://www.secardiologia.es/ |
| Swedish Society of Cardiology | http://www.swedemedsoc.se/ |

### Journals

| | |
|---|---|
| AHA Scientific Publishing | http://journals.at-home.com/get_doc/602867/2112 |
| British Heart Journal | http://www.cityscape.co.uk/users/dl88/bmjpubs/jbhj.htm |
| Canadian Journal of Cardiology | http://www.pulsus.com/cardiol/home.htm |
| Cardiovascular Research | http://www.elsevier.nl/locate/cardiores |
| Chest | http://journals.chestnet.org/chest/ |
| European Heart Journal | http://www.hbuk.co.uk/wbs/ehj/mainmenu.htm |
| JACC | http://www-east.elsevier.com/jac/Menu.html |
| JAMA | http://www.ama-assn.org/public/journals/jama/jamahome.htm |
| Journal of Thoracic and Cardiovascular Surgery | http://www.mosby.com/Mosby/Periodicals/Medical/JTCS/tc.html |
| Lancet | http://www.thelancet.com/ |
| New England Journal of Medicine | http://www.nejm.org/ |
| PACE Abstracts | http://www.heartweb.org/heartweb/pace/index.htm |

## Virtual Journals and Weblists

| | |
|---|---|
| Cardiology Compass Home Page | http://www.cardiologycompass.com/ |
| Cardiology MedWeb | http://www.gen.emory.edu/MEDWEB/keyword/cardiology.html |
| Cardiology Websites | http://www.cardiac.org/ |
| European Society of Cardiology; Weblist | http://www.esc.be/Weblist.htm |
| HeartWeb | http://www.heartweb.org/ |

## Libraries

| | |
|---|---|
| ASIS | http://www.asis.org/ |
| BioMedNet | http://biomednet.com/ |
| Countway Library of Medicine | http://www.med.harvard.edu/countway/webref/catalog.html |
| Health Sciences Library | http://www-medlib.med.utah.edu |
| MEDLINE Advanced search (healthgate) | http://www.healthgate.com/HealthGate/MEDLINE/search-adv.shtml |
| Multimedia Medical Reference Library | http://www.med-library.com |
| U.S. National Library of Medicine | http://www.nim.nih.gov/ |

## Guidelines

| | |
|---|---|
| ACC/AHA Practice Guidelines | http://www.acc.org/clinical/guidelines/index.html |
| AHA Scientific Statements | http://www.amhrt.org/pubs/scipub!ssintro.htm |
| ESC Guidelines for Patient Management | http://www.escardio.org/Guid.htm |
| German Guidelines for Cardiac Pacing | http://www.uni-duesseldorf.de/WWW/DGK/Richtlinien/herzschr.htm |
| WHO/ISFC Task Force Report Cardio-myopathy | http://cardiorepair.uni-marburg.de/cmdef1.htm |

## Specialities: Information and Education

| | |
|---|---|
| Cardiac Rhythm Management (Delos) | http://www.studio-delos.com/ |
| Computer Simulation and Visualization in the Cardiovascular System | http://www.ncsa.uiuc.edu/SCMS/DigLib/text/biology/Cardiovascular-System-Clark.html |
| Computers in Cardiology | http://www.cinc.org/ |
| EKG Quiz | http://www.voicenet.com/~kosmas/ekg.htm |
| Guide to Cardiac Pacemaker | http://DroegeComputing.com/guide.htm |
| Implantable Pacemakers and Defibrilla-tors | http://www.implantable.com/ |
| Med Files:Pacemaker and AICD | http://meded.com.uci.edu/~uci-anes/pacemaker.htm |
| Pacemaker Registry of Germany | http://www.med.uni-giessen.de/technik/ |

# Glossary

| | |
|---|---|
| A | NBG code: Atrium (see foldout table at back of book) |
| Active electrode | Cathode, negative pole of a bipolar pacing system |
| Active fixation lead | Screw-in lead, lead with retractable fixation device, etc. |
| Adapter | Connector between otherwise incompatible pacemaker header and lead |
| Algorithm | Computation method, e.g. to convert the information of the sensor of a rate-responsive pacemaker into an appropriate pacing rate |
| AMC | Automatic mode conversion (AAI/DDD) |
| Amplitude | Absolute maximum amplitude of a waveform or electrocardiographic signal. In the case of a pacemaker pulse, voltage amplitude (V) or current amplitude (mA) |
| Anode | Positive (+) pole of an electric circuit or battery. In a unipolar pacing system with „indifferent" electrode: pacemaker can. In a bipolar system: proximal electrode |
| ASIC | Application-specific integrated memory, analog parts, digital-to-analog converter and operational amplifier) on a chip. The ASIC is one of the newest developments in microelectronics; its reliability is based on computer aided design (CAD) and „computer aided manufacturing" (CAM), i.e. on computer aided chip development methods |
| Asynchronous pacemaker | Fixed-rate pacemaker. Pacemaker that paces continuously at the set rate, regardless of the spontaneous cardiac activity |
| Asystole | Absence of cardiac systole. Cardiac standstill |
| Atrial lead | Lead inserted in the atrium, often with a „J"-shaped curve (J-lead) |
| Atrioventricular crosstalk | AV crosstalk: In dual chamber pacing, AV crosstalk consists of sensing of atrial pacing in the ventricle, which may cause inhibition of the pacemaker with risk of ventricular asystole and syncope in a pacemaker dependent patient; see also: Blanking |

| | |
|---|---|
| Autocapture | The device performs threshold testing automatically and is capable of autoreprogramming its pacing output by continuously remeasuring the capture threshold (by continuously analyzing the evoked potential or evoked response (= depolarization signal) and adjusting the pacing output e.g. at 0.6 V above the threshold) |
| Automatic focus | Focus of spontaneous depolarization needed for cardiac activity. One distinguishes between a primary focus (sinoatrial node: 60–100 min$^{-1}$), and subsidiary foci situated at the AV junction/His bundle region (40–60 min$^{-1}$) or in the distal conduction system/ventricle (20–40 min$^{-1}$) |
| Automatic rate-related AVD shortening | AVD shortening according to the increasing atrial rate: to reproduce the normal physiologic adaptation of the PR interval with exercise, to maintain as optimal as possible an AVD over the entire range of sinus rates, to shorten the total atrial refractory period, which also raises the 2 : 1 pacemaker AV block rate |
| Automatic stimulus threshold test | Activation of a dedicated programmer key to measure the pacing threshold (monitored on the surface ECG) |
| Autosensing | Continuous automatic adaptation of the sensitivity setting to the various physiologic and pharmacologic conditions which may influence sensing and its safety margin; self-adaptive tuning of the device's sensitivity, as a function of changes in signal amplitude. |
| Autothreshold | See: Automatic stimulus threshold test |
| AV block | Atrioventricular conduction disorder of variable severity (degree) |
| AV correction | Shortening of the AV delay after a sensed atrial event (PV) versus the AV delay after a paced atrial event (AV) |
| AV crosstalk | See: Atrioventricular crosstalk |
| AV delay | Programmed time interval between a paced or sensed atrial event, and the corresponding paced or sensed ventricular event |
| AV interval | Time interval between a sensed or paced atrial electrogram and the following sensed or paced ventricular electrogram. The intracardiac electrograms correspond to the PQ (or PR) interval on the surface ECG |
| AV search hysteresis, (AVD scanning) | After every certain number of cycles, the programmed AVD lengthens by a given or programmable amount of ms. In absence of ventricular sensing, the next AVD returns to the original programmed value. In presence of a sended ventricular event, the AVD remains lengthened by the amount of hysteresis as long as a ventricular event is sensed after each atrial event (see p. 397). |

| | |
|---|---|
| AV-sequential pacemaker | Dual-chamber pacemaker which paces the atrium and ventricle in a coordinated fashion (usually based on DVI mode, i.e. R wave inhibited, sensing only in ventricle) |
| AV synchrony | Behavior of a „physiological" pacemaker by which the atrial and ventricular activities are coordinated (synchronized) |
| AV-universal pacemaker | Optimized AV-sequential pacemaker. Dual-chamber pacemaker capable of pacing and sensing in both the atrium and the ventricle (DDD) |
| B | ICHD code: Burst and burst pacing (5th letter) |
| Back up interval | See: Lower rate interval, Back up pacing cycle |
| Back up pacing cycle | See: Back up interval, Pacing interval |
| Back up pulse interval | See: Back up interval |
| Back up rate | See: Lower rate |
| Battery | In pacemakers one or more chemoelectric energy cells, today only with a lithium anode and usually with a iodine cathode (final product: lithium/iodide battery) |
| Battery capacity | Total charge of battery, dependent on the type of battery, expressed in ampere-hours (Ah) |
| Battery voltage | One distinguishes between a no-load voltage and an operating voltage; the pacemaker contains normally a voltage doubler for pacing voltage. In some pacemakers with telemetry a replacement indicator can be identified as a corresponding dip in the operating voltage |
| Bifocal pacemaker | Dual-chamber pacemaker with a lead in the atrium and a lead in the ventricle |
| Bifocal pacing | Pacing at two sites, usually the right atrium and the right ventricle |
| Bifurcated connector | In older generation bipolar leads the anode and the cathode interfaced with the pacemaker header via two separate connectors. See also: In-line connector |
| Binodal disease | Disease of the sinoatrial node and the AV node |
| Biofeedback system | Pacing and sensing system, the control of which is based on feedback between the pacemaker and biological signals |
| Biological pacemaker | Term seldom used for „rate responsive pacemaker" |
| Biosensor | Sensor of biological signals: in pacing, these sensors include, but are not limited to, ventilation, intracardiac pressure, pH, QT interval, oxygen saturation, cardiac volumes, central venous temperature, etc. |
| Biphasic pulse | Pulse with a positive phase followed by a negative phase or vice versa. See also: Recharge pulse |

| | |
|---|---|
| Bipolar lead | Pacing lead with the anode and the cathode within the heart. Their conductors lead to a distal ring (see also: Ring electrode, Anode) and to the lead tip (cathode), respectively |
| Blanking | *Ventricular blanking period*: brief period, after the atrial stimulus, during which the ventricular sensing amplifier of a dual-chamber pacemaker is turned off to eliminate erroneous sensing of the atrial stimulus or its afterpotentials as an R wave. See also: Atrioventricular crosstalk. *Atrial blanking period*: brief period, after the ventricular stimulus, during which the atrial sensing amplifier of a dual-chamber pacemaker is turned off to eliminate erroneous sensing of the ventricular stimulus or its afterpotentials as an P wave. See also: Ventriculoatrial crosstalk |
| Block | Interruption or delay of conduction of a stimulus or a wavefront |
| B.O.L. | Beginning of life (of the battery). See B.O.S |
| B.O.S. | (Often called B.O.L) Start of the functional duration of the pacemaker when put in service; preferably called „B.O.S." (beginning of service). By a consensus of the ISO/IEC working group „life" is to be reserved for patients, and „service" for devices |
| BPM | Beats per minute |
| Bradycardia | Slow heart rate. If severe, it may be the cause of symptoms at rest or during exercise |
| Bradycardia-tachycardia syndrome | Alternating bradyarrhythmias and tachyarrhythmias due to dysfunction or complete failure of the sinoatrial node and of the atrial electrical activity. See also: sick sinus syndrome (SSS) |
| Burst pacing | Salvo of usually rapid pulses which may be used to attempt pace-termination of a tachyarrhythmia |
| C | NBG code: Communication, telemetry (see foldout table at back of book) |
| CapSure lead | Company trade name. See: Steroid lead |
| Capture threshold | Pacing threshold |
| Cardioversion | Termination of tachyarrhythmias (e.g. atrial fibrillation) by an R wave synchronous DC shock. See also: Defibrillation |
| Carotid sinus syndrome | Complex of symptoms, including near syncope and syncope, caused by bradycardia and/or hypotension due to hypersensitivity of the carotid sinus |
| Cathode | Negative (−) pole of an electric circuit or battery. In pacemakers, the active electrode (lead tip) |
| Chest wall stimulation | Control of an implanted pacemaker through the chest wall using an external pulse generator |

| | |
|---|---|
| Chronaxie time | Pulse duration at a pulse strength equal to twice the rheobase. See also: Rheobase |
| Circuit | Electronic circuit. See also: Discrete circuit, integrated circuit |
| Closed-loop system | Regulation system which responds to changes that it has itself induced in a „closed circuit" fashion. See also: Biofeedback system |
| CMOS IC | Complementary Metal-Oxide Semiconductor Integrated Circuit. Integrated circuit with particularly low power consumption, high temperature stability and high resistance to voltage fluctuations. Bipolar CMOS (BI-CMOS) and normal CMOS are now used in hybrid technologies. In these fast circuits, gallium-arsenic compounds permit memory access times as low as 5 – 10 ns. See also: IC |
| Coaxial lead | Bipolar lead with two conductors, one as a coil within the core, the second within an insulator, used in combination with in-line connectors instead of the parallel design of the lead conductors with bifurcated connectors of older generation leads |
| Coil | Helix. Spiral. Modern designs of pacing lead conductors frequently consist of coils |
| Committed operation | Committed pacing. An atrial pulse is always followed by a ventricular stimulus with a fixed AV duration, regardless of the spontaneous ventricular activity |
| Committed pacing | See: Committed operation |
| Connector | The part of the lead (usually a pin) that interfaces with the pacemaker header |
| C.P.U. | See: Microprocessor |
| Crosstalk | Phenomenon by which electrical activity (sensed or paced) occurring in one chamber is sensed in the other chamber. See also: Blanking, Atrioventricular crosstalk, Ventriculoatrial crosstalk |
| CSNRT | See: Sinus node recovery time, corrected |
| D | NBG code: Dual (see foldout table at back of book) |
| Defibrillation | High energy asynchronous DC shock delivered to terminate life-threatening ventricular arrhythmias, usually ventricular fibrillation or polymorphous ventricular tachycardia. See also: Cardioversion |
| Defibrillation protection | Protective circuit with Zener diode to protect the pacemaker against DC shocks or other high voltage sources |
| Delay | Interval |

| | |
|---|---|
| Demand function | Also: demand mechanism. Functional unit of the pacemaker circuit which inhibits pacing until a spontaneous interval exceeds the programmed escape interval (the spontaneous rate falls below the programmed demand rate) |
| Demand pacemaker with negative control | Stimulation is inhibited when the spontaneous signals occurs at a shorter interval (higher rate) than the programmed escape interval (demand rate). Only when the escape interval is exceeded (the demand rate is not reached) does the pacemaker begin pacing |
| Demand pacemaker with positive control | Triggered pacemaker. A pacemaker stimulus is delivered into the QRS complex in synchrony with the spontaneous signals. Only when the spontaneous cardiac cycle exceeds the programmed escape interval (the spontaneous rate falls below the programmed demand rate) does the pacemaker pace at the programmed lower rate |
| Demand rate | Also: standby rate. Rate below which the demand pacemaker begins pacing; see also: Lower rate |
| Demand sensitivity | Trigger threshold of the demand function for a test signal |
| Depletion indicator | Battery depletion indicator |
| Depolarization | Discharge or charge reversal; electrical excitation of the myocardium (which leads to contraction) |
| Digital | Expression of measured data as discrete numbers (digits) as opposed to continuous values (analog). Analog signals are converted into a digital form by an „analog-to-digital (A to D) converter" |
| Diode | Electronic semiconductor element a with rectifier effect |
| Dislodged lead | Dislodgment of a pacemaker lead. Even microdislodgments, not visible on fluoroscopy, can cause exit and/or entrance block, with corresponding symptoms |
| Dual-chamber pacemaker | Pacemaker with one lead for the atrium and one for the ventricle. See also: also AV sequential pacemaker, AV-universal pacemaker |
| E | ICHD code: External (5th letter) |
| Electrode impedance | Lead impedance. Combined electrode-myocardium resistance (total impedance) |
| Electrode-myocardium impedance | Electrode impedance, consisting of electrode impedance resistance, polarization resistance and tissue resistance, through which the pulse current must flow |
| E.L.T. | Endless-loop tachycardia. Form of pacemaker mediated tachycardia associated with retrograde conduction |

| E.M.C. | Electromagnetic compatibility. In pacemakers a shield against electromagnetic fields interferences or a protection by dedicated circuits |
| --- | --- |
| E.M.I. rate | Electromagnetic interference rate; rate of the pacemaker when influenced by electromagnetic interference |
| Endocardial | Apposed to the endocardium from the inside of the cardiac chamber |
| Endocardial lead | Transvenously implanted lead to the right atrium or right ventricle |
| Energy compensation | Prolongation of the pulse duration as the pulse amplitude decreases |
| Entrance block | Failure of the sensing function in demand pacemakers. The intracardiac A or V signal are insufficient to control or inhibit the pacemaker. Caused either by insufficient signals or reduced sensitivity. Demand pacemakers generally revert to asynchronous pacing |
| E.O.L. | End of life (of the battery). See: E.O.S |
| E.O.S. | (Often called E.O.L.) Predetermined end of operation of a pacemaker, preferably called „E.O.S." (End of service). By a consensus of the ISO/IEC working group „life" is to be reserved for patients, and „service" for devices |
| Escape interval | In pacing: the time interval (in ms) from the last spontaneous or paced event to the next paced event |
| Evoked potential (EP) | See: Auto capture |
| Evoked response (ER) | See: Auto capture |
| Exit block | Ineffectiveness of the pacemaker pulse due to insufficient energy delivery, an excessively high pacing threshold, or a lead fracture („exit" from the point of view of the pacemaker system) |
| External | Extracorporeal, outside the body |
| Fallback rate | Programmed rate (in dual-chamber pacemakers) to which the ventricular pacing rate falls back when the upper atrial rate limit has been exceeded due to atrial tachyarrhythmia, to exercise |
| Far-field sensing | A signal coming from a „distant area" is sensed, e.g. the QRS complex by the atrial lead. An interpretation of the QRS complex as an atrial signal leads to dysfunction of the pacemaker |
| Fast recharge | Fast recharge of the pulse through the output circuit (see: Recharge pulse) to avoid inappropriate inhibition of dual-chamber pacemakers, optimize the sensing function in the ventricle, and allow the full delivery of the stimulus energy, even at high rates |

| | |
|---|---|
| Fixed-rate pacemaker | Pacemaker without rate responsiveness (this term is still used inconsistently, sometimes meaning „asynchronous") |
| Flywheel | A sudden rate drop or sinoatrial pause (or a few isolated P waves), as frequently occurs in the sick sinus syndrome, is compensated by appropriate pacing near the preceding spontaneous rate (Vitatron pacemaker) |
| Fusion beat | Coincidence of a spontaneous electrocardiographic event with a pacemaker pulse |
| Glass fiber-carbon lead | Pacemaker lead with glass fibers and carbon fibers as the conducting material |
| Grommet | Insulated ring at the pacemaker-lead interface |
| Hardware pacemaker | Pacemaker without programmable function |
| Hexagon socket screw | Set screw connecting the lead to the pacemaker header |
| High-output pacemaker | Pacemaker with high pacing output for patients with a high pacing threshold |
| High-rate pacing | Pacing at high rates (e.g. overdrive, burst pacing), which may be used to terminate tachyarrhythmias |
| His bundle | Segment of the conduction system situated between the distal end of the AV node and the bifurcation of the bundle branches |
| Holter function | Long-term ECG recording included in some pacemaker software |
| Hybrid circuit | Electronic circuit with components from several technological sources (discrete and integrated components together on a ceramic substrate) |
| Hysteresis | Difference between the pacing interval (automatic interval) and the escape interval, or between the pacing rate and the demand rate, i.e. the rate at which the pacemaker begins pacing. If it is programmable hysteresis is normally positive, i.e. the escape interval is longer than the pacing interval, or the demand rate at which the pacemaker begins to pace is slower than the rate at which it continues to pace |
| I | NBG code: Inhibited (see foldout table at back of book) |
| IC | See: Integrated circuit |
| ICHD code | Intersociety Commission for Heart Disease resources code: prior to 1988, the five-letter international cardiac pacemaker code. Now the NBG code is used |
| Impedance | Sum of actual resistances (ohms) and reactive resistances (e.g. capacitors) |

| | |
|---|---|
| Implantation | Usually transvenous introduction of the lead(s), their placement in the heart and the implantation (subcutaneous, subfascial, submuscular) of the pulse generator connected to it/them |
| Indicator pulse | Marker pulse: Below-threshold electric pulse that triggers no pacing. Intracardiac events (paced or sensed) are transmitted to the surface ECG via the marker channel of the pacemaker for analysis of the pacemaker function. It is used in transtelephonic pacemaker monitoring, to display retrograde P waves, verify programmed settings or, in some pacemaker models in the past (Biotec), as replacement indicator |
| Indifferent electrode | Extra- or intracardiac opposite pole (anode) of the pacing lead tip (cathode). Pacemaker can in unipolar systems |
| Inhibition | Pulse suppression in demand pacemakers when spontaneous or extraneous signals are sensed |
| In-line connector | Serial alignment of the conductors of a bipolar lead into a single pin connector via separate insulators. This new design has replaced the older generation bifurcated connectors which interfaced with two separate receptacles in the pacemaker header. This term is sometimes extended to newer unipolar connectors with the same outside dimensions. See also: Coaxial lead |
| Input sensitivity | Minimal sensitivity to sensed electric voltages of spontaneous or other signals, expressed as the measured threshold relative to a test signal |
| Integrated circuit | Abbreviated: IC. Electronic component with transistors mounted on a chip. See also: CMOS IC |
| Interference | 1. The coexistence of two wavefronts occurring at different rates, e.g. coming from different automatic foci, or the coexistence of spontaneous and paced rhythms. 2. Scrambling of signals caused by the reception of unwanted electrical activity |
| Interference measuring time | Time interval at which interference signals are measured |
| Interference rate | Also: safety rate. Asynchronous pacing rate to which a demand pacemaker switches when sensing electromagnetic interference |
| Internal resistance | Resistance within the power source (accumulator, circuit, battery). Increase in the internal battery resistance. See: Replacement indicator |
| I.P.G. | Implantable pulse generator: implantable pacemaker for permanent pacing, i.e. the type of pacemakers currently in use |

| | |
|---|---|
| IS-1 | International standard norm (no. 1): current internationally standardized system for connecting lead connectors to the pulse generator (3.2 mm diameter, special dimensions and arrangements of the sealing rings, applicable to unipolar and bipolar systems) |
| Large scale integration (L.S.I.) | High integration density of semiconductor modules in an IC, particularly a complex IC of a pacemaker |
| Lead | Conductor establishing the transfer of electrical current between a solid medium with n-type conduction and a different medium with ionic conduction. In pacing: insulated conductor for the purposes of pacing or sensing between the pulse generator and the the heart, consisting of a pin connector, one or more conductor coils, and one or more tip electrodes. More precisely, „electrode catheter" |
| Lead insulation | Thin-walled, coating material (e.g. silicone, rubber, polyurethane) insulating the metal conductors of a pacing lead |
| Lead pin | Lead connector to the pacemaker header |
| Lead tip | Tip of lead with a passive (tined lead) or active fixation system (screw-in lead) made of biocompatible material and establishing the electrical contact with the heart |
| Leak current | Direct current flowing unintentionally through a high-impedance connection (battery, capacitor). Also: shunt |
| Longevity reporting | Statistical analysis of the de facto functional life of pacemakers |
| Lower rate (limit) | Basic pacing rate; rate at which the pacemaker begins pacing when the spontaneous rate of the heart falls below this limit |
| Lower rate interval (LRI) | Time interval between two pacing stimuli at the lower rate |
| L.S.I. | See: Large scale integration |
| M | NBG code: Multiprogrammable; three or more functions (see foldout table at back of book) |
| Magnet rate | Pacing rate during magnet application. In most demand pacemakers an asynchronous pacing mode is activated by applying a test magnet over the pulse generator. Depending on the pacemaker model, the magnet test rate is different or the same as programmed the pacing rate. In many types of pacemakers it is used as a replacement indicator |
| Magnet test rate | See: Magnet rate |
| Magnetic switch | Also: reed switch. Switch within the pulse generator which is activated by the external application of a magnet turning off the sensing function |
| Mandrin | See: Stylet |

|  |  |
|---|---|
| Nominal setting | Electrocardiographic examination and recording of multiple endocardial sites by means of a multipolar electrode catheter |
| Noncommitted | Capability of telemetric transmission of intracardiac signals (sensed by the pacemaker) to the surface ECG as a marker signal |
| | See: Indicator pulse |
| Operating voltage | Unit of measurement of weak electrical currents. 1 µA = $10^{-6}$ A. Commonly used pacemakers constantly load their |
| Orthorhythmic stimulation | batteries with 6–30 µA |
| Output | Unit of measurement for small amounts of energy. 1 µJ = $10^{-6}$ J. Commonly used pacemakers consume between 20 and 50 µJ at normal load |
| Output capacitor | C.P.U. (Central Processing Unit), integrated central control unit of computers characterized by small size and high efficiency |
| Overdrive | Integrated circuit with components from single technological source, as opposed to a hybrid circuit |
| Overdrive, dynamic | See: Sinus node recovery time, maximum |
| | Pacing in another chamber than in the right atrium or ventricle as biatrial pacing, biventricular pacing, four-chamber |
| Oversensing | pacing |
| | Suppression of pacing by signals of muscular origin in demand pacemakers. See also: Myosignals |
| P | Special screw-in or fish hook lead for implantation into the myocardium (via thoracotomy) |
| Pacemaker | See: Myosignals |
| Pacemaker action | Weak endogenous electric signals of muscular origin which may be sensed by the pacemaker and interpreted as intrinsic cardiac events (Often called – rather imprecisely – myopoten- |
| Pacemaker artifact | tials |
| Pacemaker can | |
| | ICHD code: Normal-rate antitachycardia function. See also: Underdrive |
| Pacemaker change | North American Society of Pacing and Electrophysiology/ British Pacing and Electrophysiology Group; see also foldout table at back of book |
| Pacemaker check | Automatic focus in charge of spontaneous cardiac rhythm; normally the sinus node |
| Pacemaker input sensitivity | NASPE/BPEG generic pacemaker code (used after 1988 as international pacemaker code) |
| | Battery voltage with no load. See also: Battery voltage |

| | |
|---|---|
| | Standard settings of the various pacemaker functions as provided by the manufacturer |
| Nominal setting | |
| Noncommitted | Also: noncommitted pacing. Function of an AV-sequential pacemaker in which an atrial pulse is not necessarily followed by a ventricular pulse (as opposed to committed pacing) which, instead, is inhibited by a spontaneous ventricular event |
| | See: Battery voltage |
| Operating voltage | |
| Orthorhythmic stimulation | Antitachycardia pacing whereby the pacing interval is set on the basis of the preceding spontaneous rate |
| Output | In pacing: strength of the electric stimulus delivered by the pacemaker |
| Output capacitor | Discharge capacitor by which the pacemaker delivers current to the lead, to prevent the direct delivery of current through the heart |
| Overdrive | Also: overdrive pacing: antitachycardia pacing at a higher rate than the spontaneous rate |
| Overdrive, dynamic | Overdrive pacing to suppress ectopic beats: Programming option by which the pacing rate of the pacemaker remains just above the spontaneous rate in order to suppress ectopic beats (Vitatron pacemaker) |
| Oversensing | Excessively high sensitivity setting at which myosignals, T waves, electromagnetic interferences, etc., are adversely sensed by the pacemaker |
| P | NBG code: (see foldout table at back of book) 1. In fourth position: Programmable up to 2 functions. 2. In fifth position: Pacing, i.e., antitachycardiac pacing |
| Pacemaker | Also: cardiac pacemaker, pulse generator, See also: I.P.G |
| Pacemaker action | Cardiac activity caused by the pacemaker (as opposed to spontaneous action) |
| Pacemaker artifact | Pacemaker pulse on the surface ECG |
| Pacemaker can | Dense, highly biocompatible case containing the pulse generator and its energy source with one or two receptacles for the lead(s) |
| Pacemaker change | Replacement of the pulse generator when indicated, usually upon battery depletion |
| Pacemaker check | Periodic testing of the pacemaker to verify its proper function and correct programming |
| Pacemaker input sensitivity | Setting of the sensing function |

| | |
|---|---|
| Pacemaker mediated tachycardia (PMT) | The term pacemaker mediated tachycardia (PMT) includes two types of pacemaker related tachyarrhythmias: 1. Those due to tracking of atrial arrhythmias or extracardiac interferences sensed by the pacemaker atrial channel, and expressed as an acceleration of the ventricular pacing rate. 2. „Endless-loop" tachycardia (ELT), a form of reentrant tachycardia mediated by the pacemaker. The term PMT, which is more encompassing, is often used instead of ELT, but not the reverse. See also: E.L.T. |
| Pacemaker mode | Operating mode of a pacemaker. See also: NBG code (foldout table at back of book) |
| Pacemaker output circuit | Circuit of the pacemaker that regulates the discharge of the output capacitor during the pulse delivery (the discharge of this capacitor is partly modulated by the cardiac impedance) |
| Pacemaker parameters | The several parameters of the pacemaker functions, such as pulse delivery, sensing, AV synchrony, etc. |
| Pacemaker pocket | Surgically created pocket of tissue in which the pulse generator is buried (subcutaneous, subfascial, sub- or intramuscular, usually in the subclavicular area) |
| Pacemaker probe | Also: pacing probe. Lead passed transvenously to the inside of the heart (temporarily or permanently) |
| Pacemaker syndrome | Constellation of symptoms, ranging from weakness to syncope, in pacemaker patients, due to ventricular pacing without AV synchrony (e.g. improper choice of pacing mode such as VVI pacing in presence of retrograde conduction) |
| Pacemaker system | Pulse generator and leads |
| Pacemaker voltage | Measured operating voltage, averaged over the pulse duration; corresponds to the value at 1/2 the pulse duration |
| Pacing mode | Pacemaker operating mode. Pacemaker modes can be identified and decoded with the aid of the International Pacemaker Code (see NBG code in foldout table at back of book) |
| Pacing System Analyzer (PSA) | Electronic device for perioperative measurements of the patient's pacing characteristics |
| Parasystole | Simultaneous activity of two or more rhythmic foci in the heart, or coexistence of spontaneous and paced rhythms |
| Passive fixation lead | Lead without active fixation mechanisms such a screw or a hook (e.g. tined lead) |
| PEA | Peak Endocardial Acceleration; sensor for rate responsive pacemaker (Sorin) |
| Period | See: Pulse interval |
| Permanent lead | Pacing lead for permanent use |

| | |
|---|---|
| Permanent-rate pacemaker | Obsolete type of pacemaker with a fixed, nonprogrammable pacing rate |
| Phantom reprogramming | Unwanted reprogramming of the pacemaker (e.g. by electromagnetic interferences or use of an improper programmer); this has become relatively rare with new pacemaker models with coded radiofrequencies and pulsed magnetic fields |
| Physiological pacemaker | AV synchronized pacemaker which preserves the normal sequence of atrial and ventricular activity, with its hemodynamic advantages. See also: AV-sequential pacemaker, AV-universal pacemaker |
| Pin | Also: lead pin, pin connector, pacing lead connector |
| PMT | See: Pacemaker mediated tachycardia |
| Pocket stimulation | Undesirable stimulation of the muscles (twitching) in the immediate vicinity of the pacemaker pocket, caused by the electric field at the edges of the indifferent electrode (pacemaker can) |
| Polarization voltage | Voltage that is detectable in a direct current circuit at the interface between a solid and liquid conductor (in pacemakers at the lead tip and at the can) |
| Potential | Term used in medicine for a voltage deflection, (e.g. an intracardiac potential such as P or R wave recorded at the endocardium), preferably called „signal". It is, more precisely, a change in voltage |
| P potential | Depolarization signal measured within the atrium, See also: Potential |
| Primary cell | Also: primary element. Electrochemical cell. One or more cells form the battery |
| Programmable pacemaker | Pacemaker whose parameters can be modified by an external programmer |
| Programmer | Electronic device used to effectuate transcutaneously noninvasive changes in the pacemaker settings, such as pacing rate, pulse amplitude, pulse duration and other parameters (in programmable pacemakers), by means of electromagnetic signals or pulses |
| PSA | See: Pacing System Analyzer |
| Pseudofusion | Simultaneous occurrence of a pacing stimulus with a spontaneous complex on the surface ECG. Unlike in true fusion, the stimulus makes no contribution to the myocardial depolarization |
| Pseudopseudofusion | Coincidental occurrence of the atrial spike and a spontaneous QRS complex on the surface ECG |

| | |
|---|---|
| PU | Polyurethane; used for lead insulation |
| Pulse amplitude | Amplitude of the pacing pulse. See also: Amplitude |
| Pulse duration | Duration of the pacing pulse (in milliseconds) |
| Pulse generator | Pacemaker (exclusive of the lead system) |
| Pulse interval | Interval between the onset of two consecutive pacemaker pulses |
| Pulse width | See: Pulse duration |
| Purkinje fibers, network | Branching of the specialized conduction system, in the right and left ventricle, from the bundle branches to the working myocardium |
| P wave | 1. Waveform of atrial depolarization on the surface ECG<br>2. Electrogram recorded from the atrial endocardial surface |
| QRS complex | Also: R wave. ECG recording of ventricular depolarization |
| R | 1. NBG code: Rate responsiveness; also referred to as „ rate modulation „ or „adaptive pacing rate" (see foldout table at back of book). 2. Reverse. See also: Reversion. Formerly used as the third letter in the ICHD code; now abandoned |
| RAM | Random Access Memory; write-read memory |
| Rate adaptation | Ability of a pacemaker to adapt its pacing rate (lower rate) to sensed physiologic changes during exercise |
| Rate responsive | See: Responsive rate |
| Real-time measurement | Simultaneous recording and display of measurements. Pulses are recorded and presented (e.g. on the ECG) in the real, uncompressed and unexpanded time domain, and displayed in their original form. This is in contrast with the compressed or expanded modes of display used by high-speed analyzers |
| Real-time telemetry | Telemetric interrogation of an actual value in real time |
| Recharge pulse | Reversal of the current through the lead after delivery of a pulse (biphasic pulse). This recharges the output capacitor of the pacemaker and prevents an electrolytic shift at the lead tip. See also: Fast recharge |
| Redundancy | Supplementary components of electronic circuits in interconnected IC units which can replace others (e.g. if defective). In some pacemaker models used as a standby pacemaker after the replacement indicator has been reached, or as a response to interference (e.g. pacemaker from Intermedics) |
| Reed relay | Also: reed switch. Mechanical switch within the pacemaker which can be activated by an external magnet. See: Magnetic switch |

| | |
|---|---|
| Reentry | Reentrant mechanism. Term applied to tachyarrhythmias that are due to a self-perpetuating, recirculating wavefront (as opposed to an abnormal automatic mechanism) |
| Refractory period | 1. In classic electrophysiology: the time interval following the onset of depolarization and during which the cardiac tissue (atrium, conduction system and ventricle) is inexcitable (absolute refractory period) or less than fully excitable (relative refractory period and functional refractory period) 2. In pacing: the time interval following sensing (post sensing refractory period) or pacing (post pacing refractory period) during which an input signal has no effect on the timer circuit (escape and pacing intervals) of the pacemaker |
| Replacement indicator | Change in the measurement of a pacemaker parameter (usually decrease in magnet rate) which indicates the impending end of the functional life of the pacemaker |
| Reset | Reset to original position |
| Responsive rate | Dynamic rate, rate adaptation. In some pacemaker models used as a parameter for the speed of rate adaptation |
| Retrograde conduction | Ventriculo-atrial conduction |
| Reversion | (In former models) Automatic termination of the pacemaker inhibition in the presence of external interference influences (See also: R). The pacemaker works at a fast heart rate (or when there are interference signals) and does not stimulate at a low heart rate |
| Rheobase | Pacing current or voltage amplitude threshold at infinite pulse duration |
| Rheograph spikes | Subthreshold, e.g. 8 Hz current pulses delivered by ventilation-based rate responsive pacemakers via a secondary electrode for thoracic impedance measurements |
| Ring electrode | Anode, generally in the form of a ring situated near the pacing cathode, situated ca. 2–3 cm proximal to the lead tip. In some older ventilation-based rate-adaptive pacemaker systems, it serves as a secondary electrode for thoracic impedance measurements, recently also used in single lead pacemaker systems |
| ROM | Read Only Memory |
| R-on-T phenomenon | Premature ventricular complex (PVC), occurring on the T wave of the preceding cardiac cycle. May trigger arrhythmias, including ventricular fibrillation |
| R wave | Ventricular depolarizations signal on the ECG |
| S | NBG code: Shock (see foldout table at back of book); ICHD code: Scanning; automatic tachycardia cycle scanning |
| SACT | See: Sinoatrial conduction time |

| | |
|---|---|
| Safety pacing | Also: safety window pacing or ventricular safety pacing. Reversion function of some dual-chamber pacemakers for the patient's safety, delivering a ventricular stimulus upon ventricular sensing of a spurious pulse during the initial part of the AV interval |
| Safety rate | See: Interference rate |
| Safety rate limit | Safety limitation of the maximum rate to between 130 and 190 BPM (depending on the pacemaker model). protects against „runaway pacemaker failure," a dangerous dysfunction in older pacemaker models |
| Safety window pacing | See: Safety pacing |
| Screw-in lead | Pacemaker lead with a cork-screw like device fixed into the myocardium |
| Search hysteresis | Brief interruption of pacing following delivery of a series of stimuli to determine („search") whether the spontaneous rate has risen above the „hysteresis rate", i.e. the spontaneous cardiac cycle has become shorter than the escape interval, i.e. the hysteresis interval |
| Secondary element | Energy storage medium that can be electrically recharged. Accumulator |
| Sensing | Detection, by the pacemaker, of cardiac and other electrical signals and pulses. See also: Demand function |
| Sensing circuit | Component of the pacemaker electronics which senses incoming electrical signals |
| Sensing threshold | Limit of sensitivity at which the spontaneous cardiac signals (P and R wave) are sensed, expressed as the amplitude of the signal tested.(in mV) |
| Sensitivity | Setting of the sensing level in demand pacemakers |
| Sensitivity threshold | See: Sensing threshold |
| Sequential pacemaker | Dual chamber pacemaker which paces the atrium and ventricle in a sequential fashion. See also: AV-sequential pacemaker |
| Set screw | Screw used to secure and connect the lead to the pacemaker header |
| Sick sinus syndrome | SSS. Syndrome generally describing the coexistence of sinus node insufficiency and atrial arrhythmias. Term often used instead of „bradycardia-tachycardia syndrome" |
| Silicone | Synthetic rubber-like compound used as lead insulator |
| Single-chamber pacemaker | Pacemaker with a single lead to pace either the atrium or the ventricle |

| | |
|---|---|
| Sinoatrial conduction time (SACT) | Measurement of the conduction time interval between the sinus node and the right atrium, used to evaluate sinus node function |
| Sinoatrial node | Natural pacemaker of the heart. Primary focus of cardiac automaticity |
| Sinus arrest | Temporary interruption (pause) or cessation (asystole) of impulse formation in the sinoatrial node |
| Sinus bradycardia | Sinus rhythm at a rate < 60 BPM |
| Sinus node recovery time (SNRT) | Measurement of the sinus escape interval following a period of right atrial pacing, used to evaluate the function of the sinoatrial node |
| Sinus node recovery time, corrected (CSNRT) | Measurement of the sinus node recovery time corrected for the ambient sinus heart rate |
| Sinus node recovery time, maximum (MSNRT) | Longest measurable sinus node recovery time at various pacing rates |
| Skeletal muscle signal | Low amplitude signals of muscular origin which may inhibit pacing. See also: Myosignals |
| Sleep rate | Programming option by which the lower rate can be reduced during sleeping hours |
| Sleeve | Cylindrical segment of synthetic tubing sometimes used to repair or adapt leads |
| Slew rate | Rise time (time between maximum and minimum) of a spontaneous intracardiac signal (P or R wave) as recorded via the pacing leads; change in voltage per unit of time (dV/dt in mV/ms) |
| Slow response | Term sometimes used to describe the automatic behavior of cardiac tissues associated with slow impulse propagation (e.g. the sinoatrial and AV nodes) |
| S/N | Serial number |
| SNRT | See: Sinus node recovery time |
| Spike | Inscription of the pacemaker stimulus on the surface ECG |
| SSI | Single-Single-Inhibited. Single chamber demand pacemaker. May be used in the atrium or in the ventricle. See also: NBG code (fold out table at the end) |
| SSS | See: Sick sinus syndrome |
| Standby pacemaker | See: Demand pacemaker with positive control |
| Steroid lead | Pacing lead with a reservoir mounted at its tip, capable of slowly eluting small amounts of corticosteroids into the adjacent cardiac tissue over a few months period. Used to minimize the early increase in pacing threshold |

| | |
|---|---|
| | Pacemaker pulse |
| Stimulus | |
| Stimulus threshold | Minimum strength of the pacemaker stimulus required to depolarize (capture) the myocardium. Expressed as the voltage (V) or current (mA) stimulus threshold |
| Stokes-Adams attack | Also: Morgagni-Adams-Stokes (MAS) attack. Transient insufficiency of the cerebral blood flow, due to bradyarrhythmia, and resulting in syncope. Stokes-Adams attacks were the initial indication for implantation of pacemakers |
| Stylet | Steel guide wire (shapable) temporarily introduced inside the pacing lead to facilitate its maneuvering inside the heart and through the blood vessels |
| Supernormal phase | Brief period of increased excitability near the end of the refractory period (downslope of the T wave) during which a „subthreshold" stimulus may capture the heart |
| SVT | Supraventricular tachycardia |
| T | NBG code: Triggered (see foldout table at back of book) |
| Tachycardia | Heart rate above 100 BPM |
| Telemetry | Interrogation of the pacemaker by radiofrequency data and signal transmission from the pacemaker to the external programmer |
| Telephone telemetry | Use of telemetry to interrogate pacemakers over telephone lines via a dedicated communication device |
| Temporary lead | Transvenous or (rarely) epicardial lead interfaced with an external pacing device for short-term use |
| Temporary pacing | Short-term pacing using an external pacing device |
| Test signal | Preconditioned pulse to measure and set the sensitivity of a demand pacemaker |
| Threshold | See: Pacing or sensing threshold |
| Tined electrode | Pacing lead with synthetic whisker-like protrusions at its tip to promote attachment to the endocardial surface |
| Tip electrode | Electrode located at the lead tip (normally the cathode) in bipolar leads (as opposed to „ring electrode") |
| Torsades de pointes | Distinct form of polymorphous ventricular tachycardia occurring usually in the context of prolongation of the QT interval |
| Tracking | Pacemaker function by which ventricular pacing is triggered, at a fixed AV interval, by a sensed atrial signal |
| Tracking signal | Also: tracking pulse or marker pulse. See: Indicator pulse |
| Transesophageal pacing | Temporary pacing of the heart by an electrode catheter introduced into the esophagus |

| | |
|---|---|
| Transvenous lead | Electrode catheter placed inside a heart chamber from a venous access |
| Trigger | Triggering of a stimulus by a sensed signal |
| Triggered pacemaker | See: Trigger |
| T wave sensing | Incorrect resetting of the pacemaker by a sensed T wave |
| Twiddler syndrome | Rotational repositioning of the pulse generator by transcutaneous manipulation (usually by the patient) of the can. This may result in excessive coiling and dislodgment of, and damage to, the lead system, as well as transient sensing or pacing failure from loss of contact between the pacemaker and the surrounding tissues |
| Underdrive | Also: underdrive pacing. Fixed rate pacing at a rate slower than the tachycardia rate in an attempt to terminate a tachyarrhythmia |
| Undersensing | Failure to sense P or R waves causing the inappropriate delivery of pacing stimuli (e.g. at a fixed rate) |
| Unilead | (In an older model:) Single lead including pacing electrodes and a separate electrode system for ventilation sensing via measurement of the thoracic impedance |
| Unipolar lead | Electrode catheter with a single conductor and single pacing electrode. The cathode is at the lead tip, and the anode („indifferent" electrode) is the pacemaker can |
| Upper rate | Upper limit, maximum tracking rate, maximum (atrial) synchronous rate. Upper rate limit of ventricular pacing in dual-chamber pacemakers with atrial tracking function |
| Use-before date | Date of expiration of a product. Deadline recommended by the manufacturer for implantation of a pacemaker or a lead |
| V | NBG code: Ventricle (see foldout table at back of book) |
| VA crosstalk | See: Ventriculoatrial crosstalk |
| VA interval | In dual-chamber pacemakers: time interval between sensing or pacing in the ventricle and the next sensed or paced atrial event |
| Vario function | Automatic pacing threshold test (Siemens pacemakers) performed by magnet application when „Vario" has been programmed „on" |
| Ventriculoatrial | Conduction from the ventricle to the atrium; retrograde conduction |
| Ventriculoatrial crosstalk | Only encountered with pacemakers that include an atrial lead. The spontaneous (in pure atrial modes) or paced (afterpotentials or depolarization signals) ventricular QRS complex is sensed by the atrial sensing amplifier and incorrectly interpreted as spontaneous atrial signal. See also: Farfield sensing |

| | |
|---|---|
| Voltage doubler | Electronic circuit reconfiguration which doubles the voltage when the pacemaker battery voltage is below the desired output value |
| VS-1 | Voluntary standard (no. 1). Precursor of the IS-1 lead connectors standard (3.2 mm diameter). The VS-1 standard is not universally compatible with the IS-1 standard |
| Vulnerability | See: Vulnerable phase |
| Vulnerable phase | Phase of atrial or ventricular repolarization during which a spontaneous or paced event may trigger a tachyarrhythmia, including ventricular fibrillation |
| Wenckebach point | Atrial rate at which the AV relationship is no longer 1 : 1 due to AV block. The Wenckebach point is measured by gradually increasing the atrial pacing rate until the occurrence of a blocked P wave |
| Wenckebach response | In dual-chamber pacemakers: gradual prolongation of the AV interval (P-ventricular stimulus) when the spontaneous atrial rate exceeds the upper rate limit. Further increases in the atrial rate are associated with increasing AV block (i.e. 3 : 2, 2 : 1. 3 : 1 etc.) |
| X-ray identification | Pacemaker identification using an radiologically visible code in the pacemaker can |
| Zener diode | Semiconductor diode that allows conduction at predetermined voltages. Provided as a protective element which passes intracardiac signals, but blocks high voltage pulses (e.g. in cardioversion or defibrillation). See also: Defibrillation protection |

# Subject Index

# NBG-Code
## NASPE/BPEG Generic Pacemaker Code

| First letter | Second letter | Third letter | Fourth letter | Fifth letter |
|---|---|---|---|---|
| Chamber(s) paced | Chamber(s) sensed | Mode of response | Programmability | Antiarrhythmic functions |
| 0 = none | 0 = none | 0 = none | 0 = none | 0 = none |
| A = atrial | A = atrial | T = triggered | P = simple programmability | P = antiarrhythmic pacing |
| V = ventricular | V = ventricular | I = inhibited | M = multiple programmability | S = shock |
| D = dual (A-V) | D = dual (A-V) | D = dual (T+I) | C = telemetry (communicating) | D = dual (P + S) |
| | | | R = rate responsiveness (rate modulation) | |

### Standby mode (inhibited by spontaneous activity)

| | |
|---|---|
| VVI | Ventricular pacing, sensing in the ventricle |
| AAI | Atrial pacing, sensing in the atrium |
| DDD | Atrial and ventricular pacing, sensing in A and V, V pacing triggered by A sensing |
| VDD | same as DDD without atrial pacing |
| DDI | same as DDD without triggering of V pacing by A pacing |
| SSI | same as VVI and AAI depending on lead location |

### Standby modes with rate responsiveness

| | |
|---|---|
| VVIR | same as VVI with rate responsiveness |
| DDDR | same as DDI with rate responsiveness |
| VDDR | same as VDD with rate responsiveness (only in ventricular mode =VDD/VVIR) |
| DDIR | same as DDI with rate responsiveness |

### Asynchronous modes: no sensing; magnet mode

| | |
|---|---|
| V00 | Ventricular pacing only |
| A00 | atrial pacing only |
| D00 | atrial and ventricular pacing only |